Association François-Xavier Bagnoud

arranged funding for this research project

Editorial Advisory Board of *AIDS in the World*

. . . .

AIDS in the World

The Global AIDS Policy Coalition

Jonathan M. Mann, M.D., M.P.H.
  General Editor
Daniel J. M. Tarantola, M.D.
  Scientific Editor
Thomas W. Netter
  Managing Editor

Harvard University Press
Cambridge, Massachusetts, and London, England
1992

Library of Congress Cataloging-in-Publication Data

AIDS in the world / Jonathan M. Mann, Daniel J. M.
Tarantola, and Thomas W. Netter, editors.
    p.   cm.
    Includes bibliographical references and index.
    ISBN 0-674-01265-8 :   ISBN 0-674-01266-6
    1. AIDS (Disease)—Epidemiology. 2. World health.
I. Mann, Jonathan M. II. Tarantola, Daniel J. M. III.
Netter, Thomas W., 1949– .
    [DNLM: 1. Acquired Immunodeficiency Syndrome. 2.
World Health.   WD 308 A2883193]
    RA644.A25A36358 1992
    614.5′993—dc20
    DNLM/DLC
    for Library of Congress   92-1545
                                                   CIP

I hope that one day, when death finally comes, by chance or by any infection caused by the virus, nobody says that I was defeated by AIDS. I have succeeded in living with AIDS. AIDS has not defeated me.

> *From "The Soul of a Citizen," by Herbert Daniel, 1946–1992, Brazilian poet, AIDS activist, and member of the Global AIDS Policy Coalition*

To Herbert Daniel and the many others who have died and who live, undefeated by AIDS.

The Global AIDS Policy Coalition

The Global AIDS Policy Coalition (GAPC) was founded in 1991 with the support of the Association François-Xavier Bagnoud. The Coalition is committed to tracking the evolving HIV/AIDS pandemic, critically analyzing the global response, and encouraging policy analysis and advocacy activities. One of the Coalition's first projects has been the development of this book, *AIDS in the World*, which the GAPC hopes will stimulate discussion and debate about the pandemic in its full societal context. In future editions, *AIDS in the World* will focus on specific themes in order to continuously monitor and assess the pandemic, the response, and the evolving global vulnerability to HIV/AIDS.

The Coalition expresses gratitude to the many colleagues around the world who have made this book possible through their contributions, reviews, and support.

Global AIDS Policy Coalition Steering Committee

Peter Aggleton, United Kingdom

Dennis Altman, Australia

Kapita Bila, Zaire

Albina du Boisrouvray, Switzerland

Herbert Daniel, Brazil (1946–1992)

Daniel Defert, France

Eka Esu-Williams, Nigeria

Noerine Kaleeba, Uganda

Maureen Law, Canada

Hans Moerkerk, Netherlands

Jan-Olof Morfeldt, Sweden

Gloria Ornelas Hall, Mexico

June Osborn, United States

Anthony Pinching, United Kingdom

Richard Rector, Denmark

Katarina Tomasevski, Yugoslavia

Debrework Zewdie, Ethiopia

Global AIDS Policy Coalition Secretariat

Jeff O'Malley, Executive Director
Daniel J. M. Tarantola, Scientific Editor, *AIDS in the World*
Thomas W. Netter, Managing Editor, *AIDS in the World*
Jonathan M. Mann, Coalition Coordinator

Association François-Xavier Bagnoud

A young Swiss pilot flew a fatal helicopter mission on January 14, 1986, in the desert near Gao, in Mali, West Africa. The Association François-Xavier Bagnoud bears his name and the commitment to continue his joyful spirit of self-giving. The Association was founded by his family and friends in 1989, and offers financial and personal support for projects that reflect François-Xavier's special interests, including humanitarian assistance, aerospace, and community life in the Valais region of Switzerland. The Association funds projects and programs whose proven structures will ensure their endurance, allow for the Association's continued involvement, and attract the participation of other benefactors and contributors. Expanding such public outreach is one of the Association's active goals.

In the Valais, Switzerland, the Association supports a wide range of activities, including education, sports, music, flight, and rescue operations. In the field of aerospace, the Association helped to finance the University of Michigan's new aerospace engineering building and funds fellowships there in the name of François-Xavier Bagnoud. It has also established the François-Xavier Bagnoud Aerospace Prize to recognize outstanding contributions of those in the aerospace field to the advancement and benefit of humanity. Humanitarian assistance activities include the promotion of children's rights, especially the rescue of sexually abused children; the provision of care and support to children infected with the HIV virus and to those with AIDS; and other AIDS-related activities.

In its AIDS work, the Association is committed to a global and innovative strategy, integrating information, research, training, prevention, and care. Countess Albina du Boisrouvray, the President of the Association, is a founding member of the Steering Committee of the Global AIDS Policy Coalition. Other Association AIDS activities include the François-Xavier Bagnoud Chair in Pediatric Allergy, Immunology and Infectious Diseases at the University of Medicine and Dentistry of New Jersey, UMDNJ–New Jersey Medical School; the François-Xavier Bagnoud International Pediatric HIV Training and Support Program at the Children's Hospital of New Jersey; the publication and international distribution of *Jo*, a comic book providing AIDS information and support to teenagers; and a network of care and support facilities for orphaned and abandoned children with HIV and their mothers in Thailand, Uganda, Kenya, India, and the United States, and for drug-addicted HIV-infected mothers and their children in Switzerland. The Association also established a care facility in the suburbs of Bangkok for young HIV-infected commercial sex workers from Thailand who have been rejected by their families and from other Asian countries who are awaiting repatriation. Projects in development include the organization of regional conferences on AIDS and children in developing countries; creation of an international training center for managers of children's care services; establishment of additional François-Xavier Bagnoud care facilities for children with AIDS in Latin America, India, Switzerland, France, and Thailand.

The Association is financed by the personal contributions of the founding members, who actively seek the projects and programs it supports. It does not solicit outside requests and proposals, but it does accept corporate sponsorship.

Contents

Preface

The HIV/AIDS pandemic is entering a new, more dangerous phase. As the global threat increases, there are many signs of growing complacency, persistent denial, and resurgent discrimination. What is wrong? Why is it so difficult to mobilize nations against AIDS? And what is to be done?

A creative revitalization of efforts against AIDS is needed. As the pandemic expands and intensifies, the work against it is threatened by a loss of confidence and direction. There are many reasons for confusion: the status quo of institutions can bureaucratize even the most dynamic programs; many of the people working against AIDS are tired after years of struggle; many of our colleagues and friends have died.

Information can help liberate us from this confusion and uncertainty. When we began planning *AIDS in the World* a year ago, we were impressed by the unavailability of information about many key aspects of the pandemic—not only about its impact but also about the response: how much is being spent, what has worked, what common features determine success or failure.

A decade of extraordinary effort at community, national, and international levels is behind us. What have we learned? Where are we today? What are the emerging challenges for the years ahead?

AIDS in the World has a clear mission to provide information about the current status of the pandemic and the global response to it, to stimulate discussion, and to help shape understanding—all for the sake of action yet to come. We present this information from the vantage point of the Global AIDS Policy Coalition, which is independent of specific national or organizational interests. Although this has reduced our access to some sources of precious information, it has also allowed us to analyze critically. Hundreds of colleagues around the world—health workers, scientists, educators—have helped to collect previously unassembled information and present it coherently.

This first edition of a global report on AIDS—*AIDS in the World*—covers the period from the recognition of AIDS in the early 1980s through mid-1992, and thus contains both a retrospective and a current analysis of the pandemic's dimensions, shape, and impact, as well as the range of societal responses. Further editions of *AIDS in the World* will update this information base, offer further analyses, and contribute to acquiring a global vision of our world confronting AIDS. If *AIDS in the World* helps increase understanding of the challenge and of the right questions to ask—even as we yet lack definitive answers—it will have fulfilled its purpose.

We owe thanks to many people for their support and confidence. The Association François-Xavier Bagnoud provided founding support for the Global AIDS Policy Coalition and the development of *AIDS in the World;* it has continued to be generous with its resources to help ensure our progress against the great foe—the press of time. Through its members and its work, the Global AIDS Policy Coalition has been instrumental in making the book possible. Our families have been understanding of distance and frustration; together with friends and colleagues, they have made the journey one of solidarity.

And the friends whom we have lost, even in the few months involved in producing this book, have been our source of strength for the project.

AIDS in the World

. . . .

CHAPTER ONE

. . . .

A Global Epidemic out of Control?

In the first decade of response to AIDS, remarkable successes in some communities contrast dramatically with a sense of threatening collective global failure. The course of the pandemic within and through global society is not being affected—in any serious manner—by the actions taken at the national or international level. This represents not only a problem of program development, but even more a failure of creativity and vision. An adequate response to AIDS requires reaching beyond traditional approaches to protecting public health; it engages—and challenges—the health and social system itself. Looking toward the mid-1990s and beyond, we see global vulnerability to the human immunodeficiency virus (HIV) increasing—not decreasing. We see, in fact, a failure to mobilize and respond to a common threat as a united global community. As we enter the second decade of AIDS, it is time to ask: Is the AIDS pandemic now out of control?

It is extraordinary that we still lack basic information about this global epidemic and the worldwide response. More than 10 years into the pandemic and 6 years after AIDS was proclaimed to the world as a new health threat of massive proportions, future vulnerability to HIV/AIDS is becoming more pronounced each day. The purpose of *AIDS in the World* is to provide information, much of it previously unavailable or inaccessible, to help develop a global perspective on the HIV/AIDS pandemic, the response to it, and where we are headed. *AIDS in the World* is a guide, not a textbook; its goal is to provide a coherent picture and essential understanding of the pandemic, the response, and the concept of vulnerability. A global vision of AIDS is as important to the local, national, and international future as is global thinking about the Earth's physical environment. Indeed, if we were unaware how interdependent our world has become in the past 25 years—in political, economic, and social terms—AIDS would have taught us this great lesson.

▬▬▬▬ · · ·

A PANDEMIC OUT OF CONTROL?

The global HIV/AIDS epidemic is volatile, dynamic, and unstable, and its major impacts are yet to come. By early 1992, 12.9 million people around the world (including 4.7 million women, 7.1 million men, and 1.1 million children) had been infected with HIV. About one-fifth (2.7 million; 21 percent) have thus far developed AIDS; of these, over 90 percent (nearly 2.5 million) have died. The numbers become increasingly uncertain as we look ahead. Yet the basic features of the pandemic are now clear.

1. *No community or country in the world already affected by AIDS can claim that HIV spread has stopped.* In 1991, an estimated 75,000 new HIV infections occurred in Europe. Among adults in Abidjan, capital of the Côte d'Ivoire in West Africa, HIV prevalence increased from about 1 percent in 1987 to over 7 percent in 1991. Among pregnant women in São Paolo, Brazil, the rate of HIV infection increased over sixfold in just three years (1987–1990). In the United States, at least 40,000 to 80,000 new HIV infections are anticipated during 1992.

2. *HIV is spreading—sometimes quite rapidly—to new communities and countries around the world.* In Poland, the first HIV-infected drug user was detected in late 1988; by early 1991, 70 percent of HIV-infected people in Poland were drug users. Ominously, HIV is spreading from urban to rural Africa, where most of the African population lives. An explosion of HIV has recently occurred in Southeast Asia, in Thailand, Burma, and India, where within only a few years more than 1 million people have already been infected. HIV/AIDS is now reported from areas that had earlier been left relatively untouched, such as Paraguay, Greenland, and the Pacific island nations of Fiji, Papua New Guinea, and Samoa. *The global*

lesson is that HIV will reach most, if not all, human communities: geography may delay, but it will not protect against, the introduction and spread of HIV.

3. *The epidemic becomes ever more complex as it matures: the global epidemic is composed of thousands of smaller, complicated epidemics.* Most important, the impact of the pandemic on women—both directly and indirectly—is increasing dramatically. For example, in Mexico, the rate of HIV-infected men to women decreased from 25:1 in 1984 to 4:1 by 1990. In the United States, HIV/AIDS among women is growing more rapidly than among men. Within each community, HIV exploits every potential avenue for spread; in Brazil, the proportion of HIV infections linked with injection drug use has increased over tenfold since the early 1980s; in the Caribbean, heterosexual transmission is becoming the major mode of HIV spread. In one large metropolitan area in the United States, Dade County, Florida (in which Miami is located), at least five distinct subepidemics of HIV/AIDS are now under way. *Thus, HIV has repeatedly demonstrated its ability to cross all borders—social, cultural, economic, political—and the conditions that foster HIV spread are complex and changing.*

Against this background of a dynamic, evolving worldwide epidemic, the major impacts of HIV/AIDS are yet to come. By 1995, an additional 6.9 million people will become infected with HIV (5.7 million adults and 1.2 million children). In this short period, the cumulative total of adults infected with HIV will increase nearly 50 percent; during the same period, HIV infections among children will more than double (112 percent increase).

From 1992 to 1995, 3.7 million more people will develop AIDS than during the entire history of the pandemic through January 1, 1992. This 140 percent increase in the number of people with AIDS will include 2.8 million adults and over 900,000 children.

Projecting to the year 2000, the most conservative *AIDS in the World* estimates suggest that a minimum of 38 million adults will have become HIV infected: a more realistic projection is that this figure will be higher, perhaps up to 110 million. An increase to 108 million adults means that over six times more adults will have become HIV infected from 1995 to 2000 than became infected from the beginning of the pandemic until 1995. In this scenario, the number of cumulative AIDS cases by the year 2000 would reach nearly 25 million. Of great importance, the largest proportion of HIV infections by the year 2000 would be in Asia and Oceania (42 percent), compared with 31 percent in sub-Saharan Africa and 14 percent in Latin America and the Caribbean.

The impact—as illustrated in *AIDS in the World*—goes far beyond these statistics. AIDS is a unique pandemic. Unlike malaria, measles, or polio, it principally affects young and middle-aged adults; AIDS is a disease of human groups—families, households, couples—and its demographic and social impacts multiply from the infected individual to the group. In the most affected areas, infant, child, and adult mortality is rising, and life expectancy at birth is plummeting. The cost of medical care for each infected person—roughly estimated as equal to or greater than the annual per capita gross national product—overwhelms individuals and households.

███████   ·   ·   ·

RESPONDING TO THE GLOBAL EPIDEMIC

The global response to HIV/AIDS is inadequate and uncoordinated. Yet there is a fundamental dichotomy in this response: relative success at individual and community levels is coupled with threatened collective failure at national and international levels.

A decade of global experience at the community level has demonstrated that HIV prevention is entirely possible, but only if three key elements are in place: information/education, health and social services, and a supportive social environment. Programs with homosexual men, injection drug users, commercial sex workers, adolescents, and runaway youth have all produced dramatic increases in both knowledge about HIV/AIDS and behavior changes. As one example, a program for sex workers in Kinshasa, Zaire, reduced HIV incidence from 18 percent to 2 percent a year through a combination of education, peer support, counseling, condoms, and treatment for concurrent sexually transmitted diseases.

Yet these *pilot programs*, or projects, face two major challenges: to sustain their work despite dramatic increases in demand and often static (or declining) levels of resource: and to see their efforts expanded to larger groups.

In contrast to the successes posted by communities—though limited and sometimes fragile—national AIDS programs have been unable to demonstrate the same level of success. From delays in responding to AIDS when it already existed, to complacency in still relatively untouched areas of the world, the global record is not bright. Of the 37 countries surveyed in depth by *AIDS in the World*, the head of state has still said nothing publicly about AIDS in 13 (35 percent); in an additional 13 countries, the first statement about AIDS by the head of state was not made until 1989 or later.

Even when effective prevention can be achieved through the application of existing technology, it is not a viable option in many countries—especially in the developing world. Blood transfusion services provide an example. Seven years after the development of HIV diagnostic tests, unscreened blood is still being transfused in most developing countries. Even in countries where major efforts have been made to ensure that blood is safe, the long-term sustainability of such actions remains in doubt. Once again, there is a major gap between what is achievable and what is obtainable. However, inadequacies in program response can also be found in many industrialized countries, where counseling, for example, is not offered systematically and where socially disadvantaged persons and communities lack access to prevention and care.

National AIDS programs are still too narrowly conceived as government or official programs rather than as combining the efforts of government, nongovernmental organizations, and the private sector. Classic management problems and resource constraints bedevil government AIDS programs: in the *AIDS in the World* survey, one-third of national AIDS programs had never been evaluated; two-thirds of national AIDS program managers had been replaced in the past two years.

International leadership and coordination are also deficient. From 1986 to 1991, a global total of about $848 million, or about $140 million per year, was made available by the industrialized nations for HIV/AIDS prevention and care in the developing world. In 1991, these resources plateaued, and in some cases even declined, for the first time. In 1990–91, only about six percent of the total global spending for HIV prevention was in the developing world; North America spent eight times more and Europe spent nearly six times more for prevention than the entire developing world. The per capita amount spent on prevention in 1990 ranged from $2.71 in North America, $2.23 in Oceania, and $1.18 in Europe, to only $0.07 per person in sub-Saharan Africa and $0.03 in Latin America. Similarly, the global cost of AIDS care, estimated by *AIDS in the World* to be at $3.5 billion in 1990 (more than twice that of prevention), is also disproportionately spent in the industrialized world.

Policy leadership is as important as financial support: today, wealthy nations are showing a growing preference to work independently, on a bilateral basis, with developing countries. In the meantime, international organizations have difficulties reaching agreement on allocation of responsibilities and coordinating mechanisms to control AIDS. A global ethic of caring has not been developed, and the global vision is dimming as HIV/AIDS is depicted as a "developing country" problem. As a result, global leadership is declining.

New challenges for policy and leadership continue to emerge: the increasing spread of multi-drug resistant tuberculosis; concerns about HIV infections among health workers; the inequitable distribution of resources and benefits of new scientific research; resurgent threats to human rights and the need to develop a comprehensive human rights–public health alliance; and the battle against denial and complacency.

Against this backdrop of a worsening global epidemic, *AIDS in the World* analyzed the global response to HIV/AIDS and concluded that following the period of global mobilization against AIDS in the late 1980s, complacency and a lack of coordinated and strategic national and international leadership have stalled the response in the second decade of the AIDS pandemic. A new concept of *vulnerability* has been developed by *AIDS in the World* to help guide our understanding of the pandemic, its history, and its future. Analysis of the preconditions for personal vulnerability to HIV infection demonstrates that personal *empowerment* is the critical issue, and is the antithesis of vulnerability. National and community vulnerability to future HIV spread—independent of current levels of HIV—can be pragmatically assessed by considering both the nature and the quality of the AIDS program and the broad societal influences that increase, sustain, or reduce personal empowerment. Through this analysis, *AIDS in the World* identifies 57 countries as high risk for HIV spread—including countries that have thus far escaped the brunt of the pandemic, such as Indonesia, Egypt, Pakistan, Bangladesh, and Nigeria.

An additional 39 countries at substantial risk include 11 Latin American countries, eight from the South East Mediterranean, 7 from Asia—including China—4 from the Caribbean, and 9 from other regions.

<h2>. . .</h2>

A GLOBAL PERSPECTIVE: HOPES AND FEARS

Information is liberating. It helps us to ask the right questions, even where immediate answers are lacking. Information also improves accountability, not only in individual governments and international organizations, but also in our responses as a global community to the health and societal challenges of the HIV/AIDS pandemic.

Therefore, as people confront HIV/AIDS at the individual, community, and national levels, a clear global picture, a sense of how each part fits into the whole, is critical.

This global perspective, this capacity to sustain both a local and worldwide vision, is not an abstraction. First, local creativity and action inspire and motivate, even as we learn by observing others. Each affected community, each community responding to AIDS, is a laboratory of discovery in HIV/AIDS prevention and care. The capacity for accelerated global learning among communities is central to progress against AIDS, just as international sharing of scientific information from different research centers is fundamental to scientific advances.

Second, a series of global issues are now, or will become, critical to progress against HIV/AIDS. New drug developments, vaccine research, the role and status of women, and the reemerging tuberculosis pandemic are all issues of profound global and local significance.

Third, a global understanding helps us to escape the boundaries of our local environment—to recognize that our work against AIDS has the capacity to transcend our immediate horizon, linking people in distant cultures as colleagues.

Finally, the relative success of community organizations and the threatening collective failure of national and international leadership and institutions provide important insights about health and society. In confronting AIDS, national and international institutions are necessary but not sufficient. The societal implications of the definition of health promulgated by the World Health Organization—"a state of complete physical, mental and social well-being and not merely the absence of disease or infirmity"—have yet to be translated into a coherent vision of health and society.

This first edition of *AIDS in the World* describes a global epidemic spinning out of control. The tone is pessimistic—and realistic, for the contradiction between the dynamic pace of the expanding pandemic and the plateauing of efforts against it dominates the global picture. *AIDS in the World* brings together facts, figures, and analyses to alert the public that the world is lagging behind in its response to AIDS. But beyond this harsh reality are hope and confidence. Individual knowledge, commitment, and action *can* make a difference. For AIDS is an intensely personal and local as well as national and global problem. The AIDS pandemic requires a new vision of health, not only to respond to an epidemic disease, but to guide and inspire individual, community, and global work for health into the next millennium.

PART ONE

· ·

The Impact of
the Epidemic

CHAPTER TWO

· ·

The HIV Pandemic: Status and Trends

s chapter was
pared by the Editors,
n epidemiological
ormation and analysis
tributed by Karen
necki, M.P.H., and
er O. Way, Ph.D., of
Center for
ernational Research,
. Bureau of the
nsus, and Robert
nstein, M.D., M.P.H.,
he AIDS Division, U.S.
ency for International
velopment in
shington, D.C. Work
HIV/AIDS estimations
d projections was
ordinated by Carsten
ntel, M.D., M.P.H., of
Department of
demiology, Harvard
ool of Public Health.
Lepisto, and other
earch assistants at the
vard School of Public
alth in Boston,
ssachusetts,
tributed to this work.

Extensive worldwide spread of HIV started in the mid- to late 1970s. In less than two decades—during the first of which it was unknown and unsuspected—HIV became the first modern pandemic. Today, in 1992, there are signs that the pandemic of HIV/AIDS may be out of control—that is, a pandemic whose broad course through and among societies has yet to be influenced in any substantial way by policies and programs mounted against it.

This chapter of *AIDS in the World* provides a global view of this extraordinarily complex—and continuously evolving—infectious disease phenomenon. The emphasis is on shape and meaning, rather than on an encyclopedic listing. The reader is invited to discern and discover the fundamental realities of the whole, avoiding becoming lost within the overwhelming amount of data about its many parts.

Once described, the pandemic's impact is assessed, along with the specific challenges—often old, yet sometimes new—that have arisen in its wake. In turn, this broad view of the shape, status, and projected future of the pandemic sets the stage for a critical analysis of the response to HIV/AIDS—individual, community, national, and global. Together, these three elements—the pandemic, its societal impacts, and the worldwide response—describe the difficult and dangerous reality of AIDS in the world in 1992.

An important problem facing AIDS work during the 1980s was the lack of a coherent, comprehensible global framework for understanding the HIV/AIDS pandemic. In the absence of an appropriate picture or set of concepts about the pandemic, the public and professionals alike were left to their own devices and imagination. Older images, resurrected from past epidemics, were blended with prevailing stereotypes about gender, race, and geography into an inaccurate image of the world. Confusion and oversimplification were the nearly inevitable results: inaccurate and misleading images fostered extremes of denial, complacency, or panic. Never before has the importance of articulating a clear image of health problems, and the dire consequences of fuzzy or simplistic thinking, been so clearly demonstrated.

The traditional approach to describing an infectious disease epidemic provided information that was necessary and useful, but not sufficient. The usual description relies on three elements: place, time, and person.

For HIV/AIDS, in the typical *geographical approach*, a global total of HIV/AIDS would be provided, followed by a breakdown by continent, or for a few selected countries. Maps were sometimes used to

---

Box 2.1: Incidence and Prevalence: A Glossary

Incidence is defined as "the number of new events (e.g., new cases of a disease) in a defined population, within a specified period of time."[a] As an example, from a population of 1,000 people, if 50 people develop AIDS in 1991, the incidence would be 50 per 1,000 per year, or five percent per year. The key to incidence is that it involves *new* events during a specific period in a given population.

Prevalence generally refers to "the number of persons in a given population with a disease or an attribute at a specified point in time."[b] Thus, taking the example above, if there are already 100 people living with AIDS in a population of 1,000 people, and if 50 new cases develop this year, then the prevalence of AIDS in the population would be 150 per 1,000 population, or 15 percent. More specifically, this would be the so-called *point prevalence,* that is, the prevalence at a specific moment (e.g., January 1, 1992). Prevalence counts already existing cases as well as new cases: in other words, all cases existing at the specified time.

To describe the total number of people having developed AIDS during a ten-year period or longer, either the cumulative cases could be listed (e.g., 3,489 cases to date) or a cumulative incidence could be used, which expresses the number of cases divided by the total population at risk (e.g., 56.6 cases per 100,000 population).

It is important to distinguish carefully between prevalence and incidence for

portray seemingly irresistible geographical spread: countless lecture slides have shown the pandemic starting in Central Africa (without conclusive evidence), with arrows leading dramatically outward in all directions.

The *temporal approach* used graphs showing changes over time in the numbers of people infected or ill, for any particular community, country, or continent, or for the entire world. These images are useful, yet have consistently led to confusion about what exactly was being shown: incidence (e.g., new AIDS cases per unit of time); prevalence (e.g., number of people alive with AIDS at that time); or cumulative prevalence (e.g., total number having developed AIDS up to that time). Interpretation is important; each of these measures carried different meanings for an assessment of the past and current situation (see Box 2.1).

The *population approach* described the pandemic by focusing on the prevailing characteristic modes of transmission (risk groups) and on such demographic variables as age and gender. Typical of this

they have different meanings. For example, if the prevalence of HIV infection among injection drug users (IDUs) rises dramatically and then plateaus, what does this mean? In the first period, rising prevalence means that the cumulative number of HIV-infected people in this population is increasing. Each month, for example, at least some new infections are occurring, thereby adding to the total number—rising prevalence. Then, the proportion of HIV-infected IDUs in the population remains constant. Yet this does not necessarily mean that no new infections are occurring. Suppose that a certain number of HIV-infected IDUs start to die, or leave the area, or fail to return for HIV testing (for any reason); any or all of these factors would cause the prevalence to fall. Now, if the number of new HIV infections per month is equal to the number of already HIV-infected people who die of AIDS each month, a steady state will be reached, so that the prevalence will remain steady. In theory, it could mean that the epidemic is over; if no new infections occurred, prevalence would gradually fall as the already infected people died of AIDS. However, unless the specific details are known, it could also mean simply that the number of new infections is balancing out the number of people leaving the population for any reason.

a. International Epidemiological Association, *A Dictionary of Epidemiology,* ed. J. M. Last (New York: Oxford University Press, 1983).
  b. Ibid.

approach were pie charts illustrating the relative importance of the different modes of HIV transmission in a given population. A very common approach has been to describe the prevalence (and, more rarely, the incidence) of HIV infection or AIDS in a particular sub-population, defined by profession (military recruits, commercial sex workers, truck drivers), sexual preference (homosexual men), risk activities (injection drug users), preexisting health conditions (people with hemophilia), or groups participating in various kinds of health care activities (pregnant women, blood donors, clients of sexually transmitted disease clinics). The common denominator for such descriptions was generally the ready availability of data.

Each of these approaches—geographical, temporal, and population—is useful; each in its own way is illuminating and yet also misleading. Maps cannot readily display complex evolution over time and treat large populations—including national populations as complex as the hundreds of distinct ethnic groups in Zaire or the former USSR—as homogeneous for HIV/AIDS risk and experience. Most important, the audience—public, professional, or media—is usually ill-informed or unaware of how the data have been collected. The data's critical limitations, including how changes in AIDS definitions and methods and completeness of reporting strongly influence the shape of the curve, are not usually recognized.

Frustration with the complexity of the pandemic is appropriate; it is difficult to sustain a coherent image with even three variables—person, place, and time—constantly evolving, expanding, and changing all at once. The global HIV/AIDS epidemic is composed of thousands of epidemics—both separate and interdependent—occurring in communities literally around the world. The spread of HIV and the occurrence of AIDS are separated by years, so that at any specific moment in any area, these two epidemics may be evolving in very different ways. Even in a single city or population area, several different epidemics are usually underway, each with its own rate of spread, intensity, and special characteristics. Adjacent countries, districts, and even villages may have quite different HIV/AIDS histories and current profiles. Finally, each established epidemic evolves over time, new epidemics spin off from the main, and new communities become affected, continuously changing the national, regional, and even global picture.

Thus, professionals and the public have sometimes reacted as if any numbers were better than no numbers; and that numbers would tell the story—the avidity of the media for numbers is well known.

In the mid-1980s, the World Health Organization (WHO) adopted a framework that reflected the dynamics of the pandemic as they were gradually discovered. Although the modes of HIV transmission—through sexual contact, blood, or from mother to fetus/infant—were similar worldwide, geographical differences in current intensity and distribution of HIV infection served as the basis for delineating three broad epidemiological patterns (I, II, and III) (see Box 2.2). The major positive contribution of this scheme was its fundamental assumption that HIV/AIDS was already a global phenomenon, reinforcing the view of HIV/AIDS as a global problem.

However, by the late 1980s, the severe limitations of this global classification became apparent. Significantly, the pattern classification became a static reality, even while the pandemic continued to evolve rapidly. For example, in the Caribbean, whereas the majority of HIV spread in the early 1980s was through homosexual contact, by the late 1980s heterosexual sex had become a nearly equal, if not predominant, HIV transmission route. In addition, although Pattern I was characterized by transmission among homosexual men and injection drug users (IDUs), in Southeast Asia heterosexual and IDU transmission became dominant. Finally, and perhaps most important, the WHO classification inevitably lent itself to static thinking and global complacency. In least-affected areas (Pattern III), complacency was intensified by the so-called official WHO categorization of countries as low prevalence areas (Thailand, India, and Burma). In North America and Western Europe (Pattern I), the dominance of transmission among homosexual men and IDUs resulted in denial of the realities of heterosexual transmission—falsely considered an African (Pattern II) phenomenon. By 1990, the WHO classification scheme was outdated and needed replacement.

■■■■■■ · · ·

THE SHAPE OF THE PANDEMIC

AIDS in the World proposes a dual approach to describing the pandemic. First, core concepts are presented: numbers, rates, and distributions acquire meaning with this framework. Second, *AIDS in the World* proposes a new global geography of HIV/AIDS. These two approaches, although more useful than simplistic images of tidal waves or spreading colors on a world map, and more accurate than existing schemas, nevertheless represent only way stations toward more effective concepts and images. Thus, each approach should be a stimulus to creative thought and refinement.

Core Concepts

The HIV/AIDS epidemic is a new global phenomenon, still highly dynamic and unstable, whose major impacts are yet to come, and

---

Box 2.2: The Patterns of the AIDS Pandemic

In 1986–87, three broad but distinct patterns of HIV infection in the world were described. Although the modes of HIV transmission everywhere were fundamentally the same, the details of personal and social risk behaviors in different areas influenced the relative frequency and expression of these modes of spread.[a]

In Pattern I areas, HIV began to spread extensively during the mid- to late 1970s. Sexual transmission of HIV occurred predominantly among homosexual and bisexual men; over 50 percent of homosexual men in some urban areas had been infected. Heterosexual transmission also occurred in these areas and was increasing. Transmission through blood contact in Pattern I areas of the world principally involved persons with drug-injection behavior, as blood for transfusion and blood products had been made essentially safe. Perinatal transmission was uncommon because relatively few women had thus far been infected, but it was expected to increase as heterosexual transmission increased. Pattern I was predominant in North America, Western Europe, Australia, New Zealand, and many urban areas in Latin America.

In Pattern II areas, HIV also began to spread extensively during the mid- to late 1970s. Here, sexual transmission was primarily heterosexual. Up to 25 percent of the 20-to-40-year-old age group in some urban areas were already infected, along with up to 90 percent of female sex workers in some areas. Transmission through HIV-contaminated blood transfusions continued in the many places where HIV screening of blood had not yet become routine. While drug-injection behavior was rare in Pattern II, the use of unsterile needles or other skin-piercing instruments contributed to HIV spread. Perinatal transmission was a major problem; in some areas 5 to 15 percent or more of pregnant women were HIV infected. Pattern II areas included sub-Saharan Africa and, increasingly, Latin America, especially the Caribbean.

In Pattern III areas, HIV began to spread extensively throughout the 1980s. By 1987, however, only one percent of AIDS cases officially reported to WHO were from Pattern III countries. Early AIDS cases were

whose current shape and future depend exclusively on individual and collective human behavior.

First, *HIV/AIDS is a pandemic,* affecting all inhabited continents; AIDS cases have been officially reported by 164 countries, and HIV infection has been documented in virtually all countries.

Second, *the HIV/AIDS pandemic is new;* it is a very recent phenomenon in historical terms. Although the virus itself is old, and perhaps very old, its significant worldwide spread appears to have started only in the mid-1970s. By 1981, when AIDS was first de-

---

generally associated with contact with Pattern I and II areas or imported blood or blood products. Even though HIV infection had not yet penetrated into the general population of Pattern III countries, indigenous transmission was occurring, and HIV infections were increasingly recognized among persons with risk behaviors, such as commercial sex workers and persons with drug-injection behavior. Pattern III areas included Eastern Europe, the Middle East, North Africa, and most countries in Asia and the Pacific.

Although these patterns applied generally, they were not immutable; different patterns coexisted within a single country or some large cities. Although certain clear limits were set by the limited modes of transmission of HIV, the range, pattern, timing, and extent of transmission depended on a blend of individual behavior, social practices, and possible biological co-factors. Other influencing factors, such as social evolution, political unrest, economic disruption or success, also modified over time the social context within which risk behaviors flourished or receded.

The provisional nature of these global patterns was emphasized by

rapid changes in HIV epidemiology, particularly in Latin America and the Caribbean. The predominance of male homosexuals and bisexuals among HIV-infected people in the Caribbean in the early 1980s (typical of Pattern I) was succeeded by an increasing shift to heterosexual transmission (typical of Pattern II). Similar shifts were occurring in selected parts of Latin America. Therefore, by 1988–89, a new area (Pattern I/II) was designated for Latin America and parts of the Caribbean. As the epidemic in Southeast Asia progressed, the descriptive value of Pattern III also rapidly declined. As useful as the patterns were for developing initial understanding of differentiation within the global epidemic, the WHO nomenclature of 1987 rapidly grew out of date and needed replacement.

---

a. Institute of Medicine, National Academy of Sciences, *Confronting AIDS. Directions for Public Health, Health Care and Research* (Washington, D.C.: National Academy Press, 1986); J. Chin and J. M. Mann, "The global patterns and prevalence of AIDS and HIV infection," *AIDS* 2(suppl. 1)(1988):S247–S252.

scribed, HIV infections were occurring in about 20 countries, with an estimated 100,000 people worldwide HIV infected. The newness of the pandemic has two major consequences: *it is still very dynamic, unstable, and volatile;* and *its major impact is yet to come.*

The pandemic is dynamic and unstable. HIV/AIDS is not an established, settled health problem whose boundaries and future course remain constant and predictable from year to year. Rather, the HIV/AIDS pandemic is extremely mobile; at this stage, neither the geographical nor societal boundaries of HIV/AIDS are fixed. Regardless of the current status of the pandemic in any country, community, or societal group, this status must be considered provisional, not static or permanent. Change, instability, and volatility are essential features of the global HIV/AIDS pandemic.

The pandemic's dynamic quality expresses itself in three ways:

- HIV/AIDS continues to expand and intensify in all already affected areas and communities;
- HIV/AIDS is spreading—sometimes quite rapidly—into areas and communities previously spared by the pandemic; and
- Within each affected community, the epidemic evolves and becomes more complicated with time.

The second important consequence of the newness of the HIV/AIDS pandemic is that its major impact is yet to come. The long biological delay between infection with HIV and onset of HIV-related disease, combined with the global expansion of the pandemic, means that the burden of HIV disease is cumulative and building rapidly. The impact of already HIV-infected people gradually developing HIV disease, combined with new HIV infections, means that by whatever measure selected—numbers of HIV-infected people, number of men, women, and children developing AIDS, or number of AIDS orphans—the decade of the 1990s will be much more difficult than the 1980s.

Finally, *the pandemic is composed of two elements: a virus and people.* More is known about HIV than any other virus affecting human beings. No insects, food, or water mediate between the virus and humanity. Everywhere in the world, HIV spreads through the same basic and narrowly circumscribed routes of transmission—sex, blood, and mother-to-fetus/infant.

People, and specifically individual and collective human behavior, constitute the key dimension—enormously diverse and barely understood—in the HIV equation. For the specific details of HIV spread depend on the broadest imaginable range of personal behavior and societal customs, which surround and condition those highly personal and special interactions in which sex occurs, blood may be exchanged, and children are born and nurtured. Thus, human behavior—individual and collective—has determined the shape of the pandemic thus far and will determine its future course.

The New Global Geography of HIV/AIDS

The new geography of HIV/AIDS involves a division of the world into ten Geographic Areas of Affinity (GAA). Each GAA has been identified by considering four factors: the evolving epidemiology of HIV/ AIDS in each country; the type and level of response to the pandemic; societal vulnerability to further spread of HIV; and the relevant geographical realities (see Table 2.1).

The 10 Geographic Areas of Affinity are presented in Box 2.3. Appendix 2.1 contains a list of countries per GAA.

Despite its utility, the Area of Affinity system is still based on generalizations and assumptions. For example, Japan is included in Area 9, together with China and other North East Asian countries. In this GAA, the current patterns of spread, involving a low rate of heterosexual transmission and a relatively low prevalence of HIV, favored including Japan in GAA 9, in spite of the clear disparity between the level of economic development of this country and the others with which it was grouped. Likewise, all countries in Latin America were included in GAA 4, even though some evolving features of the pandemic, including diverging trends in gender ratio and the predominant modes of transmission in 1990 (see Chapter 3 on AIDS) would provide a basis for disaggregating this GAA into several subareas. (These could be distinguished as Andean, Southern Cone, Central American countries, Brazil, and Mexico, as was done by WHO/PAHO in their *1990 AIDS/HIV/STD Surveillance Report*.) Likewise, Eastern/Central Europe remains as a GAA: the course of the pandemic will be closely linked with the profound societal changes occurring in each

Table 2.1: Indicators for Geographic Areas of Affinity (GAAs)

Factors	1 North America	2 Western Europe	3 Oceania	4 Latin America	5 Sub-Saharan Africa	6 Caribbean	7 Eastern Europe	8 South East Mediterranean	9 North East Asia	10 Southeast Asia
Epidemiological[a]										
Year of HIV spread	1978	1978	1979	1978–79	1977–78	1979	1982–83	1982	1982–84	1983–84
Year first AIDS case diagnosed[a]	E80	E80	M80	E80	M80	E80	E80	L80	E80	M80
Availability of HIV/AIDS data	H	H	H	M	H	M	L	L	L	M
Major modes of HIV transmission[b]										
blood/blood products	L	L	L	M	M/L	L	L	L	L	M
homosexual/bisexual men	M	M	M/H	M	L	L	H	L	L	L
injection drug use	H	H	L	M	L	M	M/L	M/H	M/H	H
heterosexual	M/L	M/L	L	M	H	H	L	L	M/L	M/H
Urban:rural ratio	3.2:1	5:1	3.3:1	2.3:1	3.6:1	3.6:1	3.2:1	12:1	5:1	6:1
Prevalence of HIV in the general population[c]	0.005–3.0	0.007–2.8	0.03–0.2	0.0007–0.8	0.9–7.3	0.5–20	0.0001–0.003	0.0001–0.5	0.0001–0.002	0.01–0.29
Gender (male:female) ratio in populations currently infected with HIV	8:1	5:1	7:1	4:1	1:1	1.5:1	10:1	5:1	5:1	2:1
Operational/Programmatic										
Mean year of national response[d]	82	86	84	86	86	87	89	87	86.5	87.5
Level of external financing of AIDS programs	L	L	L	L	H	L	L	L	L	M/H
% of GNP spent on health services (1986)[e]	H	H	H	M	L	M	M	M/H	M/H	M/H

Societal

Mean Human Development Index (HDI)[e,f]	0.98	0.97	0.97	0.82	0.26	0.62	0.90	0.38	0.83	0.51
Mean total female score[g]	81.5	76.3	79.5	63.2	37.0	55.8	76.5	35.0	63.5	50.5
Mean Human Freedom Index (HFI)[e,h]	H	H	H	M	M/L	M	L	L	L[j]	M
Urban population annual growth rate (1990–2000)[e,k]	1.0	0.6	1.0	2.5	5.3	2.5	1.4	3.9	4.0	4.1

Source: Unless otherwise noted, the values above have been estimated by *AIDS in the World, 1992.*

Note: H = high; M = medium; L = low.

a. Because reporting of AIDS cases to the World Health Organization did not begin until 1985–86, dates of diagnosis are approximate. E80 = before 1985; M80 = 1985–1987; L80 = after 1987.

b. Estimated HIV prevalence rates in 1990 were obtained for each mode of transmission from the modified Delphi Survey.

c. For each region, the prevalence in the general population was provided by the Delphi Survey. The rates represent a range for 1991 from the lowest estimates for rural areas to high estimates for urban populations.

d. The mean year of first response to the AIDS epidemic reflects the first occurrence of two variables—the year of a national leader's address on AIDS or the year in which a national AIDS program was created.

e. *Source:* United Nations Development Programme (UNDP) Report, 1991.

f. In order to quantify a country's development beyond GNP and to capture more fully how economic growth translates into human well-being, the UNDP Human Development Index (HDI) combines annual income per capita, life expectancy, adult literacy, and mean years of schooling. Scoring ranges from 0 to 1.00, with 1.00 being the highest HDI.

g. The total female score combines several indicators to measure the overall condition of women in individual countries. Of the maximum score of 100, 75 points are based on women's status and 25 points reflect the gender gap. *Source:* Population Crisis Committee, 1988.

h. The UNDP Human Freedom Index is comprised of 40 separate indicators, including freedom from arbitrary rule, illegal arrest, and unwarranted attack on person or property; right to life, liberty, security, ethnic and gender equality, and rule of law; freedom of assembly, movement, thought, religion, and speech; right to work, free choice of jobs, and adequate standard of living; right to participate in community life and organize opposition parties or trade union groups. L = 0–10; M = 11–30; H = 31–40.

j. Even though GAA 9 has a *low* mean score, it is important to note that, alone, Japan scores *high* on this index.

k. The annual urban population growth rate should be interpreted as a surrogate indicator for urban migration.

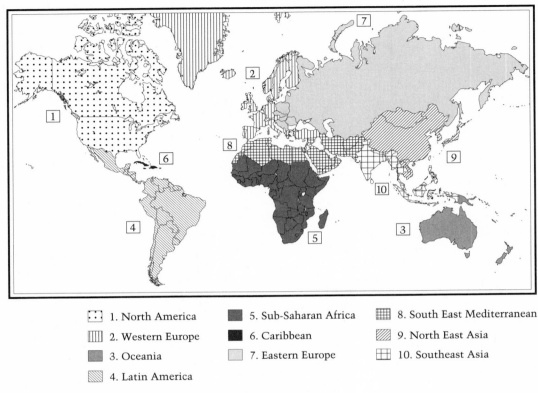

[:] 1. North America	■ 5. Sub-Saharan Africa	▦ 8. South East Mediterranean
‖‖ 2. Western Europe	■ 6. Caribbean	▨ 9. North East Asia
■ 3. Oceania	☐ 7. Eastern Europe	⊞ 10. Southeast Asia
▧ 4. Latin America		

Figure 2A. Geographic Areas of Affinity.
Source: AIDS in the World, 1992.

country in the Area. (Until recently, these countries were seen as comprising a uniform epidemiological pattern.)

The present delineation of 10 areas is, therefore, intended as an interim classification. The Global AIDS Policy Coalition is commissioning work to develop a more sophisticated classification system, taking a broader range of relevant factors (e.g., societal, behavioral) into account and drawing on modern techniques for graphic display of complex data. The goal is to develop a framework capable of incorporating change and diversity and to demonstrate local, national, and regional variability and evolution, while sustaining a coherent global vision of the pandemic and progress against it.

A Final Concept: The Continuum of Space, People, and Time

The HIV/AIDS pandemic is a complex and evolving phenomenon, with both somewhat predictable and unpredictable elements. In this pandemic, what has already occurred (HIV infections and disease) continues to exist (people living with HIV infection and disease), evolves (as those infected develop disease and die), and also influences the future (through further spread of HIV and impacts of disease and death); new events also occur (entry of HIV into new populations or areas). A composite picture is created of superimposed images, each of which continues to evolve. Reality at any moment—the still photograph—captures each element in its separate and interconnected process of evolution. Metaphors are difficult to find; human experi-

---

Box 2.3: The New Geography of HIV/AIDS

AIDS in the World has developed a new framework to facilitate tracking of the HIV/AIDS pandemic, analyze its impact, and monitor the response to it. The world has been divided into 10 Geographic Areas of Affinity (GAAs). The diversity of these areas is large enough to accommodate variability in modes of transmission of HIV, yet small enough to facilitate analysis (Figure 2.A). Appendix 2.1 contains the distribution of countries by GAA. These GAAs are based on two major factors: evolving HIV epidemiology, and the operational and programmatic characteristics of the response to the HIV epidemic. The degree of societal vulnerability to the further spread of HIV is an important underlying element.

Despite its utility, however, it is important to note that the GAA system is still based on generalizations and assumptions. The present delineation of the 10 GAAs is therefore only intended

as an interim classification. The Global AIDS Policy Coalition is commissioning work to develop a more sophisticated classification system, which will seek to take into account an even broader range of relevant factors. The goal is to understand better the local, national, and regional features of the pandemic. This information is critical for generating a more robust and focused global response.

The indicators used in defining the GAAs are presented in Table 2.A. The combination of criteria uniquely defines each of the 10 areas. For example, 2 GAAs may share certain epidemiological characteristics, yet differ in the magnitude of the response to the HIV/AIDS pandemic. This can be seen when comparing Eastern Europe and North East Asia, or the Caribbean and sub-Saharan Africa.

Fourteen indicators were selected within 3 broad categories. They were then applied to countries in order to justify their inclusion in one GAA or another.

Table 2.A: Definition of indicators for Geographic Areas of Affinity (GAAs)

1. Epidemiological factors

1.1 Presumed year of wide spread of HIV: This gives an indication of the chronology of the pandemic.

1.2 Year of first report of AIDS to WHO: This indicates the formal acknowledgment of AIDS being diagnosed in the GAA.

1.3 Availability of HIV/AIDS data: This is an indication of surveys having been completed or the existence of surveillance systems. The paucity of data from certain GAAs severely limits understanding of the dynamics of the pandemic and development of an appropriate response.

1.4 Major modes of HIV transmission: The dynamics of the pandemic are closely linked to its progression in certain population groups. This has implications for defining populations at higher risk of acquiring HIV infection and the necessity of programs to focus interventions accordingly.

1.5 Current spread to rural areas: The spread of HIV from urban to rural areas has implications in terms of the increased size of the population at risk and the need for programs to decentralize services.

1.6 Prevalence of HIV in the general population: As estimated from surveys of pregnant women or of blood donors, the extent of HIV infection within the population reflects progression of the pandemic and provides information for monitoring and planning.

1.7 Gender ratio in populations currently infected with HIV: Generally reflecting the role played by heterosexual transmission in the current spread of HIV, this ratio is also an indicator of the necessity to reinforce prevention and control programs involving women.

2. Operational/Programmatic factors

2.1 Year of response: The year a national AIDS program was created is an indicator of the rapidity of national response, when taking into account other information, such as the year the first AIDS case was reported.

2.2 Level of external financing of AIDS programs: This indicator reflects the magnitude of international support extended to developing countries and raises the issue of program sustainability.

2.3 Proportion of GNP spent on health: This economic indicator reflects the priority accorded to the health sector.

3. Societal factors

3.1 Human Development Index (HDI): Developed by the United Nations Development Program, this index is composed of three indicators: life expectancy, educational attainment, and income. HDI is computed as a national average. GAAs are categorized according to the geographic clustering of national HDI.

3.2 Total female score: These indicators, developed by the Population Crisis Committee, reflect the gender gap and, more broadly, the vulnerability of women to HIV/AIDS.

3.3 Human Freedom Index (HFI): This composite index, developed by UNDP, reflects the degree to which the person has the right to determine the course of his or her own life.

3.4 Urban population growth: These rates are used as a surrogate for the measurement of urban migration.

ence and learning have many of these qualities: the past is prologue to the present, but it also lives into the present; the past and present evolve as new elements are added to create the future.

■■■■■   . . .

CURRENT AND FUTURE DIMENSIONS

Data on HIV provide the best, most up-to-date picture of the progress of the pandemic. Starting with global estimates as of January 1, 1992, this chapter illustrates the core theme of epidemic dynamism, reviews current HIV incidence and/or prevalence data from national surveys and studies of particular groups from around the world, and summarizes the current status of HIV in each Geographic Area of Affinity. Finally, *AIDS in the World* projections for 1995 and the year 2000 are presented and discussed.

Methodology. Estimates as of January 1, 1992, of the number of HIV infections in the world, cases of AIDS, and deaths were made, and projections for the years 1995 and 2000 were also developed. Two methods were applied concurrently by *AIDS in the World* in order to estimate the number of HIV-infected persons and people with AIDS as of January 1, 1992 and to proceed with projections through 1995 and the year 2000. The application of a model (Epimodel) to HIV seroprevalence data, obtained from a large number of serosurveys for the period 1988–90, provided HIV and AIDS estimates up to January 1, 1992, and projections through 1995. Additionally, an expert panel survey (Delphi survey) provided adjustment factors that helped refine output from Epimodel and provided estimates for the year 2000. The Delphi method is described in Box 2.4. Two values (a low estimate and a high estimate) were derived from calculations in each case. In order to invite readers' comments, the details of each methodological approach are provided in Appendix 2.2 and the full set of low and high figures are presented in Appendix 2.3.

AIDS in the World's Best Estimates

The HIV seroprevalence rates that served as a basis for modeling were drawn from surveys conducted between 1988 and 1990; during this period the prevalence of HIV increased by 30 to 100 percent in many populations studied through repeat cross-sectional surveys. Comparison of estimates made by *AIDS in the World* with reference values, such as trends in reported AIDS cases and results from more recent HIV serosurveys (1991–92), showed that high estimates were all conservative and low estimates clearly understated.

Furthermore, the curves which were chosen to best fit the reference points (year of widespread HIV, adjusted AIDS cases, and prevalence of HIV in 1990) assumed that HIV incidence (new infections occurring each year) will peak before the end of the present decade in all GAAs, an assumption that, unfortunately, is most unlikely to materialize. The application of other curves would have provided different (possibly higher) projections but would have necessitated additional, largely speculative assumptions on the part of *AIDS in the World* as to the future rate of spread of HIV. This resulted in conservative estimates and projections, particularly in the case of Southeast Asia, where the epidemic may, in fact, be more likely to follow an exponential curve with a much higher rate of growth in the early to mid-1990s than what the application of the model predicts. In this particular case, the estimation of 675,000 HIV infections by January 1, 1992, may only represent 50 to 75 percent of the number of infections which Thailand and India alone estimate to have already occurred.

Box 2.4: The Delphi Method

The Delphi method was developed as a technique for reaching expert consensus on estimates for which no correct answer can be ascertained. For example, the number of HIV-infected people in Latin America in the year 2000 can only be guessed. However, it is assumed that collecting the best estimates of recognized experts will provide the best available projection. The details of Delphi methodology revolve around the desire to avoid interpersonal deformations of the so-called expert guesses. Thus, each expert is contacted directly by the survey organizer; the experts do not know the identity of the other participants. Each expert is provided with a written series of questions for which a quantitative answer is requested (e.g., How many people will be infected with HIV in Latin America by the year 2000?). The experts' responses are collected and provided back to all participants in summary form (e.g., 7.6 million). Each expert is requested to review the data and provide a second estimate (of course, he or she may repeat the first). The purpose of this second round is to narrow the range of responses. Finally, the results can be expressed either by a measure of central tendency (mean, median) or, more usually, by providing the range of second-round responses.

Of course, the Delphi is only a form of collective educated guess and should be taken as such.

Table 2.2: Cumulative HIV infections in adults and children by Geographic Area of Affinity (GAA) as of January 1, 1992

GAA	Total no. of infections (millions)	% of global total HIV infections
1 North America	1.18	9.2
2 Western Europe	0.73	5.7
3 Oceania	0.03	0.2
4 Latin America	1.04	8.1
5 Sub-Saharan Africa	8.77	68.0
6 Caribbean	0.33	2.6
7 Eastern Europe	0.03	0.2
8 South East Mediterranean	0.04	0.3
9 North East Asia	0.04	0.3
10 Southeast Asia	>0.70	5.4
Total	12.89[a]	100.0

Source: AIDS in the World, 1992.
a. Figure differs from total shown in Table 2.4 because of rounding.

For the above reasons, *AIDS in the World* considers the high values resulting from estimations and projections as its best estimates; they are used in further discussions and analyses throughout this report. For 1992 and 1995, a single best estimate (of HIV infections, of AIDS cases, and of deaths) is provided; however, for the year 2000, given the great uncertainties that surround longer-term projections, both the low and high estimates are presented. The number of HIV infections, AIDS cases, and deaths in adults and children estimated to have occurred in the world by January 1, 1992, and projections for 1995 and the year 2000 are shown in Appendix 2.3.

Global Estimates

As of January 1, 1992, an estimated 11.8 million adults and 1.1 million children—a total of 12.9 million people worldwide—have been infected with HIV. Table 2.2 and Figure 2.1 show the distribution of this cumulative number of HIV-infected people for each GAA.

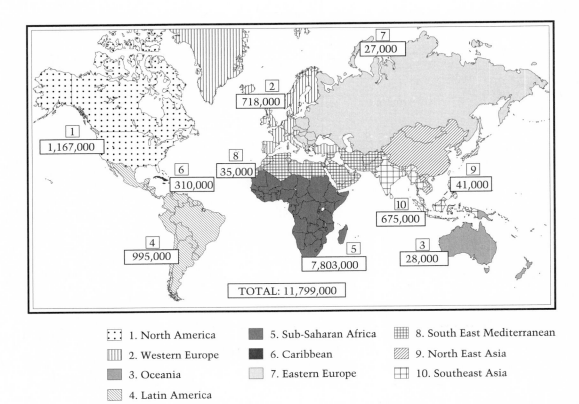

Figure 2.1. Estimate of HIV infections in adults as of January 1, 1992 for each Geographic Area of Affinity (GAA).
Source: AIDS in the World, 1992.

Table 2.3 illustrates the geographic diversity of the pandemic. Of adults infected with HIV as of January 1, 1992, two-thirds (66 percent) were from sub-Saharan Africa, which contained only 8.8 percent of the global adult population. The three other GAAs with a relative excess of cases compared with population were North America (9.9 percent of adult HIV infections, 5.4 percent of world adult population), Latin America (8.4 percent of HIV, 7.8 percent of global population), and the Caribbean (2.6 percent of HIV, 0.6 percent of global population). All other GAAs had a smaller proportion of HIV infections than of global adult population.

Table 2.3 also shows the wide range in rates of cumulative HIV infection per million population, from 51 per million in North East Asia to 32,433 per million in sub-Saharan Africa. On a population basis, the most heavily infected GAAs are sub-Saharan Africa, the Caribbean, North America, and Latin America.

In 1980, an estimated 100,000 people worldwide were infected with HIV; during the intervening 11 years, the number of HIV-infected people worldwide increased approximately 120-fold.

Of the 11.8 million HIV-infected adults, 4.7 million are women, representing 40 percent of the global total (Table 2.4). The ratio of HIV-infected men and women was estimated through the Delphi survey and applied to the overall estimate of HIV-infected adults. The

Table 2.3: Cumulative number and rate of HIV infections in adults (age 15–49 years) by Geographic Area of Affinity (GAA) as of January 1, 1992

GAA	Cumulative no. of infections	% of all infections	% of total adult population	Rate:[a] Cumulative HIV infections/adult population
1 North America	1,167,000	9.9	5.4	7,921
2 Western Europe	718,000	6.1	8.1	3,241
3 Oceania	28,000	0.2	0.5	2,095
4 Latin America	995,000	8.4	7.8	4,630
5 Sub-Saharan Africa	7,803,000	66.1	8.8	32,433
6 Caribbean	310,000	2.6	0.6	17,840
7 Eastern Europe	27,000	0.2	7.4	134
8 South East Mediterranean	35,000	0.3	6.5	196
9 North East Asia	41,000	0.3	29.5	51
10 Southeast Asia[b]	>675,000	5.7	25.4	967
Total	11,799,000	99.8	100.0	4,303

Source: AIDS in the World, 1992.
a. Expressed as X/million.
b. Conservative estimate based on limited available data.

Table 2.4: Estimated adult HIV infections by gender and pediatric infections by Geographic Area of Affinity (GAA) as of January 1, 1992

GAA	Men	Women	Total adults	Children	Total
1 North America	1,038,500	128,500	1,167,000	16,000	1,183,000
2 Western Europe	596,000	122,000	718,000	8,000	726,000
3 Oceania	24,500	3,500	28,000	500	28,500
4 Latin America	796,000	199,000	995,000	40,500	1,035,500
5 Sub-Saharan Africa	3,901,500	3,901,500	7,803,000	969,500	8,772,500
6 Caribbean	186,000	124,000	310,000	16,000	326,000
7 Eastern Europe	24,500	2,500	27,000	200	27,200
8 South East Mediterranean	29,000	6,000	35,000	1,000	36,000
9 North East Asia	34,000	7,000	41,000	750	41,750
10 Southeast Asia[a]	>452,000	>223,000	>675,000	>24,000	699,000
Total	7,082,000	4,717,000	11,799,000	1,076,450	12,875,450

Source: AIDS in the World, 1992.
a. Conservative estimate based on limited available data.

estimated gender ratio of adult HIV infections by GAA is shown in Table 2.5. In 1980, an estimated 80 percent of HIV-infected people were men; accordingly, the number of HIV-infected men increased about 90-fold from 1980 to 1991; the number of HIV-infected women increased more than 225-fold during this period.

AIDS in the World asked the Delphi group to estimate the proportion of HIV transmission attributable to different modes of spread in each GAA (Table 2.6). The results demonstrate once again the heterogeneity of the epidemic. The proportion of HIV infection associated with heterosexual transmission ranged from ten percent or less in North America, Oceania, and Eastern Europe to 70 percent or more in sub-Saharan Africa, the Caribbean, and Southeast Asia. Homosexual transmission was more common than heterosexual transmission

Table 2.5: Estimated male-to-female ratio, adult HIV infections by Geographic Area of Affinity (GAA) as of January 1, 1992

GAA	Male-to-female ratio[a]
1 North America	8.5
2 Western Europe	5
3 Oceania	7
4 Latin America	4
5 Sub-Saharan Africa	1
6 Caribbean	1.5
7 Eastern Europe	10
8 South East Mediterranean	5
9 North East Asia	5
10 Southeast Asia	2
Overall global	1.5

Source: Delphi survey, *AIDS in the World, 1992.*
a. Number of infections in men to one in women.

in six GAAs: North America, Western Europe, Oceania, Latin America, Eastern Europe, and the South East Mediterranean. Transmission through blood accounted for 5 percent or fewer of HIV infections in each area except Latin America (6 percent), the South East Mediterranean (18 percent), North East Asia (10 percent), and Southeast Asia (6 percent). Finally, the role of injection drug use in HIV transmission ranged widely from a low of 0.5 percent in sub-Saharan Africa to 20 percent or over in North America, Western Europe, the South East Mediterranean, and North East Asia. Figure 2.2 shows the global importance of each major route of HIV infection: sexual transmission was responsible for 86 percent of HIV infections (with a 5:1 heterosexual-to-homosexual ratio).

Of the 1.1 million pediatric HIV infections during this period

Table 2.6: Percentage of HIV-infected people by mode of transmission in adults (15–49 years) by Geographic Area of Affinity (GAA) as of January 1, 1992

GAA	Mode of transmission				
	Heterosexual	Homosexual	Blood	Injection drug use	Other/ unknown
1 North America	9	56	3	27	5
2 Western Europe	14	47	2	33	4
3 Oceania	6	87	2	3	2
4 Latin America	24	54	6	11	5
5 Sub-Saharan Africa	93	<1	4	<1	1
6 Caribbean	75	10	5	9	1
7 Eastern Europe	10	80	2	5	3
8 South East Mediterranean	20	35	18	22	5
9 North East Asia	50	20	10	20	0
10 Southeast Asia	70	8	6	14	2

Source: Delphi Survey, *AIDS in the World, 1992.*

(Table 2.4), the vast majority (90 percent) have occurred in sub-Saharan Africa; of the remainder, most were accounted for by Latin America (4 percent), Southeast Asia (2 percent), and North America (1.5 percent).

The Core Theme—Epidemic Dynamism: As of January 1, 1992, the pandemic remains highly dynamic. The three dimensions of epidemic dynamism are each clearly and increasingly evident: continued spread in already affected areas; spread to new communities and areas; and increasing epidemiological and societal complexity of maturing epidemics.

Spread in already affected areas: There is no already HIV-affected community, area, or country in which HIV infection has stopped. In

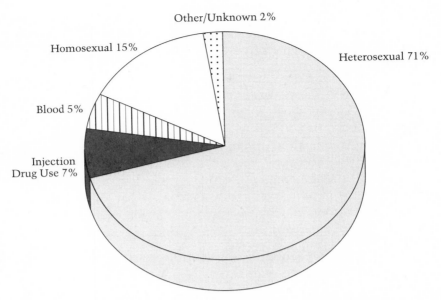

Other/Unknown 2%

Homosexual 15%

Heterosexual 71%

Blood 5%

Injection
Drug Use 7%

Figure 2.2. Proportion of cumulative adult HIV infections by mode of transmission.
Source: AIDS in the World, 1992

the United States, at least 40,000 to 80,000 new HIV infections are estimated to have occurred during 1991,[1] and 1992 estimates are at least as high. In Europe, 75,000 new HIV infections are estimated to have occurred in 1991.[2] Estimates made by *AIDS in the World* would suggest that in 1991 60,000 to 100,000 adult HIV infections occurred in North America and 90,000 to 100,000 in Europe. The issue of whether HIV and AIDS have peaked as problems in the industrialized world is addressed in Chapter 15. Clearly, if incidence (the occurrence of new infections) is declining in certain highly vulnerable groups, the incidence in the population that did not identify with high-risk behavior continues to increase. As more people in this larger population become infected, a rebound of the epidemic is seen, growing gradually toward a second peak of incidence, the timing of which cannot be set with any degree of assurance at this time.

In the developing world, many examples of continued spread in already affected areas can be provided. These examples include increases in HIV seroprevalence:

- Among men attending sexually transmitted disease clinics in Nairobi, Kenya, from 3 percent in 1981 to 23 percent in 1990.[3,4]
- Among women sex workers in San Pedro Sula, Honduras, from 19 percent in 1989 to 35 percent in 1990.[5]
- Among all adults in Abidjan, Côte d'Ivoire, from about 1 percent in 1987 to over 7 percent in 1991.[6]
- Among pregnant women in São Paulo, Brazil, from 0.2 percent (1 per 500) in 1987 to 1.3 percent (1 per 75) in 1990.[7]
- Among pregnant women in Nairobi, Kenya, from 2 percent in 1985 to 13 percent in 1991.[8,9]

However, increases in HIV seroprevalence are not universal. Studies conducted over several years in Kinshasa, Zaire,[10] Port-au-Prince, Haiti,[11] and among IDUs in New York City[12] have documented a stable HIV seroprevalence. Unfortunately, the meaning of these findings may be obscured by likely resurgences of HIV infection in Zaire and Haiti, as a consequence of political and social turmoil. It is also important to recall that a stable prevalence is compatible with continued, ongoing HIV transmission. For example, the unchanging HIV seroprevalence in Zaire was occurring in the context of an annual incidence (rate of new infections) of about 0.5 to 1.5 percent. Similarly, among IDUs in New York City, stable seroprevalence coexisted with a seroincidence of approximately 10 percent, which, although still remarkably high, represented a major decline since the early 1980s.

Spread of the pandemic to new areas: During 1991, as in previous years, HIV continued to spread—sometimes quite rapidly—into previously unaffected or little affected communities and areas. Examples include:

- In Poland, the first HIV-infected IDU was reported in November 1988; by February 1991, 829 of 1,178 (70 percent) known HIV-infected people in Poland were infected through injection drug use.[13] In Czechoslovakia, 62 percent of reported HIV infections involved homosexual men, whereas in Bulgaria, 68 percent of known HIV infections involved heterosexual transmission. As of December 21,

1990, of all central and eastern European countries, the largest number of reported HIV infections was from Yugoslavia (2,023 infections, of which 1,511 were IDUs); second largest was Romania, with 1,406 infections, reflecting the available data from institutionalized children.[14]

- There is an increasing spread of HIV into rural Africa. In the Zairian province of Bas-Zaire, HIV seroprevalence in 1989–90 ranged from 7.6 percent in large towns, to 4 percent in small towns, to 2 percent in rural villages.[15] In the Côte d'Ivoire, HIV seroprevalence among rural adults was 2.8 percent, which was higher than adult seroprevalence in Abidjan, the capital city, in 1986.[16] Although there have been some heavily affected rural areas (Rakai district, Uganda; Kagera district, Tanzania), the rural HIV epidemic is generally several years behind the urban epidemics.
- A 1991 report from Paraguay found a 9 percent seroprevalence among homosexual men in the capital city of Asuncion.[17]
- Recent reports have documented the arrival and spread of HIV in Greenland.[18]
- HIV infections have been documented in many Pacific island nations, including the Federated States of Micronesia, Fiji, French Polynesia, Guam, Kiribati, Marshall Islands, New Caledonia, Northern Mariana Islands, Papua New Guinea, Samoa, and Tonga.[19]
- In Nigeria, HIV seroprevalence among blood donors increased from zero in 1987 to 1.5 percent during 1990.[20] In Lagos, ten percent of women sex workers were found to be HIV infected.[21] Once considered an area of minimal HIV spread between the West African and Central African epicenters, Nigeria is now estimated to have at least 500,000 HIV-infected people.

Southeast Asia provides the most striking illustrations of epidemic volatility. In India:

- HIV prevalence increased among STD clinic patients in Bombay, from 4.3 percent in 1989–90 to 32.1 percent in 1991.[22,23]
- HIV prevalence among IDUs in the east Indian state of Manipur increased from zero in 1986 to 54 percent in 1990.[24]
- Among pregnant women in the south Indian city of Madras, HIV seroprevalence rose from zero in 1988 to 1.3 percent in 1990.[25]
- Among women sex workers in Bombay, HIV seroprevalence was

1.3 percent in 1987, but increased to 18.1 percent in 1990 (with some studies documenting an HIV seroprevalence of 60 percent or greater).[26]

In Thailand:

- From 1990 to 1991, HIV seroprevalence increased among blood donors in northern and central Thailand from 1.1 percent to 1.7 percent and from 0.6 percent to 1 percent, respectively.[27]
- Among patients at STD clinics in northern Thailand, HIV seroprevalence rose from 8.8 percent in 1990 to 13.2 percent in 1991; in central Thailand, the prevalence increased from 4.4 percent to 7.1 percent during the same period.[28]

Global experience has repeatedly demonstrated that even though geography may delay the arrival of HIV, it is not protective. HIV is in the process of reaching all human communities; it is not a question of if, but of when.

Increasing complexity of the pandemic: Regardless of which persons, with whatever behaviors, are first affected by HIV in a community, HIV will spread through all available routes. Time and again, countries and communities have reassured themselves by believing that HIV will remain within assumed boundaries—whether geographical, social, economic, religious, or political.

The reality is otherwise. For example:

- In Brazil from 1980 to 1984, only 1 percent of HIV infections were linked with injection drug use; by 1988, it exceeded 9 percent.[29]
- In 1984 in Mexico, there were an estimated 25 HIV-infected men for every HIV-infected woman; by 1990, this ratio had declined to 4:1.[30]
- In San Francisco, significant differences in HIV seroprevalence have been documented between white, African-American, and Latino homosexual and bisexual men.[31]
- Wars and internal conflicts can facilitate HIV spread (see Box 2.5).
- Men and women IDUs in Baltimore, Maryland, USA, have different HIV incidence rates (and risk factors for becoming HIV infected).[32]
- In Bangkok, at least eight distinct subgroups of commercial sex workers have been described, from pavement-dwelling street-based women to hotel call girls; the HIV experience of each group differs.[33]

- In the United States, of the 189 AIDS cases reported in 1981, 97 percent were men and three-fourths came from two states—New York and California. However, of the 43,000 AIDS cases reported in 1990, 11 percent were women, 800 were children, and cases came from all 50 states.[34]
- In a single large metropolitan area, like Dade County, Florida (where Miami is located), at least five distinct subepidemics of HIV infection are occurring, each with its own dynamic and special population characteristics.[35]

As the epidemic matures in any community, it continues to evolve in response to opportunities for spread. Individual and collective vulnerability to further spread of HIV remains large (see Chapter 14).

In sum, the HIV pandemic continues to be dynamic, unstable, and volatile. Based on current information, it is clear that so-called explosive HIV epidemics may not occur in many—even most—populations. Yet the data from 1990 and 1991 emphasize once again that no geographical area, population, or social group can consider itself immune to HIV, especially as the conditions that lead to vulnerability—and that foster HIV spread—are complex and changing.

· · ·

CURRENT HIV INCIDENCE AND PREVALENCE DATA

This section examines the current status of the HIV pandemic by presenting selected and illustrative HIV prevalence and incidence data, summarized in large part from the U.S. Bureau of the Census's data bank.* Particular attention is given to HIV prevalence in specific populations, including commercial sex workers, homosexual men, IDUs, STD clinic patients, pregnant women, and blood donors. These individual snapshots, along with a brief summary from each GAA, provide detail to complete the general picture of a dynamic, volatile worldwide epidemic.

---

*References to studies and surveys which provided data presented here can be found in the *U.S. Bureau of Census Periodic Update on HIV/AIDS Surveillance Data Base.*

Data Sources and Issues

Knowledge of the infection and spread of HIV and AIDS in countries around the world is based on a variety of reports and studies that are known to be incomplete and nonrepresentative. AIDS case reporting, for example, from African countries to WHO has been estimated to be about 10 to 30 percent complete, due to a variety of factors, including inadequate reporting systems within countries and, particularly in the early years of the AIDS epidemic, a reluctance on the part of countries to report AIDS cases at all. A knowledge of AIDS cases alone, moreover, is not sufficient for an understanding of the dynamics of the epidemic, due to the extended incubation period between initial

---

Box 2.5: Low-Intensity Wars and HIV Transmission

What is the impact of war and conflict on AIDS? Most of the attention has focused on patterns of individual behavior rather than their social context. Yet war, and its resulting social and economic disruption, can have a strong impact on HIV/AIDS, as it does on sexually transmitted and other diseases. An attempt to measure this impact examined the effects of low-intensity wars in Southern Africa and found a new and disturbing social model for HIV/AIDS transmission.[a]

The HIV/AIDS pandemic has spread in a number of Southern African countries—including Mozambique, Angola, and Zimbabwe—already devastated by prolonged regional military conflicts. These protracted conflicts can be characterized as low-intensity wars, in which "open military conflict alternates with civil strife, economic sabotage, destruction of vital infrastructures (including health and education services), and banditry."[b] Since the late 1970s,

low-intensity wars have devastated rural economies and displaced massive numbers of people in Southern Africa. Civilians flee areas disturbed by fighting and insecurity, and rural populations shift to towns or to be near army barracks for trading. At the same time, regular armies and groups of bandits are continuously on the move.

These population movements create opportunities for HIV/AIDS to penetrate previously less affected populations. The shift to towns or settlements near army barracks places rural populations at increased risk of exposure to HIV/AIDS, as they join the circle of poverty and marginality that includes prostitution and street children. Certain groups generated by these same social processes may play the role of a bridge between HIV-infected people and the general population. These include nonprofessional sex workers (e.g., young school girls in large towns), members of armed forces, migrant workers, long-distance truck drivers, and street children. All tend to have a high number of heterosexual

infection and later development of HIV-related illness. Thus, even the most accurate AIDS case data would only provide a picture of the epidemic of infection as it existed as many as ten years ago.

As a result, considerable attention has been paid to the collection of data on HIV infection among various population groups. In the early years of the epidemic, many of these studies were conducted in a nonscientific manner and may have provided results that were not representative even of the population group targeted by the study. More recently, increasing attention has been paid to such issues as increased sample sizes, representativeness of the sample selection, geographic coverage, and confirmatory testing of HIV-positive results. Consequently, both the quantity and the quality of seroprevalence

---

partners, links with the family or circle of friends and relatives, and large geographical diffusion. Additionally, they often share biological co-factors for HIV/AIDS, such as a high prevalence of STDs.

The consequences of war may also have significant implications for HIV/AIDS prevention efforts, by affecting the way a person understands and processes information and translates it into practice. Psychological effects, such as increased selective inattention, evasive skepticism, and desire for revenge, can have lasting impact on those who may never personally witness an armed confrontation, particularly children. The understanding of such concepts as *risk, protection, steady partner, control,* and *health* is influenced by the effects of war, and by feelings of fear and loss of control over one's life typical in a war situation. This has been interpreted as a more acute version of the powerlessness experienced by the poor all over the world; this experience, it is argued, structures the

concept of risk and health for millions of people.

Low-intensity wars provide an example of the changing social determinants of AIDS, and the need for culturally and situationally responsive solutions. AIDS research, as well as information, education, and communication activities, must account for the unique social and psychological pressures affecting people living in war and in other high-risk situations.

Low-intensity wars are underway around the world today. Each in its own way creates a special vulnerability to the introduction and spread of HIV.—The Editors

---

a. M. Baldo and A. J. Cabral, "Low intensity wars and social determination of the HIV transmission: The search for a new paradigm to guide research and control of the HIV/AIDS pandemic." In *Action on AIDS in Southern Africa. Maputo Conference on Health in Transition in Southern Africa, April 1990*, ed. Z. Stein and A. Zwi (New York: Committee for Health in Southern Africa, 1991).

b. Ibid.

data have improved markedly in recent years. Nevertheless, many biases still remain, and caution must be used in the interpretation of results.

Nationally representative seroprevalence surveys have not generally been conducted, largely due to concerns regarding cost, diversion of skilled personnel, and an understanding that a nationally representative sample may not provide much useful information about the groups at greatest risk for HIV infection. Thus, in recent years sentinel surveillance programs have been developed to monitor defined populations for changes in HIV infection levels. For example, countries may develop programs that monitor infection among antenatal women attending government clinics, patients receiving treatment for STDs, blood donors, and women engaged in commercial sex activities. Results from these studies can provide rapid feedback on infection levels and trends in populations at various levels of risk without the time and effort required to mount a national survey.

Data presented in the following discussion are taken from the *HIV/AIDS Surveillance Data Base,* developed and maintained at the U.S. Bureau of the Census, with funding support from the U.S. Agency for International Development. Data are regularly compiled from the scientific and technical literature as well as from presentations at major international conferences. The *HIV/AIDS Surveillance Data Base* currently contains more than 11,000 data records drawn from more than 1,500 publications and presentations (see Box 2.6).

General Population Surveys

Large-scale, population-based national HIV seroprevalence surveys have been conducted in only a few countries. Among these are Uganda, Rwanda, Côte d'Ivoire, and the former Soviet Union. In addition, population-based sample surveys have been undertaken in a variety of nonnational settings (i.e., Bissau in Guinea-Bissau; Bangui, Central African Republic; the Rakai district of Uganda; Cameroon). Data from the national surveys have provided, to some extent, a more complete picture of the epidemic in the country. However, it has become increasingly recognized that such surveys leave many important questions unanswered. These questions have become the motivation and focus both of sentinel surveillance efforts as well as of surveys targeted on specific geographic areas or population groups.

Uganda. Uganda's national survey[36-38] was conducted over the period of September 1987 to January 1988, with a cluster sample design using 100 clusters, stratified into rural, urban, and capital-city strata. Initially, a sample of 15,000 was targeted. A portion of the country, in the north and the east, could not be included due to logistical problems. Data from the survey have not only provided national estimates of the number of Ugandans infected, but also contributed to the understanding of age and gender patterns of infection and of the geographic variation in infection levels.

According to this survey, approximately 800,000 adult Ugandans were HIV infected; of a total population of 16.2 million, overall seroprevalence was 4.9 percent. Among the results were estimates of the HIV-infected population in rural and in urban areas. Despite consistently higher HIV seroprevalence in the urban samples, the total rural

---

Box 2.6: The HIV/AIDS Surveillance Database: What's in the Bank?

aren Stanecki, U.S. Bureau
the Census

The Center for International Research (CIR), of the United States Bureau of the Census, compiles HIV seroprevalence data for population groups in developing countries into the HIV/AIDS Surveillance Database. This database was developed and has been maintained at the Bureau since 1987, with funding support from the United States Agency for International Development. Data presented at major conferences are regularly incorporated into the database, along with information published in the scientific literature.

Currently, the database contains more than 11,000 records drawn from more than 1,500 publications and presentations. It is CIR's goal to incorporate all available data from seroprevalence studies conducted in developing countries. The data,

however, are imperfect and may be incomplete.

The database is distributed in both hardcopy and computer-readable form, along with microcomputer software for the retrieval and printing of user-selected data. In addition to distribution of the database itself, the CIR has prepared various summaries and analyses of HIV seroprevalence data for distribution to interested researchers and policy makers, for publication, and for presentation at international meetings on AIDS.

CIR welcomes comments and suggestions from readers. It also welcomes copies of articles or references to information that may not yet be in the database. Inquiries regarding the database should be addressed to:

HIV/AIDS Surveillance Database
Center for International Research
Scuderi Bldg., Rm. 604
United States Bureau of the Census
Washington, DC 20233 U.S.A.

HIV Seroprevalence (percent)

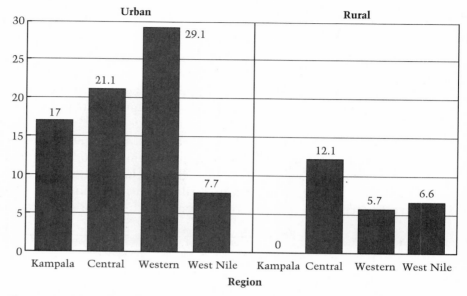

Figure 2.3. HIV seroprevalence for the population of Uganda, by region, 1987-1988.
Source: Figures compiled by the Center for International Research, U.S. Bureau of the Census.

infected population (626,091) was estimated to be approximately four times the number of infected urban inhabitants (164,439) due to differences in the population size. The seroprevalence of adult women overall was around 16 percent, compared to about 12 percent for males.

The prevalence by age and gender in Uganda, based on this national survey (shown later in this chapter), displays a tendency for women to become infected at younger ages than men. Compared to other countries, the high level of infection and the diffusion of infection into nearly all adult ages suggest an exposure to infection from HIV over a prolonged period of time.

Available data for regions show the variation in overall infection level within Uganda at this point in time (Figure 2.3). Urban areas consistently exhibited higher infection levels than did their rural

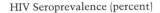

HIV Seroprevalence (percent)

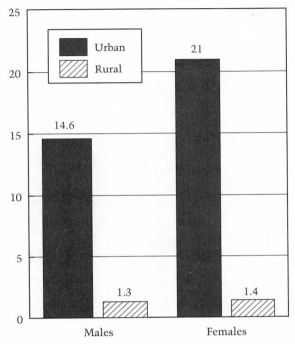

Figure 2.4. HIV seroprevalence for the population of Rwanda, by gender and residence, 1986.
Source: Figures compiled by the Center for International Research, U.S. Bureau of the Census.

counterparts, with the lowest rural rates in the West and West Nile regions.

Rwanda. In December 1986, researchers in Rwanda conducted a nationally representative serosurvey using a clustered sample design stratified into 30 urban and 30 rural clusters.[39] Results indicated more than one-fifth of urban women and about one-seventh of urban men were HIV infected (Figure 2.4). In rural areas, infection levels were much lower, as only 1.4 percent of rural women and 1.3 percent of rural men were infected. (Data by age from this survey are shown in Figure 2.5).

Despite being a relatively small country, Rwanda in 1986 exhib-

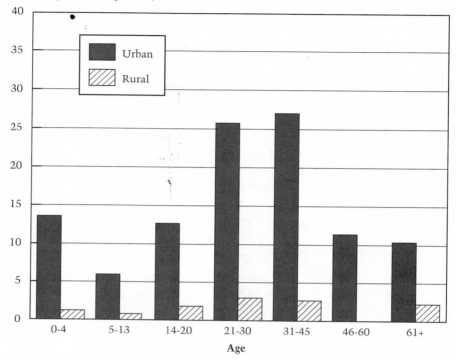

Figure 2.5. HIV seroprevalence for the population of Rwanda, by age and residence, 1988.
Source: B. Godifroid, N. Augustin, N. Didace, et al., "Etude sur la séropositivité liée à l'infection au Virus de l'Immunodéficience Humaine au Rwanda," *Revue Médicale Rwandaise* 20(54)(1988): 37-42. (Figures compiled by the Center for International Research, U.S. Bureau of the Census.)

ited considerable variation by geographic area (Figure 2.6). In all prefectures, a consistent pattern of higher urban seroprevalence was found, although the relationship between the two areas varied greatly.

Côte d'Ivoire. Several widescale, population-based surveys have been conducted in Côte d'Ivoire.[40-42] The latest for which data are available was fielded in February 1989. A total of 4,899 subjects were recruited between the ages of 15 and 65 years in a cluster sample design stratified by urban (more than 10,000 inhabitants) and rural areas. Due to the presence of HIV-2 in the population, testing included

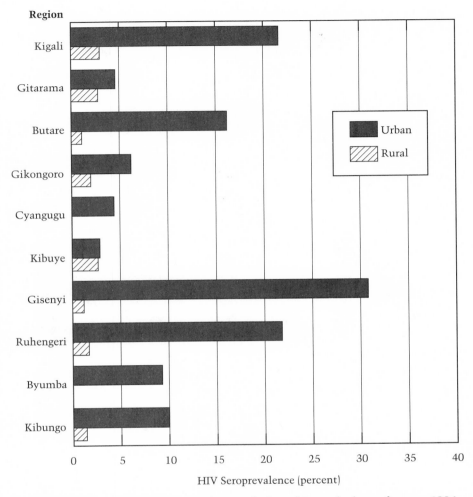

Figure 2.6. HIV seroprevalence for the population of Rwanda, by prefecture, 1986.
Source: Figures compiled by the Center for International Research, U.S. Bureau of the Census.

HIV Seroprevalence (percent)

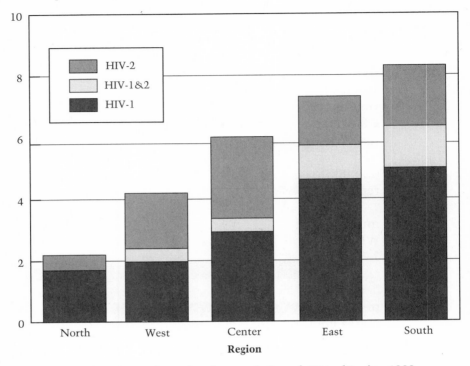

Figure 2.7. HIV seroprevalence for the population of Côte d'Ivoire, 1989.
Source: Figures compiled by the Center for International Research, U.S. Bureau of the Census.

the identification of HIV-1, HIV-2, and dual infection patterns. Based on the results of the survey, the researchers estimated that there were about 400,000 HIV-infected adults in Côte d'Ivoire at the time of the survey. This figure does not include the infected population under age 15, including infants infected through perinatal transmission.

Results showed that HIV infection has spread across all regions in Côte d'Ivoire, with over eight percent of the adult population in the south infected by HIV-1, HIV-2, or both (see Figure 2.7). Infection levels in other regions varied, with the lowest infection noted in the north. Similarly, the distribution of total HIV infection varied between the viruses, with HIV-2, for example, more important in the center region than in other areas. Overall, however, more than one-half of those infected in all regions were infected with HIV-1.

General Population Estimates: Europe, United States

In most industrialized countries, formal national HIV seroprevalence studies have been considered but consistently rejected on a combination of logistic, cost, and ethical grounds. Nevertheless, many industrialized countries have sought to generate, and subsequently refine, national estimates of the number of HIV-infected people. Estimates have been based on extrapolations from surveillance data, serosurveys (including anonymous unlinked testing), and back-calculations from reported AIDS cases.

In Europe, national authorities reported their minimum, maximum, and best estimates of the number of HIV-infected people to the WHO-EC Collaborating Center in Paris in January 1992 (see Table 2.7). The table compares the best estimate offered at a WHO consultation in February 1988 with more recent estimates. Estimated numbers of HIV-infected people ranged from zero for Albania to 150,000 in France. Of the fourteen countries whose 1988 and 1992 best estimates could be compared, seven raised their estimate for 1992 compared with 1988, six reduced their 1992 estimate compared with 1988, and one estimate remained unchanged. Spain reported the largest up-scaling, from a best estimate of 24,000 in 1988 to 100,000 in 1992; France lowered its best estimate from 200,000 in 1988 to 150,000 in 1992.

In the United States, a complex and extensive national sentinel surveillance system, the Family of HIV Seroprevalence Surveys, was created through national and state cooperation, starting in 1988. The use of standardized protocols permits useful comparisons among sites and over time (see Box 2.7).

Technical, Financial, and Ethical Issues

A variety of technical, financial, and ethical concerns have operated collectively to limit the number of national general-population surveys being conducted. These concerns have motivated the movement toward more targeted surveys.

Survey universe: General population-based surveys, by definition,

Table 2.7: Prevalence: Estimates of the total number of HIV seropositive persons in 31 European countries, February 1988 and January 1992

Country	1988 estimates[a]			1992 estimates[b]			Date of estimate
	Minimum	Maximum	Best estimate	Minimum	Maximum	Best estimate	
Albania	—	—	—	0	0	0	Oct. 1991
Austria	—	—	—	8,000	12,000	10,000	Oct. 1991
Belgium	2,500	15,000	7,000	8,500	23,000	15,000	1991
Bulgaria	100	300	200	200	600	300	Oct. 1991
Czechoslovakia	100	>1,000	>1,000	300	1,500	500	Oct. 1991
Denmark	5,000	20,000	10,000	4,000	7,000	5,000	Oct. 1991
Finland	500	1,000	500	450	600	500	Oct. 1991
France	150,000	250,000	200,000	100,000	200,000	150,000	1990
Germany	30,150[c]	120,300[c]	50,200[c]	40,000	90,000	55,000	Oct. 1991
Greece	4,000	9,000	7,000	—	—	—	Nov. 1991
Hungary	1,000	5,000	2,500	700	2,000	1500	Oct. 1991
Iceland	—	—	—	150	250	200	1991
Ireland	678	1,500	1,000	1,020	2,275	1,900	Feb. 1990
Israel	305	4,700	2,200	1,000	5,000	2,500	Oct. 1991
Italy	20,000	100,000	50,000	55,000	100,000	70,000	
Luxembourg	—	—	—	—	—	—	Oct. 1991
Malta	24	—	—	50	100	50	June 1991
Monaco	—	—	—	—	—	—	
Netherlands	15,000	20,000	—	6,000	12,000	10,000	Begin. 1990
Norway	2,000	4,500	3,200	1,200	1,700	1,500	1990
Poland	3,000	10,000	5,000	—	—	2,000	Oct. 1991
Portugal	500	5,000	—	—	—	—	Oct. 1991
Romania	16	—	—	2,700	3,800	3,200	Dec. 1991
San Marino	7	40	—	—	—	—	
Spain	24,000	—	24,000	—	—	100,000	Oct. 1991
Sweden	—	—	—	3,200	4,000	3,600	Oct. 1991

Table 2.7 (cont.): Prevalence: Estimates of the total number of HIV seropositive persons in 31 European countries, February 1988 and January 1992

Country	1988 estimates[a]			1992 estimates[b]			
	Minimum	Maximum	Best estimate	Minimum	Maximum	Best estimate	Date of estimate
Switzerland	5,000	30,000	25,000	12,000	24,000	18,000	Jan. 1992
Turkey	—	—	—	—	—	182[d]	Jan. 1992
United Kingdom	24,000	40,000	—	14,250	39,400	24,000	End 88/89
USSR	100	250	—	3,000	7,000	5,000	Nov. 1991
Yugoslavia	1,500	4,000	2,500	4,000	6,000	5,000	Oct. 1991

Sources: The European Center for the Epidemiological Monitoring of AIDS (WHO-EC Collaborating Centre on AIDS) and the national surveillance correspondents of the respective European countries.

a. Estimates given at WHO Euro consultation, Tatry Poprad, Czechoslovakia, 17–19 February 1988.

b. Estimates reported to WHO-EC Collaborating Centre on AIDS, Saint Maurice (Paris), France, January 1992.

c. Including data from the German Democratic Republic.

d. Turkey: number of reported HIV+ persons.

reach people who are not at above-average risk for infection. In settings with relatively low prevalence, however, this may be the wrong focus for data collection efforts. Findings that show the general population to be infected at a low level may serve to downplay the *potential* risk for future spread of HIV. Instead, surveys of the population at elevated risk can focus attention on the populations within which the epidemic is spreading most rapidly.

Scarce human resources: Large-scale survey research involves thousands of hours of effort in the design stage, field operations, logistics, laboratory work, and analysis. Such an undertaking can divert scarce human resources from other important activities, such as intervention and treatment programs. National programs have had to balance the desire to do all projects with a realistic assessment of their capabilities.

Distribution of HIV and optimal sample design: Standard sample designs incorporate cluster sampling to reduce costs. Because HIV is itself highly geographically clustered, the optimum sampling strategy involves a larger number of sample clusters with smaller size, thus increasing costs. If HIV has a low prevalence in a population, the sample size required to estimate the prevalence within a specified degree of accuracy is also increased. In addition, the determination of a cost-effective sample design without advanced knowledge of the geographic distribution of HIV is problematic.

Subnational geographic interest: Data from national surveys are seldom used solely at the national level. Interest in geographic (i.e., urban/rural and/or provincial) estimates means that, in effect, the national sample is composed of a number of subnational samples. All of these considerations lead to larger samples with higher costs.

Measuring change over time: National surveys with large samples are not well suited to rapid assessment of short-term (e.g., annual) changes in infection levels. At a detailed geographic level, the effect

---

Box 2.7: Family of Seroprevalence Surveys of the U.S. Public Health Service

This is a national, ongoing sentinel serosurveillance system for HIV infection that was established during the period from 1987 to 1989 using anonymous unlinked samples of blood from certain sentinel populations (see Table 2.B).

Reported cases of AIDS do not accurately reflect levels of HIV infection, even in more developed countries, because the median time from HIV infection to a diagnosis of AIDS in adults is approximately 10 years and may lengthen as treatments become more effective. The Family of Serosurveys was established to provide national, state, and local levels, patterns, and trends of HIV infection by demographic subgroups. In high-prevalence areas, nonblinded surveys complement the unlinked surveillance system.

Public health surveillance systems are a means of obtaining data for decision making. Some important uses of data from the Family of Serosurveys include (1) monitoring levels and trends of HIV infection in the sentinel populations and targeting resources and program efforts accordingly; (2) detecting deviations from expected patterns of transmission and modifying prevention and control priorities and programs accordingly; (3) determining risk factors for infection; (4) defining and targeting immediate or long-range public health actions for prevention and control; (5) setting priorities for interventions and for allocation of resources; (6) indirectly estimating HIV incidence from serial cross-sectional surveys; (7) projecting future numbers of AIDS cases and use of health care facilities; and (8) planning for mitigation of the adverse socioeconomic consequences of future AIDS cases and deaths that will inevitably result from current levels of HIV infection.

Table 2.B: Sentinel populations in the family of HIV seroprevalence surveys

Sentinel population	Access to seroprevalence survey	Overall level of risk of exposure
Persons with sexually transmitted diseases (STDs)	State and local health department STD clinics	Increased
Injection drug users entering drug treatment programs	Drug treatment centers	Increased
Women seeking family-planning services, prenatal care, abortion services	Family-planning clinics, prenatal care clinics, abortion clinics	All levels
Persons treated for tuberculosis	State and local health department tuberculosis clinics	Increased
Selected hospital patients at admission for non-HIV-related diagnoses	Hospitals	All levels
Primary care outpatients	Clinical laboratory	All levels
Primary care outpatients	Physician network	All levels
Childbearing women	Neonatal screening programs	All levels
Blood donors	Blood collection agencies	Deferral of persons at increased risk
Civilian applicants to military service	Department of Defense HIV screening program	Deferral of persons at increased risk
Native Americans and Alaskan natives	Indian Health Service health clinics	All levels
Job Corps entrants	Department of Labor HIV screening program	All levels
University students	University health clinics	All levels
Prisoners	Prisons and jails	All levels
Homeless persons	Health clinics	All levels

Source: M. Pappaioanou, T. J. Dondero, L. R. Peterson, et al., "The family of HIV seroprevalence surveys: Objectives, methods, and uses of sentinel surveillance for HIV in the United States," *Public Health Reports* 105(2)(1990):113–18.

of sampling error may make fluctuations over time difficult to interpret.

Potential for differential participation: In Rwanda, researchers reported that 1.6 percent of the urban and 1.4 percent of the rural sample refused to allow their blood to be sampled. Although these levels are not high, to the extent that respondents have the option not to participate, those who consider themselves to be at elevated risk for infection may choose to exclude themselves from the survey. This process introduces a bias into the sample that can, for example, decrease the estimate of HIV prevalence in the population. Careful staff training and study design can reduce this bias, but it remains an important issue.

HIV Prevalence and Incidence in Specific Populations

The following discussion focuses on groups at varying levels of risk for HIV infection, namely, commercial sex workers, homosexual men, IDUs, patients at STD clinics, pregnant women, and blood donors. The purpose is to describe the HIV/AIDS epidemic as it has been documented in these groups. This categorization is based on a desire to track infection patterns in populations at elevated risk of infection (sex workers, homosexual men, IDUs, and STD patients), as well as to describe infection in samples that may be more representative of the general population (pregnant women and blood donors). Due to the lack of large numbers of surveys of the general population, this approach is also determined by data availability issues.

Commercial Sex Workers: Given the predominant role that heterosexual transmission plays in the HIV epidemic in many countries, it should be no surprise that sex workers and their clients have an important role in this pandemic.[43] The organization of the commercial sex industry and the availability of casual sex partners can play a key role in the spread of HIV infection in a country.[44] Modelers in the field of STDs have documented the importance of *core groups* in the spread of infection.[45] (For further discussion of this, see Chapter 5, Box 5.1, "The Core Group Concept.") Sex workers, because of the number of their sexual partners, are, in many countries, the group at greatest risk for HIV infection (e.g., with infection levels approaching 50 percent in many

African cities). Especially among sex workers of low socioeconomic status (who tend to have more clients), infection levels have become extremely high. In other regions of the world, sex workers may have rates of infection that have not reached these levels, but infection is increasing rapidly in many regions, especially Asia.

Africa. Data are available on HIV infection among samples of urban sex workers in the *HIV/AIDS Surveillance Data Base* for 22 countries in sub-Saharan Africa (Figure 2.8). In ten of these 22 countries, the most recent data show infection levels over 30 percent. In several countries, more than half of the women are infected. As with data from other population groups, infection levels in many countries are increasing, and there is no guarantee that, for example, the five countries in Figure 2.8 with infection levels under ten percent will continue at such low levels for long. Although data on commercial sex workers are not available for all countries, it can be safely said, based on these 22, that infection levels in this population group are much higher than in the general population.

Latin America. Available data from Latin America and the Caribbean show high infection levels among commercial sex workers in several regional settings, reaching above 40 percent in samples from Haiti and Martinique. In samples from Central and South America, infection levels recorded over the past several years are lower. Several of the samples from South America had infection levels below one percent.

Asia. Despite high rates of sexual contact, HIV infection had been generally slow to spread to sex workers in Asia. For example, the latest data from South Korea, the Philippines, and Taiwan show levels of infection among commercial sex workers below 1 percent. In recent years, however, the increase in infection in this population group in two countries, India and Thailand, has been quite dramatic and raises the specter of future levels of infection in countries of the region approaching those in some African countries.

Data from India and Thailand are shown in Figure 2.9. In Bombay, infection increased nearly tenfold over a three-year period, reaching nearly 20 percent of a sample of commercial sex workers in 1990. In Thailand, data from the national sentinel surveillance system document the rapid increase in infection among commercial sex workers working in brothels throughout the country.

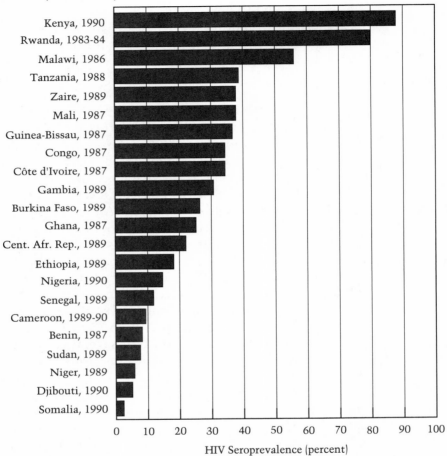

Figure 2.8. HIV seroprevalence for commercial sex workers in sub-Saharan Africa, circa 1990.
Source: Figures compiled by the Center for International Research, U.S. Bureau of the Census.
Note: Includes infection from HIV-1 and/or HIV-2.

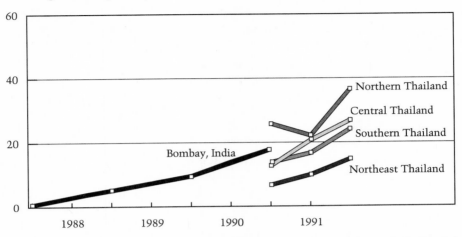

HIV Seroprevalence (percent)

Figure 2.9. HIV seroprevalence for commercial sex workers, India and Thailand, 1987-1991.
Source: Figures compiled by the Center for International Research, U.S. Bureau of the Census.

Homosexual Men: Few studies have been conducted among homosexual men outside of Europe and North America. Around 1980, HIV infection began to spread extensively among homosexual men in North America, Europe, Australia, and New Zealand. In Western Europe, the large majority of AIDS cases in the north have occurred in homosexual men.

In Latin America and the Caribbean, the epidemic affected homosexual men early, yet by the mid-1980s, heterosexual transmission of HIV had become a major if not the primary mode of HIV spread. In Mexico, Argentina, and Brazil, the levels of HIV infection in homosexual men range from around 20 to 35 percent. In some of the other countries in Latin American (Colombia, Costa Rica, and Peru) the levels of HIV infection hover around 5 percent.

In Africa, heterosexual transmission of HIV continues to be the predominant mode of spread. And in Asia, homosexual activity does not appear to be a predominant mode of HIV transmission, but there is very little information on this group. In Asia, the few studies conducted among homosexual men show the levels of HIV infection to be low. In Hong Kong and Taiwan, studies report levels of HIV infection between 5 and 10 percent. In Japan, Singapore, the Philippines, and India, the rates were well below 5 percent.

Injection Drug Users (IDUs): IDUs, in general, are an important but difficult group to study the world over. In both the industrialized and certain areas of the developing world, injection drug use has been a major factor in HIV transmission. In southern Europe, particularly Spain and Italy, IDUs make up more than half of reported cases.[46]

In Latin America, the HIV infection rates among IDUs have generally reached or exceeded 30 percent. For example in Brazil, HIV infection rates among injection drug users of 40 percent have been reported in Rio de Janeiro, along with 54 percent in São Paulo and 57 percent in Santos.

In Asia, the HIV infection rates among IDUs vary widely. In some countries (Thailand, Burma, India) the rates have increased dramatically over a short period of time. In one study in Thanyarak Hospital in Bangkok, HIV infection rates among IDUs increased from 1 percent in August 1987 to 29 percent in July 1988. Further studies found infection rates between 30 and 40 percent in various sites, or even higher in Bangkok IDU treatment clinics (see Figure 2.10). India, Burma, and parts of China now have high rates of HIV infection among IDUs. At this time, HIV infection rates for IDUs in Taiwan and Malaysia appear relatively low.

In the United States, the Family of Serosurveys system includes HIV seroprevalence testing in drug treatment centers; in 1990, 105 such centers in 40 cities participated. The median HIV seroprevalence was 3.9 percent, with a range from zero to 49.3 percent. Men attending these centers had a higher HIV seroprevalence than did women (4.8 percent vs. 3.5 percent). A major geographical difference was noted, with highest rates in the Atlantic (east) coast states; for example, HIV seroprevalence in New York and New Jersey ranged from 21.4 to 49.3 percent, whereas in the Pacific coast states seroprevalence was much lower, ranging from 2.1 to 7.9 percent (Figure 2.11).

STD Clinic Patients: Knowledge of levels of HIV infection among the population with frequent casual sexual contacts is of high priority. But the selec-

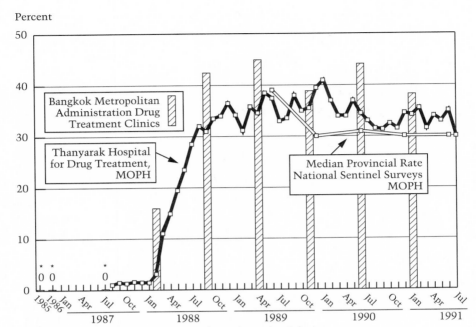

Percent

* Early *ad hoc* surveys in 1985, 1986, and 1987 detected no infections.

Figure 2.10. HIV-1 infection rates among injection drug users in Bangkok, and national median rates, 1985-1991.

Source: Reproduced with permission fron B.G. Weniger, et al., "The epidemiology of HIV infection and AIDS in Thailand," *AIDS* 5 (Suppl. 2) (1991): 571-85. (Published by Current Science, Ltd.)

Note: A total of 36,788 patients were admitted and tested for HIV at Thanyarak Hospital from August 1987 through July 1991, for a mean of 766 patients per month during the period.

tion of such a sample is understandably problematic. However, patients attending STD clinics can be considered a sample of that population, because they or their partners are likely to have had sexual contact with other people. They are at elevated risk of HIV infection due both to the presence of multiple partners as well as to the potentially enhanced risk of HIV infection among people with other STDs.[47] Various studies, for example, have estimated that people with a recent STD are at several times higher risk for HIV infection compared with those having no STD.

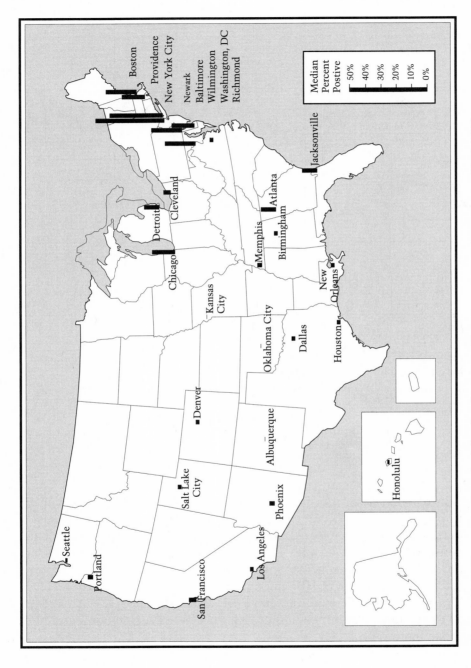

Figure 2.11. HIV seroprevalence in injection drug users. Drug treatment center surveys, 1988–1990.
Source: National HIV Surveillance through 1990. U.S. Public Health Service, Centers for Disease Control, 1992.

HIV Seroprevalence (percent)

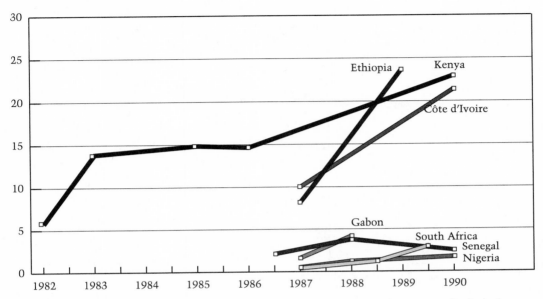

Figure 2.12. HIV seroprevalence for STD patients in urban areas of selected African countries, 1982-1990.
Source: Figures compiled by the Center for International Research, U.S. Bureau of the Census.
Note: Includes infection from HIV-1 and/or HIV-2.

Several factors, on the other hand, may lead to the data on HIV infection among STD patients not being representative of the total population with casual sex behavior. Among these factors are biases in the propensity to seek treatment at public facilities and variation (e.g., by gender) in the presence of symptomatic infections. Nevertheless, such studies provide valuable information on a potentially large population at high risk of HIV infection at a time when surveys of AIDS knowledge, attitudes, behaviors, and practices (KABP) are beginning to shed some light on sexual contacts outside of marital partnerships.[48]

Africa. Patterns of increase in HIV infection among large samples of STD patients for several sub-Saharan Africa countries are shown in Figure 2.12. Quite rapid increases were noted recently in Kenya, Côte

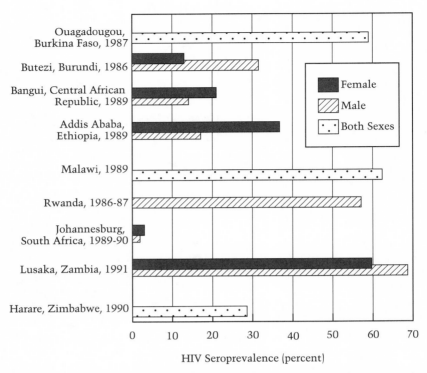

Figure 2.13. HIV seroprevalence for STD patients by gender in selected African countries.
Source: Figures compiled by the Center for International Research, U.S. Bureau of the Census.
Note: Includes infection from HIV-1 and/or HIV-2.

d'Ivoire, and Ethiopia. Infection levels in the capital cities of these countries has reached over 20 percent for STD patients. Although both Gabon and South Africa (results for black African women) show relatively low levels of infection, the increases noted in the most recent data are ominous. In contrast with these other countries, Nigeria has documented only a slow increase in infection among this population group.

Studies of STD patients in several other African countries have documented HIV infection levels over 50 percent (Figure 2.13). Patterns of sex differentials in HIV infection are inconsistent. In some

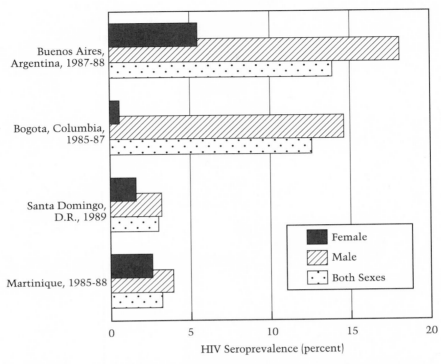

Figure 2.14. Seroprevalence for STD clinic patients by gender in selected Latin American sites.
Source: Figures compiled by the Center for International Research, U.S. Bureau of the Census.

cases (e.g., Burundi, Zambia), men have higher HIV infection levels than do women; in others (Central African Republic, Ethiopia, South Africa), the reverse situation was found. The stage of the epidemic or patterns of treatment in public facilities may contribute to these observed differences.

Latin America and the Caribbean. Available data on HIV infection levels by gender for STD patients in Latin America and the Caribbean consistently show higher levels for men than for women (Figure 2.14). Homosexual activity and possibly injection drug use among men in the region may contribute to some of these observed differences. However, as heterosexual infection has taken an increas-

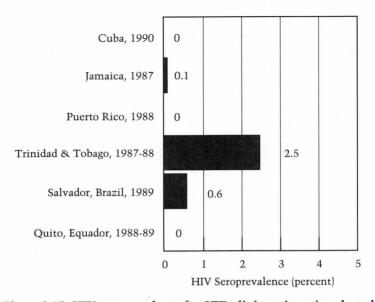

Cuba, 1990 — 0

Jamaica, 1987 — 0.1

Puerto Rico, 1988 — 0

Trinidad & Tobago, 1987-88 — 2.5

Salvador, Brazil, 1989 — 0.6

Quito, Equador, 1988-89 — 0

HIV Seroprevalence (percent)

Figure 2.15. HIV seroprevalence for STD clinic patients in selected Latin American sites.
Source: Figures compiled by the Center for International Research, U.S. Bureau of the Census

ingly important role in the region, these patterns will be subject to change.

Data for men attending STD clinics in Bogota and Buenos Aires in the late 1980s showed levels of HIV infection between 14 and 18 percent, respectively, with a high male-to-female infection ratio. In Martinique and the Dominican Republic, on the other hand, infection was below five percent, while male/female ratios were lower.

In various other settings in the region, HIV infection levels vary (Figure 2.15), with studies in Cuba, Puerto Rico, and Quito, Ecuador, not detecting any HIV infection.

Asia. Although the coverage of studies is far from complete, data on STD clinic patients from India and Thailand confirm the spread of HIV infection in these countries (Figure 2.16). The most recent data from both countries show considerable variation of infection levels, with some sites having infection levels over 20 percent. In Bombay, HIV-2 and dual infection of HIV-1 and HIV-2 were also reported.

HIV Seroprevalence (percent)

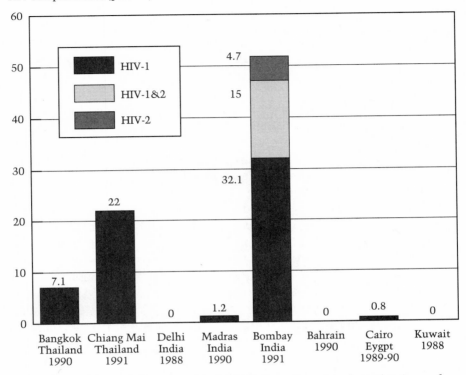

Figure 2.16. HIV seroprevalence for STD clinic patients in selected Asian and Middle Eastern countries.
Source: Figures compiled by the Center for International Research, U.S. Bureau of the Census.

South East Mediterranean. A low level of infection was reported for STD clinic patients in Cairo, Egypt, and no infection was reported for samples of this type in Bahrain or Kuwait.

United States. In the United States' Family of Serosurveys, from mid-1988 through 1990, nearly 400,000 blood samples were tested from clients of STD services from 107 clinics in 44 metropolitan areas. The overall median seroprevalence was 2.1 percent (range: 0–39 percent). Among men attending these STD clinics who reported having sex with other men, median seroprevalence was 32.4 percent (range: 15–61 percent). Among STD clinic attendees who were also IDUs, seroprevalence varied by gender: the median among men was 5.1 percent, compared with 2.6 percent among women. Finally, among STD clients who reported no specific other risk behavior, a median of 1.1 percent of men and 0.7 percent of women were HIV-seropositive. As with IDUs generally, HIV seroprevalence was higher in the eastern United States than in the western parts of the country.

Pregnant Women: Samples of pregnant women are often used as surrogates for the general population. This is convenient because, in many countries, women attend government clinics to receive antenatal care. To some extent, pregnant women can be considered to be at somewhat higher risk than is the general population because they are evidently sexually active. On the other hand, they also are drawn from a limited age range, may be biased toward those in marital (either formal or informal) unions, and they tend to be younger than adult women in general, given typical age-specific fertility rate patterns. Nevertheless, for many countries, data on pregnant women provide the most representative picture of HIV infection in the general population. This is particularly true when testing is conducted in a way that results cannot be linked individually to the person tested (anonymous, unlinked method), with voluntary testing and pre-/post counseling for the purpose of individual diagnosis being offered separately.

Africa. Since 1985, HIV seroprevalence studies of pregnant women have been conducted in many African countries. Seroprevalence data from those studies provide an initially confusing picture of regional trends (Figure 2.17). A variety of studies over the past six or more years in Uganda, Zambia, and Malawi show a consistent and rapid increase in HIV infection levels among pregnant women in the capital cities of these countries. By 1990, more than 20 percent of pregnant women tested for HIV in those areas were infected, whereas in 1986, infection levels in both Lusaka, Zambia, and Lilongwe, Malawi, had been well below 10 percent. Kigali, Rwanda (not shown in Figure 2.17), with a reported infection rate of over 30 percent in 1989, is another major urban area with high levels of infection.

In contrast, moderate increases in HIV seroprevalence have been documented among pregnant women in Nairobi, Kenya, and Bangui, Central African Republic, and infection levels in Kinshasa, Zaire, have remained relatively stable at around 5 to 6 percent. Infection levels

HIV Seroprevalence (percent)

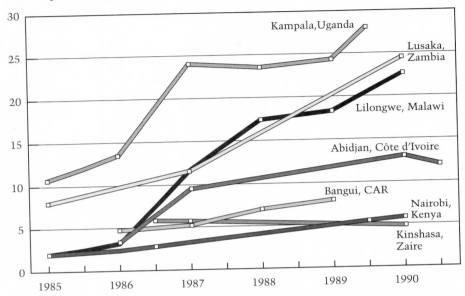

Figure 2.17. HIV seroprevalence for pregnant women in selected urban areas of Africa, 1985-1990.
Source: Figures compiled by the Center for International Research, U.S. Bureau of the Census.
Note: Includes infection from HIV-1 and/or HIV-2.

for pregnant women in Abidjan, Côte d'Ivoire, increased rapidly to around 10 percent by 1987, but appear to have reached a plateau by 1990.

Latin America and Caribbean. Available data for Latin America and the Caribbean are insufficient to judge trends in pregnant women over time. Figure 2.18 shows the prevalence in three settings: Cite Soleil, Haiti; Martinique; and São Paulo state, Brazil. In Haiti, the level of infection among pregnant women in this lower socioeconomic urban setting has fluctuated since 1986, but it appears to be relatively stable. In contrast, the prevalence in both Martinique and in São Paulo state is rising, although still at a relatively low level at the time period covered by the data.

Asia. As with other population groups, infection levels for preg-

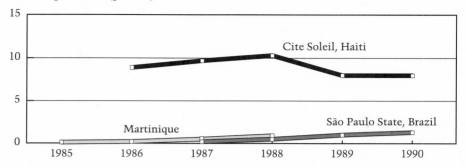

HIV Seroprevalence (percent)

Figure 2.18. HIV seroprevalence for pregnant women in selected Latin American and Caribbean countries, 1985-1990.
Source: Figures compiled by the Center for International Research, U.S. Bureau of the Census.

nant women in Thailand and India are on the rise. In Thailand's Changwat, the median HIV prevalence among pregnant women increased from zero to 0.7 percent between June 1990 and June 1991. In Madras, India, HIV prevalence for pregnant women increased from zero in 1988 and 1989 to over 1 percent in 1990. Data collected in Bombay over the period 1986–1990 showed 0.4 percent of pregnant women to be infected.

United States. The U.S. Family of Serosurveys has also examined blood specimens taken from newborns, which provides a surrogate measure of HIV seroprevalence among childbearing women. Through unlinked anonymous testing of specimens taken for other reasons (routine metabolic and other screening programs), about 4 million babies from more than 40 states were tested from 1988 to 1990; this represented about one-third of all live births in the United States during that period. In 1989–90, the national seroprevalence (among childbearing women) was 0.15 percent, or 1 of 667 women. Applied to national data, this suggested that approximately 6,000 births occurred in 1989 and also in 1990 to HIV-infected mothers. As with IDUs, higher seroprevalence rates were found in the Atlantic Coast states. In general, seroprevalence rates (ranging among states from 0–0.66 percent) were higher in large metropolitan areas, but infections were also found in both smaller urban and rural areas. Finally, the stability of seroprevalence per state from 1989 to 1990 provided further evidence of continuing HIV infection among childbearing-age women.

Three additional efforts to document HIV experience among women of childbearing age were included in the U.S. Family of Serosurveys. The first focused on women attending reproductive health clinics (family planning, prenatal, and abortion clinics) in 40 metropolitan areas. Among 146 clinics from 1988 to 1990, the median HIV seroprevalence was 0.2 percent (1 of 500); again, highest rates were in the Atlantic Coast area. Among African-American women, median clinic-specific seroprevalence was 0.4 percent, compared with 0.1 percent among both white and Hispanic women.

The second effort involved screening of applicants to the Job Corps, a program for disadvantaged youth 16 to 21 years old. In contrast to other studies in the Family of Serosurveys, women's seroprevalence was equal to men's: from 1987 to 1990, HIV seroprevalence was 0.31 percent among women applicants and 0.36 percent among men. From 1988 to 1990, HIV seroprevalence among women applicants increased, while it remained essentially unchanged or declined among men.

Finally, women and men applying for military service (voluntary in the United States) have been tested for HIV since October 1985. As applicants are aware that HIV testing is required and that HIV-infected people will not be accepted into military service, the sample is clearly biased against inclusion of people with risk behaviors and known HIV-seropositive status. During the period 1985–90, the cumulative HIV seroprevalence among women was 0.06 percent (or 1 per 1,667 applicants), which was about one-half the prevalence among men (0.13 percent). A general pattern of higher HIV seroprevalence among African-Americans and geographical patterns similar to those for IDUs and childbearing women were noted.

Blood Donors: HIV seroprevalence data from blood donors represent, for many countries, a readily accessible sample for use in monitoring changes in HIV infection in the population. However, comparisons with general-population samples in several areas raise questions regarding the representativeness of the blood donor samples.[49] Donors tend to be predominantly young adult men. In addition, women donors appear

HIV Seroprevalence (percent)

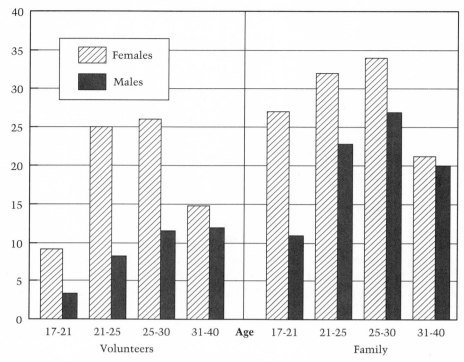

Figure 2.19. HIV seroprevalence for blood donors by age, gender, and type of donor, Uganda, 1990.
Source: Figures compiled by the Center for International Research, U.S. Bureau of the Census.

to be a higher-risk group than are the general population or men donors. Screening and self-selection processes may act to further bias the sample.

Africa. An example of such screening and self-selection processes can be seen in data from blood donors in Uganda (Figure 2.19). Female volunteer donors are about twice as likely to be HIV-positive as are their male volunteer counterparts, whereas family donors, perhaps more representative of the population, are more evenly balanced. Studies in Zaire and other African countries have confirmed this tendency for family donors to be more likely to be infected than volunteers.

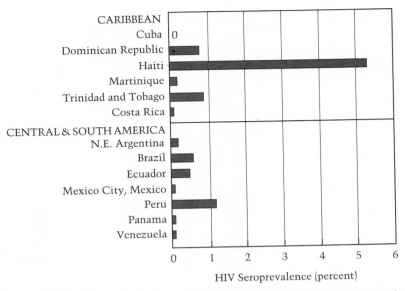

Figure 2.20. HIV seroprevalence for blood donors in Latin America and the Caribbean, 1989-1990.
Source: Figures compiled by the Center for International Research, U.S. Bureau of the Census.

Latin America and the Caribbean. Recent seroprevalence data for blood donors from Latin America and the Caribbean are shown in Figure 2.20. Most of the countries represented in this figure have HIV seroprevalence levels below 1 percent. Exceptions are Haiti, with over five percent seroprevalence in 1990, and Peru with 1.2 percent in 1989.

Asia. The tendency for some types of donors to have a higher seroprevalence than do volunteer donors is illustrated by recent data from Asia. Figure 2.21 contrasts HIV seroprevalence levels for volunteer donors with data for paid donors in India and in Thailand. In every situation in which HIV infection was detected, prevalence for paid donors was at least twice as high as for volunteer donors. In Chiang Mai, Thailand, HIV seroprevalence for all donors increased rapidly between 1988 and 1989, but the ratio between paid and volunteer donors remained relatively constant.

Obviously, issues related to the quality of the blood supply influence decisions regarding the monitoring of blood donors. From the

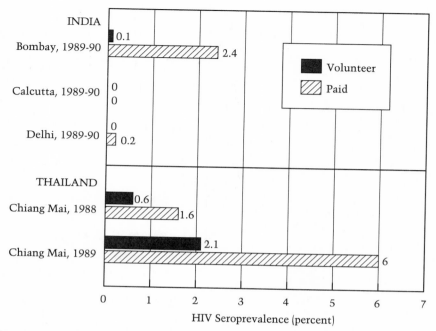

Figure 2.21. HIV seroprevalence for Asian blood donors, by type, 1988-1990.
Source: Figures compiled by the Center for International Research, U.S. Bureau of the Census.

available data to date, it does not appear that this group is sufficiently representative of the general population. These data also raise questions regarding the use of paid donors. In high-prevalence countries, family donors may represent more of a risk for HIV infection than do volunteer donors.

United States. Routine HIV testing of blood donors started in the United States in 1985, when the HIV-antibody test was commercialized. Because blood donors are prescreened to eliminate those with risk behaviors, HIV prevalence is lower than would be expected from a general population. Data from the American Red Cross (which supplies about half the blood collected in the United States) show that from 1985 to late 1990, overall HIV seroprevalence declined from 1 per 4,500 donors (0.022 percent) to about 1 per 20,000 donors (0.005 percent). First-time donors are especially important to monitor, as

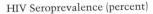

HIV Seroprevalence (percent)

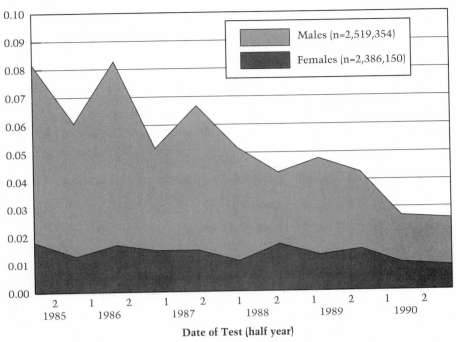

Date of Test (half year)

Figure 2.22. HIV seroprevalence in first-time blood donors by sex and date of donation, United States, July 1985-December 1990.
Source: American Red Cross.

new trends in HIV infections (reaching people who are unaware of their risk and therefore do not self-select themselves out of donating blood) could be identified in this manner. From 1985 to 1990, HIV seroprevalence among male first-time donors declined from 1 per 1,240 donors to 1 per 4,310 donors; among female first-time donors, the rate fell from 1 per 5,600 to 1 per 13,700 donors (Figure 2.22).

Trend Analysis

Correlation of HIV Seroprevalence among Various Groups: What have we learned from the existing data regarding trends in the epidemic? Are there correlations in the rates of HIV infection among various population

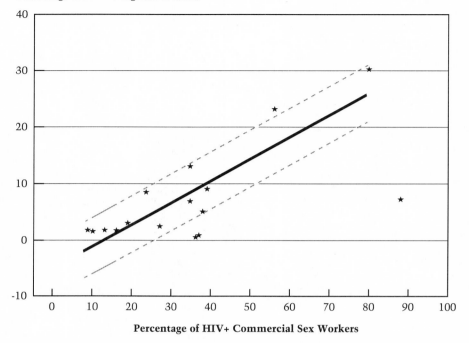

Percentage of HIV+ Pregnant Women

Percentage of HIV+ Commercial Sex Workers

Figure 2.23. HIV seroprevalence – percentage of infected commercial sex workers/pregnant women, Africa, circa 1990.
Source: Figures compiled by the Center for International Research, U.S. Bureau of the Census.

groups, such as pregnant women and blood donors, pregnant women and commercial sex workers, or commercial sex workers and STD patients? Knowing the HIV seroprevalence rate in one risk group, can we estimate what the seroprevalence might be in other risk groups?

Africa. At first glance, a correlation is apparent between rates of HIV infection in pregnant women and commercial sex workers in Africa (Figure 2.23).* However, when viewed more closely, the corre-

---

*The figure shows both the regression line (**bold**) and the 95 percent confidence interval (dashed lines). A confidence interval (C.I.) is a statistical expression of variability around an estimated point. Thus, a 95 percent confidence interval is the range within which an actual value would be expected to fall 95 percent of the time.

Percentage of HIV+ Commercial Sex Workers

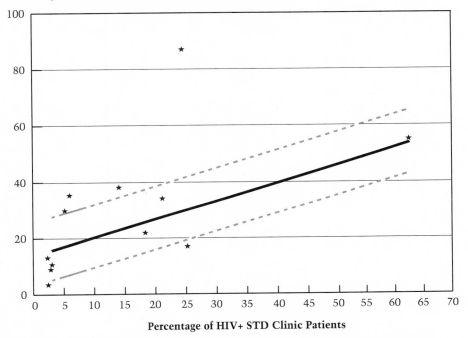

Percentage of HIV+ STD Clinic Patients

Figure 2.24. HIV seroprevalence – percentage of infected STD clinic patients/ commercial sex workers, Africa, circa 1990.
Source: Figures compiled by the Center for International Research, U.S. Bureau of the Census.

lation shows a great deal of variability. Among the countries in which the observed rates of HIV infection in commercial sex workers are between 30 and 40 percent, the observed HIV-seroprevalence rates in pregnant women range between 0.1 and 13 percent. In countries in which the observed HIV seroprevalence rates in commercial sex workers are between 5 and 15 percent, the observed HIV-seroprevalence rates in pregnant women range between 1 and 2 percent.

Figure 2.24 looks at the relationship in HIV seroprevalence rates between STD clinic patients and commercial sex workers. Once again, there is considerable variability in the relationship; the 95 percent confidence interval is plus or minus 10.6 percent. In countries in which the HIV seroprevalence rates in STD clinic patients are below

5 percent, the HIV seroprevalence rates in commercial sex workers range from 5 to 15 percent. In the countries presented here with rates in STD clinic patients ranging around five percent, the observed rates of HIV infection in commercial sex workers range from 26 to 37 percent.

In both of these figures, the rates in Kenya are unusual. In Figure 2.23 the HIV-seroprevalence rate in pregnant women is seven percent, while the rate in commercial sex workers is nearly 90 percent. In Figure 2.24, the rate in STD clinic patients is 23 percent. The study of commercial sex workers in Kenya, however, was limited to those from the lower socioeconomic class.

Thailand. In Thailand, sentinel surveillance sites reported HIV seroprevalence rates in June 1990, December 1990, and June 1991. The data in Figure 2.25 are for the 6 different regions at each of these times.

Evidence of strong trends emerge from this data. However, the predictive value of the trends is limited, again due to variability in the relationship. The stronger trends evident in this figure compared with data for Africa may be due to the fact that all the data come from the same country and may not be as confounded by different sexual behaviors.

The correlation in HIV seroprevalence is strongest between STD clinic patients and commercial sex workers, with HIV seroprevalence rates approximately three times higher among commercial sex workers than among STD clinic patients. Knowing the HIV seroprevalence in STD clinic patients, one could estimate the prevalence among commercial sex workers within 3 percent.

However, the relationship between the rates of HIV infection among commercial sex workers and pregnant women is not as strong. HIV infection rates in commercial sex workers are from 17 to 120 times higher than the rates among pregnant women.

These data demonstrate a clear relationship between the levels of HIV infection in various groups at a particular point in a geographic area. Strong trends and relatively high correlations were evident. Clearly, variations in levels of risk of infection are reflected in the observed levels of HIV seroprevalence.

However, the practical usefulness of these observations is limited by variability within these data. Knowledge of the level of HIV infection among commercial sex workers in Africa, for example, still leaves

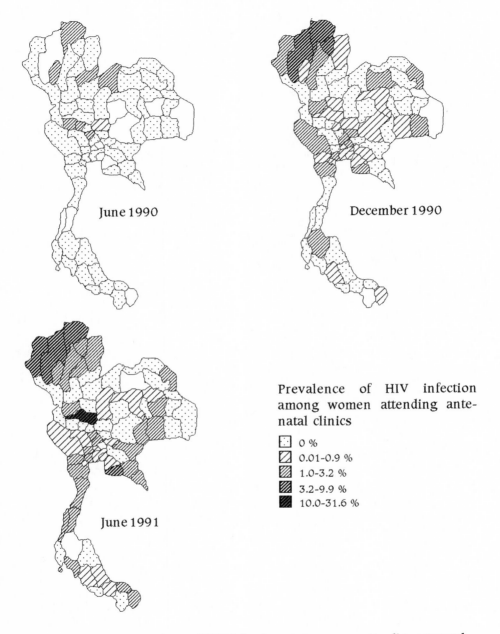

June 1990

December 1990

June 1991

Prevalence of HIV infection among women attending antenatal clinics

- ⬚ 0 %
- ▨ 0.01-0.9 %
- ▨ 1.0-3.2 %
- ▨ 3.2-9.9 %
- ■ 10.0-31.6 %

Figure 2.25. Prevalence of HIV infection among women attending antenatal clinics in Thailand, June 1990; December 1990; June 1991.

Source: Ministry of Public Health, National Sentinel Surveillance. In U. Brinkmann, "Features of the AIDS epidemic in Thailand," Harvard School of Public Health, Department of Population and International Health, Working Paper no. 3 (1992).

us with an estimated range of more than ten percentage points around our point estimate of the infection level for pregnant women. Therefore, although sentinel surveillance among high-risk groups can serve as an early warning measure for infection in lower-risk groups, it cannot replace the need for careful surveillance and monitoring of levels and trends of HIV infection.

Age and Sex Patterns of Infection: Although the precise values are not yet known, there is increasing evidence that women are more at risk of HIV infection when considered either on a *per contact* or *per partnership* basis. In this respect, HIV is similar to other STDs. On the population level, however, the risk of HIV infection for women will be a result of the sexual behavior of those women and the behavior of their sexual partners. Available data from several African countries in the latest round of sexual behavior surveys suggest that a differential in sexual behavior exists, such that males are more likely to engage in casual sexual contacts than are females. This will tend to counterbalance the female's biologically higher susceptibility to infection. The result is that the overall sex ratio of HIV-infected population in Africa is close to 1:1.

This does not mean that one can expect equal levels of infection in every African country, as the timing of the epidemic and sexual behavior patterns will differ. Several serosurveys in Uganda, for example, found a male-to-female sex ratio of 1:1.4.[50] In Côte d'Ivoire, on the other hand, nationally representative rural seroprevalence levels applied to the population, by age and sex, suggest a nearly 2:1 male-to-female ratio.

Another important factor is age-mixing—the tendency for males to choose a younger female as a spouse (and also as a casual sexual partner). This behavior results in the tendency for HIV infection levels in younger women to be higher than that in men in the same age cohort, whereas older men tend to have higher infection levels than do women of the same age. This pattern is shown in Figure 2.26 for Uganda and in Figure 2.27 for Côte d'Ivoire.

Urban-Rural Differentials: Available data from sub-Saharan Africa have tended to show a large differential in HIV infection levels between urban and rural areas of a country. A representative population survey in Rwanda

HIV Seroprevalence (percent)

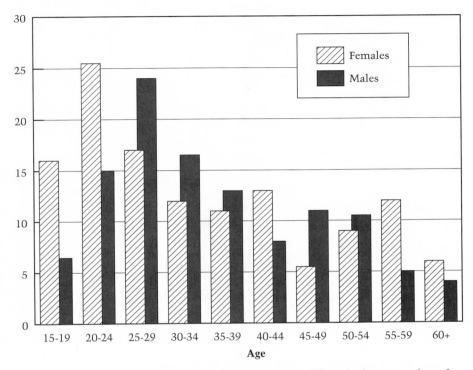

Figure 2.26. HIV seroprevalence for the population of Uganda, by age and gender, 1987-1988.
Source: Figures compiled by the Center for International Research, U.S. Bureau of the Census.

in 1987, for example, found 17 percent of the adult population in the capital city of Kigali to be infected, compared with only 2.1 percent of the rural population. Data from Côte d'Ivoire demonstrate both the typical age pattern of infection and urban-rural differentiation in infection levels (see Figure 2.27).

Such patterns are likely to result from differences in the timing of the introduction of HIV into the population and, perhaps, differences in patterns of sexual behavior between urban and rural populations. However, many exceptions to this generalization can be identi-

HIV Seroprevalence (percent)

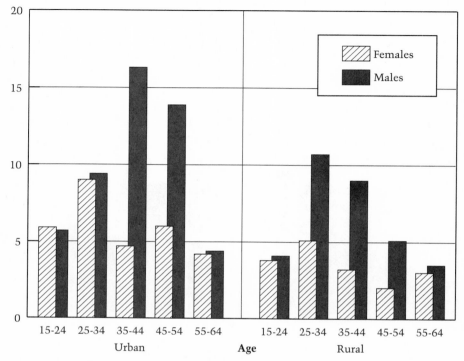

Figure 2.27. HIV seroprevalence for the population of Côte d'Ivoire, by age, gender, and urban/rural residence, 1989.
Source: Figures compiled by the Center for International Research, U.S. Bureau of the Census.
Note: Includes infection from HIV-1 and/or HIV-2.

fied. For example, the Rakai district in rural Uganda has recorded HIV infection levels that equal those in the capital, Kampala. Across the border in Tanzania, the Bukoba district has a higher HIV seroprevalence than does Dar es Salaam. However, within the Bukoba district, urban areas exhibited higher rates of infection than did rural areas (24 percent and 5 percent, respectively). The availability of adequate transportation routes to and through rural areas and the level of rural-urban migration both contribute to the speed of the spread of HIV infection to these areas. Thus, countries with well-developed transportation infrastructures and high levels of rural-urban migration may experience more rapid spread of HIV infection to rural areas.

In other regions of the world, similar differences would be expected between levels of infection in urban and rural areas. Exceptions to these patterns will, however, exist where behavior patterns may place selected rural populations at higher risk for HIV infection.

Geographic Variation: Results from seroprevalence surveys presented earlier have tended to highlight the trends in particular population groups and focus on the differentials among populations at different levels of risk. It is equally important to emphasize the geographic variation in current levels of HIV infection, both between and within countries, based on a comparison of urban population groups. General population samples and pregnant women are used as low-risk samples, with occasional inclusion of blood donors when other samples are not available.

Africa. Figure 2.28 shows the most recent available data on HIV-1 infection by country for Africa, based largely on rates for low-risk groups such as pregnant women and blood donors.* High levels of infection are evidenced in many countries in Central and Eastern Africa, along with Côte d'Ivoire in West Africa. Relatively lower levels of infection of HIV-1 occur generally in Southern, West, and North Africa.

Factors that can be shown or hypothesized to contribute to the observed variation include the timing of HIV entry into the population, sexual practices before and outside of marriage, prevalence of STDs in the population, and male circumcision. The geographic pattern of infection will change over time.

The geographic pattern of HIV-2 infection shows higher prevalence in West Africa, along with other African countries with a Portuguese colonial history. Troops movements among these former Portuguese colonies and travel facilitated by cultural ties may have contributed to the spread of HIV-2 infection in these select countries. Several countries bordering those with substantial HIV-2 infection as yet show little evidence of an HIV-2 epidemic.

Thailand. The foregoing discussion has demonstrated the geo-

---

*Data, in tabular form, for high- and low-risk population groups in urban areas and outside of urban areas are provided in Appendix 2.2.

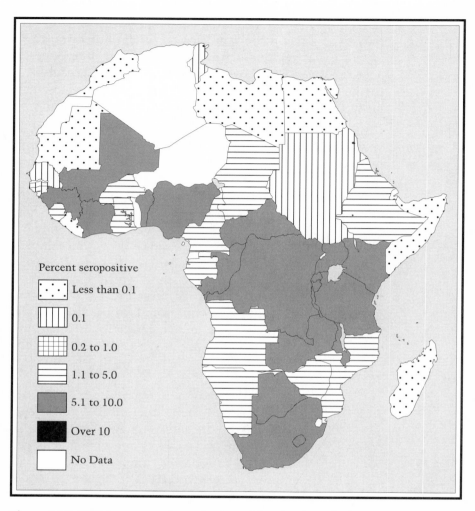

Figure 2.28. HIV-1 seroprevalence for low-risk urban populations.
Source: Figures compiled by the Center for International Research, U.S. Bureau of the Census.

graphic variation of HIV infection between countries. Levels of HIV infection also vary widely within a country, even beyond the urban-rural variation discussed above. Thailand illustrates this potential for dramatic variation in infection levels even within a single population group. HIV seroprevalence for pregnant women within Thailand in December 1990 varied from a low of zero to a high 4.5 percent in Chiang Mai, in the north. Indeed, the northern region as a whole shows high rates of infection, even relative to the central region (which includes the Bangkok metropolitan area).

Multiple Epidemics: The spread of HIV infection within a country can be visualized, at least in part, as multiple epidemics that reach population groups characterized by progressive prevalence of HIV risk behaviors. The availability of sentinel surveillance data for Thailand enables tracking the spread of HIV infection in a country from a very early stage of the epidemic. Figure 2.25 shows data from the surveillance system as well as from other sources prior to 1990.

This figure gives a picture of the spread of HIV infection among various groups at progressively lower risk for infection. What is not clear from this picture is the ultimate level of infection that will prevail among different groups when HIV infection becomes endemic. However, from the available data there appear to be differences between the risk groups in the rate of spread of infection following its introduction. For example, the explosive spread among IDUs in early 1988 can be contrasted with the slower, steady growth among commercial sex workers in more recent years. Trends among pregnant women may in turn be characterized by a generally slower growth in infection levels, although HIV seroprevalence had already exceeded 3 percent in this group in certain provinces.

The Leveling Off of HIV Prevalence and/or Incidence Rates

Given the variation in observed levels of infection and epidemic growth rates described here, a series of questions relating to the epidemic naturally follow. How rapidly will HIV continue to spread in the future? At what point in current high-prevalence countries will HIV infection become endemic, that is, stabilize? Will countries with currently low levels of infection inevitably progress to HIV prevalence levels currently recorded in such areas as Kampala, Uganda, or Kigali, Rwanda, or is a plateauing at a lower level likely to occur?

Although crystal ball technology continues to lag, valuable insights can be obtained from the available seroprevalence data as well as from results of mathematical modeling, described below. These data suggest the following tentative responses to the above questions:

- Variation in the speed of increase in HIV infection and in the endemic level of infection will result from variations in sexual behavior, presence of STDs and other cofactors, and perhaps other unknown factors;

- Although by no means definitive, available studies have not found infection levels above 30 percent in general populations or among pregnant women. This raises the question of how much above this level HIV infection can spread in the general population. However, infection levels in several high HIV prevalence sites appear to be increasing. Studies conducted over the next several years in high-infection areas may help to shed light on possible upper limits to infection levels in the general population.

- Results from several settings have shown relatively stable and moderate levels of infection in some general population samples over a period of several years, for example, in Kinshasa, Zaire (at least until recent political and social turmoil intervened).

- Infection levels in rural populations will generally lag behind urban prevalence levels and may plateau at lower levels.

Has the Epidemic Peaked in Industrialized Countries? One of the most common questions about the pandemic is whether it has already peaked in some populations and areas. The article on HIV/AIDS trends in the United States and Europe (Chapter 15), and the projections for the industrialized countries for 1995 and the year 2000, suggest that any declaration of victory in stemming the HIV/AIDS pandemic would be premature, at best.

Geographic Areas of Affinity: Status Report

In this section, the 10 Geographic Areas of Affinity are examined individually, with attention to area-specific particularities. The numbers of HIV infections, AIDS, and deaths estimated to have occurred in each of the GAAs and in the world through January 1992, and projections through 1995, are shown in Figures 2.29 through 2.48.

GAA 1—North America:[51-53] In the United States, a countrywide serosurveillance system has been in operation since 1988 (Family of Serosurveys). Although results from the Family of Serosurveys indicated a widespread distribution of HIV in the country, marked variations in seroprevalence rates existed in different risk groups. The highest rates were found among those reporting high-risk behavior and among tuberculosis patients. Nationwide, seroprevalence rates among men who reported having sex with men ranged from 15 to 61 percent, with a median seroprevalence of 32 percent. Other results included a range of zero to 58 percent (median 6 percent) among tuberculosis (TB) patients; zero to 49 percent (median 4 percent) in IDUs; and an overall nationwide rate of 0.15 percent in childbearing women. Prevalence rates were generally higher in urban areas than in rural areas and in the Middle Atlantic, southeastern states, and Puerto Rico. African-Americans and Hispanics tended to have higher prevalence rates than did whites.

Although from 1988 to 1990 no evidence of changing trends in HIV-infected women of childbearing age surfaced, certain factors indicated that a shift was occurring in the population as a whole. The Centers for Disease Control noted a marked decline in the gender ratio of reported AIDS cases, from 14:1 in 1984 to 7:1 in 1991. This trend, in conjunction with the finding of an almost equal gender distribution of HIV seroprevalence in certain groups (Job Corps applicants, for example), indicated a disproportionate increase of HIV-infected women. These findings highlight the increasing role played by heterosexual transmission in the spread of HIV.

AIDS in the World estimated that by the end of 1991, in North America, 1.2 million adults were HIV infected; of these, approximately 130,000 were women; in addition, about 16,000 pediatric HIV infections had occurred (see Figures 2.29 and 2.30).

GAA 2—Western Europe:[54] France, Italy, and Spain have reported the largest number of AIDS cases in Western Europe, accounting for 62 percent of all European cases reported as of January 1, 1992.

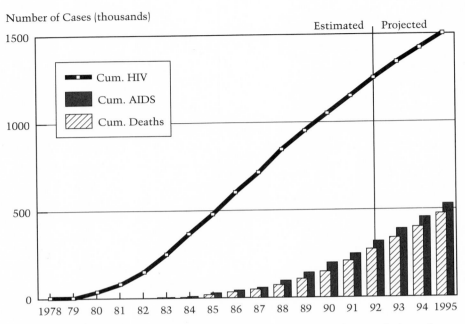

Number of Cases (thousands)

Figure 2.29. Cumulative adult HIV, AIDS cases, and deaths for North America (GAA 1), 1978-1995.
Source: AIDS in the World, 1992.

Blinded serosurveys have been conducted in several European countries. Among pregnant women, surveys have documented seroprevalence rates of 0.41 percent in pregnant women in Paris and from 0.06 to 0.70 percent in the greater London area. Among neonates, 0.27 percent seroprevalence was documented in Paris (1990) and 0.13 percent in London. These rates reflect an increasing trend between 1988 and 1990.

Mirroring the trend for women, upward seroprevalence trends have been noted in IDUs in several countries, particularly those in Southern Europe, whereas a decline in HIV incidence has generally been noted in men who have sex with men. The continuing spread in certain groups of reproductive-age women and men signals the vulnerability of young adults and newborns to the pandemic.

By January 1, 1992, *AIDS in the World* estimates that approxi-

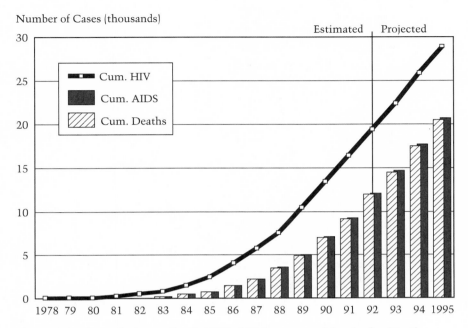

Number of Cases (thousands)

Estimated | Projected

Figure 2.30. Cumulative pediatric HIV, AIDS cases, and deaths for North America (GAA 1), 1978-1995.
Source: AIDS in the World, 1992.

mately 720,000 adults have become HIV-infected, including 122,000 women. In Western Europe, the gender ratio among HIV-infected adults was 5:1, significantly lower than that in North America and Oceania. In addition, an estimated 8,000 pediatric HIV infections have occurred in Western Europe (see Figures 2.31 and 2.32).

GAA 3—Oceania:[55] By early 1992, almost half of the HIV-infected people in Australia were men who had sex with men. The prevalence of HIV among IDUs remained lower than in Western Europe or North America, a success that can be attributed, at least in part, to the early availability of sterile injection equipment. Similarly, in New Zealand and Papua New Guinea, most HIV infections have been among homosexual and bisexual men. Overall in this region, by January 1, 1992,

Number of Cases (millions)

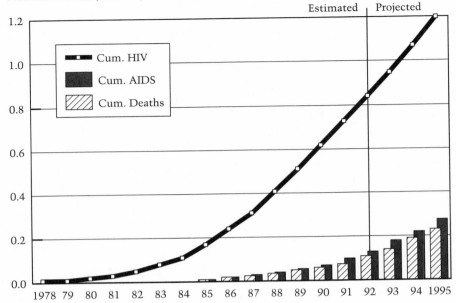

Figure 2.31. Cumulative adult HIV, AIDS cases, and deaths for Western Europe (GAA 2), 1978–1995.
Source: AIDS in the World, 1992.

Number of Cases (thousands)

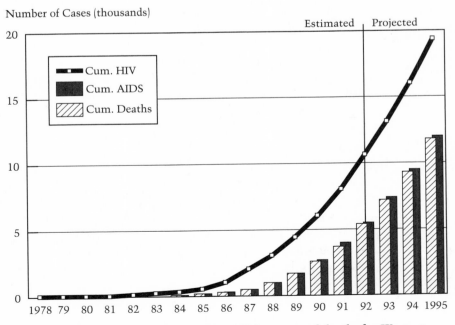

Figure 2.32. Cumulative pediatric HIV, AIDS cases, and deaths for Western Europe (GAA 2), 1978-1995.
Source: AIDS in the World, 1992.

Number of Cases (thousands)

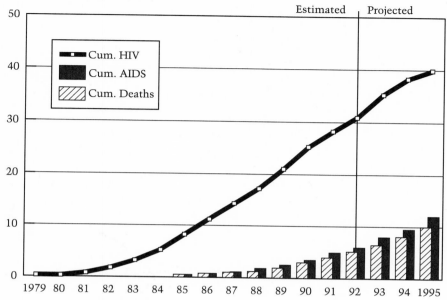

Figure 2.33. Cumulative adult HIV, AIDS cases, and deaths for Oceania
(GAA 3), 1979-1995.
Source: AIDS in the World, 1992.

11 of the 21 island countries and territories with small populations
in the Pacific had reported AIDS cases or HIV infections.

AIDS in the World estimates that cumulatively in this region,
28,000 adults have been infected with HIV. Here, the gender ratio
among infected adults is approximately 7:1, indicating a lower degree
of heterosexual transmission than that observed in North America.
As a result, the number of cumulative pediatric HIV infections is low,
estimated to total 500 (see Figures 2.33 and 2.34).

GAA 4—Latin America:[56] In the early 1980s, when HIV began to spread in Latin
America, most people infected were homosexual and bisexual men,
IDUs, and recipients of blood products. Though the numbers in the

Number of Cases

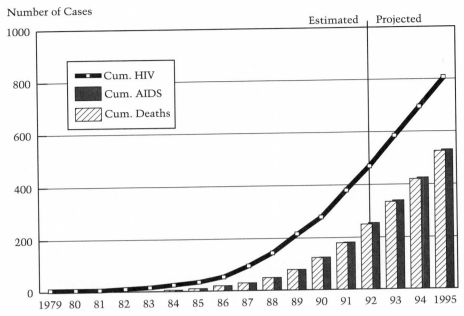

Figure 2.34. Cumulative pediatric HIV, AIDS cases, and deaths for Oceania (GAA 3), 1979-1995.
Source: AIDS in the World, 1992.

lattermost group have decreased as a result of the (partial) introduction of more effective blood safety measures, the pandemic is taking a different shape in three geographic subareas. In the Southern Cone countries and in Brazil, 20 to 76 percent of IDUs are HIV infected. Concurrently, there is a marked increase in heterosexual and mother-to-child transmission.

Due to the paucity of information on the progression of the pandemic from urban to rural areas, calculating HIV prevalence for Latin America is problematic. *AIDS in the World* estimates that as of January 1, 1992, a cumulative total of nearly 1 million adults had become HIV infected, including approximately 200,000 women; slightly more than 40,000 pediatric HIV infections have also occurred in Latin America (see Figures 2.35 and 2.36).

Number of Cases (thousands)

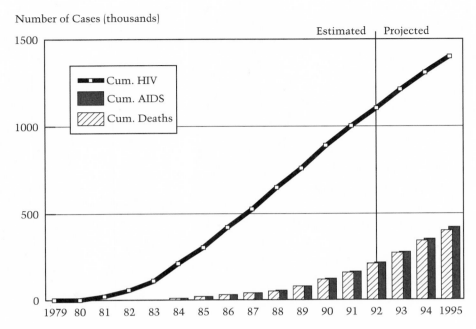

Figure 2.35. Cumulative adult HIV, AIDS cases, and deaths for Latin America (GAA 4), 1979-1995.
Source: AIDS in the World, 1992.

GAA 5—Sub-Saharan Africa:[57–59] With only 10 percent of the world's population, sub-Saharan Africa accounts for 2 out of every 3 HIV infections among adults, 83 percent of HIV infections among women worldwide, and 90 percent of the world's burden of pediatric HIV infection.

Since the beginning of the pandemic, the transmission of HIV in this area has been predominantly heterosexual, with a gender ratio that approximates 1:1, although with important intra- and intercountry differences. Detailed descriptions of African HIV and AIDS distribution and epidemic evolution are provided in earlier sections.

The available data further underscore the severity of the HIV-1 pandemic in Central, Eastern, and Southern Africa and reveal the existence of a concurrent epidemic in West Africa, where HIV-2 plays a major role although the frequency and impact of HIV-1 infections is steadily increasing.

Number of Cases (thousands)

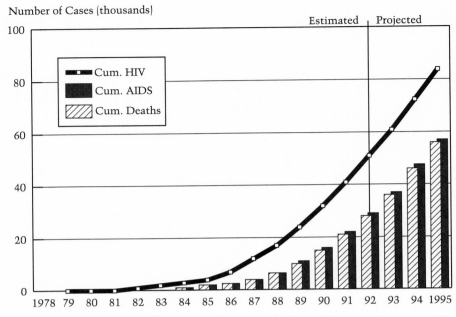

Figure 2.36. Cumulative pediatric HIV, AIDS cases, and deaths for Latin America (GAA 4), 1978-1995.
Source: AIDS in the World, 1992.

The HIV pandemic has taken its toll on whole families. Young, productive adults/parents become ill and die, and many of their children, born infected, are confronted with disease, disability, and death. Approximately 1.1 to 1.6 million children have already been orphaned by this disease. Given the intense impact of the pandemic on this region, family and community supports are weakening. Throughout this book, considerable attention is given to describing the impact and response to HIV/AIDS in sub-Saharan Africa. This deliberate emphasis is motivated by the hope that the facts and testimonies presented here will stimulate global solidarity between the developed world and a region that, more than others, is struggling to fight this pandemic in a context of dramatic economic recession.

According to *AIDS in the World* estimates, by January 1, 1992, 7.8 million adults, half of whom are women, and nearly 970,000

Number of Cases (millions)

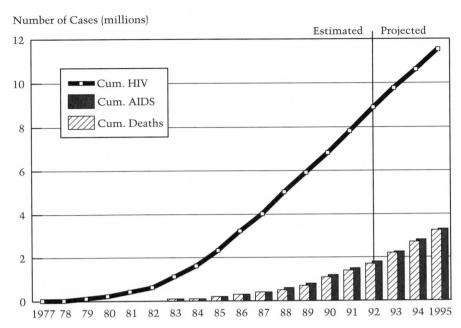

Figure 2.37. Cumulative adult HIV, AIDS cases, and deaths for sub-Saharan Africa (GAA 5), 1977-1995.
Source: AIDS in the World, 1992.

children have been infected with HIV in sub-Saharan Africa (see Figures 2.37 and 2.38).

GAA 6—Caribbean:[60] In the Caribbean, where HIV began to spread in the early 1980s, the heterosexual mode of transmission now predominates with an estimated male-to-female ratio of 1.5:1.

In Haiti, one of the countries most affected by the epidemic, prevention and control efforts were intensified in the late 1980s. However, now faced with political and social unrest, the future of the Haitian HIV epidemic is unclear. Cuba's strategy of mass screening and quarantine of infected persons continues, still awaiting a much desired international evaluation of its purported effectiveness.

Based on sparse serosurvey information, it is conservatively estimated that by January 1, 1992, the best estimate of cumulative adult

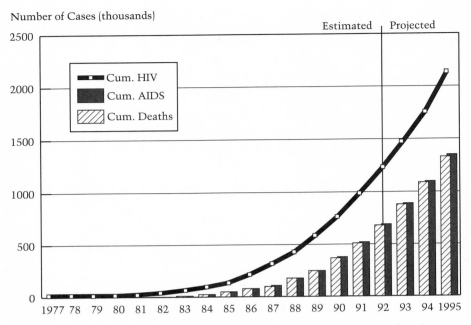

Number of Cases (thousands)

Figure 2.38. Cumulative pediatric HIV, AIDS cases, and deaths for sub-Saharan Africa (GAA 5), 1977-1995.
Source: AIDS in the World, 1992.

HIV infections in the Caribbean was 310,000, of whom 124,000 are women. An estimated 16,000 pediatric HIV infections have occurred in this GAA (see Figures 2.39 and 2.40).

GAA 7—Eastern Europe:[61] This GAA includes eight countries in Central and Eastern Europe that, until 1990–91, had a centrally planned economy and a socialist political system. At that time, the notification of AIDS cases as well as of HIV infections was compulsory, and mass HIV testing was performed: by January 1991, 91 million people, or 30 percent of the population, had been screened in the USSR, and 45 percent of the population had been HIV screened in Bulgaria. By March 1991, a cumulative total of only 523 HIV infections had been reported in the USSR and 90 in Bulgaria: truly a meager yield of unproven public value for a one-time massive effort.

Number of Cases (thousands)

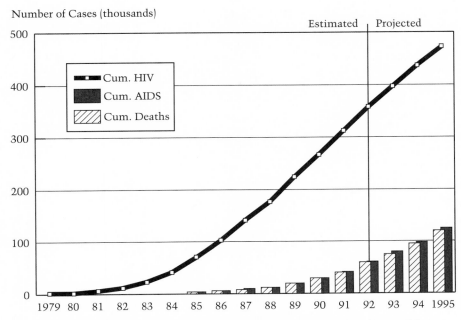

Figure 2.39. Cumulative adult HIV, AIDS cases, and deaths for the Caribbean (GAA 6), 1979-1995.
Source: AIDS in the World, 1992.

Romania, and then the USSR, reported a large-scale epidemic of HIV transmission through blood transfusion, plasma, and injection equipment in health care settings. These epidemics, which occurred in the late 1980s, resulted in several thousand HIV infections; more than 1,400 HIV infections were reported in Romania alone.

Other modes of transmission were reported in the region. Several countries in the area, including Poland and Yugoslavia, reported a major rise in the prevalence of HIV infection in IDUs; in Czechoslovakia, the predominant modes of transmission were through homosexual contact, and in Bulgaria, through heterosexual contact.

AIDS in the World conservatively estimates that as of January 1, 1992, 27,000 adults had become HIV infected, of whom only 2,500 were women. Among children, approximately 200 had become HIV infected perinatally, along with an unascertained number of nosocomial infections.

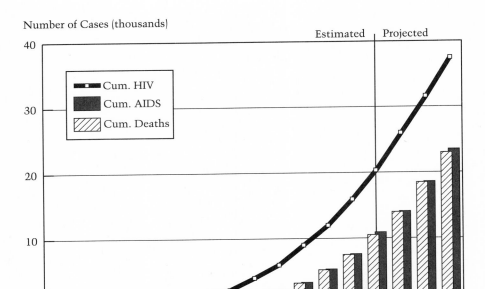

Figure 2.40. Cumulative pediatric HIV, AIDS cases, and deaths for the Caribbean (GAA 6), 1979-1995.
Source: AIDS in the World, 1992.

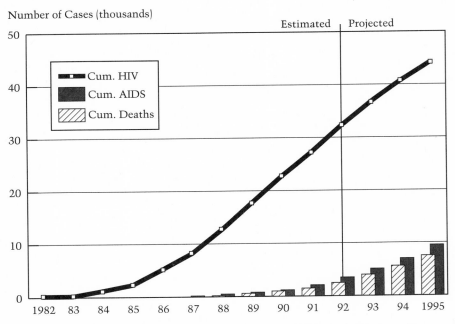

Figure 2.41. Cumulative adult HIV, AIDS cases, and deaths for Eastern Europe (GAA 7), 1982-1995.
Source: AIDS in the World, 1992.

Number of Cases

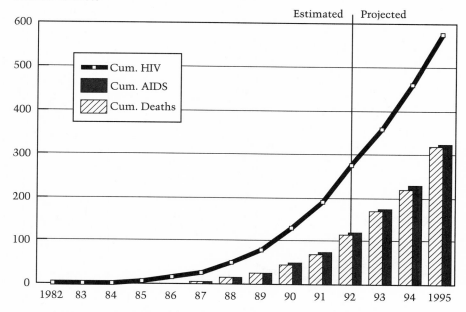

Figure 2.42. Cumulative pediatric HIV, AIDS cases, and deaths for Eastern Europe (GAA 7), 1982-1995.
Source: AIDS in the World, 1992.

By mid-1991, with major political and social changes sweeping through Central and Eastern Europe, the potential for the spread of HIV within and across communities increased sharply. The future course of the pandemic in this region will largely depend on the capacity of societies now undergoing vast reforms to create stable social and economic systems and rapidly restore (or create) viable public health services (see Figures 2.41 and 2.42).

GAA 8—South East Mediterranean: Little epidemiological and seroprevalence information is available from countries in this GAA, although virtually all have national HIV/AIDS programs. AIDS in the World estimates that by January 1, 1992, a best estimate of 35,000 cumulative adult HIV infections have occurred, of whom 6,000 are women. An estimated 1,000 pediatric HIV infections have also occurred in this GAA.

Number of Cases (thousands)

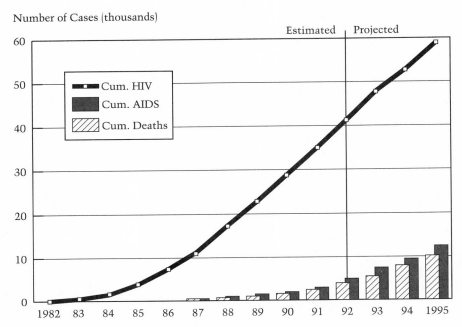

Figure 2.43. Cumulative adult HIV, AIDS cases, and deaths for South East Mediterranean (GAA 8), 1982-1995.
Source: AIDS in the World, 1992.

In this area, the predominant modes of transmission are believed to be through heterosexual contact and injection drug use. The transmission of HIV was partially facilitated in the mid-1980s by migratory movements between North Africa and Europe. In this area, the HIV pandemic has now acquired its own dynamic. The availability of heroin, which has been transported through the region's war-torn countries in recent years (Lebanon, Iran, and Afghanistan), has created another risk of HIV spread.

Before it is assumed that cultural patterns and social mores have limited the spread of HIV in the area, more data are required to document the current epidemiological situation (see Figures 2.43 and 2.44).

GAA 9—North East Asia: As with the South East Mediterranean, the scarcity of epidemiological data from the most populated country in the world—

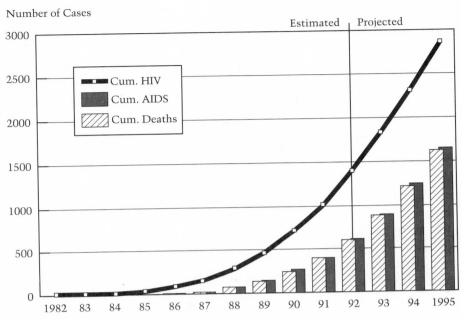

Number of Cases

Figure 2.44. Cumulative pediatric HIV, AIDS cases, and deaths for South East Mediterranean (GAA 8), 1982-1995.
Source: AIDS in the World, 1992.

China—makes the assessment and projection of the pandemic difficult to predict. Reports in 1990 cited the use of injection drugs among poppy-growing tribal communities in the province of Yunnan, along the Burmese border. The spread of HIV in Chinese provinces adjacent to Hong Kong illustrates how borders cannot stop the spread of the virus. In Japan, where, imported blood products received by persons with hemophilia initially represented the main mode of transmission, sexual transmission is now the main contributor to infections acquired both within the country and abroad. Recent reports on the low awareness and widespread misperceptions about HIV/AIDS in the country may increase vulnerability of Japan and the entire GAA to HIV epidemics.

Since HIV began to spread in the mid-1980s, *AIDS in the World* estimates that 41,000 adults have become HIV infected, including

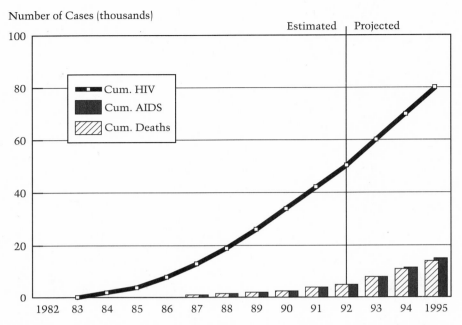

Number of Cases (thousands)

Figure 2.45. Cumulative adult HIV, AIDS cases, and deaths for North East Asia (GAA 9), 1982-1995.
Source: AIDS in the World, 1992.

7,000 women; fewer than 1,000 perinatal HIV transmissions are likely to have occurred thus far in this GAA (see Figures 2.45 and 2.46).

GAA 10—Southeast Asia:[62,63] In Thailand and Burma, in the mid- and late 1980s, the initial spread of HIV was largely attributed to injection drug practices. However, the face of the pandemic evolved with extraordinary rapidity, and today, heterosexual transmission is dominant in most areas. Thus, in Burma today, exposure to HIV results from both injection drug use and patterns of commercial sex work.

Since 1986, India has been screening blood donations, testing certain sectors of its population, and performing surveillance activities. Most of these activities have focused on large urban areas that included the cities of Bombay, Madras, and Calcutta. In a subsample of 4,565 HIV infected people, the male-to-female ratio was close to

Number of Cases

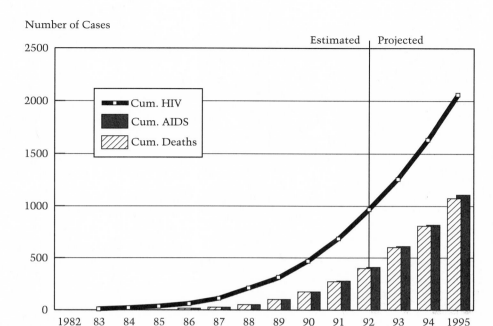

Figure 2.46. Cumulative pediatric HIV, AIDS cases, and deaths for North East
Asia (GAA 9), 1982-1995.
Source: AIDS in the World, 1992.

2:1. For women, the main mode of infection was through heterosexual
transmission. Among the men, however, most of the infections were
attributed to injection drug use, heterosexual transmission, and contaminated blood collection equipment in blood donation centers in
that order. Although resulting from a biased sample, these results
illustrate the multiplicity of modes of spread of HIV in India.

It is clear that the pandemic has a high velocity in Southeast Asia.
AIDS in the World considers its best estimate of the cumulative
number of HIV-infected adults as of January 1, 1992, to be very conservative, at 675,000. This total includes 223,000 women; an estimated 24,000 pediatric HIV infections have also occurred in the
Affinity Area. Many estimate that by mid-1992 there were over 1.5
million HIV infections in Southeast Asia, a sign of the dramatic
velocity of the pandemic in this area.

Number of Cases (thousands)

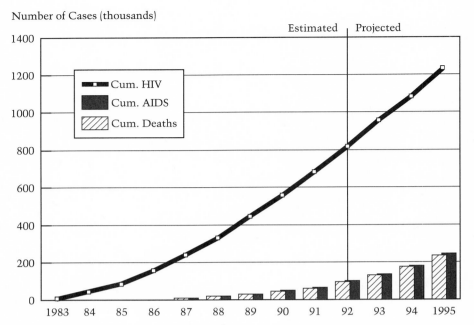

Estimated | Projected

Figure 2.47. Cumulative adult HIV, AIDS cases, and deaths for Southeast Asia (GAA 10), 1983-1995.
Source: AIDS in the World, 1992.

Number of Cases (thousands)

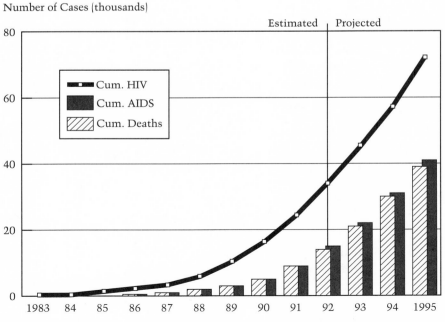

Estimated | Projected

Figure 2.48. Cumulative pediatric HIV, AIDS cases, and deaths for Southeast Asia (GAA 10), 1983-1995.
Source: AIDS in the World, 1992.

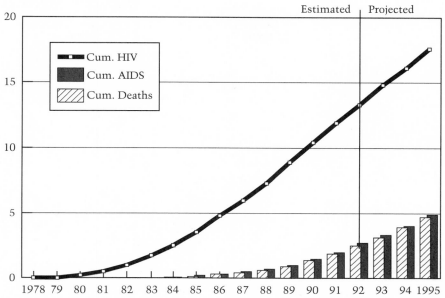

Number of Cases (millions)

Figure 2.49. Cumulative HIV, AIDS cases, and deaths for adults worldwide, 1978-1995.
Source: AIDS in the World, 1992.

Tragically, the remainder of the 1990s will witness a major pandemic wave, fueled by new infections in this GAA. Following earlier HIV spread in North America, Western Europe, and sub-Saharan Africa, HIV has now found multiple entry points into densely populated and highly vulnerable Southeast Asia (see Figures 2.47 and 2.48).

The number of HIV infections, AIDS cases, and deaths estimated to have occurred worldwide in adults and children by January 1, 1992, and projections for the year 1995 are shown in Figures 2.49–2.53.

HIV Infections in the World: Projections to 1995

According to *AIDS in the World* projections, an additional 5.7 million adults and 1.2 million children, or a total of 6.9 million people, will become newly infected with HIV by 1995. This represents an average annual increase of 1.7 million people (1.4 million adults and 0.3

Number of Cases (thousands)

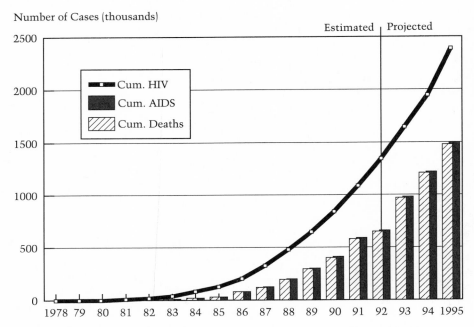

Figure 2.50. Cumulative pediatric HIV, AIDS cases, and deaths worldwide, 1978-1995.
Source: AIDS in the World, 1992.
Note: Pediatric infections/cases refer only to mother-fetus/infant transmission.

Number of Cases (millions)

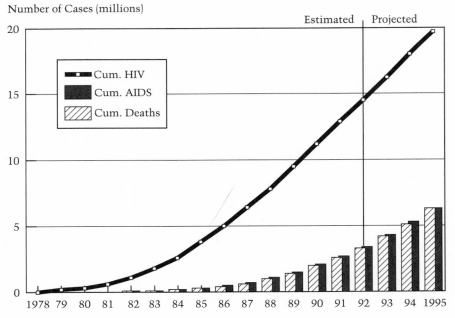

Figure 2.51. Cumulative adult/pediatric HIV, AIDS cases, and deaths worldwide, 1978-1995.
Source: AIDS in the World, 1992.
Note: Pediatric infections/cases refer only to mother-fetus/infant transmission.

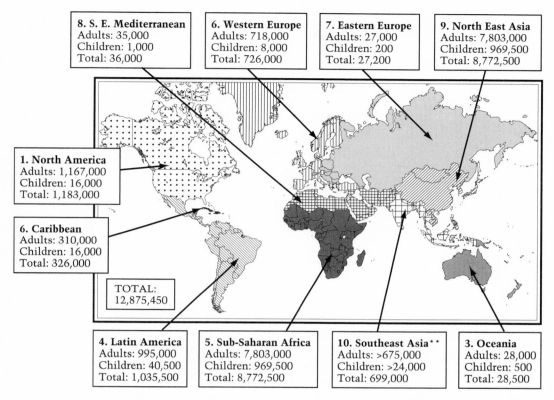

8. S. E. Mediterranean
Adults: 35,000
Children: 1,000
Total: 36,000

6. Western Europe
Adults: 718,000
Children: 8,000
Total: 726,000

7. Eastern Europe
Adults: 27,000
Children: 200
Total: 27,200

9. North East Asia
Adults: 7,803,000
Children: 969,500
Total: 8,772,500

1. North America
Adults: 1,167,000
Children: 16,000
Total: 1,183,000

6. Caribbean
Adults: 310,000
Children: 16,000
Total: 326,000

TOTAL:
12,875,450

4. Latin America
Adults: 995,000
Children: 40,500
Total: 1,035,500

5. Sub-Saharan Africa
Adults: 7,803,000
Children: 969,500
Total: 8,772,500

10. Southeast Asia**
Adults: >675,000
Children: >24,000
Total: 699,000

3. Oceania
Adults: 28,000
Children: 500
Total: 28,500

Figure 2.52. Cumulative HIV infections in adults (men and women) and children by Geographic Area of Affinity, January 1, 1992.*
Source: AIDS in the World, 1992.
*AIW estimate.
**conservative estimate based on limited available data.

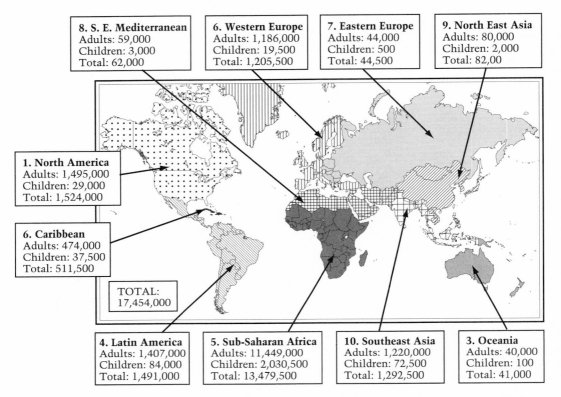

8. S. E. Mediterranean
Adults: 59,000
Children: 3,000
Total: 62,000

6. Western Europe
Adults: 1,186,000
Children: 19,500
Total: 1,205,500

7. Eastern Europe
Adults: 44,000
Children: 500
Total: 44,500

9. North East Asia
Adults: 80,000
Children: 2,000
Total: 82,00

1. North America
Adults: 1,495,000
Children: 29,000
Total: 1,524,000

6. Caribbean
Adults: 474,000
Children: 37,500
Total: 511,500

TOTAL:
17,454,000

4. Latin America
Adults: 1,407,000
Children: 84,000
Total: 1,491,000

5. Sub-Saharan Africa
Adults: 11,449,000
Children: 2,030,500
Total: 13,479,500

10. Southeast Asia
Adults: 1,220,000
Children: 72,500
Total: 1,292,500

3. Oceania
Adults: 40,000
Children: 100
Total: 41,000

Figure 2.53. Cumulative HIV infections in adults (men and women) and children by Geographic Area of Affinity, 1995.
Source: AIDS in the World, 1992.

Table 2.8: Cumulative adult HIV infections by Geographic Area of Affinity (GAA) as of January 1, 1992, and 1995

GAA	January 1, 1992, estimate	1995 estimate	No. of new infections, 1992–1995	% increase, 1992–1995
1 North America	1,167,000	1,495,000	328,000	28
2 Western Europe	718,000	1,186,000	468,000	65
3 Oceania	28,000	40,000	12,000	43
4 Latin America	995,000	1,407,000	412,000	41
5 Sub-Saharan Africa	7,803,000	11,449,000	3,646,000	47
6 Caribbean	310,000	474,000	164,000	53
7 Eastern Europe	27,000	44,000	17,000	63
8 South East Mediterranean	35,000	59,000	24,000	69
9 North East Asia	41,000	80,000	39,000	95
10 Southeast Asia	675,000	1,220,000	545,000	66
Total	11,799,000	17,454,000	5,655,000	48

Source: AIDS in the World, 1992.

million children). Thus, by 1995, the cumulative total of HIV-infected adults is projected to be nearly 17.5 million, along with 2.3 million children.

Table 2.8 shows the cumulative estimates of HIV infection among adults, by GAA as of January 1, 1992, and 1995. The overall increase in the cumulative number of HIV-infected adults during this period is 48 percent, and the median percentage increase is 58 percent, ranging from a low of 28 percent in North America to a high of 95 percent in North East Asia. The largest number of new HIV infections is projected to occur in sub-Saharan Africa (3.6 million) and the smallest in Oceania (12,000). Of all new HIV infections among adults during this period, the largest proportion is in sub-Saharan Africa (64 percent), followed by Southeast Asia (10 percent), Western Europe (8 percent), Latin America (7 percent), and North America (6 percent). All to-

Table 2.9: Cumulative pediatric HIV infections by Geographic Area of Affinity (GAA) as of January 1, 1992, and 1995

GAA	January 1, 1992, estimate	1995 estimate	No. of new infections, 1992–1995	% increase, 1992–1995
1 North America	16,000	29,000	13,000	81
2 Western Europe	8,000	19,500	11,500	144
3 Oceania	500	1,000	500	100
4 Latin America	40,500	84,000	43,500	107
5 Sub-Saharan Africa	969,500	2,030,500	1,061,000	109
6 Caribbean	16,000	37,500	21,500	134
7 Eastern Europe	200	500	300	150
8 South East Mediterranean	1,000	3,000	2,000	200
9 North East Asia	750	2,000	1,250	167
10 Southeast Asia	24,000	72,500	48,500	202
Total	1,076,450	2,279,500	1,203,050	112

Source: AIDS in the World, 1992.

gether, by 1995, the developing world is projected to account for 84 percent of the cumulative global total of HIV infections.

The overall increase in the cumulative number of HIV-infected children from January 1, 1992, to 1995 is 112 percent (see Table 2.9). Large increases are projected for all GAAs; only in North America is the expected increase less than 100 percent. Of all new HIV infections among children during this period, 88 percent (1,061,000 of 1,203,050) are in sub-Saharan Africa.

Projections of Global HIV Infection: To the Year 2000

For the year 2000, only adult HIV infections are estimated, using the Delphi method. The inherent difficulties of projecting beyond a few years are reflected in the widely varying estimates; as shown in Table

Table 2.10: Cumulative adult HIV infections by Geographic Area of Affinity (GAA): Projections for the year 2000

GAA	Low estimate	High estimate
1 North America	1,811,000	8,150,000
2 Western Europe	1,188,000	2,331,000
3 Oceania	22,000	45,000
4 Latin America	1,599,000	8,554,000
5 Sub-Saharan Africa	20,778,000	33,609,000
6 Caribbean	536,000	6,962,000
7 Eastern Europe	>2,000	20,000
8 South East Mediterranean	893,000	3,532,000
9 North East Asia	>6,000	486,000
10 Southeast Asia	11,277,000	45,059,000
Total	>38,112,000	108,748,000

Source: Delphi Survey, *AIDS in the World, 1992.*

2.10, the range is quite large within each GAA and, therefore also for the global total, which was between a minimum of 38 million and a high estimate of about 109 million (which can be approximated at 110 million).

Projections by *AIDS in the World* are substantially higher than the projections of the World Health Organization. The most conservative estimate by *AIDS in the World* was at the high range of the WHO projections for the year 2000 (30–40 million), and the higher *AIDS in the World* estimate is 2.8 to 3.6 times higher than the WHO estimates.

According to the higher Delphi estimates, by the year 2000, 42 percent of cumulative HIV infections will have occurred in Asia and Oceania (GAAs 3, 9, and 10); Africa will have accounted for 31 percent of infections; and Latin America and the Caribbean will have contributed 14 percent to the global total. Overall, by the year 2000, 90

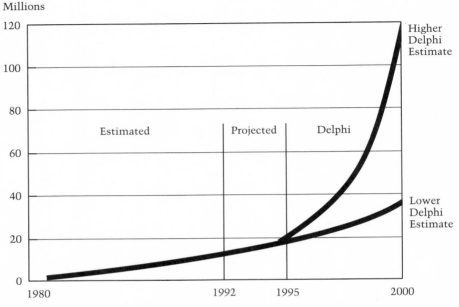

Figure 2.54. Cumulative HIV infections in the world, 1980-2000.
Source: AIDS in the World, 1992.

percent of all HIV infections will have occurred in the developing world.

The epidemic curve, including the January 1, 1992, estimates projections for 1995 (based on the application of Epimodel), and Delphi estimates for the year 2000 (Figure 2.54) suggest a sharp increase in HIV infections worldwide in the middle of the decade. This increase is the combined result of two forces: continued spread in already affected areas (North and Latin America, the Caribbean, Western Europe, sub-Saharan Africa) and expected major increases in thus far less affected populations in Southeast and North East Asia. The future course of the pandemic will largely depend on the ability to prevent HIV transmission among the large, vulnerable populations of Asia, including the most populated Asian countries: Bangladesh, China, India, and Indonesia.

CHAPTER THREE

· ·

The AIDS Pandemic

According to *AIDS in the World* estimates, more than 2.6 million people have developed AIDS as of January 1, 1992. Of these people, 2.02 million are adults and nearly 575,000 are children.

As shown in Table 3.1, the largest proportion of adult AIDS cases (67.7 percent) have occurred in sub-Saharan Africa, followed by North America with 12.8 percent of adult cases and Latin America with 8.6 percent. Together, Africa and the Americas (including the Caribbean) account for over 90 percent of all adult AIDS cases to date. Among children with AIDS, 9 of 10 (91 percent) are from sub-Saharan Africa; the Americas (including the Caribbean) account for nearly 7 percent.

With adjustments made for underreporting and delays in reporting, a striking geographical disparity emerges (see Table 3.2). Although Africa has only 9 percent of the world's adults, it bears 67.7 percent of the global adult AIDS burden; similarly, the Americas and the Caribbean have 14 percent of the adults and 23.5 percent of the world's adult AIDS cases. Conversely, North East and Southeast Asia together have 55 percent of the world's adults but only a small fraction (3.4 percent) of the world's adult AIDS cases as of January 1, 1992.

━━━━━━━ · · ·

AIDS AND REPORTED AIDS CASES

The official reports of AIDS cases are issued by the World Health Organization, based on voluntary reporting by national authorities (see Appendix 3.1). It is clear that officially reported AIDS cases represent only a fraction of actual cases; on a worldwide basis, only about

Table 3.1: Cumulative adult and pediatric AIDS cases by Geographic Area of Affinity (GAA) as of January 1, 1992

GAA	Adult cases No.	Adult cases %	Pediatric cases No.	Pediatric cases %	Total cases No.	Total cases %
1 North America	257,500	12.8	9,000	1.6	266,500	10.3
2 Western Europe	99,000	4.9	4,000	0.7	103,000	4.0
3 Oceania	4,500	0.2	200	—	4,700	0.2
4 Latin America	173,000	8.6	21,500	3.7	194,500	7.5
5 Sub-Saharan Africa	1,367,000	67.7	520,500	90.7	1,887,500	72.8
6 Caribbean	43,000	2.1	8,000	1.4	51,000	2.0
7 Eastern Europe	2,500	0.1	100	—	2,600	0.1
8 South East Mediterranean	3,500	0.2	400	0.1	3,900	0.1
9 North East Asia	3,500	0.2	300	0.1	3,800	0.1
10 Southeast Asia	65,000	3.2	9,500	1.7	74,500	2.9
Total	2,018,500	100.0	573,500	100.0	2,592,000	100.0

Source: AIDS in the World, 1992.

Table 3.2: Comparison of adult population (age 15–49 years) and cumulative AIDS cases, by Geographic Area of Affinity (GAA), as of January 1, 1992

GAA	% of world adult population, 1991	% of cumulative adult AIDS cases (Reported)	% of cumulative adult AIDS cases (adjusted)
1 North America	5.4	45.2	12.8
2 Western Europe	8.1	13.1	4.9
3 Oceania	0.5	0.7	0.2
4 Latin America	7.8	8.6	8.6
5 Sub-Saharan Africa	8.8	29.9	67.7
6 Caribbean	0.6	1.6	2.1
7 Eastern Europe	7.4	0.5	0.1
8 South East Mediterranean	6.5	0.2	0.2
9 North East Asia	29.5	0.1	0.2
10 Southeast Asia	25.4	0.1	3.2
Total	100.0	100.0	100.0

Source: AIDS in the World, 1992.

one of five AIDS cases (including both adults and children) is reported to WHO. Yet, as the WHO data represent the only system of routine reporting on AIDS worldwide, it is important to derive whatever information possible from these reports (see Box 3.1). Particularly, once reporting starts and becomes systematized, trends over time may give some indication, however limited, of the true picture of AIDS in a country.

Officially Reported AIDS Cases: 1985 to 1992

As of April 3, 1992, a total of 484,163 AIDS cases had been reported to WHO. The annual and cumulative numbers of reported cases are

---

Box 3.1: Reporting AIDS to WHO

WHO receives reports of AIDS in many different formats from ministries of health throughout the world. These reports come to WHO directly from countries or through WHO's six regional offices. This type of data collection is well known to be incomplete and sometimes quite misleading.

First, there are obvious problems, such as the ability of countries to collect accurate information from health workers, delays in communicating this information, problems in diagnosis (particularly when testing facilities are inadequate), and varying definitions of what constitutes a case of AIDS.

In addition, there are political distortions of data (not surprising in a world where reports of cholera have been suppressed by countries to protect their tourist industry). Thus, Zaire refused to report AIDS cases officially to WHO until 1988, yet an active AIDS research program had presented data at International Conferences since 1985, describing hundreds of confirmed cases! Similarly, Saudi Arabia refused to report until 1990–91, while articles on confirmed cases in that country had appeared in the medical literature since 1986. Thus, one must also wonder about the 25 remaining countries that have yet to report any AIDS case as of January 1, 1992, including, Albania, Bahrain, Burma (where a major HIV epidemic is underway), and Yemen.

When a ministry of health does make the decision to report to WHO, the number of cases suddenly increases from zero, giving the impression that AIDS has only recently appeared. This happened in Uganda, when the number of reported cases rose from 126 in 1986 to 3,477 (still a vast undercounting) in 1987.

Problems in completeness of reporting are not restricted to the developing world. In Europe, estimates vary among countries, but range from perhaps 60 to 90 percent complete; in the United States, concern has recently been raised about further decreases in completeness of reporting.

Number of Cases (thousands)

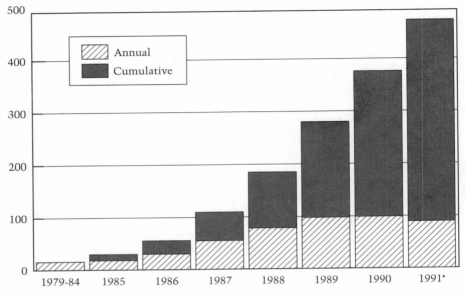

Figure 3.1. Annual and cumulative AIDS cases reported to WHO as of January 1, 1992.
Source: World Health Organization, Geneva Switzerland, 1992.
*Reported as of April 3, 1992. Figures for 1991 are not yet complete.

shown in Figure 3.1. The number of new cases reported each year increased nearly sevenfold from 1985 to 1990, from 15,252 to 102,818.

Reports from very recent years (1991, and to some extent 1990) are known to be incomplete due to delays in reporting at local, national, and international levels. Delays in reporting of AIDS cases by ministries of health vary from country to country and, within the same country, from one period to another. For example, the dates of the last reports received by WHO as of January 1, 1992, averaged less than six months for over 90 percent of the countries in North America, Western and Eastern Europe, South East Mediterranean, and Oceania. In contrast, the majority of countries in Latin America, North East Asia, and sub-Saharan Africa had not submitted a report in the previous six months. Twenty-five countries (13 percent) in the world had not reported for more than a year (see Table 3.3). Therefore, the

Table 3.3: Delay in reporting AIDS to WHO as of January 1, 1992 (190 countries/territories)

GAA	No. of countries/ territories reporting	No. of countries/territories with reporting delay of:		
		≤6 months	7–12 months	>12 months
1 North America	2	2 (100%)		
2 Western Europe	22	21 (96%)	1 (4%)	
3 Oceania	23	21 (90%)	2 (10%)	
4 Latin America	21	4 (19%)	17 (81%)	
5 Sub-Saharan Africa	48	14 (29%)	14 (29%)	20 (42%)
6 Caribbean	22	17 (77%)	2 (9%)	3 (14%)
7 Eastern Europe	8	8 (100%)		
8 South East Mediterranean	21	19 (90%)	2 (10%)	
9 North East Asia	11	3 (27%)	6 (52%)	2 (21%)
10 Southeast Asia	12	8 (70%)	4 (30%)	
Total	190 (100%)	117 (62%)	48 (25%)	25 (13%)

Source: Adapted from the *WHO Weekly Epidemiological Record,* January 1992.

apparent drop-off in the increase of cases from 1989 to 1990, and particularly the decline in the total number of officially reported cases from 1990 to 1991, should be considered as an artifact of the data collection and reporting process. (Appendix 3.1 contains a complete listing of reported AIDS cases, by country and year.)

The diagnosis of AIDS in children is more complex than for adults. In many developing countries, where the majority of the world's pediatric AIDS occurs, symptoms and signs of AIDS are quite similar to those of common conditions, such as malaria, failure to thrive, malnutrition, or diarrheal disease. Even when laboratory diagnostic facilities are available, AIDS is difficult to confirm until the child is one year of age or older. Therefore, on a global basis, WHO has assumed that pediatric AIDS cases are very infrequently reported, so that the reports nearly exclusively involve adults.

GEOGRAPHICAL OVERVIEW

AIDS cases have been reported to WHO from 164 countries, including 52 countries in Africa, 45 in the Americas, 28 in Asia, 28 in Europe, and 11 in Oceania.

Sub-Saharan Africa: A total of 144,522 cases (30 percent of the world total) have been reported from sub-Saharan Africa, and only one country (Seychelles) has yet to report a single AIDS case. Nine countries, mainly in Central and East Africa, have reported more than 5,000 cases each (in descending order: Uganda [30,190], Tanzania [27,396], Zaire [14,762], Malawi [12,074], Zimbabwe [10,551], Kenya [9,139], Côte d'Ivoire [8,297], Rwanda [6,578], and Zambia [5,802]) (see Figure 3.2). Together, these 9 countries accounted for 86 percent of all reported AIDS in Africa. Eighteen countries, mainly in North Africa, Southern Africa, and the island nations, have reported fewer than 100 cases to WHO.

The Americas: A cumulative total of 268,477 AIDS cases (55 percent of the global total) have been reported from the Americas. All 45 countries in the Americas have reported AIDS cases, ranging from one case in the tiny island nation of Montserrat to 213,641 in the United States (80 percent of all cases in the Americas, and 44 percent of the global total). In addition to the United States, three other countries have reported more than 5,000 cases each: Brazil (22,583), Canada (5,348), and Mexico (9,073). Together, these four countries account for 93 percent of all reported AIDS cases in the Americas. Eighteen countries reported fewer than 100 cases each, including 13 Caribbean nations, 2 from Central America (Belize and Nicaragua), and 3 from South America (Bolivia, Paraguay, and Suriname).

Asia and the Middle East: Fewer than 1 percent (0.3 percent) of all reported AIDS cases have been from Asia and the Middle East; only 28 of 40 countries in this region have officially reported any AIDS cases. Japan reported the largest number of cases (453); in addition to Japan, 5 countries have each reported more than 50 AIDS cases: Israel (169), Thailand (179), India (102), Turkey (62), and the Philippines (53). These 6 coun-

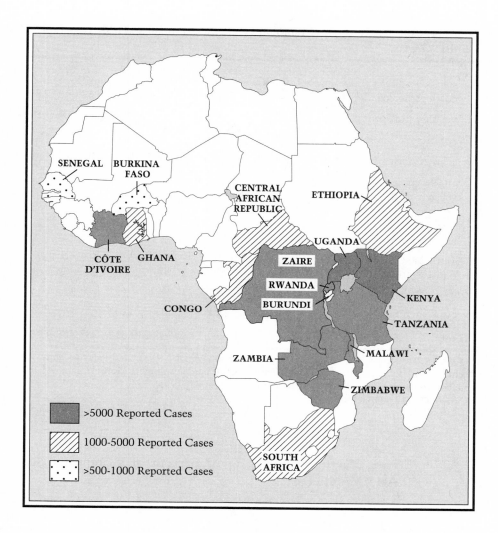

Figure 3.2. Cumulative reported AIDS cases to WHO from Africa, by country as of January 1, 1992.*
Source: World Health Organization, Geneva, Switzerland, 1992.
*Reported as of April 3, 1992.

Table 3.4: Cumulative total of reported AIDS cases through 1991[a] by Geographic Area of Affinity (GAA)

GAA	<1985	1985	1986	1987	1988	1989	1990	1991[a]
1 North America	10,805	22,477	41,479	69,819	104,123	142,812	180,337	218,989
2 Western Europe	1,251	3,087	6,812	13,879	23,301	37,504	51,527	63,659
3 Oceania	61	195	439	847	1,425	2,077	2,763	3,509
4 Latin America	326	1,096	2,791	6,763	13,062	20,187	28,850	41,603
5 Sub-Saharan Africa	207	785	4,344	18,195	42,137	77,899	116,568	144,522
6 Caribbean	500	723	1,262	2,416	3,947	5,554	7,161	7,885
7 Eastern Europe	0	8	25	63	133	528	1,708	2,236
8 South East Mediterranean	18	31	87	182	284	446	592	813
9 North East Asia	0	15	29	72	113	222	427	516
10 Southeast Asia	2	5	18	44	93	159	273	431
Total	13,170	28,422	57,336	112,280	189,618	287,388	390,206	484,163

Source: Reports from the World Health Organization (April 3, 1992) and Pan American Health Organization (1992), and the European Center for the Epidemiological Monitoring of AIDS (WHO-EC Collaborating Centre on AIDS), St. Maurice (December 31, 1991).

a. As reported through January 1, 1992.

tries together account for 67 percent of all reported AIDS cases in Asia/Middle East.

Europe: With the exception of Albania, every European country has reported AIDS. Europe has reported 66,126 cases, representing 14 percent of the world total. The largest number of reported cases are from major Western European countries: France (17,836), Italy (11,609), Spain (11,555), Germany (7,533), the United Kingdom (5,451), Switzerland (2,228), and the Netherlands (2,017). Together, they account for 88 percent of all reported European cases. With the dramatic exception of Romania (1,704 cases), most Central and Eastern European countries have reported fewer than 100 AIDS cases: Bulgaria (13), Czechoslovakia (26), Hungary (82), Poland (87), and Russia (70).

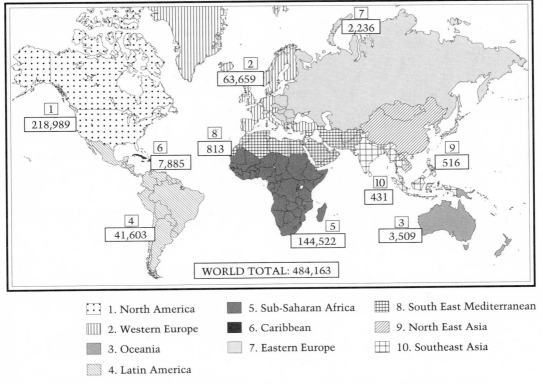

Figure 3.3. Cumulative number of reported adult AIDS cases worldwide by Geographic Area of Affinity, through January 1, 1992.*
Source: World Health Organization, Geneva, Switzerland, 1992.
*Reported as of April 3, 1992.

Oceania: The Pacific Ocean countries have reported only 0.7 percent of world AIDS cases, with only two countries—Australia (3,137) and New Zealand (274)—accounting for the vast majority (97 percent) of all reported cases. Eleven of the 21 island countries in this region have not reported any AIDS cases to WHO. Of these island nations, the largest numbers of reported cases are from Papua New Guinea (37), French Polynesia (27), and New Caledonia (18).

Geographic Trends

Table 3.4 and Figure 3.3 show the cumulative reported case total for each of the 10 GAAs through 1991. During this period, 97 percent of reported AIDS cases have been from four GAAs: North America (45 percent of total); sub-Saharan Africa (30 percent); Western Europe (13 percent); and Latin America (9 percent).

The relative contribution of these GAAs to the cumulative total of reported cases has changed substantially during the period from 1985 to 1991. The proportion of cases reported from North America decreased from 79 percent of all cases in 1985 to only 45 percent of reported cases in 1991 (see Table 3.4). During this time, the proportion of reported cases for sub-Saharan Africa increased nearly tenfold, from 3 percent of reported cases in 1985 to 30 percent in 1991. Thus, for the first time in 1990, the number of newly reported AIDS cases from Africa exceeded the number from North America.

In Europe, the United States, and Canada, official reporting does include the probable route of exposure to HIV.

Europe: In Europe, AIDS cases in 1985 were substantially more likely to have been infected through homosexual contact compared with 1990 (64 percent vs. 47 percent); in contrast, a larger percentage of cases in 1990 were associated with injection drug use (30 percent vs. 5 percent in 1985) (see Figure 3.4). The proportion of cases linked with heterosexual contact decreased from 17 percent in 1985 to 10 percent in 1990, associated with a substantial decrease in the proportion of foreign-born (African, Caribbean) people with AIDS during this period. Among women with AIDS in 1985 in Europe, the largest single exposure category was heterosexual (55 percent), whereas among the cases in 1990, injection drug use accounted for nearly 50 percent and heterosexual transmission for only 30 percent (see Figure 3.5). This same trend, of decreasing relative importance of sexual transmission and the increasing role of injection drug use, was observed to a lesser extent among men with AIDS in Europe (see Figure 3.6).

The United States: Similar data are available for the United States (see Figure 3.7). Overall, the role of homosexual/bisexual transmission has decreased since 1985, while the proportion of cases associated with injection drug use and heterosexual transmission has increased.

For women, the proportion of AIDS cases linked with heterosexual transmission has increased from 26 percent in 1985 to 36 percent in 1991 (see Figure 3.8); for men, heterosexual transmission has also

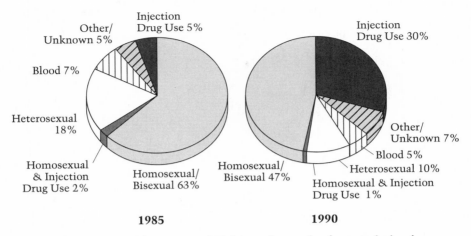

Figure 3.4. Proportion of European AIDS cases by mode of transmission in adults, 1985 and 1990.
Source: The European Center for the Epidemiological Monitoring of AIDS, Paris (WHO-EC Collaborating Centre on AIDS).

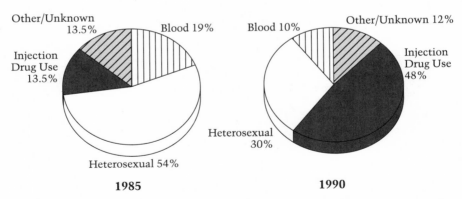

Figure 3.5. European AIDS cases in women by mode of transmission, 1985 and 1990.
Source: The European Center for the Epidemiological Monitoring of AIDS, Paris (WHO-EC Collaborating Centre on AIDS).

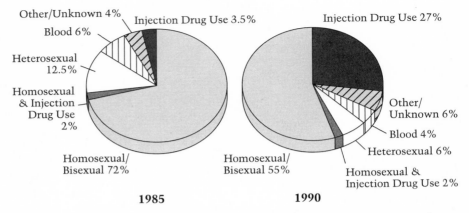

Figure 3.6. European AIDS cases in men by mode of transmission, 1985 and 1990.
Source: The European Center for the Epidemiological Monitoring of AIDS, Paris (WHO-EC Collaborating Centre on AIDS).

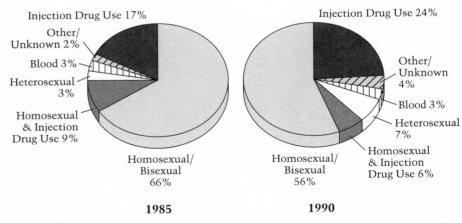

Figure 3.7. Proportion of AIDS cases in United States by mode of transmission in adults, 1985 and 1990.
Source: 1990 AIDS/HIV/STD surveillance report, Pan American Health Organization, Regional Office of the World Health Organization, Washington, DC.

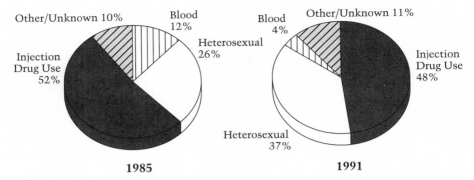

Figure 3.8. Cases in United States in women by mode of transmission, 1985 and 1991.
Source: 1990 AIDS/HIV/STD surveillance report, Pan American Health Organization, Regional Office of the World Health Organization, Washington, DC.

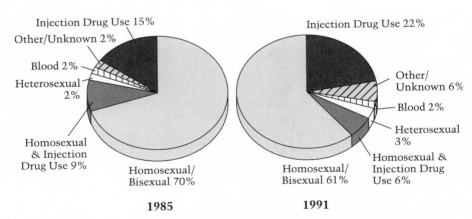

Figure 3.9. AIDS cases in United States in men by mode of transmission, 1985 and 1991.
Source: 1990 AIDS/HIV/STD surveillance report, Pan American Health Organization, Regional Office of the World Health Organization, Washington, DC.

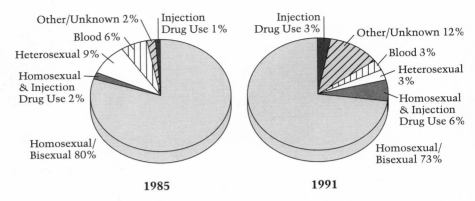

Figure 3.10. Proportion of AIDS cases in Canada in adults by mode of transmission, 1985 and 1991.
Source: 1990 AIDS/HIV/STD surveillance report, Pan American Health Organization, Regional Office of the World Health Organization, Washington, DC.

increased slightly as a proportion of all cases, from two percent in 1985 to 3.3 percent in 1991 (see Figure 3.9).

Canada: Despite its geographical proximity to the United States, a strikingly different pattern has emerged in Canada (see Figure 3.10). For all AIDS cases, the proportion attributed to homosexual/bisexual transmission has remained nearly constant from 1985 to 1991 (80 percent vs. 73 percent), the proportion of cases linked with heterosexual transmission has decreased (9 percent to 3 percent), and injection drug use remains a minor contributor (3 percent of cases in 1991). However, sources of exposure for men and women with AIDS are strongly divergent (see Figure 3.11).

Central America, the Caribbean, and South America: The Pan-American Health Organization (PAHO) has compared the sources of exposure for AIDS cases in 1987 and 1990 in Mexico, Central America, the Caribbean, Brazil, the Andean Region (Venezuela, Colombia, Peru, Bolivia, Ecuador, Paraguay), and the Southern Cone (Chile, Argentina, Uruguay). As shown in Table 3.5, each subregion is epidemiologically distinct. Nevertheless, the contribution of homosexual/bisexual transmission is declining in all areas, although most markedly in Central America,

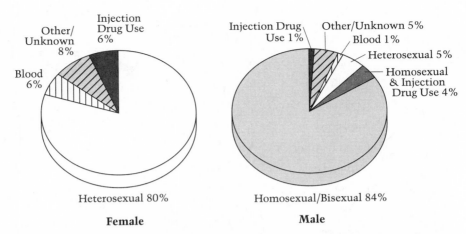

Figure 3.11. Proportion of AIDS cases in Canada by mode of transmission for each gender, up to July 1, 1991.
Source: 1990 AIDS/HIV/STD surveillance report, Pan American Health Organization, Regional Office of the World Health Organization, Washington, DC.

Table 3.5: Percentage of AIDS cases by mode of transmission, 1987 and 1990, the Americas

Region	Homo/bisexual		Heterosexual		Injection drug use	
	1987	1990	1987	1990	1987	1990
Andean	84	73	13	23	1	2
Southern cone	78	51	9	14	7	29
Brazil	69	43	7	19	12	27
Central American isthmus	61	25	30	67	1	1
Mexico	75	54	8	19	1	2
Caribbean	28	21	52	71	17	6
Latin Caribbean	21	6	60	80	1	2
North America	68	62	3	5	19	25

Source: Pan American Health Organization/WHO, *1990 AIDS/HIV/STD Annual Surveillance Report.*

Table 3.6: Male-to-female ratios of reported AIDS, 1985, 1987, and 1990[a]

Region	1985	1987	1990
Europe	7.3	8.3	5.8
United States	14.8	10.7	7.3
Canada	11.4	17.0	23.7
Mexico		9.5	5.1
Central America		4.0	2.3
Caribbean		2.5	2.2
Latin Caribbean		2.2	1.7
Brazil		9.9	9.4
Southern cone		12.9	16.2
Andean area		7.0	7.0

Source: Pan American Health Organization/WHO, *1990 AIDS/HIV/STD Annual Surveillance Report.*
a. Number of AIDS cases in men to one in women.

Mexico, Brazil, and the Southern Cone. From 1987 to 1990, the role of heterosexual transmission increased substantially in all areas. Compared with 1987, injection drug use made a smaller contribution to AIDS in 1990 in the Caribbean, but made a larger contribution in the Southern Cone, and particularly in Brazil.

Gender Ratio of AIDS Cases

In general, AIDS cases reported to WHO are not classified by gender. However, data on male-to-female ratio of AIDS cases is available from several areas (see Table 3.6). Comparing 1985 or 1987 with 1990, the male-to-female ratio of reported AIDS cases is generally declining, with the exception of Canada and South America.

■■■ . . .

AIDS MORTALITY BY JANUARY 1, 1992

By January 1, 1992, nearly 2.5 million people had died of AIDS, including 1.9 million adults and more than 550,000 children (see Table

Table 3.7: Cumulative adult and pediatric deaths from AIDS by Geographic Area of Affinity (GAA) as of January 1, 1992[a]

GAA	Adult deaths		Pediatric deaths		Total deaths	
	No.	% of total	No.	% of total	No.	% of total
1 North America	214,500	11.4	9,000	1.6	223,500	9.1
2 Western Europe	78,500	4.2	4,000	0.7	82,500	3.4
3 Oceania	3,500	0.2	200	—	3,700	0.2
4 Latin America	166,000	8.8	21,000	3.7	187,000	7.6
5 Sub-Saharan Africa	1,312,000	69.6	511,000	90.8	1,823,000	74.5
6 Caribbean	41,000	2.2	7,500	1.3	48,500	2.0
7 Eastern Europe	2,000	0.1	100	—	2,100	0.1
8 South East Mediterranean	2,500	0.1	400	0.1	2,900	0.1
9 North East Asia	3,500	0.2	300	0.1	3,800	0.2
10 Southeast Asia	61,500	3.3	9,000	1.6	70,500	2.9
Total	1,885,000	100.1	562,500	99.9	2,447,500	100.1

Source: AIDS in the World, 1992.
a. Figures in percent column do not add to 100.0 because of rounding.

3.7). Of all AIDS deaths, three-fourths have been in Africa and nearly 20 percent in the Americas.

Of the adult AIDS deaths, 70 percent were in Africa, 11 percent in North America, and 9 percent in Latin America. Together, these GAAs accounted for 90 percent of all adult AIDS deaths to date.

AIDS is now among the 10 leading causes of deaths in 35- to 44-year-old men in a growing number of industrialized countries (see Table 3.8). In 1988, mortality reports submitted to WHO by Australia, Canada, France, Italy, the Netherlands, and the United States, for example, showed AIDS among major causes of mortality in this gender and age group, together with diseases of the cardiovascular system, cancer, and violence. In New York City, in 1988–89, AIDS was the leading cause of death among women 25 to 39 years old, and the fourth leading cause of death among women 15 to 24 years old. Mortality

Table 3.8: Absolute numbers of cause-specific deaths from AIDS in men, 35–44 years, in industrialized countries, in comparison with other cause-specific mortality, 1988.

Country and cause of death	No. of deaths	Country and cause of death	No. of deaths
Australia		5. Acute myocardial infarction	671
1. Accidents	769	6. Chronic liver disease and cirrhosis	637
2. Diseases of the circulatory system	562	7. Mental disorders	386
3. Malignant neoplasms	444	8. AIDS	367
4. Suicide and self-inflicted injury	388	9. Epilepsy	102
5. Acute myocardial infarction	251	10. Infectious and parasitic diseases	99
6. Mental disorders	86		
7. Homicide	61	**Italy**	
8. AIDS	54	1. Malignant neoplasms	1,686
9. Infectious and parasitic diseases	33	2. Diseases of the circulatory system	1,486
10. Pneumonia	21	3. Accidents and adverse effects	1,201
		4. Acute myocardial infarction	663
Canada		5. Chronic liver disease and cirrhosis	536
1. Diseases of the circulatory system	777	6. Suicide and self-inflicted injury	373
2. Accidents and adverse effects	728	7. Homicide	186
3. Malignant neoplasms	654	8. AIDS	105
4. Suicide and self-inflicted injury	506	9. Mental disorders	103
5. Acute myocardial infarction	359	10. Diabetes mellitus	59
6. AIDS	233		
7. Chronic liver disease and cirrhosis	110	**Netherlands**	
8. Mental disorders	68	1. Diseases of the circulatory system	494
9. Homicide	64	2. Malignant neoplasms	450
10. Pneumonia	27	3. Acute myocardial infarction	267
		4. Accidents and adverse effects	172
France		5. Suicide and self-inflicted injury	167
1. Malignant neoplasms	2,396	6. Chronic liver disease and cirrhosis	67
2. Accidents and adverse effects	1,940	7. AIDS	56
3. Diseases of the circulatory system	1,658	8. Diabetes mellitus	46
4. Suicide and self-inflicted injury	1,578	9. Mental disorders	18
		10. Homicide	16

Table 3.8 (cont.): Absolute numbers of cause-specific deaths from AIDS in men, 35–44 years, in industrialized countries, in comparison with other cause-specific mortality, 1988.

Country and cause of death	No. of deaths	Country and cause of death	No. of deaths
United States		6. Homicide	2,962
1. Diseases of the circulatory system	10,879	7. Chronic liver disease and cirrhosis	2,597
2. Accidents and adverse effects	8,871	8. Mental disorders	1,626
3. Malignant neoplasms	6,913	9. Infectious and parasitic diseases	1,073
4. AIDS	5,656	10. Pneumonia	888
5. Suicide and self-inflicted injury	3,975		

Sources: AIDS mortality: WHO, Global Health Situation Assessment and Projections; other mortality: WHO, *World Health Statistics Annual 1990,* 1991.

reports from developing countries, in particular those where the incidence of AIDS is high, are too incomplete to allow for such an analysis.

Among children dying of AIDS, over 90 percent were in Africa, with important yet smaller numbers from North America, Southeast Asia, Latin America, the Caribbean, and Western Europe.

PROJECTIONS OF AIDS: 1995

The number of people with AIDS is expected to more than double by 1995, from 2.6 million to 6.4 million. Of the 6.4 million AIDS cases by 1995, 77 percent will be adults (4.9 million) and 23 percent will be children (1.5 million) (see Table 3.9).

Thus, a total of 3.8 million people will develop AIDS from 1992 to 1995, which is 150 percent more than developed AIDS from the beginning of the pandemic through January 1, 1992. These new AIDS cases developing between 1992 and 1995 will include 2.9 million adults and more than 900,000 children. The geographical distribution of AIDS in 1995 will continue to reflect the progression of the pandemic to the developing world (see Table 3.9). By 1995, more than 4.6 million Africans will have developed AIDS, or more than 8 times the

Table 3.9: Cumulative adult and pediatric AIDS cases by Geographic Area of Affinity (GAA) as of January 1, 1992, and 1995

GAA	January 1, 1992			1995		
	Adult	Pediatric	Total	Adult	Pediatric	Total
1 North America	257,500	9,000	266,500	534,000	21,000	555,000
2 Western Europe	99,000	4,000	103,000	279,500	12,000	291,500
3 Oceania	4,500	200	4,700	11,500	500	12,000
4 Latin America	173,000	21,500	194,500	417,500	56,000	473,500
5 Sub-Saharan Africa	1,367,000	520,500	1,887,500	3,277,500	1,338,500	4,616,000
6 Caribbean	43,000	8,000	51,000	121,000	23,500	144,500
7 Eastern Europe	2,500	100	2,600	9,500	300	9,800
8 South East Mediterranean	3,500	400	3,900	12,500	1,500	14,000
9 North East Asia	3,500	300	3,800	14,500	1,100	15,600
10 Southeast Asia	65,000	9,500	74,500	240,500	40,500	281,000
Total	2,018,500	573,500	2,592,000	4,918,000	1,494,900	6,412,900

Source: AIDS in the World, 1992.

number of North Americans, nearly 10 times the number of Latin Americans, and nearly 16 times the number of West Europeans.

Among adults, the cumulative number of AIDS cases will increase 2.3-fold from January 1, 1992, to 1995, from 2.1 to 4.9 million (see Table 3.10). The proportional increase varies substantially among GAAs, from a 2.1-fold increase in North America to a stunning 4.1-fold rise in North East Asia; the median proportional increase from 1992 to 1995 is projected to be 2.8-fold.

Among children, an overall 2.6-fold increase from 0.6 million AIDS cases in 1992 to 1.5 million cases in 1995 will be observed among all GAAs (see Table 3.11).

PROJECTIONS OF AIDS: TO THE YEAR 2000

Projections of the number of people with AIDS in the year 2000 are based on the Delphi estimates of HIV-infected people. Therefore, the

Table 3.10: Cumulative adult AIDS cases by Geographic Area of Affinity (GAA) as of January 1, 1992, and 1995

GAA	January 1, 1992	1995	Proportional increase, 1992–1995
1 North America	257,500	534,000	2.1
2 Western Europe	99,000	279,500	2.8
3 Oceania	4,500	11,500	2.6
4 Latin America	173,000	417,500	2.4
5 Sub-Saharan Africa	1,367,000	3,277,500	2.4
6 Caribbean	43,000	121,000	2.8
7 Eastern Europe	2,500	9,500	3.8
8 South East Mediterranean	3,500	12,500	3.6
9 North East Asia	3,500	14,500	4.1
10 Southeast Asia	65,000	240,500	3.7
Total	2,018,500	4,918,000	2.4

Source: AIDS in the World, 1992.

Table 3.11: Cumulative pediatric AIDS cases by Geographic Area of Affinity (GAA) as of January 1, 1992, and 1995

GAA	January 1, 1992	1995	Proportional increase, 1992–1995
1 North America	9,000	21,000	2.3
2 Western Europe	4,000	12,000	3.0
3 Oceania	200	500	2.5
4 Latin America	21,500	56,000	2.6
5 Sub-Saharan Africa	520,500	1,338,500	2.6
6 Caribbean	8,000	23,500	2.9
7 Eastern Europe	100	300	3.0
8 South East Mediterranean	400	1,500	3.8
9 North East Asia	300	1,100	3.7
10 Southeast Asia	9,500	40,500	4.3
Total	573,500	1,494,900	2.6

Source: AIDS in the World, 1992.

Table 3.12: Cumulative adult AIDS cases by Geographic Area of Affinity (GAA) as of 1995 and 2000

GAA	2000[a]		Proportional increase, 1995–2000	
	Low	High	Low	High
1 North America	671,000	3,603,000	1.3	6.7
2 Western Europe	268,000	536,000	—[b]	1.9
3 Oceania	11,000	20,000	—[b]	1.8
4 Latin America	175,000	1,883,000	—[b]	4.5
5 Sub-Saharan Africa	5,505,000	10,583,000	1.7	3.2
6 Caribbean	156,000	2,505,000	1.3	20.7
7 Eastern Europe	>1,000	>3,000	—[b]	—
8 South East Mediterranean	150,000	711,500	12.0	56.9
9 North East Asia	>1,000	51,000	—[b]	3.5
10 Southeast Asia	1,051,000	4,111,000	4.4	17.1
Total	8,000,000	24,000,000	1.6	4.9

Source: AIDS in the World, 1992.
a. Numbers are to the nearest 100,000.
b. The Delphi Survey provided more conservative low estimates for these GAAs for the year 2000 than those derived from Epimodel through 1995.

projections in this section are extremely conservative, because only adult AIDS cases are included; separate AIDS case estimates have been made for the low and high Delphi figures of HIV-infected people in the year 2000.

By the year 2000, from 8 to 24 million adults will have developed AIDS. Therefore, from 1995 to 2000, the total number of adults with AIDS will increase from 1.6-fold to about 5-fold (see Table 3.12). In this period (1995–2000), from 3 to 19 million new AIDS cases will develop worldwide (see Tables 3.10 and 3.12). As in the past, the geographic variations are important; proportional increases from 1995 to 2000 (according to the high Delphi estimate) will range from

Table 3.13: Adult and pediatric deaths from AIDS by Geographic Area of Affinity (GAA) as of January 1, 1992, and 1995

GAA	January 1, 1992			1995			Proportional increase of total
	Adult	Pediatric	Total	Adult	Pediatric	Total	
1 North America	214,500	9,000	223,500	475,500	20,500	496,000	2.2
2 Western Europe	78,500	4,000	82,500	238,000	12,000	250,000	3.0
3 Oceania	3,500	200	3,700	10,000	500	10,500	2.8
4 Latin America	166,000	21,000	187,000	406,000	55,000	461,000	2.5
5 Sub-Saharan Africa	1,312,000	511,000	1,823,000	3,184,000	1,320,500	4,504,500	2.5
6 Caribbean	41,000	7,500	48,500	117,000	23,000	140,000	2.9
7 Eastern Europe	2,000	100	2,100	7,500	300	7,800	3.7
8 South East Mediterranean	2,500	400	2,900	10,500	1,500	12,000	4.1
9 North East Asia	3,500	300	3,800	14,000	1,100	15,100	4.0
10 Southeast Asia	61,500	9,000	70,500	231,000	40,000	271,000	3.8
Total	1,885,000	562,500	2,447,500	4,693,500	1,474,400	6,167,900	2.5

Source: AIDS in the World, 1992.

1.8/1.9-fold (Oceania/Western Europe) to greater than 5-fold (North America, Caribbean, South East Mediterranean, and Southeast Asia).

■ • • •

AIDS DEATHS AMONG ADULTS AND CHILDREN: 1995–2000

From 1992 to 1995, 3.7 million people are expected to die of AIDS; this includes 2.8 million adults and more than 900,000 children (see Table 3.13). Therefore, more AIDS deaths are projected between 1992 and 1995 alone than occurred during the entire pandemic to date. Although overall, a 2.5-fold increase in cumulative deaths (adult plus pediatric) will occur from 1992 to 1995, there is some variation according to GAA.

Table 3.14: Adult AIDS deaths as of January 1992, 1995, and 2000

| | 1992 | 1995 | 2000[a] | |
			Low	High
Cumulative adult AIDS deaths	1,885,000	4,693,500	5,881,000	20,406,000
Interval number of new deaths				

| (1992–1995) |
| 2,808,500 |

| (1995–2000 low) |
| 1,187,500 |

| (1995–2000 high) |
| 15,712,500 |

| (1992–2000 low) |
| 3,996,000 |

| (1992–2000 high) |
| 18,521,000 |

Source: AIDS in the World, 1992.
a. High and low Delphi Survey projections are based on 85% mortality of AIDS cases to date.

A conservative estimate of adult AIDS deaths by the year 2000 can be made. Applying current survival rates, it is assumed that 85 percent of AIDS cases by that time will have died. According to this calculation, between 5.9 million and 20.4 million adults will have died of AIDS by the year 2000 (see Table 3.14). Thus, from 1995 to 2000, between 2.1 and 15.7 million new AIDS deaths will occur among adults worldwide. Compared with 1992, the number of deaths from AIDS among adults will increase by 4.9 to 18.5 million, or from 4-fold to 11-fold.

. . . .

CHAPTER FOUR

Interactions of HIV
and Other Diseases

AIDS is a unique disease; no other known infectious disease causes its damage through a direct attack on the human immune system. Because the immune system is the final mediator of human host-infectious agent interactions, it was anticipated early on that HIV infection would complicate the course of other important human diseases.

This has proven to be the case, particularly for tuberculosis and certain sexually transmitted infections, such as syphilis and the genital herpes virus. Yet the search for relationships between major diseases and HIV has been complicated. For example, the discovery of AIDS in Africa between 1982 and 1984 raised fears that malaria, a hyperendemic parasitic disease on that continent, would be exacerbated or accelerated in people already infected with HIV. Indeed, early serological studies (with techniques of inadequate specificity) suggested an association between malaria and AIDS. Now, as succinctly summarized in the section in this chapter by Alan Greenberg, the major interaction has been shown to be indirect; children needing blood transfusions due to acute malaria risk becoming HIV infected if they receive unscreened blood.

The importance of these disease interactions is enormous—both for individual health and public health. For example, the strong association between HIV and tuberculosis is in the process of complicating the management of both tuberculosis (the most important single cause of infectious disease mortality in the world) and HIV/AIDS.

Similarly, the interactions between HIV and other sexually transmitted infections (discussed in several sections of *AIDS in the World*) is of major importance, particularly as the control of each is inextricably linked with that of the others.

This chapter discusses several of these critical interactions between major diseases and the HIV/AIDS pandemic. Unfortunately, with longer experience with HIV and more knowledge, and particularly as HIV spreads into new ecological environments (Southeast and North East Asia, Oceania), it is highly likely that new disease interactions will be discovered. None of these are likely to be beneficial; most, if not all, will result in a net increase in illness, suffering, and premature death.

HIV's focused attack on the human immune system calls to mind the Hydra, a mythical creature whose many heads increased its danger. The lesson from the Hydra myth is that while we must fight the many different heads, we must not lose sight of the need to attack and control the central element—the expanding HIV pandemic.

■■■■■ . . .

AIDS AND CANCER

Prepared by Robert J. Biggar, M.D., Viral Epidemiology Section, National Cancer Institute, Bethesda, Maryland; and Ramnik J. Xavier, M.D., Massachusetts General Hospital, Boston, Massachusetts

Cancer has been linked with AIDS since 1981, when the increased occurrence of a highly unusual malignancy, Kaposi's sarcoma, led physicians and other investigators to recognize that a new health problem had emerged. Since then, HIV infection has been associated with a second malignancy, non–Hodgkin's lymphoma. People infected with HIV are at much higher risk of developing either of these cancers than are people without HIV infection—from 100 times as likely with non–Hodgkin's lymphoma to up to 40,000 times as likely in the case of Kaposi's sarcoma. Other cancers have been found in HIV-infected people, but thus far no more than would be expected by chance alone.[1,2]

The following section provides detailed information about cancers and AIDS. From a global perspective in 1992, cancers associated with HIV infection add only slightly to the overall worldwide burden from cancer. Yet with more global experience, longer survival of people with AIDS, and more HIV-infected people, additional forms of cancer will probably be found to be associated with HIV infection.

Table 4.1: Evolving features of Kaposi's sarcoma (KS) in sub-Saharan Africa[a]

	Before the HIV/AIDS pandemic: Endemic KS		During the HIV/AIDS pandemic: Atypical KS
Age	Early childhood (2–3 years)	Adults 25 years and older	Adults
Sex ratio	1:1	Male predominance	Slight female predominance
Clinical signs/ evolution	Involves lymph nodes Rapidly fatal	Clusters of indolent cutaneous nodules involving extremities	General symmetrical lymphadenopathy Aerodigestive tract involvement Systemic involvement Skin lesion on face, trunk, and genitalia

Sources: A. G.-M. I. Lulat, "African Kaposi's sarcoma," *Transactions of the Royal Society of Tropical Medicine and Hygiene* 83 (1989):1–4. A. C. Baley, et al., "HTLV-III serology distinguishes atypical and endemic Kaposi's sarcoma in Africa," *Lancet* 1 (1985):359–61.

a. In sub-Saharan Africa, evolving features of Kaposi's sarcoma have been observed concurrently with the spread of the HIV/AIDS pandemic. These features involve age and gender of persons affected, clinical signs, and evolution.

This must be monitored particularly closely in parts of the world where HIV infection has more recently arrived, such as in North East and Southeast Asia, Latin America, and the South East Mediterranean Geographic Areas of Affinity.

Kaposi's Sarcoma

This disease was first recognized as a malignant tumor of the inner walls of the heart, veins, and arteries in 1873 in Vienna, Austria. Prior to the AIDS epidemic, Kaposi's sarcoma (KS) was a rare tumor (1973–78 incidence in the United States: 0.29 in men and 0.07 in women, per 100,000, age-adjusted[3]) that mainly affected older people and that was reported more commonly in people of Mediterranean and Jewish origin. The past thirty years have seen a higher incidence among Africans, particularly those from East and Central Africa. Clinically, these pre–AIDS KS patients usually had nodular disease of the extremities, and the cancer had an indolent clinical course, although a more

Percentage of AIDS Diagnoses

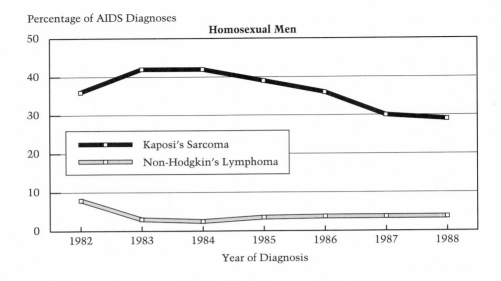

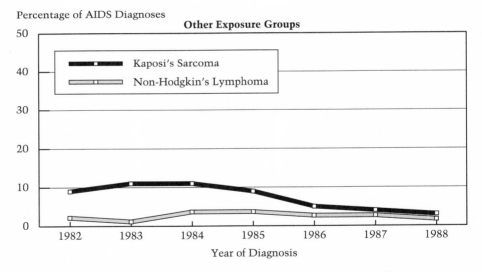

Figure 4.1. Proportion of KS and NHL by exposure group among primary diagnoses in European AIDS cases.

Source: Casabona, et al., "Kaposi's sarcoma and non-Hodgkin's lymphoma," *International Journal of Cancer* 47 (1991): 49-53.

Note: The declining proportion of KS as the first diagnosis of AIDS has also been observed in the United States. These declines are attributed to an increasing likelihood that non-KS AIDS diagnoses will present first in persons with severe immunosuppression (see Figure 4.2).

aggressive form involving lymph node dissemination was also observed, particularly in younger African patients (see Table 4.1). People whose immune systems had been artificially suppressed to control transplant rejection were recognized to have a high incidence of KS, and in some cases, the tumor spontaneously regressed when the immunosuppressive regimen was reduced.

Because KS had been so rare in young people, its sudden appearance among otherwise apparently healthy, young homosexual men was one of the first indicators of the AIDS epidemic in 1981. Its relationship to immunosuppression was quickly appreciated, and further testing soon confirmed that these people were markedly immunodeficient. Subsequent studies found that homosexual men infected with HIV were 20,000 to 40,000 times more likely to have KS than were men of the same age in the pre–AIDS era.[4] In the United States, based on reports available through 1987, 9,000 AIDS-related KS cases are projected to occur in 1992.[5]

How HIV infection and/or HIV-related immunodeficiency contributes to the onset of KS is unknown. The origin of the KS tumor cells is not well established, but it is known that HIV does not infect the malignant cells. One clue is that the incidence of KS varies in different HIV-exposure groups. Kaposi's sarcoma is at least six times more common in homosexual men compared with other HIV-exposure groups in North America and Europe,[6,7] even though all groups have the same degree of immunosuppression (see Figure 4.1). Yet in Africa, areas with a high incidence of KS unrelated to HIV also have a high proportion (10 to 20 percent) of AIDS patients whose condition was first indicated by KS, even though HIV in Africa is spread almost entirely by heterosexual routes.[8] These observations argue that environmental factors are involved.[9] Sexually transmitted viruses, chemicals, and genetics have been postulated to act both directly and through release of growth factor intermediaries; but at present, there is insufficient evidence for any specific hypothesis.

Furthermore, the proportion of cases in which AIDS is manifested first as KS is clearly declining in all areas in which trends have been examined. Analyses of these trends is complicated because any increase in the risk of other diseases will independently lower proportions for KS[10] (see Figure 4.2). In any case, the incidence of KS in HIV-infected people continues to rise the longer they have been in-

Percent

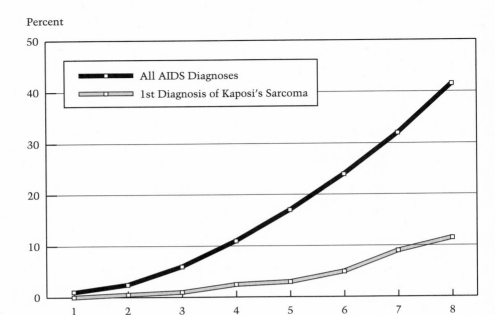

Figure 4.2. Cumulative risk (by year) of Kaposi's sarcoma and all AIDS diagnoses in 1,231 homosexual men.

Source: R.J. Biggar and International Registry of Seroconverters, "AIDS incubation," *AIDS* 4 (1990):1059-66.

Note: By the onset of the ninth year, the cumulative risk of all AIDS diagnoses approaches 50 percent. The cumulative risk of a first diagnosis of Kaposi's sarcoma increases steadily, although not so rapidly as the risk of other AIDS diagnoses.

fected. However, as the immune system weakens, the risk of opportunistic infections increases more rapidly than does the risk of KS. This may not be so in the future; with better control of opportunistic infections, the proportion of cases for whom KS (and lymphoma) represents the first manifestation of AIDS may increase.

Clinically, KS in HIV-infected, immunodeficient persons occurs most often as plaque lesions of the trunk and head. The mouth and many internal organs (especially of the gastrointestinal and respiratory tracts) may be involved either symptomatically or subclinically. In people infected with HIV, the mere presence of KS says little about how the cancer will progress in an individual because that depends more on the status of the immune system. People who die of AIDS usually succumb to opportunistic infections rather than to KS. Furthermore, patients with KS but with only modest degrees of immunosuppression usually have a more restricted distribution of KS and may survive for years even with minimal therapy.[11]

Non–Hodgkin's Lymphoma

Non–Hodgkin's lymphoma (NHL) is a relatively common malignancy worldwide (1973–74 incidence in the United States: 10.2 in men and 7.5 in women, per 100,000, age-adjusted [12]). Incidence rises markedly with age, and blacks have a lower incidence than do whites. Notably, NHL incidence has increased steadily (on average, 3 to 4 percent per year) in almost all areas of the world during the past several decades in which registry data have been collected. This increase has been seen in men and women for all age groups and in all races. The reasons for the pre–AIDS increases are unclear, but during the 1980s, a dramatic increase in NHL incidence among young men was also observed in association with the AIDS epidemic (see Figure 4.3).

Approximately 3 percent of AIDS diagnoses in all risk groups and in all areas originate through discovery of NHL.[13] Risk increases with age.[14] HIV generally infects T cells, but NHL tumors are almost always of B-cell origin; analyses of genetic material from these tumors confirms that HIV is not present in the genome. The little variation by risk group and region (see Figure 4.1) suggests that, in contrast to KS, immunodeficiency is the major causative factor and that strong environmental cofactors are unlikely.[15]

Among HIV-infected homosexual men in 1987, the relative risk of developing NHL was 100 times higher compared with noninfected men of the same age.[16] This relative risk is much lower than with KS because NHL's background incidence is much higher. Among American and European homosexual men with AIDS, the ratio between KS and NHL was approximately 3:1 in 1987. However, this ratio will decrease in the future, for several reasons. Kaposi's sarcoma is more common among homosexual men, but there are relatively fewer new HIV infections in this population. Among nonhomosexual HIV-infected people, the incidence of KS and NHL is similar (Figure 4.1). Furthermore, NHL incidence appears to increase as the immune sys-

Incidence per 100,000 (log scale)

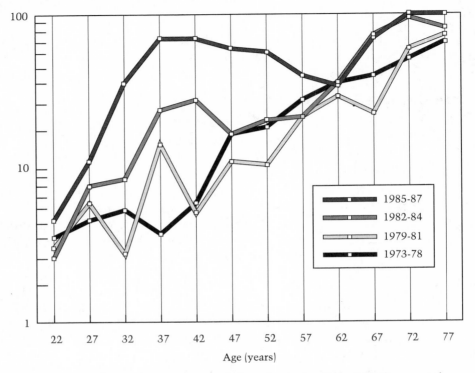

Age (years)

Figure 4.3. Incidence of NHL among adult males in San Francisco, by age and year groups, 1973-1987.

Source: C.S. Rabkin, et al., "Increasing incidence of cancers associated with the human immunodeficiency virus epidemic," *International Journal of Cancer* 47 (1991): 692-96.

Note: The steady rise with age is apparent in all years, but marked increase in NHL incidence among young men in association with the increasing AIDS epidemic between 1982 and 1987 is striking documentation of the changing pattern of NHL incidence occurring as a result of the AIDS epidemic.

tem weakens. As the epidemic matures in a given population, an increasing fraction of the HIV-infected population is becoming severely immunodeficient, and the risk of NHL should, therefore, increase. Prophylactic therapy for opportunistic infections will also contribute to the AIDS-free survival of patients with severe immunodeficiency, thereby putting them at greater risk of NHL.[17]

In the United States, 3,000 to 4,000 AIDS-related NHL cases are

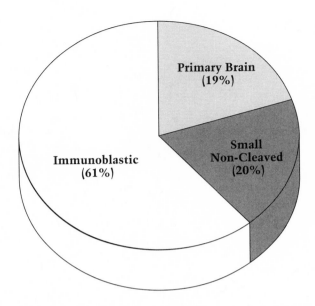

Figure 4.4. Distribution of AIDS-related lymphomas in the United States.

Source: U.S. Centers for Disease Control, Atlanta, GA.

Note: Data from 4,337 patients reported in the United States (through 6/1990) were obtained from the Centers for Disease Control. AIDS-associated tumors have been aggressive (high grade) B-cell tumors. The most common histological subtype is large cell immunoblastic lymphoma (61%), but small non-cleaved cell lymphoma, often called Burkitt's or Burkitt-like lymphoma, constitutes 20 percent. Primary brain lymphomas (19%) are usually immunoblastic but may also be of the small non-cleavedcell subtype.

expected to occur in 1992 constituting about 10 percent of all NHL seen in this year.[18,19] These lymphomas are generally B-cell malignancies of high-grade (aggressive) types. The two most common forms are large-cell immunoblastic lymphomas, which usually involve lymph nodes as well as other sites, and small non-cleaved-cell lymphomas (often called Burkitt's or Burkitt-like lymphomas), which are usually seen as abdominal masses and/or lymphadenopathy (see Figure 4.4). About 81 percent of AIDS-related lymphomas involve sites outside the lymph nodes (including bone marrow), which is twice the expected frequency; 19 percent are within the central nervous system, a very rare site of lymphomas in the pre–AIDS era.[20,21] In diagnosis, primary brain lymphomas can be easily confused with toxoplasmosis

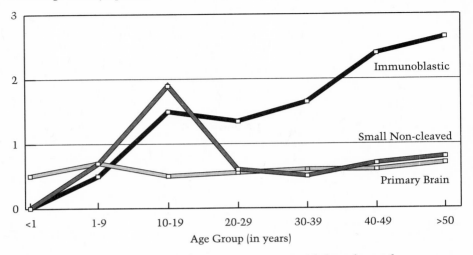

Percentage with Lymphoma

Figure 4.5. Percentage of United States AIDS cases with lymphoma, by age group.

Source: V. Beral, et al., "AIDS-associated non-Hodgkin's lymphoma," *Lancet* 337 (1991): 805-9.

Note: Except in the >1 age group, the proportion of AIDS diagnosed as NHL is 3-4 percent. However, NHL subtype patterns differ by age; immunoblastic tumors increase with age whereas brain lymphomas are fairly constant and small non-cleaved cell lymphomas have an age peak in adolescents.

of the central nervous system, a potentially treatable condition. The risk of NHL subtypes varies with age (Figure 4.5). Often, NHL diagnoses are only made at autopsy, and current rates probably underestimate the true risk of NHL. Although Burkitt's lymphoma is endemic in tropical Africa and New Guinea, no evidence suggests that lymphoma is a more common presenting diagnosis of AIDS among these populations than among other groups.

These malignancies are difficult to treat because patients often cannot tolerate the further immunosuppression that treatments cause. As with KS, prognosis depends largely on the initial level of immunity. Patients with adequate immune reserves may tolerate therapy and respond reasonably well. However, in people with severe immunodeficiency, survival is only 4 to 7 months on average. Patients diagnosed with HIV-related brain lymphomas have a very poor prognosis, often surviving only one to two months.[22]

Other Tumors

Among the more commonly reported tumors seen in AIDS patients are Hodgkin's disease and cervical cancer (see Box 4.1). However, studies of population-based registry data do not support an increased incidence of these malignancies in AIDS patients. Nevertheless, a small increase in the relative risk might have been overlooked among particular subgroups, such as injection drug users. Other tumors sometimes mentioned as occurring in excess are testicular cancers, anal and anal rectal cancer (which may be unrelated to HIV because the association with male homosexuality was observed in the pre–AIDS era), and leukemias of various types. However, there is little or no evidence that the incidence of these tumors increases in HIV-infected persons.[23,24]

People with HIV infection and these unrelated tumors will differ in the degree of their immunodeficiency. If they are mildly immunosuppressed, they may tolerate therapy well and have a good response to chemotherapy. However, severely immunosuppressed persons tolerate systemic cytotoxic chemotherapy poorly and often die of complicating opportunistic infections. Management of such patients can be very difficult and should involve nonsystemic therapy if possible. Prognosis will depend largely on the level of immune function when therapy begins.

HIV AND MALARIA

red by Alan E.
nberg, M.D., Division
/AIDS, National
r for Infectious
ses, Centers for
ses Control, Atlanta,
jia

The epidemic of HIV-1 in malaria-endemic areas of the world has generated serious concerns about possible interactions between HIV and malaria. The investigation of this relationship is necessarily complex, as numerous clinical, epidemiologic, and immunologic issues need to be explored. To date, most studies on HIV-1 and malaria have been conducted in sub-Saharan Africa, where the transmission of *Plasmodium falciparum* (the most virulent malaria species) is most intense, and where both HIV-1 and malaria are major causes of disease and death. This section reviews current knowledge of the interrelationship between these two major public health challenges in developing countries.

Is There an Association between HIV-1 and Malaria?

Early serologic surveys appeared to support the existence of an association between HIV-1 and malaria. One study found a strong correlation between HIV-1 seropositivity and high titers of antibodies to *P. falciparum* among outpatients in rural Zaire.[25] HIV-1 seropositivity was also found to be more prevalent in patients infected with *P. falciparum* and *P. vivax* than in healthy blood donors in Venezuela.[26] However, these findings may have resulted from the nonspecificity of earlier laboratory tests;[27, 28] in fact, one study subsequently demonstrated an absence of strong serologic cross-reactivity between antibodies to HIV-1 and *Plasmodium* species.[29]

A series of cross-sectional field investigations were then conducted to further assess whether there was an association between

---

Box 4.1: Cervical Cancer

Carola Marte, M.D., Beth Israel Medical Center, New York, New York

Unusual or unusually severe gynecologic conditions can be an indication of immune compromise in HIV-infected women. Many HIV-infected women suffer unnecessarily from conditions that could be treated or prevented because the gynecologic effects of HIV infection have not been well characterized and are often omitted from health care protocols. Conversely, women and their health care providers are often unaware that a gynecologic abnormality may be an important clue to unsuspected HIV infection.

Cervical carcinoma is of particular concern because, with Papanicolaou (PAP) screening, preinvasive (also called cervical dyplasia or cervical intraepithelial neoplasia-CIN) and most early stage (microinvasive) carcinomas can be successfully treated, whereas lesions that are untreated and spread may become life threatening. Formal studies investigating whether cervical cancer occurs with greater frequency or is more aggressive in HIV-infected women are only now starting, but reports suggest this may be an important problem.

Human papillomavirus (HPV) is thought to be the agent responsible for most cervical carcinoma, although the degree of association varies geographically. Other HPV-related conditions, cervical dysplasia and condylomata acuminata (genital warts), are known to occur more frequently in HIV-infected individuals. Unusually profuse condylomata and frequent recurrences despite therapy are well described in HIV-infected individuals. These are analogous to the unusual lesions of the other viruses potentiated by HIV infection, for example, the persistent or ulcerating lesions of severe genital herpes.

All studies of cervical dyplasia, the

HIV-1 and malaria. In these studies, single blood samples were obtained from various populations and screened for both HIV-1 antibodies and *P. falciparum* parasites. Multiple investigations conducted among adults, children, and pregnant women in Zaire,[30–34] Zambia,[35,36] Uganda,[37] and Rwanda[38] consistently demonstrated no association between HIV-1 and malaria.

Several studies have begun to explore the immunologic relationship between HIV-1 and malaria. No differences in the levels of antibodies to *P. falciparum* were found in HIV-1-infected and uninfected patients in Zaire[39] and in Zambia.[40] Additionally, HIV-1-infected patients were found to have generally lower levels of antibodies to specific blood-stage malarial antigens than did uninfected controls.[41]

Is Malaria More Severe in HIV-1-Infected People?

Because the cellular immune system is believed to be critical to protection against malaria,[42,43] it is plausible that malaria could be

---

precursor of cervical carcinoma, have documented unusually high rates of occurrence in HIV-infected women. However, these studies, like those of other HIV-related gynecologic conditions, are limited due to inadequate controls and small numbers of subjects. Most are reports from individual clinics. Therefore, results of a meta-analysis of CIN studies published from 1986 to mid-1990 are of special interest. In studies with adequte controls, risk of cervical dysplasia in HIV-infected women was 3 to 10 times higher than that for non HIV-infected women, a risk that averaged 4.9 times (95% confidence interval when the studies are combined 3.0 to 8.2).[a]

Similar risk behaviors for HPV and HIV transmission and high background rates of HPV in the same communities where HIV is prevalent are confounding factors that seriously complicate studies on the association between cervical disease and HIV. This is true also for research on interactions between other sexually transmitted diseases (STDs) and HIV. Women at risk for contracting HPV and other STDs are at higher risk for contracting HIV as well. Socioeconomic and behavioral, as well as medical, determinants will need to be considered in studying cervical carcinoma and other manifestations of HPV in HIV-infected individuals.

Because cervical dyplasia often seems to recur soon after treatment in HIV-infected women, it is anticipated that many of these preinvasive lesions will progress to invasive carcinoma if careful monitoring and follow-up care are not available. However, the exact relationship between stage of HIV infection and stage of cervical dysplasia or rate of progression to carcinoma remains to be clarified. Nor is it known whether standard therapies for CIN and cervical carcinoma are more severe in people infected with HIV-1. However, studies of malaria-infected patients in Zaire,[44] Zambia,[45] and Uganda[46] found no significant differences in mean parasite densities between HIV-1-infected and -uninfected patients. Similarly, no differences were found in the HIV-1 seropositivity rates of Rwandan women with increasing densities of *P. falciparum* parasitemia.[47] In one study, the mean parasite density was higher in children infected with HIV-1 than in uninfected children, but only six HIV-1-infected children were included in this analysis.[48]

Studies examining the clinical severity of malaria in patients with and without HIV-1 infection found no significant differences in the symptoms that malaria produces either in Ugandan children and adults[49] or in Zairian children with AIDS.[50] Similarly, no differences were found in the rates of malaria-related hospitalizations and deaths in HIV-1-infected and uninfected Zairian children with AIDS com-

---

adequate for treatment of severely immunocompromised HIV-infected women, and whether ongoing maintenance therapy after initial treatment is needed to suppress recurrence.

That so much vital information is missing for a lethal disease like cervical carcinoma illustrates the inadequacy of our understanding of HIV infection in women. It is sobering that even if all these issues are rapidly addressed by research, many women will die of an easily preventable cancer because they do not have access to the services that research has proven they need. The HIV epidemic threatens to repeat a long history of neglect for the health needs of women. This is just one dimension of women's *triple jeopardy* in the HIV epidemic.[b]

Across all cultural and geographic boundaries, women share two realities: primary responsibility as caretakers for their families and inferior socio-economic status. In both wealthy and impoverished nations, poverty places a person at risk for AIDS.[c] AIDS, like poverty, is becoming feminized; it increasingly affects women and women heads of household. The challenge for all of us—professionals, political leaders, and communities at risk—is to turn our attention to women in order to learn about the natural history of their disease, how it affects their daily lives and social roles, and how their suffering can be alleviated and shared or, better, prevented.

---

a. J. S. Mandelblatt et al., "Association between HIV infection and cervical neoplasia: Implications for clinical care of women at risk for both conditions," *AIDS* 6 (1992):173–78.

b. The PANOS Institute, *Triple Jeopardy: Women and AIDS* (London: The PANOS Institute, 1990).

c. E. M. Ankrah, "AIDS and the social side of health," *Social Science and Medicine* 32 (1991):967–80.

pared to uninfected children.[51] Finally, no increase in the incidence of admissions for cerebral malaria was observed in a large Ugandan hospital from 1985 to 1989, a period during which there was a dramatic increase in admissions for patients showing symptoms of HIV-1-related disease.[52]

The Impact of HIV-1 on the Response to Antimalarial Therapy

Among patients with *P. falciparum* infections, no difference in the efficacy of chloroquine and pyrimethamine-sulfadoxine,[53] or in the efficacy of quinine,[54,55] has been found between those infected with HIV-1 and those uninfected. Furthermore, no significant difference in the response to therapy of malaria was found among Zairian children with AIDS compared to HIV-1-infected children or uninfected controls.[56]

The Effect of HIV-1 on the Incidence of Malaria

Two separate investigations seemed to indicate that the incidence of malaria was higher in children infected with HIV-1 than in those who were uninfected, but this observation was confounded by the significantly higher incidence of fever in HIV-1-infected than in uninfected children.[57,58] The proportions of fevers that were caused by malaria were not significantly different in HIV-1-infected and uninfected children; thus, the elevated incidence of malaria in HIV-1-infected children was probably due to the fact that these children were more likely to have blood smears performed, which led to the detection of malarial infections that would otherwise have gone undiscovered. In summary, the incidence of malaria is probably unaffected by HIV-1 infection.

The Influence of Malaria on the Course of HIV-1 Infection

It has been postulated that repeated malarial infection could accelerate the progression of HIV-1 related disease,[59-61] because malarial antigens can activate T lymphocytes and induce their proliferation, and because malaria can cause a transient decrease in CD4 lymphocytes.[62,63] The only study that has addressed this issue showed that the incidence of malaria in HIV-1-infected children who later developed AIDS was not significantly different from those who did not.[64]

However, the number of patients in this analysis was small, and these findings need to be confirmed.

From Malaria to Anemia to Blood Transfusion to HIV Infection

An indirect association between HIV-1 and malaria that has profound implications for public health involves the use of blood transfusions in the treatment of the severe anemia frequently caused by *P. falciparum* malaria.[65] In areas of high prevalence of HIV-1 infection where HIV-1 antibody screening of blood is either limited or unavailable, patients with severe malaria-related anemia are at high risk of becoming infected with HIV-1 through blood transfusions at health care facilities. Therefore, it is imperative that HIV-1 antibody screening of blood products be widely available in malaria-endemic areas.

Conclusion

The scientific evidence that has been collected to date has consistently failed to demonstrate a direct, biologic association between HIV-1 and *P. falciparum* malaria. Further studies are needed in other geographic areas, notably in West Africa where the relationship between HIV-2 and *P. falciparum* can be assessed, and in South America and Asia where the relationship between HIV-1 and *P. vivax* (the most prevalent, though less virulent, malaria species) can be explored. Lastly, in vitro studies of the cellular response to malarial antigens may provide important insights into why people infected with HIV-1 seem to preserve their protection against malaria.

. . .

AIDS AND TUBERCULOSIS: A DANGEROUS SYNERGY

Prepared with the participation of Dr. Ramnik J. Xavier, Massachusetts General Hospital, Boston, Massachusetts

The dynamics and magnitude of the HIV/AIDS pandemic cannot be understood without considering the critical interaction between HIV and tuberculosis (TB). This relationship is synergistic, so the combined effect of both—for individuals and for public health—is worse than their separate effects added together. HIV multiplies the problems of tuberculosis for individuals and entire communities; tuberculosis complicates the management and course of HIV infection.

The HIV-TB link is already having a dramatic impact, particularly in the developing world where 95 percent of people with dual tuberculosis and HIV infection live. In countries and cities around the world with higher levels of HIV infection, "the HIV/AIDS pandemic is having a devastating effect on tuberculosis control programs."[66]

Just a few years ago, tuberculosis was considered a stable, endemic health problem. Now, in association with the HIV/AIDS pandemic, tuberculosis is resurgent. The recent emergence of multi-drug resistant TB—which has reached epidemic proportions in New York City—has created a serious and growing threat to the capacity of tuberculosis control programs around the world. Thus, the interaction of TB and HIV provides a view of a future of rapidly worsening epidemics, each intensifying the other.

AIDS has become one of the most highly visible diseases in the world. Yet worldwide, tuberculosis is the single most important microbial pathogen and is responsible for one-quarter of avoidable deaths.[67] In 1990, approximately 8 million new cases of clinical tuberculosis occurred worldwide, and an estimated global total of 1.7 billion people—one-third of the world's population—are infected with *Mycobacterium tuberculosis.*

Of HIV infections, the large majority also occur in regions with high prevalence of *M. tuberculosis* infection. Therefore, any interaction between HIV and TB would be potentially important; in fact, the HIV-TB link is the most important interaction between HIV and another disease yet demonstrated.

To understand the mechanisms of interaction between the old pandemic of tuberculosis and the new pandemic of HIV/AIDS, this section reviews current tuberculosis trends worldwide, explores the clinical links between HIV and TB, evaluates the observed and projected impact of the HIV/AIDS-TB interaction, and examines the responses available.

Epidemiology of HIV and Tuberculosis

A global review for the World Health Organization (WHO) estimated that, in 1990, over 75 percent of the 1.7 billion people infected with the TB bacterium lived in developing countries (see Table 4.2).[68] Worldwide, one in every three people is infected, with a prevalence ranging from 44 percent in the Western Pacific to 19 percent in the Eastern Mediterranean. This rate varies enormously by age, depending on an individual's cumulative risk of exposure to infection. In devel-

Table 4.2: Worldwide prevalence of tuberculosis infection, 1990

Region	Prevalence (%)	No. infected (millions)	% of total
Africa[a]	33.8	171	9.9
America[b]	25.9	117	6.8
Eastern Mediterranean	19.4	52	3.0
Southeast Asia[a]	34.3	426	24.7
Western Pacific[c]	43.8	195	11.3
China	33.7	379	22.0
Europe and others[d]	31.6	382	22.2
All regions	32.8	1,722	100.0

Source: P. Sudre, et al., "Tuberculosis in the present time: A global overview of the world situation,"*Bulletin of the World Health Organization* 3(1992).
a. Includes all countries of WHO region.
b. Includes all countries of WHO American Region except the United States and Canada.
c. Includes all countries of WHO Western Pacific Region except China, Japan, Australia, and New Zealand.
d. United States, Canada, Japan, Australia, and New Zealand.

oping, tropical sub-Saharan countries, the largest number of TB infections occurs among young adults who also have the highest prevalence of HIV infection. In Western Europe (see Figure 4.6), older people had been the major group with TB infection, but this may be changing in the context of the HIV/AIDS pandemic. Nevertheless, the prevalence of tuberculosis infection only provides a view of the situation at one point in time. It does not tell us about the dynamics of spread or about the severity of infection. Projecting the number and distribution of tuberculosis infections estimated by the World Health Organization, and combining them with *AIDS in the World* estimates of HIV infection, by early 1992 there were more than 4.6 million people with both infections, 81 percent of them in Africa (see Table 4.3 and Figure 4.7).[69]

Reported cases of tuberculosis in the United States decreased each year from 1953 until they leveled off in 1985 and then increased by three percent in 1986.[70] By 1990, there were 28,000 newly reported

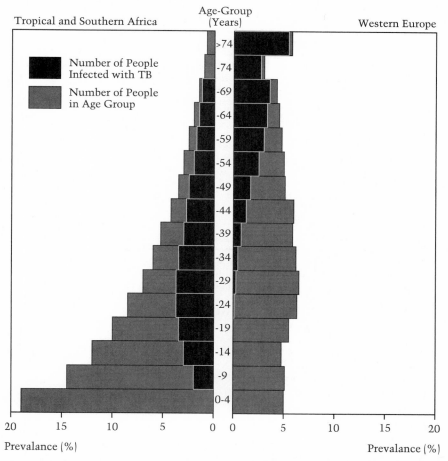

Figure 4.6. Prevalence of tuberculosis infection by age in Tropical and Southern Africa, and in Western Europe.

Source: P. Sudre, G. ten Dam, and A. Kochi, "Tuberculosis: A global overview of the situation today," *Bulletin of the World Health Organization* 70 (2) (1991).

Note: In Tropical and Southern Africa, TB infection occurs more among adolescents and young adults, which coincides with the period of highest vulnerabilities in their lives.

Table 4.3: Current distribution of individuals 15–49 years old infected with tuberculosis and HIV estimated for late 1991

Region	No. of HIV infected (thousands)	% of TB infected	HIV/TB infected No. (thousands)	% of total
Africa[a]	7,800	48	3,744	80.6
Americas[b]	1,305	30	392	8.4
Eastern Mediterranean[a]	35	23	8	0.2
Southeast Asia[a] and Western Pacific[c]	716	40	286	6.2
Europe[a] and others[d]	1,940	11	213	4.6
All regions	11,796	34	4,643	100.0

Source: Adapted from M. C. Raviglione et al., "HIV-associated tuberculosis in developing countries: Clinical features, diagnosis and treatment," *Bulletin of the World Health Organization,* 1992. The number of individuals infected with HIV is an *AIDS in the World* estimate.

a. Includes all countries of WHO region.

b. Includes all countries of WHO American Region except the United States and Canada.

c. Includes all countries of WHO Western Pacific Region except Japan, Australia, and New Zealand.

d. United States, Canada, Japan, Australia, New Zealand.

TB cases in the United States, a 9.4 percent increase over 1989[71,72] (see Figure 4.8). More alarmingly, sub-Saharan African countries have witnessed a doubling in the average number of reported TB cases over the past four to five years, with increases of 140 percent in Burundi, 154 percent in Zambia, and 180 percent in Malawi.[73] Despite underreporting, trends in case notification from sub-Saharan countries are sufficiently consistent (see Figure 4.9) to indicate that an epidemic of tuberculosis is growing alongside the HIV/AIDS pandemic.

The prevalence of HIV in tuberculosis patients also provides some indication of the interaction between the two infections. In tuberculosis clinics in 14 metropolitan areas of the United States, the average HIV seroprevalence rate was 3 to 4 percent, but it has been reported as high as 34 percent in Newark, New Jersey, and 46 percent in New

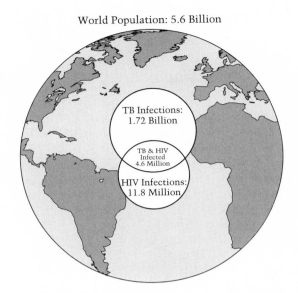

Figure 4.7. Tuberculosis and HIV infection in the world, 1991.

Source: Adapted from P. Eriki, et al., "The influence of human immunodeficiency virus infection on tuberculosis in Kampala, Uganda." *American Review of Respiratory Diseases* 143 (1991):185-87.

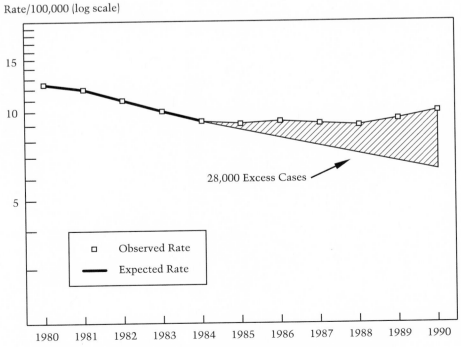

Figure 4.8. Expected and observed TB cases, United States, 1980-1990.
Source: *Morbidity and Mortality Weekly Report* 40 (ss-3) (1991):23-27.

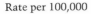

Rate per 100,000

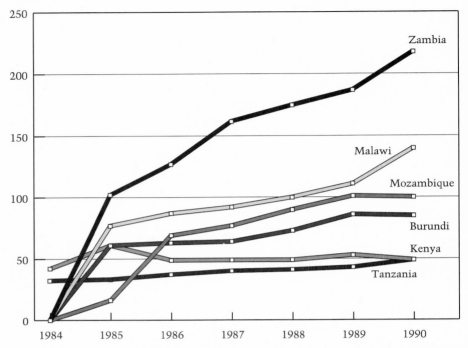

Figure 4.9. Annual TB notification rates in selected African countries, 1985-1990.
Source: Adapted from J.P. Narain, M.C. Raviglione, and A. Kochi, "HIV-associated tuberculosis in developing countries: Epidemiology and strategies for prevention." WHO/TB/92.164, Geneva, 1992.

York City.[74,75] In urban areas of the United States, the present upsurge in tuberculosis cases is occurring among young (aged 25–44) injection drug users, ethnic minorities, homeless people, and immigrants from countries with a high prevalence of TB. In the United States, tuberculosis increased by 26.5 percent from 1986 to 1989 among young black and Hispanic adults; among non–Hispanic whites, the increase was less than 0.5 percent. A twenty-nine-state survey in the United States revealed that prison inmates in many states have tuberculosis infection rates nearly four times higher than those among adults in the community aged from 15 to 64 years.[76]

In the developing world, HIV seroprevalence in patients with pulmonary tuberculosis varies from 17 to 66 percent; prevalence is even higher in those with extra-pulmonary tuberculosis (44 to 77 percent).[77-83]

Interactions between HIV and *Mycobacterium Tuberculosis*

The range of interactions can include: (1) a greater risk of developing tuberculosis in HIV-infected people; (2) increased severity of clinical tuberculosis or a diminished response to treatment of tuberculosis in HIV-infected people; (3) increased infectiousness of tuberculosis in an HIV-infected person; (4) the facilitated emergence of multi-drug resistant *M. tuberculosis* in people with HIV/AIDS; (5) a diminished safety and efficacy of BCG vaccine; and (6) an adverse impact of tuberculosis on the natural history of HIV/AIDS.

Risk of Developing Tuberculosis in HIV-Infected People

HIV-infected people have a six to thirty times greater risk of developing clinical tuberculosis compared with people not infected with HIV.[84] Tuberculosis can be either subclinical (infection) or clinical (disease). Clinical tuberculosis develops through three different pathways: progressive primary infection, reactivation of latent infection, and exogenous reinfection—sometimes with multiple drug-resistant organisms—in a host with a defective immune response.

This first major interaction between HIV and tuberculosis occurs as a result of the weakening of the immune system in association with progressive HIV infection. The vast majority of people exposed to tuberculosis are infected but not clinically ill. Their subclinical tuberculosis infection is kept in check by an active, healthy immune system. However, when a tuberculosis-infected person becomes infected with HIV, the immune system begins to decline. At a certain level of immune damage from HIV, the tuberculosis bacteria, initially dormant, can become active again and cause clinical tuberculosis.

Mycobacterium tuberculosis is a more virulent pathogen than either *Pneumocystis carinii* or *Toxoplasma gondii* and will therefore cause disease at an earlier stage of HIV infection. Pneumocystosis and toxoplasmosis are not usually seen in HIV-infected people until the CD4 count falls below 200 per microliter (μl). In contrast, HIV-infected people with tuberculosis in Barcelona and San Francisco had relatively high CD4 counts of 441/μl and 336/μl, respectively.

As mentioned above, an HIV-infected adult has a greatly increased likelihood of developing clinical tuberculosis.[85] The annual incidence of clinical tuberculosis in HIV-infected people is estimated at eight percent, with a cumulative lifetime risk of 30 percent or higher. Thus, in a study of 109 tuberculosis-infected injection drug users in New York, 7 of 49 (14%) of the HIV-infected users developed tuberculosis within a 21-month period, compared with none of the 62 HIV-negative drug users.[86] Studies from Africa show similar findings among tuberculin reactors (indicating past tuberculosis infection) who acquired HIV infection through heterosexual transmission.[87,88]

Clinical Tuberculosis and Its Treatment in HIV-Infected People

Clinical tuberculosis is often the first opportunistic infection occurring among HIV-infected people whose immune systems are less able to deal with infection. Tuberculosis may in these cases rapidly affect the lungs (pulmonary form) and other organs (extrapulmonary forms). HIV reduces the immune response to *M. tuberculosis*; thus, the clinical illness suffered in people jointly infected with HIV and TB is more devastating, and clinical management of tuberculosis is more complex.

Tuberculosis often precedes the diagnosis of clinical AIDS, but it may occur at any stage of HIV infection. Most people with AIDS and tuberculosis develop the pulmonary form of tuberculosis. In Africa, pulmonary tuberculosis occurs in 42 to 80 pecent of AIDS-TB cases;[89–91] in the United States, pulmonary involvement is seen in 74 to 93 percent of patients with dual infection.[92–94] However, tuberculosis patients with severe immunosuppression are predisposed to diffuse air space/miliary disease, enlarged hilar lymph nodes, and pleural effusions. The clinical picture traditionally seen in reactivation tuberculosis—of cavitary and upper lobe disease—is still seen, but usually in HIV-TB patients with less severely compromised immune status.

Throughout the world, extrapulmonary tuberculosis has increased fourfold over the last 5 years.[95,96] In the United States, as the AIDS epidemic progressed, extrapulmonary tuberculosis also increased by 20 percent from 1984 to 1989, compared with a rise of three percent in uncomplicated pulmonary tuberculosis.[97]

Extrapulmonary tuberculosis presents physicians, used to diagnosing tuberculosis in its pulmonary form, with a wide and potentially confusing range of symptoms. Tuberculous mycobacteremia can present as HIV-associated fever of unknown origin, lymphadenitis, tuberculous meningitis in adults, anomalous blood counts, and genitourinary tuberculosis. A recent study demonstrated that the presence of HIV infection makes TB five times more likely to affect the central nervous system.[98]

Fifty to 60 percent of people with untreated tuberculosis will die within 5 years;[99] 98 percent of these deaths will occur in the developing world. Even with good treatment, initial studies suggest increased mortality among patients with combined tuberculosis and HIV infection,[100] mainly because of HIV-associated opportunistic infections, extrapulmonary tuberculosis,[101] and progressive immunodepression. In Tanzania, for example, the TB mortality rate was 4 percent before the AIDS pandemic; now, among HIV-infected people in urban Tanzania, the TB mortality rate is 11 percent. Overall, the prevalence of HIV is 2 to 10 times higher in tuberculosis patients than in the general adult population (see Table 4.4).

Infectiousness of Tuberculosis in HIV-Infected People: Tuberculosis is the only opportunistic infection associated with HIV/AIDS that is directly transmissible to household and other contacts. Clinical tuberculosis, at least in its major forms, is transmissible to other people; therefore, each case of active tuberculosis is a threat to household and community health. For example, of thirty HIV-infected people exposed to an index case of clinical tuberculosis in a communal home in San Francisco, half developed tuberculous infection (11 with clinical disease and 4 with positive PPD reactions). However, there is no evidence that HIV-infected people with tuberculosis are more efficient transmitters of *M. tuberculosis* compared with non–HIV-infected tuberculosis cases.

Emergence of Drug-Resistant M. tuberculosis in HIV-Infected People: In several studies, HIV-infected people with pulmonary tuberculosis have responded normally to antituberculous therapy but have then experienced a higher rate of clinical relapse than non–HIV-infected cases of tuberculosis. Several reasons for emergence of multi-drug resistant *M. tuberculosis* have been proposed, including the complexities of maintaining people with tuberculosis on long regimens of tuberculosis

Table 4.4: Comparison of HIV seroprevalence among patients with tuberculosis and estimated HIV seroprevalence in adults 15–49 years old

Country	Year of study[a]	No. of studies	HIV prevalence in TB patients (%)	Estimated HIV prevalence in adults (%)
Zaire	1985–87	3	17.0–38.0	<5
Burundi	1986	1	54.0	<5
Burkina Faso[c]	1988–89	1	22.7	<10
Malawi	1988–89	2	26.0–52.0	<10
Uganda	1988–89	1	66.0	<20
Zimbabwe	1988–89	1	40.6	<20
Côte d'Ivoire[c]	1989–90	2	34.3–40.2	<10
Haiti	1989–90	2	24.0–41.9	<10
Kenya	1989–90	1	30.4	<10
United States	1989–90	2	4.0–46.0	<1

Source: Adapted from M. C. Raviglione et al., "HIV-associated tuberculosis" (1992).
a. In some studies, confirmed and suspected pulmonary tuberculosis cases were combined.
b. *AIDS in the World* estimates based on HIV seroprevalence survey data.
c. Includes HIV-2 infections.

treatment. It is important to emphasize that the appearance and spread of multi-drug resistant *M. tuberculosis* is not considered a direct effect of the HIV/AIDS-TB connection.

Observed and Projected Impacts of HIV/TB: The local, national, and global impact of HIV on tuberculosis depends on several factors: the prevalence of tuberculosis infection, the risk of new transmission, the rate at which latent infections are reactivated, and—not least—how quickly TB can be detected, treated, and cured.

Of the 2.5 to 3 million deaths caused by tuberculosis in the world during 1990, an estimated 120,000 to 150,000 were related to HIV infection.[102] Thus, the impact on mortality of two of the world's most serious public health problems will increase as the path of each pandemic takes its course, intersecting and expanding in force through the decade.

Diagnosis of Tuberculosis

The standard tuberculin test, Purified Protein Derivative (PPD), is generally used to identify people infected with *M. tuberculosis* who do not have clinically active disease. However, in people with HIV infection or AIDS, the PPD is not reliable; cross-reactions with other mycobacteria can muddle the results, and more important, the weakened immune system may simply be unable to respond to the test.[103]

As a result, with an HIV-infected person, clinicians have to interpret the PPD test differently. Whereas normally, a positive reaction to the PPD test is a 10-millimeter wide *induration*, or hardened area of skin, an induration of five millimeters or greater is considered positive for HIV-infected people.[104]

In people with HIV/AIDS, clinical TB has two basic patterns. Early, when immunosuppression caused by HIV is mild to moderate, the disease can resemble *reactivation* tuberculosis. However, because the classic clinical and radiological hallmarks of reactivation tuberculosis are less common in people with weakened immune systems, clinicians must constantly watch for TB in people with HIV/AIDS. It was once thought that the commonly used Ziehl-Nielsen smear test (sputum examination for TB bacilli) would be ineffective on the grounds that people with HIV/AIDS and TB had a lower incidence of cavitary pulmonary tuberculosis. However, it appears that people with AIDS and TB produce so many TB bacilli that the smear test is as sensitive as in people with pulmonary tuberculosis who are not infected with HIV.[105–109] Finally, in people who have developed AIDS, tuberculosis characteristically appears as "galloping consumption" of the lung and often shows up outside the lung (extrapulmonary infection).

Treatment

The WHO global objectives for tuberculosis control for the year 2000 are to detect at least 70 percent of tuberculosis cases and of these, to cure at least 85 percent.[110] The specific treatment of tuberculosis consists of different combinations of drugs. Treatment of drug-sensitive tuberculosis works equally well for people with or without HIV (although, for reasons that are not clear, TB relapse rates are higher in people with HIV).

Duration is a central issue in treatment: tuberculosis is the most common bacterial infection requiring a long period of treatment. Short-course treatment, over six to nine months, has excellent cure rates in people with and without HIV, deals better with drug-resistant organisms, and has low relapse rates.[111,112] A study in Brazil of HIV-infected people treated with short-course chemotherapy showed a 92 percent sputum conversion rate after the intensive phase of treatment.

Although studies are still underway to determine the ideal duration of TB treatment in HIV-infected people, short-course chemotherapy is clearly the first option. This normally entails combinations of 4 drugs: isoniazid, rifampin, pyrazinamide, and ethambutol. Although short-course TB treatment takes months to complete, it is feasible even under difficult conditions. For example, Tanzania, Malawi, and Mozambique have reported 85 percent treatment completion rates. In

---

Box 4.2: The Tuberculosis Epidemic in New York City

Laurie Garrett, Science and medical writer, *Newsday*

Multidrug-resistant tuberculosis has reached epidemic proportions in New York City, catching many physicians and officials by surprise. Health officials are working in crisis mode, and using the language of disaster to describe TB outbreaks in jails, court holding pens, homeless shelters, and hospitals. People infected with HIV are the most vulnerable to tuberculosis. They are at risk any time they share breathing space, even for just a few hours, with those already infected with the TB bacillus.

No multidrug-resistant strains of tuberculosis had surfaced in New York City before September, 1989, according to an unpublished Centers for Disease Control study of two unidentified teaching hospitals. Then, cases began to appear in patients (a total of 40) and staff (four), most of whom got the disease after January, 1990. Analysis of drug resistance

patterns showed that multidrug-resistant tuberculosis was largely contracted in the two hospitals, mainly from men also infected with HIV. Twenty-six of the patient cases and one health care worker died of their tuberculosis. Outbreaks have since occurred in at least seven hospitals in the city.

The problem is not limited to the hospitals. Since January, 1990, of the over 3,500 New Yorkers listed on the city's tuberculosis registry, some 600 pass through the prison system each year. In 1990, there was an outbreak of multidrug-resistant tuberculosis in the state prison system, prompting a court order to create isolation facilities for prisoners with tuberculosis. Creating these and other isolation facilities in public and private hospitals will cost the financially strapped city hundreds of millions of dollars.

Authorities blame decades of neglect and reduced government expenditures for the epidemic. Budgets for tuberculosis control and

stark contrast, a recent study of 179 patients at Harlem Hospital in New York found that 89 percent failed to complete their course—not only endangering themselves by prolonging the infection, but also contributing to the emergence of drug-resistant strains of *M. tuberculosis.*[113]

In people with AIDS, however, a different approach may be necessary. They commonly require a number of drugs for other conditions, and drug interactions are a potential hazard. Rifampin, for example, is a potent inducer of drug metabolism in the liver and can interact with and reduce the effectiveness of drugs that people with AIDS may require for other reasons, such as ketoconazole and methadone.

In developing countries, cost is the determining factor in treat-

---

basic research have declined steadily since the early 1970s. Although tuberculosis is treatable, it never fully disappeared. Lacking the resources to follow up on recalcitrant outpatients, the city simply lost track of many of them, and they, in turn, lost contact with the TB treatment system. New York City has the lowest rate of patient compliance with tuberculosis medication in the world.

Patients who did not complete treatment not only remained infectious but also contributed to the development of drug-resistant tuberculosis. As of early 1992, about 34 percent of all tuberculosis cases in the city involved strains resistant to one drug (isoniazid or rifampin). At least an additional 20 percent of the cases are resistant to two or more drugs, and patients have been identified who carry strains resistant to over seven drugs.

The conditions which have made this a crisis are not unique to New York City, and there are lessons to be learned from its experience.

- Even at high cost, it is imperative that every active tuberculosis case be followed through to the end of treatment.
- Antibiotics are often overused and overprescribed. Where this is true, their use should be monitored and curtailed if possible.
- Programs and interventions in areas which have good patient compliance rates should be assessed to see what can be learned from them.

In the early stages of the AIDS epidemic, those who were most deeply concerned about the implications of the new disease were sometimes accused of being alarmist. Many public health officials now say that the rise in multiple drug-resistant tuberculosis in New York is just the tip of a national and even global iceberg, to be ignored at great peril.

ment. In addition, severe reaction to thiacetazone—a favored anti-TB drug in the developing world—in HIV-infected people has sharply curtailed its use.[114] An emerging problem is the unavailability of therapeutic drugs—not, ironically, because they are expensive, but because their profit margins are low and there is little incentive to produce them.[115] Even in the United States, shortages of streptomycin have been reported, and the supply of isoniazid, the first-line drug, has been erratic. In economic terms, this is wasteful: a six-month course of anti-TB therapy costs about $300 in the United States; if it develops into a case of multiple drug-resistant TB, the costs, including hospitalization, may reach $180,000!

Finally, there is a growing prevalence of TB infections that resist drug treatment. Resistance to isoniazid varies from 19 percent among homeless TB patients in New York City to 32 percent in urban dwellers in Kinshasa, Zaire.[116] Multiple drug-resistant TB has already appeared in 13 states in the United States.[117] (See Box 4.2.)

Prevention

Most clinical tuberculosis in people with HIV/AIDS involves a reactivation of tuberculosis bacilli already in the body but normally held in check by the immune system. Infection with HIV is a strong risk factor for the reactivation of latent TB infection. Preventive drug therapy—given to prevent reactivation of latent TB infection—substantially reduces the risk of subsequent reactivation, and it further interrupts the cycle of TB transmission. Isoniazid is effective as a preventive drug when given for twelve months, and initial studies using rifampin and pyrazinamide for a shorter duration have suggested comparable effectiveness.[118,119]

Finally, vaccination has a role in prevention. BCG vaccine (the TB vaccine prepared from the Calmette-Guerin Bacillus) is at least 60 percent effective in preventing tuberculosis in certain populations, and it also prevents disseminated disease in children if they become infected with TB. BCG vaccine is administered shortly after birth as part of the WHO Expanded Program on Immunization. There is no evidence that healthy-appearing infants or children have an increased rate of adverse reactions or serious side effects following BCG vaccination; accordingly, WHO recommends that where BCG vaccine is part of the routine immunization program, it be continued without reference to children's possible HIV status. However, WHO recommends that children with clinical AIDS not receive BCG vaccine. There is no evidence at present regarding the efficacy of BCG vaccination in HIV-infected children (especially as BCG efficacy, in general, is a subject of active debate).

Worldwide, tuberculosis control programs have long been neglected, with declining priority and resources. In turn, this neglect has increased the vulnerability of the population to tuberculosis, and the emergence and spread of HIV has further exacerbated the situation. Populations most at risk of TB—and of HIV/AIDS—have generally been those already disadvantaged and with reduced access to quality medical care. In order to bring this resurgent public health crisis under control, tuberculosis programs must be restructured, and a major political and resource commitment is urgently needed.

Surveillance, prevention, disease containment, and ongoing program assessment and evaluation are critical components in controlling the spread of tuberculosis. Furthermore, newer technologies and programmatic approaches are needed to detect tuberculosis early, prevent active disease, and ensure completion of therapy. The commitment and knowledge of health professionals, the participation of communities in prevention and control activities, and close cooperation between tuberculosis and HIV control programs, will all be essential.

CHAPTER FIVE

HIV and Other Sexually Transmitted Diseases

section was
pared by Nancy
zin, senior editor of
pital Practice, New
, New York.

The relationship between HIV and other sexually transmitted diseases (STDs) appears to be both highly dynamic and synergistic.[1] Persons who have histories of STD are at increased risk of acquiring HIV, while HIV-infected persons are likely to have greater susceptibility to infection with other STDs and, if co-infected, may experience them in an unusually severe and protracted course. Although the rough outlines of this relationship are increasingly apparent, important details are missing. Reliable data describing the transmission dynamics of STDs are scarce, as are basic incidence and prevalence data that would permit accurate estimation of the public health and economic impacts of STDs in developing countries.

This chapter will focus on the epidemiology of STDs, the interaction of STDs and HIV, and issues for STD prevention and control.*

---

*A note about terminology: Although the traditional nomenclature has been retained in this chapter, the term *sexually transmitted infections* (STIs) is gradually replacing *sexually transmitted diseases* (STDs) as the preferred characterization for this collection of sexually transmitted infections and illnesses. The intent is to unify conceptually a field in which AIDS is often viewed as apart from the rest. In fact, like HIV/AIDS, the majority of STIs do not result from contact with partners who are obviously diseased, but rather from exposure to subclinical or barely noticed infections.

GLOBAL EPIDEMIOLOGY: 1992

Global prevalence and incidence of STDs are rising. In industrialized nations, more recently discovered second-generation STDs such as chlamydia and the viral STDs (genital herpes, human papillomavirus, hepatitis B, and HIV) have become a greater health threat than syphilis, gonorrhea, or chancroid. Both first- and second-generation STDs remain endemic and epidemic throughout the developing world. Evolution of antimicrobial-resistant pathogen strains, such as penicillinase-producing or tetracycline-resistant *N. gonorrhoeae*, has hampered control efforts in many areas.

Cross-sectional studies provide an indication of the relatively high prevalence of STDs in various population groups, as shown in Table 5.1.

In Great Britain and Canada, incidence of primary and secondary syphilis has declined steadily since 1978. By contrast, the United States has experienced a resurgence of syphilis since 1985, mainly among inner-city black and Hispanic populations. This increase has been attributed to (1) use of crack cocaine and bartering of sex for drugs; (2) possibly the widespread use of spectinomycin rather than penicillin for treatment of gonorrhea (unlike penicillin, spectinomycin is not effective against syphilis); and (3) the shifting of resources from syphilis control to AIDS. Data from developing countries are incomplete but indicate continued high prevalence of primary and secondary syphilis in many areas, as well as considerable risk/incidence of congenital syphilis.

Gonorrhea incidence has been declining in the United Kingdom since the early 1970s. In the United States, gonorrhea reached a peak in 1975 (473 cases per 100,000 population) and subsequently declined, with the greatest reductions observed after 1987, presumably in response to safer sex practices (see Figure 5.1). Although by 1990 the incidence of gonorrhea in the United States had decreased to 277 per 100,000, an increasing proportion of strains were becoming resistant to penicillin. In Sweden, gonorrhea incidence has declined almost continuously since the early 1970s (see Figure 5.2). As with syphilis, incidence figures for gonorrhea from developing countries are unreliable. However, estimates for large cities in Africa suggest an annual

Table 5.1: Prevalence of selected sexually transmitted diseases (STDs) in developing countries, 1973–1992

Region/country	Year	Study group	Ref.	% found positive		
				N. Gonorrhoeae	C. Trachomatis	Syphilis
Sub-Saharan Africa						
Cameroon	1980	Antenatal	1	15	—	—
		Family planning clinic	1	2–21	—	—
	1984	Delivery	2	14	—	—
	1991	Antenatal	3	—	—	14.6
Ethiopia	1991	CSWs	4	30.1	—	37.4
Gambia	1982	STD clinic female	5	—	15	—
	1985	Antenatal	6	22–27	35	11
Kenya	1973	Family planning clinic	7	19	—	—
	1985	CSWs	8	16–46	—	—
	1986	Delivery	9	7	29	—
	1989	Delivery	10	4–11	15	5
	1990	CSWs	11	50	25	32
	1991	Antenatal	12	—	—	6.5
Nigeria	1972	Antenatal	13	3	—	—
		Female STD	13	33	—	—
		Male STD	13	17	—	—
	1989	Antenatal	14	—	—	0.35
	1989	Family planning clinic	15	3	—	18
Senegal	1991	Antenatal	16	1.1	11.3	5.4
		OB/GYN clinic	16	1.6	13.3	15.9
		Male STD clinic	16	47	17	12
	1991	CSWs	17	15.3	19.9	26.8
South Africa	1981	STD female	18	13	—	—
	1989	Antenatal	19	6	11	12
Uganda	1965	STD clinic	20	66	—	4
	1973	Community survey	21			—
		Teso male		9.6	—	—
		Teso female		21.6	—	—
		Aukole male		4.2	—	—
		Aukole female		4.0	—	—

Table 5.1 (cont.): Prevalence of selected sexually transmitted diseases (STDs) in developing countries, 1973–1992

Region/country	Year	Study group	Ref.	% found positive		
				N. Gonorrhoeae	C. Trachomatis	Syphilis
Zaire	1988	CSWs	22	29	14	14
	1991	CSWs	22	24	24	6
	1991	Antenatal	23	1.4	4.7–7.7	1.3–6.2
Zambia	1980	Female STD clinic	24	19	—	—
	1982	Antenatal	25	—	—	12.5
		Delivery	25	—	—	6.5
Zimbabwe	1977	Antenatal	26	2	—	—
		Family planning clinic	26	12	—	—
Southeast Asia						
Bangladesh	1989	Rural female	27	0.4	2	—
India	1988	Rural female	28	0.3	—	—
Singapore	1977	CSWs	29	7		
Thailand	1988	Male STD clinic (military)	30	41	13	—
		Male STD clinic	30	24	14	—
Oceania						
Fiji	1987	Antenatal	31	2	45	9
Latin America						
Chile	1984	Antenatal	32	2	—	—
Panama	1987	Female CSWs	33	31	3	23
		"bar-girls"	33	10	2	7

Source: Adapted from R. C. Burnham and J. E. Embree, "The magnitude of reproductive tract infections in the Third World," in *AIDS and Women's Reproductive Health,* ed. L. Chen, J. Sepúlveda-Amor, and S. J. Segal (New York: Plenum, 1992).

Note: CSWs = commercial sex workers.

References:

1. B. T. Nasah, R. Nguematcha, M. Eyong, et al., "Gonorrhea, Trichomoniasis and Candida among gravid and nongravid women in Cameroon," *International Journal of Gynecology Obstetrics* 18 (1980):48–52.

2. F. P. Galega, D. L. Heymann, and B. T. Nasah, "Gonococcal ophthalmia neonatorum: The case for

Table 5.1 (cont.): Prevalence of selected sexually transmitted diseases (STDs) in developing countries, 1973–1992

prophylaxis in tropical Africa," *Bulletin of the World Health Organization* 62 (1984):95–98.

3. L. Zekeng, J. M. Garcia Andela, et al., "Trends of HIV infection among pregnant women in Yaoundé, Cameroon, from 1989 to 1991," presented at the VI International Conference on AIDS in Africa, Dakar, Senegal, 1991.

4. A. Geyid, H. S. Tesfaye, A. Abraha, et al., A study on STD pathogens in sex workers in Addis Ababa, Ethiopia, presented at the VII International Conference on AIDS, Florence, Italy, June 1991.

5. D. C. W. Mabey and H. C. Whittle, "Genital and neonatal chlamydial infection in a trachoma endemic area," *Lancet* 2 (1982):300–01.

6. D. C. W. Mabey, G. Ogbaselassie, J. N. Robertson, et al., "Tubal infertility in the Gambia: Chlamydial and gonococcal serology in women with tubal occlusion compared with pregnant controls," *Bulletin of the World Health Organization* 63 (1985):1107–13.

7. M. Hopcraft, A. R. Verhagen, S. Ngigi, et al., "Genital infections in developing countries: Experience in a family planning clinic," *Bulletin of the World Health Organization* 48 (1973):581–86.

8. L. J. D'Costa, F. A. Plummer, I. Bowmer, et al., "Prostitutes are a major reservoir of sexually transmitted diseases in Nairobi, Kenya," *Sexually Transmitted Disease* 12 (1985):64–67.

9. M. Laga, H. Nsanze, R. C. Brunham, et al., "Epidemiology of ophthalmia neonatorum in Kenya," *Lancet* 2 (1986):1145–48.

10. B. Elliott, R. C. Brunham, M. Laga, et al., "Maternal gonococcal infection as a preventable risk factor for low birth weight," *Journal of Infectious Diseases* 161 (1990):531–36.

11. J. N. Simonsen, F. A. Plummer, E. N. Ngugi, et al., "HIV infection among lower socioeconomic strata prostitutes in Nairobi," *AIDS* 4 (1990):139–44.

12. M. Temmerman, G. Maitha, J. O. Ndinya-Achola, et al., HIV-1 and syphilis infection in pregnant women in Nairobi, Kenya, presented at the VI International Conference on AIDS in Africa, Dakar, Senegal, 1991.

13. A. O. Osoba, "Epidemiology of urethritis in Ibadan," *British Journal of Venereal Disease* 48 (1972):116–20.

14. P. C. Gini, W. O. Chukudebelu, and A. N. Njoku-Obi, "Antenatal screening for syphilis at the University of Nigeria Teaching Hospital, Enugu, Nigeria—A six year survey," *International Journal of Gynecology Obstetrics* 29 (1989):321–24.

15. B. I. Nsofor, C. S. S. Bello, and C. C. Ekwempu, "Sexually transmitted disease among women attending a family planning clinic in Zaria, Nigeria," *International Journal of Gynecology Obstetrics* 28 (1989):365–67.

16. S. N. Deguene, F. van der Veen, M. Sene, et al., Programme pilote de surveillance sentinelle des MST au niveau des laboratoires périphériques du Sénégal, presented at the VI International Conference on AIDS in Africa, Dakar, Senegal, 1991.

17. I. Diaw, I. Thior, T. Siby, et al., Prévalence du VIH et MST majeures chez les prostituées nouvellement inscrites, presented at the VI International Conference on AIDS in Africa, Dakar, Senegal, 1991.

18. R. C. Ballard, H. G. Fehler, M. O. Duncan, et al., "Urethritis and associated infections in Johannesburg: The role of Chlamydia trachomatis," *South African Journal of Sexually Transmitted Disease* 1 (1981):24.

19. N. O. O'Farrell, A. A. Hoosen, B. M. Kharsany, et al., "Sexually transmitted pathogens in pregnant women in a rural South African community," *Genitourinary Medicine* 65 (1989):276–80.

20. J. W. Kibukamusoke, "Venereal disease in East Africa," *Transactions of the Royal Society of Tropical Medicine and Hygiene* 59 (1965):642–48.

21. O. P. Arya, H. Nsanzumuhire, and S. R. Taber, "Clinical, cultural and demographic aspects of

Table 5.1 (cont.): Prevalence of selected sexually transmitted diseases (STDs) in developing countries, 1973–1992

gonorrhoea in a rural community in Uganda," *Bulletin of the World Health Organization* 49 (1973):587–95.

22. M. Kivuvu, M. Tuliza, B. Malele, et al., "HIV infection and other STD among Kinshasa prostitutes: A comparison between 1988 and 1991," presented at the VI International Conference on AIDS in Africa, Dakar, Senegal, 1991.

23. K. Mokwa, V. Batter, F. Behets, et al., Prevalence of sexually transmitted diseases (STD) in childbearing women in Kinshasa, Zaire, associated with HIV infection, presented at the VII International Conference on AIDS, Florence, Italy, June 1991.

24. A. V. Ratnam, S. N. Din, and T. K. Chatterjee, "Gonococcal infection in women with pelvic inflammatory disease in Lusaka, Zambia," *American Journal of Obstetrics Gynecology* 138 (1980):965–68.

25. A. V. Ratnam, S. N. Din, S. K. Hira, et al., "Syphilis in pregnant women in Zambia," *British Journal of Venereal Disease* 58 (1982):355–58.

26. R. Weissenberger, A. Robertson, S. Holland, et al., "The incidence of gonorrhea in urban Rhodesian black women," *South African Medical Journal* 52 (1977):119.

27. J. N. Wasserheit, J. R. Harris, J. Chokraborty, et al., "Reproductive tract infections in a family planning population in rural Bangladesh: A neglected opportunity to promote MCH-FP programs," *Studies in Family Planning* 20 (1989):69.

28. R. Bang, An approach to the gynecological problems of rural women: Epidemiological study and intervention through primary health care. First Annual Meeting, Community Epidemiology/Health Management Network, Khon Kaen, Thailand, February 1–4, 1988. Quoted in J. N. Wasserheit, "The significance and scope of reproductive tract infections among third world women," *Journal of Gynecology Obstetrics* Suppl. 3 (1989):145–68.

29. R. Khoo et al., "A study of sexually transmitted diseases in 200 prostitutes in Singapore," *Asian Journal of Infectious Disease* 1 (1977):77.

30. K. Kuvanont, A. Chitwarakorn, C. Rochananond, et al., "Etiology of urethritis in Thai men," *Sexually Transmitted Disease* 16 (1989):137–40.

31. R. Gyaneshwar, H. Nsanze, K. P. Singh, et al., "The prevalence of sexually transmitted disease agents in pregnant women in Suva," *Australia New Zealand Journal of Obstetrics Gynecology* 27 (1987):213–15.

32. E. Donoso, E. Vera, P. Villaseca, et al., "Infection gonococica en el embarazo (Gonococcal infection during pregnancy)." *Revista Chilena de Obstetrica Ginecológia* 49 (1984):84.

33. W. C. Reeves and E. Quiroz, "Prevalence of sexually transmitted diseases in high-risk women in the Republic of Panama," *Sexually Transmitted Disease* 14 (1987):69–74.

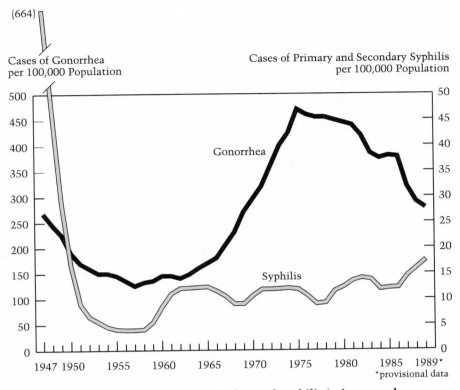

Figure 5.1. Reported incidence of gonorrhea and syphilis (primary and secondary) in the United States, 1947-89.
Source: A. DeSchryver and A. Meheus, "Epidemiology of sexually transmitted diseases: The global picture," *Bulletin of the World Health Organization* 68 (1990): 639-54.

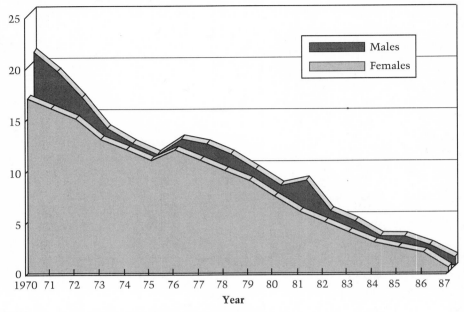

Figure 5.2. Cases of gonorrhea in Sweden, 1970-87.
Source: Adapted from the Department of Epidemiology, National Bacteriological Laboratory, Stockholm. Published in A. DeSchryver and A. Meheus, "Epidemiology of sexually transmitted diseases" (1990).

gonorrhea incidence rate of 3,000 to 10,000 new cases per 100,000 inhabitants.

Trends in the incidence of proven *Chlamydia trachomatis* infections are not well defined. However, trends in the incidence of nongonococcal urethritis (NGU) in men provide a reasonable approximation because the proportion of new cases attributable to *C. trachomatis* has remained fairly stable (around 40 percent) in industrialized countries over the past decade.

In the United Kingdom, rates of NGU in men have been rising steadily and are now 3 to 4 times higher than gonorrhea rates. Laboratory reports of genital *C. trachomatis* infection in women in the United Kingdom increased more than 5-fold (from 3,500 to 18,500) between 1981 and 1986. It is likely, however, that part of this increase

Table 5.2: Estimated annual total of sexually transmitted diseases, 1990

Disease	Total
Trichomoniasis	120 million
Genital chlamydia	50 million
Genital papillomavirus	30 million
Gonorrhea	25 million
Genital herpes	20 million
Syphilis	3.5 million
Chancroid	2 million
Human immunodeficiency virus	1 million

Source: World Health Organization, 1991.

stemmed from increased provider awareness and more widespread chlamydial diagnostic testing. Similarly, NGU is now three times as common as gonococcal urethritis in the United States. *C. trachomatis* caused approximately 4 million or more infections in the United States in 1986, affecting women more than men. Studies from Sweden have also shown significantly higher incidences of chlamydial infection in women—particularly young women aged 20 to 24 years. Although recognition of *C. trachomatis* has been slow in developing countries, prevalence among women appears to be similar to the prevalence in industrialized countries. In fact, *C. trachomatis* appears to be fast overtaking *N. gonorrhoeae* as the major etiologic agent in both pelvic inflammatory disease (PID) and ophthalmia neonatorum.

Genital herpes cases increased dramatically in both the United Kingdom and the United States during the 1970s, peaking in the mid-1980s. The number of cases has since declined slightly in the former and leveled off in the latter—presumably in response to extensive use of acyclovir to prevent recurrence. Nevertheless, an estimated cumulative total of 20 to 40 million persons in the United States have genital herpes. Reliable data are not available for developing countries.

Global epidemiology of human papillomavirus (HPV) is similar to that of genital herpes, although its magnitude is three to four times greater and its potential consequences (e.g., cervical cancer) far more severe. The incidence of genital warts increased nearly nine times (from 30 per 100,000 population to 260 per 100,000 population) in the United Kingdom between 1970 and 1988. The trend in physician visits for this condition was similar in the United States during the same period. It is generally accepted that because of the high proportion of subclinical infections and lack of a convenient diagnostic test, identified cases of HPV represent only a tiny fraction of the actual prevalence in the population.

Although chancroid is rare in industrialized nations, its global incidence exceeds that of syphilis. Improved detection methods have made identification of the causative agent (*Haemophilus ducreyi*) in developing countries more feasible, while observation of increased HIV transmission in patients with genital ulcers associated with this pathogen has added a new note of urgency to an old epidemic. Commercial sex workers (especially those from lower social strata) and their sex partners play an important role in the spread of chancroid, particularly in Southeast Asia and eastern and southern Africa. Contact with sex workers and the exchange of sex for crack cocaine have also been implicated in a number of recent outbreaks of chancroid in U.S. urban and migrant labor populations. In 1985, the number of reported chancroid cases in the United States rose above 2,000 for the first time since 1956. By 1987, that number had more than doubled.[2]

FACTORS INFLUENCING STD TRANSMISSION

A distinguishing feature of STDs is the disproportionate role played by those with multiple partners in spreading disease.[3] Recognition that even a small number of highly sexually active individuals can maintain an STD epidemic in an otherwise low-risk population has led to emphasis on targeting such *core groups* for preventive interventions.[4] Core groups are defined as segments of the population who are high frequency transmitters of STDs (see Box 5.1). Although STD core groups are likely to be found within groups with high risk sexual behavior, they should be recognized as an entity of their own, characterized by geographic, demographic, ethnic, and behavioral factors that may combine to produce high frequency of STD transmission.

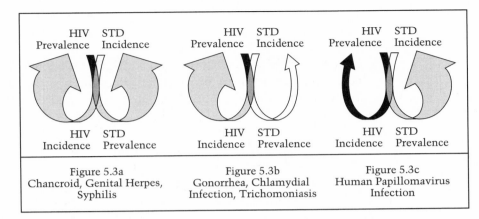

Figure 5.3. Epidemiological synergy: Inter-relationships between HIV infection and other STDs.

Source: J.N. Wasserheit, "Epidemiological synergy: Inter-relationships between HIV infection and other STDs." In *AIDS and Women's Reproductive Health*, L. Chen, et al (eds.) (New York: Plenum, 1992).

Note: The relationships between HIV infection and other STDs may differ for different STDs. Genital ulcer diseases (GUD) and HIV infection appear to reinforce each other because these STDs facilitate HIV transmission, whereas HIV infection may simultaneously prolong or augment the infectiousness of individuals with GUD (5.3a). The discharge syndromes probably interact with HIV infection in a unidirectional fashion by promoting HIV transmission without a synergistic increase in their own prevalence or incidence (5.3b). HPV infection may represent a traditional opportunistic infection, the expression and progression of which are augmented by HIV (5.3c).

Because of the difficulty in identifying core groups within a population, however, epidemiological studies and program interventions usually target individuals or communities considered at high risk as a result of their sexual practices.

Commercial sex workers and their clients represent an obvious high risk group for STDs. Other high risk groups may include members of the military, long-distance truck drivers, travelers, and homosexual men. Perhaps the most potentially significant STD high risk group consists of adolescents and young adults, who frequently change partners and engage in unprotected sexual intercourse. Young people play a critical role in the spread of STDs in developing countries, where the proportion of the population aged 15 to 30 years is much larger than in industrialized nations.[5] In addition, HIV infection, syphilis, chlamydia, genital herpes, hepatitis B, and other STDs have subclinical phases in which transmission can occur in the absence of overt symptoms.

Transmission of infectious agents in genital secretions tends to be more efficient from men to women. Presumably, this discrepancy is largely a function of anatomy, as the vagina and cervix provide a large surface area for infection and a natural reservoir for microorganisms. Women are not only more vulnerable to acquiring STDs but also less likely to seek treatment and more likely to be misdiagnosed when they seek it. Symptoms, signs, and laboratory test results may all be less reliable in women.[6] For these and other reasons, women and infants sustain a disproportionate share of major STD complications, including pelvic inflammatory disease, infertility, ectopic pregnancy, fetal wastage, neonatal blindness, and genital malignancy.

Although the data are very limited, the risk of transmission per

---

Box 5.1: The Core Group Concept

Richard Rothenberg, National Center for Chronic Disease Prevention and Health Promotion, Centers for Disease Control, Atlanta, Georgia

The concept of core groups is based on the simple notion that some segments of the population are more likely than others to transmit infections sexually. In the late 1970s, James Yorke and Herbert Hethcote created a mathematical framework to develop this idea. They posited that relatively small groups of people—definable by geographic, sociodemographic, and behavioral characteristics—were responsible for maintenance of gonorrhea endemicity. Within such groups, on average, a person with gonorrhea generates one or more new cases. Persons with gonorrhea but not within core groups, on the other hand, do not help reproduce the infection. Thus, in the absence of core groups, gonorrhea—and by extension other STDs—would not be sustained or propagated in populations. Yorke and Hethcote provided a quantitative approach to defining group interactions, supporting the hypothesis that such groups were definable, nontransitory, and small.

During the 1980s, empirical evidence emerged that such groups did in fact exist. By carefully studying reported cases, four geographic foci of gonorrhea endemicity were described in Denver, Colorado: a small neighborhood that was predominantly African-American, a small area that was more than 50 percent Hispanic, an area with a large concentration of homosexual men, and a military base. While sociodemographic characteristics and sexual behaviors were different among these four groupings, each was shown to contain substantial numbers of gonorrhea transmitters. Similar foci were demonstrated in Colorado Springs, Colorado, and in Des Moines, Iowa. The distribution of 120,000 gonorrhea cases in New York State was

partner contact appears lower for HIV than for other major STDs. For gonorrhea, transmission from an infected woman to an uninfected man is thought to be around 20 percent for a single episode of vaginal intercourse, with the rate rising to 60 to 80 percent after four episodes. Transmission from men to women is more efficient, and may be as high as 90 percent.[7] The transmission rates for chlamydia appear to be roughly comparable. The transmission rate of syphilis has been estimated to be 30 percent per act of sexual intercourse.[8] In contrast, the transmission rate for HIV in a low-risk population may be 0.1 percent or less for a single act of heterosexual intercourse. As a result of variations in infectivity, rates of co-infection with other STDs, and the impact of frequent partner exchange, HIV transmission rates are considerably higher among homosexual men and among commercial sex workers and their clients, especially in developing countries.[9]

---

particularly striking: each of 12 major metropolitan areas gave evidence of a tightly clustered central inner-city core of gonorrhea transmission, surrounded concentrically by areas of diminishing disease occurrence. Epidemic spread of Penicillinase-producing N. gonorrhoeae in Dade County, Florida, revealed the same pattern. More detailed epidemiologic examination of some of these groups has provided important information about the nature of sexual interactions within a core group, the characteristics of persons involved, and the dynamics of transmission within and between groups.

Confusion may arise from the misapplication of the term core to persons rather than to groups. The epidemiologic description of a core group—its geographic boundaries; its age, sex, and ethnic/racial makeup; its predominant sexual preferences and habits—by no means commits all its members to a life of disease transmission. In fact, like other aggregate descriptors, it provides little guidance in identifying critical individuals. A major thrust of research in this area is to explore the concept of a core group as a network. One current hypothesis suggests that importance (or centrality) in the network may identify those who are critical for disease transmission.

The public health importance of these concepts rests in their potential to permit targeting of limited resources to groups that are most critical for transmission. Some recent evidence suggests that focused case-finding and partner notification may diminish the endemicity of gonorrhea. Both the theoretical arguments and the intuitive appeal of a core group approach make it a fertile strategy to explore for controlling sexually transmitted infections, including HIV.

INTERACTION OF STDs AND HIV

Numerous studies support the role of STDs as biological cofactors with HIV. The data are strongest with respect to the genital ulcer diseases (chancroid, genital herpes, syphilis), which appear to interact with HIV in a bidirectional fashion: presence of genital ulcers fosters HIV transmission, while HIV may cause more severe clinical manifestations of STD infection. There is anecdotal evidence that HIV-infected individuals who are also infected with syphilis may experience rapid progression to neurosyphilis, and single-dose therapy with benzathine penicillin G is often inadequate. Serologic responses to *Treponema pallidum* may also be confounded in patients with HIV infection who have previously received treatment for syphilis. Likewise, the severity, persistence, and rate of recurrence of herpes simplex (HSV) lesions may increase in those who are HIV-infected, and the appearance of acyclovir-resistant HSV isolates has been noted.

Although data regarding the discharge syndromes (gonorrhea, chlamydia, trichomoniasis) are less convincing, these syndromes also appear to promote transmission of HIV. The effect appears to be unidirectional, however, as prevalence and incidence of the discharge syndromes do not seem to be altered by HIV. There is also growing evidence that HIV-induced immunosuppression may facilitate development of anogenital dysplasia and neoplasia in patients with human papillomavirus.[10]

WHERE ARE THE DATA?

The continuing scarcity of accurate incidence or prevalence data, especially from the developing world, reflects "the low level of priority assigned to classic STDs in most countries."[11] The weakness of the database is a serious handicap to global control of all STDs—including HIV—because similar sexual behavior influences transmission. Furthermore, trends in the incidence and prevalence of *some* STDs are easier to monitor than are trends in HIV seroprevalence. In an eight-year study designed to measure the impact of fear of AIDS on risk behaviors in a U.S. urban population, significant changes were noted in gonorrhea, syphilis, and hepatitis B incidence rates among homosexual men, and to a lesser extent among heterosexual men and women. The study concluded that gonorrhea incidence "remains the most accurate indicator of recent changes in sexual behavior owing to high incidence, short incubation, easy detection, and quick cures."[12]

■■■■■   .   .   .

STD PREVENTION AND CONTROL

Each year, an estimated 250 million or more new sexually transmitted infections occur around the world. Yet in the past, analyses of STDs have tended to downplay their importance relative to other infectious diseases. However, AIDS has sparked a resurgence of scientific interest in the field and drawn attention to the extensive and lasting damage caused by STDs in general, especially in developing countries which often lack adequate treatment facilities (Box 5.2). In terms of healthy and productive life-years lost per year, STDs in high prevalence urban areas of Africa, Asia, and Latin America constitute a substantial fraction of the entire disease burden in those populations.[13]

The high cost of diagnostic and treatment tools and lack of clinical services are major factors hampering STD control. Health care providers seeing patients with STDs at the point of first contact with the health system are often unable to offer adequate clinical care due to lack of training, drugs, and diagnostic means. Although the problem is most urgent in developing countries, it is hardly confined to them. In the United States, the failure to meet the health needs of the urban poor and the explosion of crack cocaine use in inner-city communities have created an STD crisis. As recently noted, "The deteriorating STD situation of the U.S. urban underclass increasingly resembles that seen in the slums of the least developed countries, where acquired immunodeficiency syndrome . . . has been spreading at epidemic rates among heterosexuals."[27]

Lack of adequate medical services for diagnosis and treatment is one factor contributing to the difficulty of controlling STDs in the developing world. Other factors that have been cited include high birth rate and relatively large proportion of the population in sexually active age groups; urbanization, male migration, and changing social structures; poverty and gender inequality fostering prostitution; war and social strife; and HIV infection and its destablizing influence on conventional STD epidemiology.[28]

Urban migration, a major demographic trend in developing countries, appears to promote the spread of STDs through a variety of interrelated mechanisms. Young people uprooted from their families and freed from the constraints of their traditional cultures may adopt new sexual habits, including casual sexual relationships, unprotected sex with a number of partners, or intercourse with commercial sex workers. In addition, urban areas in developing countries tend to have

---

Box 5.2: The Veiled Impact of STDs

The editors wish to thank Judith N. Wasserheit, M.D., Chief, Division of STD/HIV Prevention, Centers for Disease Control, Atlanta, Georgia, for assistance in the review of this article.

In a world confronted with HIV, opportunities should not be missed to achieve a major impact on the health and survival of women, men, and children through combined efforts to prevent and control other STDs. In addition to the critical role of other STDs in HIV transmission, these diseases are important because of their severe complications in women and infants.[14]

The reproductive impact of STDs is primarily mediated through the development of upper genital tract infection or pelvic inflammatory disease (PID). Infections with *Neisseria gonorrhoeae* and *Chlamydia trachomatis* are the major causes of pelvic inflammatory diseases (PID). When untreated, PID can severely compromise a woman's health, fertility, and productivity.[15] In sub-Saharan Africa, the annual incidence of PID may be as high as 1 to 3 percent among women aged 15 to 44 years living in urban areas,[16] with an annual mortality rate of 0.1 to 0.5 per 1,000. It has been estimated that annually in the United States, approximately one million women suffer from PID, of whom roughly 300,000 are hospitalized.[17] In 1979, mortality in the United States due to PID was 0.29 per 1,000 women 15–44 years old.[18] Data from other industrialized countries, including Sweden and the United Kingdom, showed that PID is often associated with STDs and is more frequent in women aged 15–24.[19]

Tubal obstruction caused by PID resulting from STDs can also lead to infertility. One third of women who have had two episodes of PID will become infertile, adding an emotional and social dimension to the course of infection and jeopardizing family planning efforts.[20]

In men, urethritis caused by gonococcal and chlamydial infections may lead to chronic epididymitis and sterility by complete obstruction of seminal ducts. In developing countries 20 to 40 percent of male infertility can be attributed to this cause.[21]

Worldwide, especially in developing countries, STDs acquired prior to or during pregnancy are probably responsible for much of the burden of spontaneous abortions, prematurity, low birth weight, and neonatal/infant

disproportionately high concentrations of young men between the ages of 20 and 45 years. This phenomenon serves as a magnet for commercial sex workers, especially if education and employment opportunities for girls and women are scarce. The concentrated sexual mixing that occurs helps explain why STD incidence and prevalence are considerably higher in the cities than in the countryside.[29] For example, the Rwandan HIV Seroprevalence Study Group reported HIV seropositivity rates were 13.7 times higher among urban dwellers (17.8%) than among rural villagers (1.3%).[30]

---

infections. In Zambia, 19 percent of spontaneous abortions were attributed to congenital syphilis.[22]

Ectopic pregnancy, another complication of STDs, not only results in fetal death, but endangers a woman's survival. In the United States in 1985, about 1.5 percent of all pregnancies were ectopic with non-white women facing a much higher risk (fourfold) of death than white women.[23] In the developing world, late diagnosis and reduced access to health care increase the impact of ectopic pregnancy on maternal mortality. Post-partum infections and ectopic pregnancy due to gonococcal and chlamydial infections may be responsible for as many as 40 percent of all maternal deaths in some areas of sub-Saharan Africa and as many as 20 percent in the United States.[24]

Even when pregnancy is carried to term, STDs may have a severe impact on the infant. Prematurity and low birth weight resulting from infection, and neonatal respiratory infections and meningitis, may compromise the infant's physical and mental

development and survival. Congenital syphilis (which was present in 7 per 1,000 live births in Bangkok and 32 per 1,000 in Addis Ababa) result in the death of 1 in every 10 infected neonates.[25]

With a transmission rate of 30 to 50 percent from mother to offspring, *Chlamydia trachomatis* and *Neisseria gonorrhoeae* infections in neonates are major causes of neonatal conjunctivitis (ophthalmia neonatorum) and, in the case of *N. gonorrhoeae* infection, may lead to blindness.[26] The incidence rate of neonatal gonococcal conjunctivitis has declined in the industrialized world but in developing countries where the prevalence of gonorrhea in pregnant women ranges between 3 to 15 percent (with half of the infections being resistant to penicillin), ophthalmia neonatorum remains a major public health problem.

The morbidity, mortality, and infertility resulting from STDs are commonly underestimated. The combined prevention of sexually transmitted diseases and HIV infection has a considerable potential for reducing severe STD associated complications.

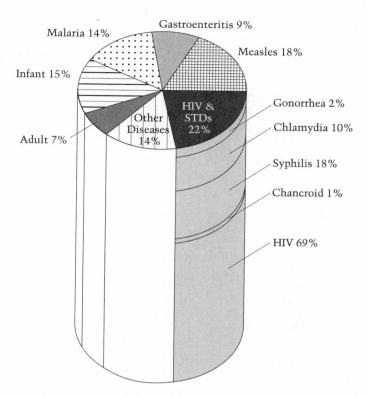

Figure 5.4. STDs' share of total disease burden in a high prevalence African city.
Source: Adapted from M. Over and P. Piot, "HIV infection and sexually transmitted diseases," Population, Health and Nutrition Division, The World Bank, Washington, D.C. (1991).

War and social strife exert an even more dramatic destabilizing effect by uprooting families, concentrating large populations of sexually active young men in confined areas, and promoting reliance on commercial sex workers (many of whom have been raped, widowed, abandoned, or otherwise deprived of economic support). Resulting social patterns may persist long after the fighting stops. The thriving sex tourism industry in Southeast Asia derived much of its momentum from the wars in Vietnam, when impoverished young women from the countryside flocked to military centers to service visiting troops on "rest and relaxation."

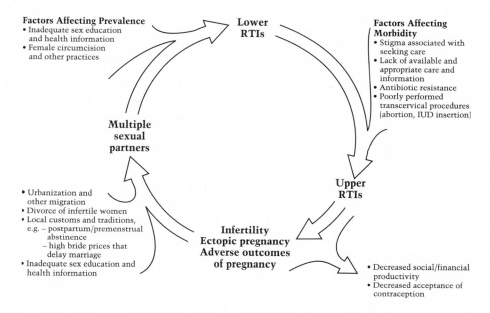

Figure 5.5. Selected societal, behavioral, and physiological factors associated with female reproductive tract infections (RTIs) in developing countries.

Source: J.N. Wasserheit, "The significance and scope of reproductive tract infections among Third World women, " *International Journal of Gynecology and Obstetrics* Suppl.3 (1989): 145-68.

Low social status and economic marginality of women in many developing countries are important contributors to high STD prevalence and morbidity. A recent comprehensive study of reproductive tract infections in women from developing countries clearly illustrates the interrelationship of societal, behavioral, and physiological factors (see Figure 5.5).[31] Women who cannot achieve economic or social self-sufficiency tend to be unequal partners in marital or sexual relationships. In such settings, females often become sexually active at an early age, whereas males tend to marry later in life after having a number of sexual partners (of which some may have been commercial sex workers). In some traditional societies, prohibitions against intercourse during the menstrual period or for a long time after giving birth contribute to male patterns of multiple-partner sex. Low levels of education of women in developing countries not only limit job access; they also promote misconceptions about disease prevention and reduce receptivity to public health messages. Female vulnerability to STDs may also be enhanced by local customs designed to increase men's sexual pleasure or by rituals such as female circumcision.[32]

Once a woman in such a setting has contracted a genital infection, her opportunities for early treatment (and, in some cases, her chances of avoiding more serious complications) are often limited by the absence of medical facilities and by the social stigma attached to seeking care for an STD. Ironically, a further deterrent to seeking care is fear of discovery of HIV infection, which could lead to abandonment by her husband or extended family. Marital abandonment may also be provoked by infertility resulting from untreated pelvic inflammatory disease (often due to *N. gonorrhoeae* or *C. trachomatis*)—a commonplace scenario in developing countries.[33] Finally, even if the woman is fortunate enough to obtain timely treatment, the duration of infection is often prolonged by the presence of antibiotic-resistant pathogens. Thus, a vicious cycle is set up in which increasing numbers of women with sexually transmitted infections are set adrift economically and migrate to cities where, because of lack of education and job skills, they may resort to commercial sex work in order to survive. A recent report for the United Nations Commission on Human Rights suggests another grim aspect of this cycle: a worldwide increase in the sale of female and, to a lesser extent, male children, who are forced into commercial sex work to satisfy customers' desires for sex partners free of HIV and other STDs.[34]

--------------- · · ·

ISSUES IN STD PREVENTION AND CONTROL

Despite improved therapies and a cluster of scientific breakthroughs that have enlarged our understanding of their natural history and pathogenesis, the world is still far from controlling STDs. Some of the societal factors contributing to the remarkable persistence of this group of infections have already been discussed. There are also important biological explanations, such as the absence of effective cures for the major viral STDs (herpes simplex, human papilloma, hepatitis B, and HIV), the ability of people to remain asymptomatic for long periods while infectious, and the tendency of even common bacterial pathogens such as gonorrhea to develop stubborn, antimicrobial-resistant strains.

By far the greatest stumbling block, however, is the human element: STDs are spread by sexual behaviors that are deeply ingrained and highly complex. They are also viewed as private—and, as the disagreement over partner notification vividly illustrates, the individual's right to privacy is often perceived to be in conflict with the goal of protecting the public from transmissible diseases. Finally, sexual customs, behaviors, and expectations are highly variable throughout society and depend on local cultural and demographic factors. Thus, an effective prevention message in one population may have no effect, or even a negative effect, elsewhere.

Because HIV/STD control is an evolving field, each new piece of information adds to our store of knowledge and raises further questions. The following section highlights several issues of concern to investigators in which changing human behavior plays a key role. (The issues involved with notifying partners of infected people are dealt with by R. Keenlyside and K. Toomey in Chapter 16.)

TARGETING INTERVENTIONS TO HIGH-RISK BEHAVIOR

The concept of the core group, referred to earlier, suggests a focus for STD prevention and control—behavioral interventions that center on high-frequency transmitters of STDs. This approach is highly cost effective: "A policy of targeting the one-time intervention at the core averts ten times as many cases as would have been averted by a policy directed at the noncore" (see Table 5.3).[35]

The largest high-risk group is composed of young people who have recently become, or are about to become, sexually active. This is a difficult audience to influence because of peer pressure and influence of social norms, as well as the sense of invulnerability that accompanies youth. A study of HIV risk behaviors among more than 2,000 16-to-24-year-olds in France, the United States, and the United Kingdom observed that despite knowledge about and perceptions of HIV/STD risk, a high percentage of young people continued to experiment with high-risk behaviors. According to the investigators, these find-

Table 5.3: The dynamic effects of preventing 100 STD cases in the core rather than the noncore group[a]

Disease	Discounted new cases averted over 10 years by:		Ratio core to noncore[b]
	Targeting the core	Targeting the noncore	
Chancroid	810	83	9.8
Chlamydia	4,096	423	9.7
Gonorrhea	4,278	426	10.0
HIV no ulcers	1,744	180	9.7
HIV ulcers	2,106	201	10.5
Syphilis	4,132	422	9.8

Source: M. Over and P. Piot, "HIV infection and sexually transmitted diseases" (Population, Health and Nutrition Division, World Bank, Washington, D.C., 1991).

a. The new cases averted over 10 years are the sum of the savings in both the core and noncore groups of an initial preventive or curative policy applied to only one group. The streams of saved cases are discounted at an annual rate of 3 percent.

b. Number of cases in the core group to one case in the noncore group.

ings "suggest that intervention programs that merely educate young people about risk behaviors are inadequate in producing behavioral change. Risk-reduction strategies are likely to succeed only if they intervene in the social networks of these risk takers to change norms and behaviors."[36]

Secondary school students may already be past the optimum age for preventive interventions. Those who should receive the highest priority are early adolescents, who need to develop the emotional maturity and persuasive skills to negotiate condom use as well as a sense of responsibility for their bodies and their sex partners. It has been noted that many of the basic skills needed to protect against STDs are also critical in nonsexual interactions. In this perspective, adolescent sex education should not be a single item on the school curriculum but rather part of an integrated program of preventive health care for young people that would include general health screening (e.g., hypertension, cholesterol), contraceptive advice, and appropriate immunizations.

Such a program of coordinated and comprehensive adolescent health care is currently available in Sweden, where compulsory sex education and extensive condom promotion have been credited with substantially lowering STD rates. Other industrialized countries have been slow to follow the Swedish example, however, and worldwide, comprehensive adolescent health care remains a rarity.

In contrast to the lack of preventive interventions for adolescents, many industrialized and developing countries encourage or require STD screening of commercial sex workers. Yet the impact on STD incidence and the cost benefit of these interventions have not been thoroughly evaluated. Questionable STD detection methods (i.e., Gram-stained blind cervicovaginal smears) are often used, and the overall approach may result in stigmatization of the patient. Furthermore, screening is not always accompanied by other primary prevention activities, such as aggressive promotion and distribution of condoms.[37]

Street-outreach interventions—in which condoms are dispensed free of charge by specially trained health workers, and commercial sex workers and their clients are provided literature on safer sex and urged to visit the STD clinic for screening and counseling—appear to have a positive impact. Following one such intervention in a small U.S. city, reported cases of gonorrhea among commercial sex workers and their sex partners declined 16 percent over a 3-year period.[38] However, because the program was not part of a randomized trial, the effect of the intervention on risk behavior could not be rigorously evaluated.

DEVELOPING POPULATION-SPECIFIC INTERVENTIONS

Although the main elements of efforts to prevent STDs—education about safer sex and sexuality, condom promotion, and provision of diagnostic and treatment services—are essentially the same in all settings, the populations needing such programs are extremely varied. Interventions that fail to consider the context in which preventive messages are received are unlikely to succeed and may even do harm. This context may be determined by health care priorities, mobility, literacy level, social customs and taboos, and local religious beliefs.

An example of misperceived health priorities concerns the use of silver nitrate eye prophylaxis for newborns, as part of STD control efforts in areas where gonorrhea is endemic. Despite the proven effectiveness and low cost of this preventive measure, it is not widely used in several developing countries with high rates of gonorrhea. Why? Is it because silver nitrate prophylaxis is no longer recommended in a number of Western European countries where the prevalence of gonorrhea among pregnant women is extremely low? Is it because, theoretically, gonorrhea ought to be detected and treated in the prospective mother prior to delivery, or merely a consequence of logistic difficulties in ensuring the sustainable supply of silver nitrate? The reality is that screening pregnant women for gonorrhea is expensive and rare in the developing world and that the administration of silver nitrate to newborns is not systematic. As a result, the incidence of gonococcal conjunctivitis in newborns in these areas may run as high as 1 to 5 percent.[39]

Priorities for behavioral interventions relating to prevention and control of STDs in developing countries have been identified within the following three categories: 1) development of health education messages appropriate to the local epidemiological situation, health care infrastructure, and sociocultural context; 2) identification of target groups and development of community-based programs; and 3) provision of clinical services and national treatment guidelines through various settings such as urban clinics, private physicians, primary care clinics, and pharmacies.[40] Unfortunately, few program planners have taken advantage of the availability of ethnographic data to design appropriate interventions for targeted high-risk groups in the developing world. Those interventions that are available tend only to address HIV infection and ignore curable STDs.

Interestingly, the same might be said of the United States, a multiethnic society in which the core heterosexual transmission groups for STDs are largely inner-city minorities. The safer sex campaigns that have reduced the spread of HIV/STD among gay men have not been equally successful in African-American and Hispanic communities. A number of explanations have been proposed, including cultural barriers against using—or even discussing the use of—condoms, the relative powerlessness of minority women in enforcing condom use, and mistrust of public health interventions based on past experiences of discrimination and economic disadvantage.[41] It has been suggested that prevention efforts which address the significance of the African-American extended family and community may be more powerful motivators of behavioral change in that community than efforts that focus only on the individual.[42]

APPROACHES TO COORDINATED HIV AND STD PROGRAMS

In industrialized as well as developing countries, insufficient systematic, long-term efforts were made to contain the spread of STDs prior to the recognition of AIDS. (It should be noted that where aggressive STD control measures were undertaken, as in the United Kingdom, Scandinavia, and the Netherlands, they were often successful.) With the advent of AIDS, HIV-specific prevention policies and programs were organized on an emergency basis. Control measures for other STDs were considered almost as an afterthought.

The obvious inefficiency of this approach has led many investigators to suggest combining the two. The concept has not been without opposition: "Resistance to combined STD/AIDS control programs can be found within both categorical STD and AIDS programs. Recent vintage AIDS program professionals often lack a background in sexually transmitted or other infectious diseases; tend to view gonorrhea, syphilis, herpes, and other STDs as commonplace and unimportant; and fear that a single program will draw away AIDS resources to STDs and dilute public concern. Categorical STD professionals, on the other hand, feel that they have long labored in an unglamorous and underfunded field that never has been given the health priority it deserves, in view of the enormous aggregate morbidity and mortality which STDs cause. They are jealous of new and generously funded vertical AIDS programs that appear to further diminish STD resources and disregard their professional experience and expertise."[43]

These reservations notwithstanding, the trend is clearly towards integrating HIV and STD programs. In a recent worldwide survey by *AIDS in the World*, more than two-thirds of the 34 nations queried reported at least partial coordination of HIV/STD services, with the majority of diagnostic and treatment facilities located in urban centers.[44] National AIDS programs created in 1990–91 were more likely to be at least partially integrated with STD programs than those

Table 5.4: Availability of sexually transmitted disease (STD) clinics and percentage of STD patients by type of facility and gender, 1991

Regions and countries	STD clinics available		% of patients					Does country practice	
	In urban areas only	In urban and rural areas	Seen in public health facilities	Seen in private facilities	Other facilities	Male	Female	STD partner notification?	HIV partner notification?
North America									
Canada	yes		30	70		60	40	yes	yes
United States		yes						yes	yes
Western Europe									
Netherlands	yes							yes	no
France	yes							yes	yes
Sweden		yes	96	4		40	60	yes	yes
Italy	yes					67	33	no	no
Germany		yes	10	85	5	80	20	no	no
United Kingdom		yes	90	10		50	50	yes	yes
Norway	yes		90					yes	yes
Switzerland	yes							no	no
Oceania									
Australia		yes						yes	yes
Latin America									
Mexico	yes		30	30	40	70	30	yes	yes
Argentina	yes		34	66		30	70	yes	yes
Colombia	N/A[a]	N/A[a]	60	10	30			no	no
Sub-Saharan Africa									
Uganda	yes		40	60		60	40	yes	yes
Tanzania		yes	50	40	10	60	40	yes	no
Côte d'Ivoire	yes		90					yes	yes

Nigeria	yes		5	90	5	70	30	yes	no
Zambia	yes					70	30	N/A	N/A
Cameroon	yes		25	5	70	70	30	no	no
Congo		yes	90	10	10	60	40	yes	no
Rwanda			65	25	10	42	58	yes	yes
Senegal		yes	45	45		50	50	yes	yes
Ethiopia	yes					50	50	no	no
Caribbean									
Trinidad and Tobago	yes	yes	100			71	29	yes	no
St. Lucia		yes	30	45	25	27	73	yes	yes
Haiti	yes		75	20	5	60	40	yes	yes
Eastern Europe									
USSR (CIS)		yes	50	0	50	56	44	yes	yes
Czech Republic		yes	100	0	0	53	47	yes	no
Slovak Republic		yes	100		0	57	43	yes	yes
Poland		yes	90	10		75	25	yes	no
South East Mediterranean									
Egypt	yes							no	yes
Morocco	yes		10	80	10	80	20	yes	yes
Pakistan	yes		35	20	45	65	35	no	yes
North East Asia									
Japan		yes	20	80		82	18	no	no
China	yes		90	10		75	25	no	yes
Southeast Asia									
Thailand		yes	25	25	50	33	66	no	no
India		yes	40	50	10	85		yes	yes

Source: AIDS in the World, 1992.
a. There are specialized clinics only for certain groups of the population.

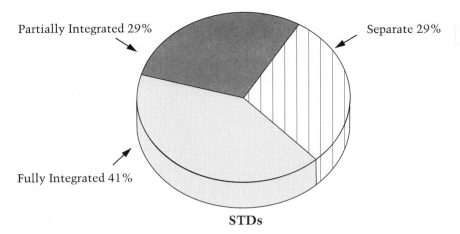

Partially Integrated 29%

Separate 29%

Fully Integrated 41%

STDs

Figure 5.6. Status of integration of national STD and HIV programs, as of January 1992, as reported by national AIDS program manager, for 34 countries.
Source: AIDS in the World survey.

created before 1990 (70 percent in 1992 versus 20 percent in 1989). (See Chapter 8, "National AIDS Programs" for more about the program survey.)

Over the next decade, more sophisticated educational interventions, greater accessibility of STD testing and treatment, and development of new diagnostic reagents and barrier methods such as the female condom (see Chapter 16) will gradually reduce transmission of STDs in countries that can afford to implement such measures. However, comprehensive STD control will remain out of reach for much of the developing world, and painful decisions about the allocation of limited resources will have to be made.

Consolidation of STD and HIV prevention and control efforts may lower the cost of some activities and permit policy planners to take advantage of both the technical expertise and clinical service infrastructure provided by traditional STD programs and the potential ability of AIDS programs to attract financial resources, mobilize mass media, and serve as advocates for the rights of individuals. The integrated primary health care (PHC) approach, using simplified treatment guidelines and standardized treatment with essential drugs, may also provide an effective and affordable option, and may be more acceptable to women than visiting STD clinics.

In conclusion, the dynamic and synergistic relationship between HIV and other STDs demands that the broadening of our base of knowledge about all STDs become a global priority for the 1990s. It is clear that successful STD control depends not only on the availability of effective technologies but also on the appropriateness of the messages used to convey them and the ability of the target population to respond. However comprehensive and well-integrated preventive services may be, they cannot easily overcome the hard economic realities and cultural barriers that foster disease spread. Societal conditions at the heart of the epidemic must be confronted and dealt with if HIV and STD prevention programs are to accomplish their goal.

CHAPTER SIX

The Demographic, Economic, and Social Impact of AIDS

Armstrong is an economist in the Eastern Africa Department of the World Bank, Washington, DC. Eduard Bos is a demographer in the Population, Health, and Nutrition Division of the World Bank's Population and Human Resources Department.

Although it is less than a decade since the virus that causes AIDS was discovered, it has become increasingly evident that this pandemic will have profound economic and social implications for both developed and developing countries. The importance of health as an input to the economic development and growth of a country is well established—a healthier population is more productive and has an increased capacity for learning. The adverse impacts of the HIV/AIDS pandemic will undermine improvements in health status and, in turn, reduce the potential for economic growth. AIDS is distinct from other diseases, and its impact can be expected to be quite severe.

Why is AIDS so different? AIDS remains an essentially fatal disease, thereby contributing to increased mortality. However, its most critical feature, distinguishing AIDS from other life-threatening and fatal illnesses, such as diarrhea (among children in developing countries) or cancer (among the elderly in developed countries), is that it selectively affects adults in their sexually most active ages, which coincide with their prime productive and reproductive years.

At the family level, an adult with AIDS will severely compromise household resources as the functional capacity to work is reduced, medical expenditures increase, and the income of both the infected

This article and its views are those of the authors and do not necessarily represent the views of the World Bank, its Board of Directors, or the countries it represents.

individual and those who care for that person is lost. Reduced income, in turn, threatens food supply, the ability to pay for the education or health of surviving family members, and the ability to invest in productive inputs, such as seeds, pesticides, machinery, and even labor. AIDS threatens more than the capability of a household to function as an economic unit; the entire social fabric of the family is potentially disrupted or dissolved. The loss of either or both parents leaves behind dependents, both the very young (orphans) and the elderly, who may have been relying on their children for support in old age. Box 6.1 depicts how AIDS can affect an agricultural household in Africa. It also illustrates the complexity and the ripple effects triggered by the death of one or more adults.

From an economic and societal perspective, HIV infection and AIDS can be considered a disease whose effects multiply far beyond the infected/ill individual. In parts of the world with high fertility, a single HIV-infected mother or father may directly and adversely affect the lives of 5 to 10 children, as well as wider circles of extended family,

Box 6.1: Impact of AIDS on a Rural Household

Adapted from A. Barnett and P. Blaikie, *AIDS in Africa: Its Present and Future Impact* (London: Bellhaven Press, 1992)

The impact of AIDS is unlike that of many other illnesses because the effects are gradual, manifesting themselves over a period of years. A compounding factor is that AIDS deaths tend to be narrowly clustered: often, more than one adult—and more than one child—will be infected with HIV within a household. Figure 6.A shows how illness and death from AIDS affect an agricultural household over time. These effects and the coping mechanisms a family might adopt in response to the resulting illness and death are portrayed. Although the pictograms are simplified, they were based on interviews conducted by researchers in the Rakai District of Uganda.

Stage 1 (Year 1): The household comprises a man and a woman, their five children living at home, and two older sons who do not live in the household but send cash home from income they earn. The family cultivates two acres consisting of the main staple (plantain) and beans, potatoes, and vegetables. Two-thirds of an acre is planted with coffee, the main cash crop. Two workers are hired for a month and a half each to weed and plant annual crops. Limited amounts of herbicide and pesticide are bought.

Stage 2 (Year 4): One son dies of AIDS, and the second falls ill and is unable to work. Remittances stop, and, although the family's labor is still intact, they are unable to hire additional workers. They also cannot afford either herbicides, which means that they must spend more time weeding, or

village, and community. The multiplier effect of HIV infection and its direct threat to survival of family and household units have not yet been sufficiently emphasized or measured.

The burden of HIV/AIDS is already being felt by individuals, households, and businesses. But over time, a much more severe impact will be seen in whole sectors of the economy and societies. Clearly, differences in epidemiological and contextual factors that shape the Geographic Areas of Affinity will give rise to differences in the scope and severity of the pandemic's impact. In particular, AIDS will pose additional strains on some less developed countries, where the social and economic infrastructure is weaker and resources—both financial and human—are more constrained, making the challenges for economic growth and improved quality of life even greater. The result is that some countries are more vulnerable in terms of their capacity to cope effectively with the consequences of existing HIV infections. Detecting or measuring this impact at an aggregate level at this time is complicated by the long incubation period between

---

pesticides, so averge yields fall. The family members spend longer days cultivating.

Stage 3 (Year 6): The husband is ill with opportunistic infections related to AIDS, and the second son dies. The husband can no longer work, and the wife must devote time to care for him. The oldest girl is taken out of school to save fees and to help on the farm. Coffee becomes neglected; as yields fall, income generated from its sale is reduced. More cassava is grown because it is less demanding of labor during peak harvest time for other crops; beans and potatoes are reduced. The plantains are neglected. The family spends some of its remaining income on medical expenses for the husband.

Stage 4 (Year 8): The husband dies, and the wife becomes ill with AIDS. Funeral expenses are substantial. The remaining children cannot attend school. Family labor is critically short—coffee is abandoned, and the plantains are infested with weeds and attacked by weevils. Food intake is reduced. The youngest child is sent to grandparents.

Stage 5 (Year 10): The wife dies. The eldest daughter spends time away from home trading to earn cash. The older sons offer their labor part time to other households. The surviving family members try to maintain subsistence crops. Clothing and food are inadequate.

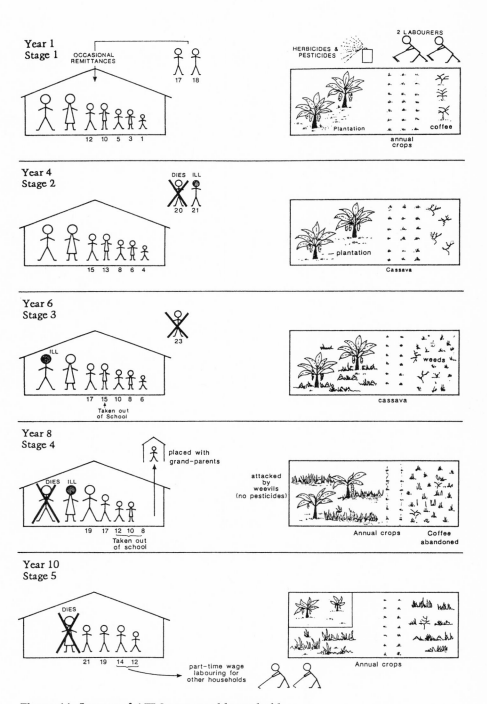

Figure 6A. Impact of AIDS on a rural household.
Source: T. Barnett and P. Blaikie. *AIDS in Africa: Its Present and Future Impact* (London: Bellhaven Press, 1992):89.

infection with HIV and the development of AIDS. This means that at a population level the true dimensions of the epidemic will be revealed only gradually as more and more HIV-infected persons progress to AIDS.

Because quantitative information on the magnitude of the economic impact is so limited,[1] this chapter articulates in a qualitative manner how AIDS is different by drawing the linkages between AIDS, demography, the economy, and society. Because the effect at the macroeconomic level is likely to be more severe for developing countries—although again, data are limited—the following discussion focuses more on those countries, although the mechanisms through which AIDS will affect economic life will be applicable to some degree in other parts of the world.

■■■■■■■ . . .

DEMOGRAPHIC IMPACT

The expected impact of AIDS on population growth and structure differs in significant ways among the Geographic Areas of Affinity. Not only do current levels of HIV infection vary from negligible to substantial, but the dominant transmission modes that distinguish the Areas of Affinity are highly relevant to demographic impact. From the perspective of population growth rate, not all individuals are equal: women starting their reproductive years have considerably more potential for affecting a population's growth and structure than do women past the reproductive years or men outside the reproductive process. In North America, for example, where the primary mode of HIV transmission so far has been through homosexual contacts, measurable demographic impact will be greatest on adult male mortality, which will have little effect on population growth. But in areas where the dominant mode of transmission is through heterosexual contacts, as in sub-Saharan Africa, women of childbearing age tend to become infected and die before having the number of children they otherwise might have had. Also, pregnant women may infect their fetuses or newborns, causing increased infant and child mortality, with measurable impact on population growth. Further differences between Geographic Areas of Affinity in the demographic consequences of AIDS result from variations in mortality from other causes—the more likely a person is to die from a cause other than AIDS, the lesser the impact of AIDS.

The demographic impact of AIDS is most immediate and serious in sub-Saharan Africa and in parts of the Caribbean, where falling life expectancy and increasing infant and child mortality have already been observed. Given the high proportion of the population already infected—up to 30 percent of young adults in some urban areas—and the high mortality resulting from the disease, a demographic impact over the next two decades is inevitable in these areas. The impact may eventually become as serious in several other Geographic Areas of Affinity, but this will depend foremost on whether the spread of HIV can be contained.

The following illustration of the projected demographic impact

---

Box 6.2: Modeling the Demographic Impact of AIDS: Overview of Approaches and Findings

Modelers have taken different approaches to show the demographic impact of HIV/AIDS. A workshop organized by the United Nations and the World Health Organization in December 1989 brought together modelers to compare approaches and results and to improve future models.[a] As part of this effort, Palloni and Glicklich identified four broad types of models, distinguished according to the data required and their complexity. Each model provides an estimate of future HIV infections and AIDS cases on which the demographic impact of the epidemic can be calculated.

The first category can be called *mathematical extrapolations*. These models fit a distribution for either the incidence of AIDS over time, or the cumulative number of AIDS cases over time, and infer future incidence from the assumed distribution. Such models are useful only for short-term projections and assume that the number of AIDS cases has been reported with the same accuracy over time. During the initial stages of the epidemic, an exponential function fits the cumulative number of cases well. Other functions that have been used or proposed are a Weibull and a cubic polynomial.

A second category of models projects HIV incidence using the reported number of AIDS cases and a mathematical function that gives the progression from infection to the onset of AIDS. This approach, used in WHO's *Epimodel,* is sensitive both to assumed incubation time as well as to the assumed functional representation. Its use is also limited to short-term projections.

A third family of models incorporates assumptions about the probability of HIV transmission in addition to assumptions regarding the incubation period (as in the second category of models). In most of these models, AIDS incidence and mortality are

of AIDS is based on a hypothetical country with fertility, mortality, and age structure typical for East Africa. The projection uses a model developed at the World Bank that has been used to forecast the course of the epidemic and its effect on population for a number of countries in sub-Saharan Africa.[2] A hypothetical East African country model is used, because it can be specified with a stable population structure and standardized vital rates that facilitate demonstrating the impact of AIDS. Several other models have been developed; their approaches and findings are summarized in Box 6.2.

In this model, HIV prevalence is assumed to have been zero in 1975, increasing to about 5 percent of the adult population in 1985 and to nearly 10 percent in 1990. It is assumed that sexual behavior and cofactors that determine the spread of HIV are unchanged in the

---

projected from a given estimate of HIV prevalence and starting year of the epidemic. These models may then link with a demographic projection model and produce estimates of the impact on demographic indicators. An example of this approach is the model developed at the Future's Group, called *Demproj*.

The fourth family of models incorporates assumptions about behavior associated with the spread of HIV. These models require that a population be divided into several risk groups characterized by specific patterns of sexual behavior. These are generally the most complex models, and they allow interaction of cofactors, such as occurrence of genital ulcers, along with behavioral characteristics. Most of the models that have generated projections of the demographic impact of HIV/AIDS belong in this category.

Other models exist, but this workshop provided the most standardized approach for evaluating the magnitude of the demographic

impact of HIV/AIDS. The results shown in the table are generated by the models on the assumption of intermediate values for the infectivity of HIV. All models listed in the table are capable of producing greater effects on demographic indicators, if infectivity is higher. A model developed by Anderson et al. in 1991 suggested that AIDS may cause population growth rates to become negative if the doubling time of the epidemic is much shorter than assumed in the intermediate scenario.[b] However, there is agreement among the more complex behavioral models that such an outcome is not likely.

---

a. *The AIDS epidemic and its demographic consequences: Proceedings of the UN/WHO workshop on modelling the demographic impact of the AIDS epidemic in Pattern II countries, December 13–15, 1989.* United Nations and World Health Organization (1989).

b. R. M. Anderson, R. M. May, M. C. Boiley, et al., "The spread of HIV-1 in Africa: Sexual contact patterns and the predicted demographic impact of AIDS," *Nature* 352 (1991):581–89.

Millions of People

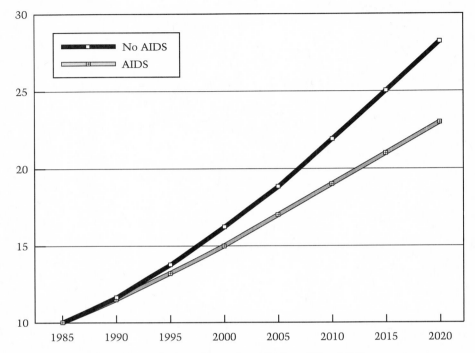

Figure 6.1. Projected population size under AIDS and No-AIDS scenarios, 1985-2020 (hypothetical country).

future, resulting in a gradually increasing percentage of HIV-infected adults. In this hypothetical model, toward the year 2000 the increase in the number of new infections flattens out, and by 2020, the end of the projection period, about 20 percent of adults are HIV-infected. These assumptions make the projection a severe scenario, perhaps consistent with an upper limit to the demographic effect to be expected in severely affected African countries. Of course, the impact could be more severe: several assumptions concerning social and cultural practices, sexual behavior, and disease parameters in the model are based on incomplete knowledge and may therefore be too optimistic. Finally, although the model has been shown to simulate the growth and the impact of the epidemic quite accurately up to the present,[3] there is no guarantee that key assumptions will remain valid in the future. A more detailed description of the model and its assumptions is provided in Appendix 6.1.

Effect on Population Growth

Starting with a population of 10 million in 1985, two scenarios were projected: the first is based on standard World Bank assumptions of the future course of fertility and mortality in the absence of AIDS;[4,5] the second scenario assumes the same trends in fertility, but incorporates mortality from AIDS.

Figure 6.1 shows the projected populations from 1985 to 2020. By the end of the projection period, the no-AIDS scenario shows over 5 million more people than the AIDS scenario. The discrepancy in population builds up very gradually and is hardly noticeable until after 1990. This result is consistent with findings from the most affected sub-Saharan African countries, such as Uganda and Malawi, where the number of AIDS cases has been increasing sharply in the past few years, but population size is not yet affected to a discernible extent. The reason is the multiplier effect of mortality of adults of reproductive age: the deficit of people at this time is almost exclusively due to AIDS mortality, which is only a small proportion of all deaths. Two or three decades from now, the reduced number of people will be due both to AIDS mortality and to births that did not occur because of the additional mortality among women of reproductive age.

Figure 6.2 shows population growth rates for the two scenarios. As fertility is assumed to be progressively reduced after 1995, both scenarios show declining growth rates. The difference between the scenarios is very steady, ranging from 0.5 percent in the early 1990s to 0.8 percent in the early years of the next century. At no point is the effect such that the population starts to decline.

It may appear odd that the effects of even severe HIV infection rates do not have a greater impact on population growth. One reason clearly is the high fertility level—and consequently, high growth rate—that are characteristic of most sub-Saharan African countries. In these above projections, the total fertility rate was initially assumed to be at 6.5 children per woman. If a woman becomes infected with HIV at age 20 and lives until age 30, she is likely to have borne enough children to replace herself before she dies of AIDS. Unfortunately,

Percentage per Year

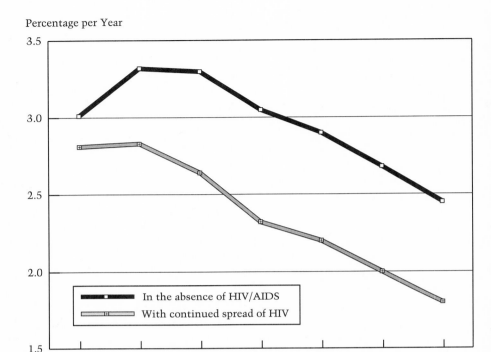

Figure 6.2. Projected population growth rate, 1985-90 to 2015-20 (hypothetical country).

detailed understanding of the interaction between HIV and fertility is very limited, and hypotheses for both a decreasing and an increasing effect of AIDS on fertility have been proposed.[6] Among the latter, it has been suggested that couples may marry earlier in order to reduce the probability of having an infected spouse; early age at marriage is known to increase fertility. In addition, women, perhaps without knowing whether they are infected may have more children to replace those that apparently die from common childhood illnesses, but were in fact HIV infected.

Effects on the Death Rate

Mortality is the demographic indicator most immediately affected by AIDS, and this is clearly noticeable in the projected crude death rate

Per Thousand

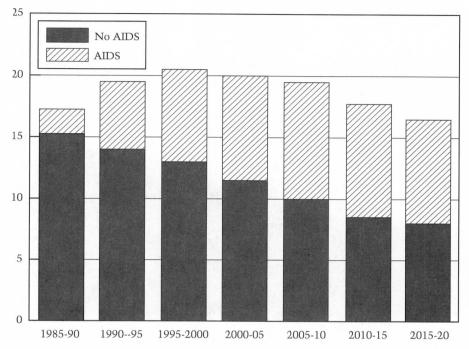

Figure 6.3. Projected crude death rate, 1985-90 to 2015-20 (hypothetical country).

(CDR—the number of deaths per 1,000 population in a given year). Instead of an expected decline, the CDR increases at first and is subsequently and persistently about 10 deaths per 1,000 population higher than without AIDS. Figure 6.3 illustrates the projected trend in the death rate (solid bars) and the additional mortality from AIDS (backslash pattern). From about 2005 on, about half of the entire CDR is attributable to AIDS. Box 6.3 discusses the implications of AIDS for adult mortality rates.

Effect on Life Expectancy at Birth

Population projections made at the World Bank assume that life expectancy at birth increases every calendar year by a given quantity, which varies with the level of life expectancy. For our hypothetical

Percentage of Deaths

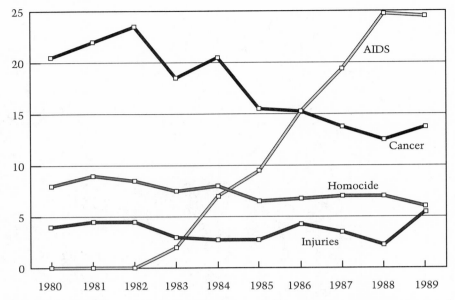

Figure 6.B. Leading causes of death among women 25-39 years, New York City, 1980-1989.
Source: New York City Department of Health Vital Statistics.

Box 6.3: The Impact on Adult Mortality

Even in regions where overall health status is poor, young adult mortality is still a rare event. For example, the probability of an adult death in sub-Saharan Africa is in the order of 5 in 1,000. Here, the impact of AIDS can be quite dramatic. Assume that 10 percent of an adult population is HIV infected. Then, on average, for every 1,000 persons, 100 will carry HIV. Assuming that 5 percent of infected people will develop AIDS each year and that survival is, on average, one year, then AIDS will cause an additional five deaths each year. Thus, at 10 percent prevalence, the adult mortality rate is doubled from 5 to 10 per thousand. Similarly, an HIV prevalence rate of 20 percent results in a trebling of the underlying adult mortality rate; 30 percent will quadruple it. Already in some population subgroups, in both developed and developing countries, AIDS is the leading cause of adult death (e.g., in Abidjan, Côte d'Ivoire) and of women aged 25 to 39 (in New York City; see Figure 6.B).

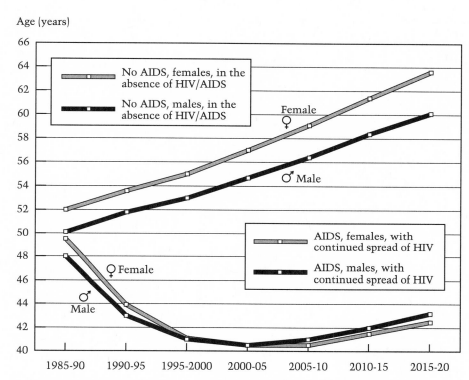

Age (years)

Figure 6.4. Projected life expectancy, male and female, 1985-90 to 2015-20 (hypothetical country).

country projection, Figure 6.4 shows that with AIDS, this trend is reversed; life expectancy at birth declines steeply before leveling off and recovering somewhat. By 2020, life expectancy for males at birth in this scenario is 17 years below projected life expectancy in the no-AIDS scenario; for women the loss in life expectancy is even greater—21 years. A second observation is that where under standard assumptions the gap in life expectancies between women and men would gradually increase, with women living longer than men, the trend is reversed in the AIDS scenario, with women having a shorter life expectancy after the year 2000. Evidence from sub-Saharan Africa suggests that women on average have as high or higher HIV infection rates than do men, which explains this diverging trend.

Per Thousand

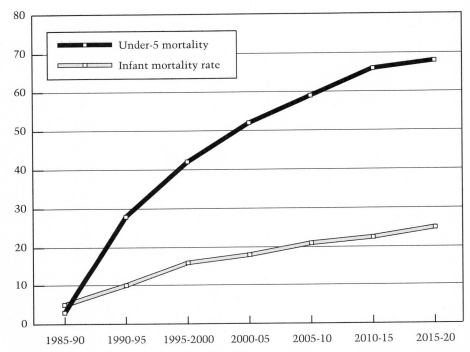

Figure 6.5. Projected relative excess infant mortality rate and under-5 mortality, 1985-90 to 2015-20 (hypothetical country).

Effect on Infant and Child Mortality

The recent gains in child survival are likely to be reversed, particularly in countries where HIV prevalence is high among pregnant women.[7] In these projections, it is assumed, based on studies from sub-Saharan Africa, that 1 out of 3 children born to an infected mother will be HIV infected. Because HIV-infected infants have a much shorter survival time than do HIV-infected adults, the effects of AIDS on infants and children are visible earlier than for adults. Figure 6.5 shows the excess in the infant mortality rate (IMR) and under-5 mortality rate (q5) resulting from AIDS mortality compared with the no-AIDS scenario. Because most HIV-infected infants survive their first year but die

Dependency Ratio (x 100)

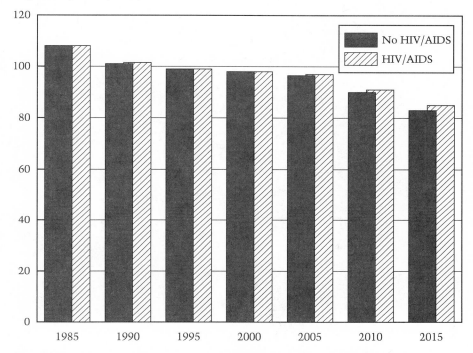

Figure 6.6. Projected dependency ratio, 1985-2015 (hypothetical country).

before reaching age 5, the effect on the under-5 mortality rate is much more pronounced than on the infant mortality rate.

Effect on Dependency Ratio

The dependency ratio is defined as the ratio of the population under age 15 and over 65 to those between 15 and 64. The dependency ratio in this model is shown to be affected only slightly (see Figure 6.6). In a typical sub-Saharan country, AIDS affects 2 age groups in particular: to the greatest extent, young adults; to a somewhat lesser extent, children under five. But the different survival times after initial HIV infection (an estimated median of 10 years for adults, 2 to 3 years for children) have the effect of keeping the dependency ratio practically unchanged. The absence of an increase in the dependency burden at

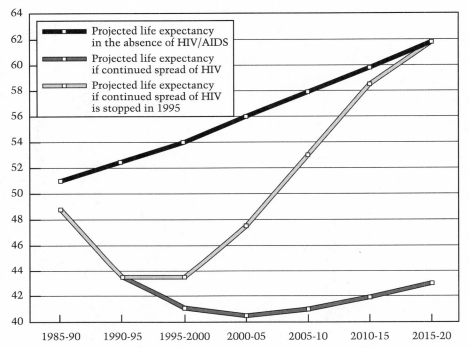

Age (years)

Figure 6.7. Projected life expectancy at birth, various scenarios, 1985-90 to 2015-20 (hypothetical country).

the aggregate level does not mean that individual families are not severely affected. Projections of the percentage of children under 15 experiencing orphanhood in a severely affected country, such as Uganda, show that this may be double as a result of AIDS mortality.[8]

Effect of Interventions

The AIDS scenario projection was made assuming no change in sexual behavior during the entire period 1975 to 2020. What would be the demographic impact if in 1995 HIV infection would stop spreading, that is, if no new infections would occur? This is clearly an unlikely scenario, but addressing this question is, nevertheless, instructive. A projection was made with no new HIV infections after 1995. Figures

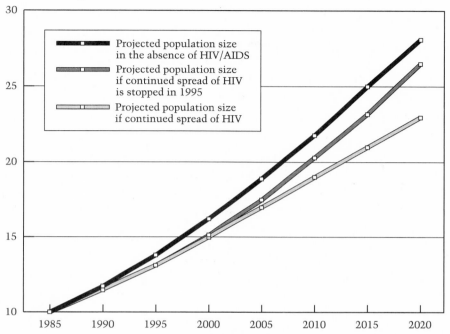

Figure 6.8. Projected population size, various scenarios, 1985-2020 (hypothetical country).

6.7 and 6.8 show the effect on life expectancy and on population size. Initially, life expectancy drops well below its no-AIDS projected levels as adults infected before 1995 develop the disease and die. It then recovers rapidly, mainly because there are fewer infected infants dying, and it regains the no-AIDS level by the end of the projection period. The deficit in total population (Figure 6.8) is shown to increase for another decade before stabilizing at about 93 percent of the no-AIDS projection. Even if the projection were to be extended further into the future with the same levels and trends in vital rates, population would remain below the numbers in the no-AIDS scenario.

Demographic indicators, such as infant and child mortality and life expectancy, are often used to monitor progress in economic development, in conjunction with such measures as Gross National

Product (GNP) per capita. The model described here, which is consistent with observed trends in the prevalence of HIV infection, demonstrates that demographic indicators are already beginning to be undermined in places where the AIDS epidemic had its start in the late 1970s. As the next section demonstrates, this has important consequences for economic development.

ECONOMIC IMPACT

The health status of the people in any country is a critical element in the growth of its economy as well as an important factor in overall quality of life. Because AIDS tends to selectively affect young adults, it will influence a wide range of social and economic factors. The specific impact of the pandemic on certain sectors and, within these sectors, on certain critical elements can be predicted with sufficient confidence to alert policy, and decisionmakers and the public. For other sectors, however, the direction and magnitude of the medium- and short-term effects of the pandemic are still unclear. They are likely to vary from one situation to another as the pandemic continues to evolve.

A conceptual framework (see Table 6.1) shows the types of impacts that the HIV/AIDS pandemic may have on various sectors: health, social, education, agriculture, and industry and trade. The impact is examined for three levels: individual; household, family, community, and production unit; and national. Within each cell in the table, key impact issues resulting from HIV/AIDS have been noted. This list of impact issues is neither exhaustive nor relevant to all situations. It can, however, be used for exploring the broad consequences of the pandemic. Specific examples are presented to illustrate the range, direction, and magnitude of the impact of the pandemic in various regions in the world.

The main channel through which AIDS will affect economic performance will be changes in the size and quality of the household or economywide labor force with its associated adverse effects on productivity levels.[9] In the developing world, not only are prevalence levels generally higher, but the epidemic is an additional burden for many countries already struggling with heavy debt loads, fragile econ-

Table 6.1: Selected sectoral impacts of HIV/AIDS

Level/sector	Individual	Household/family/ community/production unit	National
Population and health			
	Morbidity	Triage for medical care	Increased demand for services
	Mortality	Fertility trends	Need for prevention and care
	Undernutrition	Change in dependency ratios	Need to expand health infrastructure
	Disability	Change in infant/child mortality	Population movement in response to the epidemic
	Emotional trauma		
Economic			
Health	Increased expenditure	Increased expenditure	Need to expand health infrastructure
	Fewer resources per head	Lower expenditure on other preventive medicine and on public health programs	Competition for resources within health sector
	Reduced standards of care	Reduced standards of care	Need to reconsider resource allocation within the health sector
			Need to reconsider resource allocation between health and other sectors
			Displacement of people with curable illnesses
Education	Absenteeism	Decreased value of future human capital	Loss of trained people
	Reduced labor productivity	Need for duplication of training and education	Decreased value of future human capital

Table 6.1 (cont.): Selected sectoral impacts of HIV/AIDS

Level/sector	Individual	Household/family/ community/production unit	National
	Reduced resource availability	Shortage of teachers	Declining level of education
	Exclusion from international training/studies	Fewer community resources for education	Loss of educators
	Poorer standards as educator numbers decline	Lower literacy and numeracy rates	Reduced performance in education-/skill-dependent activities
Industry and trade	Loss of productivity	Increased emigration	Effects on tourism
	Reduced capacity for investment	Decreased household/family productivity	Effects on international trade and terms of trade as overall labor productivity declines
	Reduced opportunities for overseas employment	Lower industrial productivity	Impact on foreign exchange as economy is newly perceived by overseas investors
	Increased costs of foreign specialists—result of both their increased scarcity value and overheads such as insurance and medical protection plus risk premiums	Loss of community purchasing power	Possible restriction on movements of nationals by health/residence regulation in other countries
		Time costs of absenteeism, health care, funeral attendance for employees	Decline in remittances as national workers are less able to undertake labor migration
		Need to supplement locally trained work force	Additional cost of foreign specialists

Table 6.1 (cont.): Selected sectoral impacts of HIV/AIDS

Level/sector	Individual	Household/family/ community/production unit	National
Agriculture	Loss of productivity	Reduction in cultivated area	Threat to food security—particularly in already dry, eroded, or low-fertility areas
	Constraints on women's participation in food production	Possible expansion of pests in bush (e.g., tsetse)	Additional foreign exchange costs in attempt to replace lost labor by capital (e.g., rotary cultivators)
	Constraints on women's participation in cash crop production	Labor shortages	Overall reduction in national food availability
		Reduction of range of food and cash crops grown in response to labor shortage	Change in composition and value of agriculture
		Reduction in handicraft production and level of maintenance of rural infrastructure (e.g., terracing, irrigation works)	Loss of foreign exchange earnings from reduced cash crop production
		Generalized property disputes	
		Tenure disputes in relation to orphans and widows of land holders	

Table 6.1 (cont.): Selected sectoral impacts of HIV/AIDS

Level/sector	Individual	Household/family/community/production unit	National
Sociopolitical			
Differentiation	Differentiated access in employment, travel, access to health care, health/life insurance, access to credit	Increased social differentiation as effects are felt more profoundly by poor as opposed to wealthy households/families	Social and political tension associated with population movement, anomie, and reduced resource base
	Differentiated access to housing	Age becomes additionally disadvantaged as care providers die young	Problem of supporting the elderly
		Age becomes disadvantaged as orphan burden grows	Problem of caring for and educating orphans
		Increased differentiation in level of life between affected and unaffected households and communities	Intercommunal tensions
Power relations	Stigmatized widows less able to protect their livelihood strategies	Widows lose economic security, seek other income opportunities, may turn to prostitution	Increased stigmatization of women—change in women's social and political position
	Health workers gain power as they offer health favors		

Table 6.1 (cont.): Selected sectoral impacts of HIV/AIDS

Level/sector	Individual	Household/family/ community/production unit	National
Market position	Stigmatized workers less employable Differentiated access to credit	Localized unemployment and underemployment	Increased numbers of people searching for means of survival Increased national poverty decreases international resource flows and solidarity Increased dependence on donors
Kinship/family	Renegotiation of existing obligations and rights	Uncertainty about care and other rights and obligations Orphan care becomes problematic as existing coping strategies come under stress Widening age gap between men and women at first intercourse and at marriage	
Culture/beliefs	Stigmas attached to behavior and HIV/AIDS status Search for solutions—rise of millenarianism and healing cults Anomie	Stigmas on group sharing behavior—exacerbation of existing social stigma (e.g., caste, ethnicity, class) Revision of customary beliefs	

Table 6.1 (cont.): Selected sectoral impacts of HIV/AIDS

Level/sector	Individual	Household/family/ community/production unit	National
Locational	People move away from home after relatives' deaths	Depopulation	Urban-rural migration/rural-urban migration Restrictions on refugee and other cross-border movements
Groups/ organizations	Discrimination in work, educational, and other organizations—interpersonal tension in work, leisure, and other organizations	Reduced effectiveness of any organization in which human resource reduction and interpersonal suspicion exist	Reduced effectiveness of government/ administrative/ judical/legal and military structures

Source: This framework was produced by the editors and the authors of the chapter, with additional input by Tony Barnett, School of Development Studies, University of East Anglia, Norwich, England.

omies, high poverty levels, limited government resources, scarce human capital, and food insecurity. AIDS will have serious implications for the development process in countries hard hit by AIDS. For countries where the pandemic is still in its early phases, the consequences now faced by severely affected countries highlight the importance of effective prevention.

Adults in their prime sexual and most productive ages are among those most infected. Yet unlike other diseases that disproportionately strike the poor, AIDS does not spare the occupational or urban elite. In some African capitals, HIV appears to have initially spread more rapidly among higher socioeconomic classes. AIDS is already the leading cause of adult death in Abidjan, Côte d'Ivoire,[10] and about 20 percent of adults in Kampala, Uganda, are HIV infected. Although infection rates in some African urban centers may be double those in rural areas, there is increasing evidence that rural rates are increasing and catching up with urban rates. This may be attributable to improved reporting, but it is also plausible that urban-to-rural migration, especially movements of high-risk groups (for example, soldiers, or commercial sex workers in Thailand and India returning to home villages), is contributing to the spread of the virus in rural areas. Transmission along major trucking routes in Africa is noticeable, with high prevalence levels among truck drivers.[11]

SERVICE AND INDUSTRIAL SECTORS

The HIV/AIDS pandemic will pose serious challenges to economic growth through its impact on the service and industrial sectors. At the company level, HIV/AIDS morbidity is likely to reduce productivity. Recent reports from copper-mining industries—a labor-intensive sector—in central and southern Africa illustrate growing concern about the impact of AIDS on the availability of miners and trained staff, leading to declines in production.[12] HIV-related illnesses will also boost companies' medical expenditures through employee health programs. Many firms provide health and other social services not only to employees but to their dependents as well; given the high probability of heterosexual transmission in couples and infection of infants, there will be further increases in medical outlays.

Eventual mortality also entails significant costs for death benefits and funerals. In addition to the lost investment made in training employees, the costs involved in recruiting and training replacements—especially highly skilled and experienced workers—are already beginning to escalate. This could mean having to pay higher wages to attract scarce skilled workers. Ironically, the positive impact of prevention campaigns may have negative consequences for the viability of other sectors. The most notable is the tourism sector in Thailand, where the entire industry has been affected.[13]

AGRICULTURE

The rural sector will not escape the impacts of the epidemic. Although infection rates are generally lower in rural areas throughout much of the developing world, most people still live there, so that absolute numbers of people infected in rural areas will be higher. For countries where the bulk of agricultural produce is labor intensive and grown on smallholder plots, shortages of able-bodied adults may lower over-all agricultural yields. Whether farming systems are vulnerable to labor loss depends on the organization of labor and its supply.[14] On the demand side, shortages of labor will probably surface during the peak seasons of planting and harvesting. On the supply side, the age and gender composition of those most productive and their vulnerability to HIV infection (for example, women in an agricultural household) will help identify households or systems that are particularly sensitive to labor loss.

Not only will the impact of an adult AIDS death drastically curtail labor, but illness before death and the time other household members spend caring for those infected will also reduce productivity. Household resources—otherwise used to purchase agricultural inputs, such as labor or fertilizers—may be diverted for such expenses as medical treatment and, later, funeral costs.[15] Reduced inputs, in turn, mean further reductions in household resources.

The links between AIDS, nutrition, and food security are complex. Extreme weight loss is one hallmark of AIDS. But distinguishing between AIDS and malnutrition may be difficult without testing for HIV. The indirect effects of AIDS within households on the food security and the nutritional status of surviving family members are likely to be substantial. The productive capacity, purchasing power, and per capita food availability of a household are all likely to be reduced when adults die. Disruption—even dissolution—of family structures because of AIDS is likely to increase food insecurity and malnutrition: extended families that take in orphans will spread food resources more thinly.

Coping mechanisms involving decisions on labor allocation are not well understood. Children may do more of the work as families struggle to maintain current cropping patterns. Nonessential activities, such as weeding and pruning, may be curtailed. If a household becomes unable either to supply labor internally or to hire temporary workers, the composition of crops may be altered. Established patterns of many smallholders in Africa indicate that subsistence needs are usually met first, with marketable crops grown thereafter. Farmers might incrementally reduce labor-intensive or cash crops rather than drop them altogether, but that will depend on the coping mechanisms as well as on underlying factors, such as population density, soil fertility, rural infrastructure, and migration.[16]

Overall, as was the case with many plagues and epidemics in the past, the short- and medium-term socioeconomic consequences could be severe, but in the long term, families, communities, and nations will make adjustments to cope with the increased mortality. If labor becomes a truly binding constraint, technological changes to conserve or replace human labor may emerge. If AIDS is widespread and wages are increased, migration could also play an equilibrating role. What is clear, however, is that more information is needed about how the disease will alter development prospects in individual countries with differing resource endowments.

EDUCATION

Investing in people through improved health, education, and nutrition—particularly in women—is not simply a desirable end in itself; it is the key to higher productivity and growth in the long term. In many developing countries, especially where skilled labor is scarce, the AIDS epidemic poses a serious threat to the further development of human capital by potentially reversing recent gains in the quality and longevity of life.

Families with an AIDS illness or death will be less able to invest in their children's education, in part because of other expenditures on medical care and reduced disposable income.[17] Children may also be required to spend more time at home performing work normally carried out by adults. In addition, when students develop HIV-related illness, the benefits of many years of education are jeopardized.

HEALTH SECTOR

One of the most immediate and visible impacts of the AIDS epidemic in both developed and developing countries is in the health sector. As more and more HIV-infected individuals develop AIDS, the demand for health care is likely to rise at a rapid, even exponential rate. Figure 6.9 shows the incidence of AIDS cases for the hypothetical African country discussed earlier.

One obvious effect is that expenditures will rise both in absolute terms and as a percentage of overall expenditure in the health sector. Early attempts to estimate the economic consequences of the epi-

Thousands

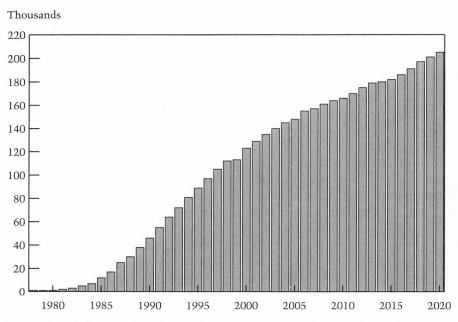

Figure 6.9. Projected AIDS incidence, 1980-2020 (hypothetical country).

demic tried to quantify how much it would cost to treat an individual with AIDS, frequently called the *direct cost* of AIDS.[18] Although the data are limited, the orders of magnitude are strikingly different for developed and developing countries when expressed as a percentage of health expenditures. In the United States, about 1 percent of total health care expenditures is spent on HIV/AIDS. The few available data on overall cost implications of the AIDS epidemic in developing countries suggest that it will consume significant amounts of current expenditures on health care.[19-22] In some sub-Saharan African countries, AIDS consumes anywhere from one-quarter to more than half of the government's spending on health.[23] Nevertheless, the incremental cost that this new epidemic poses in absolute terms is staggering. (For further discussion on the global cost of care, see Chapter 11.)

In examining the cost implications of the HIV/AIDS pandemic, a common trend has emerged in both developed and developing countries. As more and more HIV-positive individuals develop AIDS, there has been a noticeable shift away from caring for AIDS patients in a hospital-based setting toward more emphasis on hospice, home, or community-based care with outpatient support. Yet, while decentralizing care may reduce hospital costs, it is also likely to shift the cost—both financial and physical—onto the families and friends of people with AIDS.[24]

Even before AIDS, many developing countries were straining to improve the general health of their populations. Now they must also cope with growing demands for health personnel, drugs, and hospital beds—increasingly in Africa, many occupants of hospital wards are HIV infected. In Mamo Yemo Hospital in Kinshasa, Zaire, which always operates at beyond full capacity, 50 percent of internal medicine admissions are HIV infected.[25] The opportunity costs of treating illnesses in terminal AIDS patients could be enormous, compared with highly cost-effective preventive measures for treatment of patients with curable ailments. (See also Chapter 10, "Providing Care.")

In industrialized countries, the emerging issue is less about how much of health care budgets is devoted to HIV/AIDS, but rather who bears the cost. The response depends on the type of health care system, with a clear distinction between Western Europe and the United States.

In most Western European countries, health care is financed predominantly by the public sector. The United Kingdom, Denmark, and Italy, for example, have a comprehensive national health system and finance AIDS care primarily through general tax revenues. Countries such as France have a mixture of compulsory national health insurance schemes (employment based) with state support for the unemployed. Over time, an increasing share of total spending on AIDS prevention and control activities has gone to patient care, reflecting the progression of HIV-infected populations to AIDS, increased duration of survival with AIDS, and availability of new (and often expensive) therapeutic and prophylactic interventions. In the United Kingdom, for instance, where the Department of Health provides earmarked funds to health authorities for services related to HIV/AIDS, only £500,000 (less than $1 million) was spent for AIDS in 1986, all on prevention activities. By 1988, £25 million was allocated for patient care, representing 35 percent of all public expenditures for AIDS. By 1991, this share had risen to 62 percent, or £126 million—

more than $200 million.[26] However, the 1991 figures represented less than 1 percent of total public expenditure on health that year in the United Kingdom.

Estimates for other countries in Western Europe yield similar proportions. Although national health budgets in Europe are clearly not being overwhelmed by AIDS, issues have arisen over the concentration and distribution of AIDS resources. In Denmark, for example, people with AIDS are treated in only three designated hospitals, while health budgets are allocated to counties. The direct cost per AIDS patient is now being calculated in order to redistribute funds from national treatment sites to counties of residence so that care can take place within the community.[27] In other countries, such as France, access to health care—including for HIV/AIDS-related illnesses—may not be universal, even with social insurance for those unemployed. Not just the unemployed, but also the homeless and illegal immigrants may be unable, or unwilling, to seek health care through public providers.

In the United States, caring for people with AIDS has again highlighted a major underlying problem of the U.S. health care system: the lack of universal health care coverage. More than thirty million Americans have no form of public or private health insurance; most cannot afford health insurance or qualify for federally subsidized Medicaid.[28] It is estimated that approximately one-quarter of those with AIDS have no health insurance at all.[29] Thus, an increasing share of the costs of AIDS care is being assumed by public sector health facilities which are not reimbursed fully by government Medicaid/Medicare programs.

Nevertheless, the insurance industry, too, has seen the effects of AIDS. Estimated AIDS-related claims paid by the life and health insurance industry in the United States during 1990 totaled $1.2 billion, an increase of approximately 17 percent over the previous year. But the overall figure hides important differences. Life insurance claims related to AIDS in 1990 continued to rise as a percentage of total claims, while health insurance claims for AIDS remained level (approximately 1.4 percent of all claims).[30] This relatively constant share of health insurance claims supports the observation that the public sector's share of AIDS care financing is rising as HIV infection increases in lower income groups, who are less likely to be covered by private insurance, and as the incidence of new HIV infections declines among homosexual and bisexual men. Improved medical management and reduced hospitalization could also help limit increases in health insurance claims. Finally, some employees may prefer not to file claims for certain HIV/AIDS-related illnesses for fear of losing their jobs if the employers find out that they are HIV infected.

■■■■■■   .   .   .

SOCIAL IMPACT

As heterosexual contact becomes increasingly the main mode of HIV transmission worldwide, women and children will become more vulnerable, both as potential AIDS casualties and as survivors. The implications are serious, given that in many developing countries—particularly in Africa—women are not only the main care providers, but are also largely responsible for food production, agricultural labor, and the raising of children.

Another cause of deep concern is the children who are not infected with HIV, but whose mothers are HIV-infected. In addition to the nearly 2.3 million pediatric HIV infections projected worldwide by 1995, *AIDS in the World* estimates that there may be 3.7 million orphans in Africa alone. In 10 central and east African countries, it has been estimated that between 6 and 11 percent of the total population under 15 years will be orphaned by the turn of the century.[31] Often the responsibility to feed, clothe, shelter, and educate these children falls on extended families or on elderly grandparents with little means of financial or physical support. Of growing concern is the ability of widows and orphans to acquire property rights (especially land) after the death of a male head of household. Without access to means of production, widows and children may be forced into petty theft or commercial sex work to support themselves—a vicious cycle that could contribute to increased rates of HIV infection.

The AIDS pandemic has brought to the foreground, often in dramatic fashion, social inequities that otherwise might have continued to receive little attention. The issues of financing care for people with HIV and AIDS, including the need for counseling and outreach services, have highlighted underlying weaknesses in health care systems, particularly in the quality and extent of services. The pandemic has also drawn together people who are infected, affected, or otherwise concerned with the urgent need to curb the spread of HIV and to provide better care to people with HIV and AIDS. Community-based organizations—the first to respond to the HIV pandemic in industrialized countries—are playing an increasing and increasingly important role in the developing world. The mobilization of people who are exposed or opposed to inequity, prejudice, and discrimination because they are infected with HIV, are women, homosexuals, commercial sex workers, injection drug users, or prisoners, or belong to certain ethnic or socioeconomic groups, has led to the recognition that these people have their own needs and demands.

Financial and technical resources have been provided to help developing countries in their efforts to prevent HIV transmission and care for affected people. Although these resources fell short of meeting needs and may have resulted in a reallocation of globally declining international aid, they enabled many countries to improve public information, provide more effective training of health workers, and set in place better systems for blood transfusion or programs for preventing and controlling sexually transmitted diseases.

CONCLUSION

This review of the impact of HIV/AIDS on demography, economy, and society illustrates some effects of the pandemic as observed today and those that can be reasonably projected for the future. Although this review could conclude by stressing further the gravity of the global situation, rather it should stimulate an enhanced response worldwide to both expand prevention efforts and to care more effectively for persons infected and affected by the pandemic. The monitoring and evaluation of AIDS programs are still weak: there is insufficient understanding of what should be measured and how; there is also a lack of commitment to critical and objective assessment of the effects—or lack thereof—of programs or interventions. Social, behavioral, and economic research leadership and effort are desperately required, not only to improve understanding of the dynamics of the pandemic and its impact, but also to be translated, as never before, into public health and societal action and an ever more solid understanding of the inextricable relationship between the individual and public health and between health and society.

PART TWO

. . . .

The Global Response

There have been four distinct phases in the global response to the HIV/AIDS pandemic. In the first phase, from the mid-1970s until 1981, the presence of a new pandemic was not suspected. HIV spread, silently and unnoticed, to all inhabited continents. There is a great global lesson in this experience, for the modern world is uniquely favorable to global spread of infectious agents. Whether new microbiological threats to health emerge as isolated ecologies are brought into contact with the rest of the world, or old agents mutate or extend their range through changes in human behavior and ecology, or a new infectious agent emerges, the fundamental need will be to detect it as rapidly as possible so as to respond with efficiency and effectiveness. HIV illustrates that a seemingly obscure health event in one place can become, within a short time, a health crisis at home. The world was fortunate that this first, silent period of the HIV/AIDS pandemic was short; recognition of AIDS might easily have been delayed for an additional 5 or 10 years—with enormous consequences for global health.

The second phase started with the recognition of AIDS in 1981 and lasted until about 1985. This period of discovery and initial response was marked by tremendous scientific creativity and progress. The power of epidemiology was again demonstrated, as the routes oftransmission were determined—and prevention recommendations formulated accordingly—even before the etiologic agent, HIV, was identified. The scientific achievements of this period stand in stark contrast to the generally slow societal response to AIDS. From 1981 to 1985, few nations responded actively to AIDS, and international organizations were relatively passive. Therefore, HIV progressed almost unimpeded in the world during this period, despite the work of many community and nongovernmental organizations that arose to confront AIDS.

The third phase, of global mobilization, started in 1985–86. By early 1990, the world's first truly global strategy against a disease was developed; more importantly, it was implemented as a common strategy for community, national, and international action. In an unprecedented manner, with speed and intensity, national AIDS programs were created around the world, and a measure of international solidarity emerged in response to the common perception of threat. Solidarity was symbolized by the October 1987 special session on AIDS at the United Nations General Assembly—the first time that the UN General Assembly debated a disease. The resulting resolution called for coordinated and strong international action. Solidarity was also present in January 1988 in London, as more ministers of health gathered for the Global Summit on AIDS than had ever assembled before, for any purpose. Thus, between 1986 and 1989, the pace of the work against AIDS was closing the gap with the continued spread of the pandemic.

In the fourth, and current, phase, as this section will demonstrate, commitment and resources have now reached a plateau. Yet the pandemic is intensifying; the gap between the pace of the pandemic and our response to it is growing once again, and widening dangerously.

CHAPTER SEVEN

. . . .

Achievements in Research

s chapter was written
Oliver Morton, science
d technology editor of
e *Economist* magazine,
ndon, and other
ntributors.

Seen against the backdrop of history, the rapidity of the response of science to the AIDS pandemic has been remarkable. In 10 years, a causative agent—the human immunodeficiency virus (HIV)—has been identified, its genes mapped and analyzed, drugs that act against it found and tried, and vaccines developed to a preclinical stage. AIDS research has quickly approached, and often surpassed, the frontiers of traditional science, spanning the disciplines of basic biomedical, clinical, epidemiological, and social sciences. This response is all the more remarkable considering the complexity of HIV*—its *virological* variability, the fact that not one but two agents must be contended with (HIV-1 and HIV-2)[1] and the difficulties of identifying its pathogenic mechanisms.[2] It is tempting to call this kind of progress unprecedented. For the first time, activism is playing a major role as a catalyst for faster research, drug development and approval, and more resources, while also inspiring other disease-specific advocacy movements. Political and moral issues have emerged, provoking debate over whether too much or too little is being spent on AIDS. Although epidemiological and clinical research has focused primarily on men, advocates are calling for more natural history studies and clinical trials involving women and children. However, research into the so-

---

*The focus of this chapter is on HIV-1 and all references to HIV concern HIV-1 unless otherwise stated.

called soft-sciences—social, behavioral, prevention—has yet to come of age.

Thus, as AIDS research progresses, it is worth posing a series of questions: What have been the results of 10 years of work, and what is on the horizon? What is the status of development of antivirals, therapeutics for prevention and treatment of opportunistic infections and malignancies, immunoregulators, and alternate therapies? What vaccines are at what phase in clinical trials, and when might a vaccine be available and to whom? What is the role of social and behavioral research? Will there be enough funding in a time of recession and growing donor or governmental fatigue? Is a "Manhattan project" approach viable? This chapter also seeks to measure the current state of HIV/AIDS research through an analysis of funding for national and international research, allocation of resources to various research sectors, focus of cohort and behavioral studies, and the production of scientific papers.

Box 7.1: AIDS Activism: A Model for Disease-Specific Advocacy?

Excerpted from Robert Wachter, M.D., "AIDS, Activism, and the Politics of Health," adapted and reprinted with permission of the *New England Journal of Medicine* 326(2) (1992):128–33

Modeled on the remarkable success of the AIDS activist movement, new groups have come to appreciate the power of disease-specific advocacy movements in influencing health policy. Thus far, 2 groups—representing patients with breast cancer and Alzheimer's disease—have taken up the gauntlet, demanding a greater voice in policy making and a larger share of funding. We can expect that additional disease-specific advocacy movements will emerge in the future.

What effect will these groups have on overall health policy? Advocates for patients with different diseases might form powerful coalitions of health consumers, since the groups' members have a number of issues of concern in common. For example, the lobbies for AIDS, breast cancer and Alzheimer's disease may work in concert to improve access to health care for all Americans, expedite the approval process at the FDA for all drugs, and fight discrimination against victims of all diseases.

On the other hand, disease-specific activist groups may find themselves pitted against one another as they advocate their own interests. This possibility raises two matters of concern. First, it will render the players in the health policy arena increasingly fractious, making collaborative and multidisciplinary work more hazardous. Second, and perhaps more worrisome, if advocates for AIDS, breast cancer, and Alzheimer's disease succeed in garnering larger slices of the resource pie for their groups and the overall health budget remains static, smaller and smaller slices will be left for other groups that support equally deserving causes but that lack activists to argue on their behalf.

Because AIDS activists have

When the history of the first decade of the AIDS pandemic is written, research efforts may be characterized as incremental progress resulting from a series of small but significant steps. Yet while science seeks a cure or vaccine, the social disciplines of prevention and behavioral research must bear a large share of the responsibility for slowing the spread of AIDS. Still, most people today, whether already affected by AIDS or fearing the future, look to science for a cure or vaccine—a so-called magic bullet. Whether and how soon that bullet can be found are the questions of the decade, if not of this century and the next.

■■■■■■■■■■   .   .   .

THERAPEUTICS AND MEDICINES

The identification of the first AIDS cases by Los Angeles clinicians in 1981 opened a new and difficult chapter in scientific history and triggered the research effort now underway. But there is general agree-

---

demonstrated the degree of influence that a well-organized, highly motivated advocacy group can have, we can be certain that the empowerment of patients will be a major part of the American social landscape of the 1990s. In this new order, some health professionals will view a powerful consumer movement as a direct threat to their competence and power. Without question, having our patients and research subjects ask—or demand—to have an active voice in what we do and how we do it will at times be difficult, laborious, and even unpleasant. It is also undeniably right.

Rather than feel threatened, we as physicians and researchers should embrace this movement and, whenever possible, work with our patients and their advocates toward our many shared goals. Together, we form a coalition—albeit a fragile

one—with immense power to shape health policy. We have far more to gain from pooling our strengths than from emphasizing our differences.

To what extent is this movement of patient activism a U.S. phenomenon and to what extent is it becoming increasingly international? There are excellent opportunities (e.g., International AIDS Conferences) for developing transnational networks among people concerned about AIDS. Then, what about linkage with other health groups and broader health concerns? Is the current global vision of health adequate for the task? In our view, the articulation of a vision sufficiently broad and powerful to help disease-specific activists find common cause for health is urgently needed.
—The Editors

Table 7.1: AIDS medicines in development in the United States or by U.S.-affiliate pharmaceuticals, 1987–1991

	1987	1988	1989	1990	1991
Summary of survey results					
Approved medicines	1	2	9	11	14
Medicines/vaccines in development	27	46	55	62	88
Companies developing medicines/vaccines	30	39	39	40	64
Results by development status					
Phase I	15	13	22	18	28
Phase I/II	3	10	13	25	15
Phase II	2	12	11	7	22
Phase II/III	3	4	8	18	18
Phase III	2	6	6	14	16
Phase I/II/III	0	0	1	0	0
Application submitted	1	3	1	1	5
In clinical tests	1	2	3	0	0
Results by product class					
Antiviral	15	13	17	27	34
Cytokines	a	a	11	16	12
Immunomodulators	12	25	7	10	12
Anti-infectives	a	6	16	19	23
Vaccines	0	2	2	2	7
Others	a	a	2	3	8
Total research projects[b]	27	46	55	77	96

Source: Pharmaceutical Manufacturers Association (USA) (December 1991).

Note: By the end of 1991, 14 AIDS medicines had been approved in the United States, arguably the nation with the strictest regulations and the bellwether for other nations' approval of such drugs. At least 88 medicines were in development by U.S. or U.S.-affiliate pharmaceutical companies for AIDS and AIDS-related conditions, representing a 42 percent increase over 1990 and 300 percent more than in 1987.

a. Category was not included in survey that year.

b. Reflects medicines in development for more than one use.

ment that without prior decades of basic scientifc investigation, the building of a foundation for current research on AIDS would have been far more difficult.[3] HIV is a lentivirus, consisting of an RNA genome wrapped in viral protein and cellular membrane. It infects cells carrying the surface molecule CD4. That means primarily the subset of immune system cells that "help" others in their tasks, but also includes a wide range of other cell types, from the immune system to the gut and the brain. When inside the cell, the virus transcribes its genes from RNA to DNA, which can then be slotted into the cell's own genes. At some later point, it will make copies of its genes, direct the cell to make the proteins it needs, and start to reproduce itself.

Many details of the life cycle of HIV are still unclear. The roles of many of the seven regulatory genes in the viral genome are not fully understood, although one of them, the *tat* gene, is agreed to be important in starting viral replication.[4] The mechanisms by which the virus actually causes immune system damage in people with AIDS and others infected with HIV are not understood, but such studies of pathogenesis are a major research focus (see "HIV Virus Variability" later in this chapter). Answers will be needed as therapeutic issues become more complicated, for example, in order to suggest at what stage various therapies might be most effective. In addition, research into the viral life cycle is widely justified on the basis of cutting the process up as finely as possible, thus revealing its weakest links. These weak links, it is hoped, will be amenable to therapeutic attack.

Antiviral Therapy

Only one stage in the process has so far yielded to disruption on any practical scale: reverse transcription. Reverse transcriptase (RT), an enzyme carried by the virus, makes DNA copies of HIV's RNA genes. The drug zidovudine (AZT), marketed by Burroughs Wellcome as Retrovir®, appears to block this process by mimicking one of the chemicals RT has to use. Once taken up by the enzyme it is thought to block its action. AZT was approved for use in the United States in 1987 and is now the so-called "gold standard"[5] of care as an anti-retroviral treatment. It does not prolong life indefinitely, and it can have severe side effects.

In 1991, a second RT inhibitor, ddI, marketed by Bristol-Myers Squibb as VIDEX®, was approved. A third drug, ddC, Hivid®, produced by Hoffmann-La Roche, has received approval from the U.S. Food and Drug Administration for use in combination with AZT. AZT and the newcomers are not necessarily alternatives, but may be administered in tandem. For example, the side effects resulting from using ddI or ddC differ from those associated with AZT. This is useful for individuals no longer able to tolerate the first drug and may mean that taking lower doses of two, rather than high doses of one, is a useful option. Trials have shown benefits from combined AZT/ddI and AZT/ddC treatments.

A further spur in the direction of multiple-drug therapies (already common in the treatment of cancer, leprosy, and other diseases) is the problem of resistance. Reverse transcription is error prone at copying RNA into DNA, making, on average, one error every time it copies out the genome. This makes all the genes in HIV highly mutable—including the reverse transcription gene. In laboratory studies, viral strains can become resistant to AZT, presumably because they develop mutant RTs immune to its influences. This could be bad news, and although there is no firm evidence to show that this biological resistance causes clinical symptoms, it is true that virus samples from people using AZT eventually show resistance.

Other drugs are also being developed to block RT. Some are similar to the first three, while others work slightly differently. These non-nucleoside-analogue RT inhibitors do not resemble the building blocks of DNA and thus may do less harm to the host than do nucleoside analogues. In laboratory studies, they look highly promising. However, at least some appear to suffer from severe viral resistance problems. The viral enzyme mutates in such a way as to evade these drugs easily. For this reason, two of these drugs, Boehringer Ingelheim's BI-RG 587, or nevirapene, and Merck's L-697,661 were withdrawn from trials in late 1991.

Three other points in the viral life cycle have been targeted for intensive drug development so far: entry, activation, and protein processing. One has failed, the other two have yet to be proven. There was, in the mid- to late-1980s, considerable interest in using genetically engineered CD4 to decoy the virus and keep it from entering cells. Such drugs, after large investments of time, effort, skill, and money, have so far failed to show widespread and worthwhile clinical effects. Laboratory work has shown that the virus particles in patients' bodies show considerably less affinity for the synthetic CD4s than do particles of the standard viral strain used in laboratories. This has led to a change in research directions and practice in many laboratories. Although standard strains grown in cell culture are still used for much work, virus freshly isolated from infected people is preferred as a way to check key results.

Two other targets now being tried are further along in the virus's life cycle. One of them, the activation process mediated by the product of the *tat* gene, is at present causing some excitement. This is due to the course of HIV infection within the body. After an initial period marked by a brief flu-like fever, there is a latency period prior to the onset of AIDS. This latency period, during which the immune system enters decline and various illnesses can occur, appears to last on average at least 10 years in the populations studied so far. However, the latency is not complete. Although there is relatively little HIV to be found in the blood during this time, there is activity in the immune cells in the lymph nodes. Some of these cells appear to produce HIV steadily with no clear adverse effects to their own integrity.

Box 7.2: The U.S. Drug Approval Process

Adapted from a newsletter the Pharmaceutical Manufacturers Association, Washington, DC (1992)

It takes 12 years on average for an experimental drug to travel from lab to medicine chest. Only 5 in 4,000 compounds screened in preclinical testing make it to human testing, and only one of these 5 is approved. The U.S. system of new drug approvals is perhaps the most rigorous in the world. On average, it costs $231 million to get a new medicine from the laboratory to the pharmacist's shelf, according to a 1990 study conducted by the Center for the Study of Drug Development at Tufts University, Boston, Massachusetts.

Figure 7.A shows the success rate of drugs for each phase of the development process and the length of time each step takes.

New medicines are developed as follows:

Preclinical Testing: Laboratory and animal studies are done to show biological activity against the targeted disease, and the compounds are evaluated for safety. These tests take approximately three and one-half years.

Investigational New Drug Application (IND): After completing preclinical testing, the company files an IND with the Food and Drug Administration (FDA) to begin to test the drug in people. The IND becomes effective if the FDA does not disapprove it within 30 days. The IND shows results of previous experiments; how, where, and by whom the new studies will be conducted; the chemical structure of the compound; how it is thought to work in the body; any toxic effects found in the animal studies; and how the compound is manufactured. In addition, the IND must be reviewed and approved by the Institutional Review Board, where the studies will be conducted, and progress reports on clinical trials must be submitted at least annually to the FDA.

Clinical Trials, Phase I: These tests take about 1 year and involve about 20 to 80 normal, healthy volunteers. The tests study a drug's safety profile, including the safe dosage range. The

	Preclinical Testing		Phase I	Phase II	Phase III		FDA	Approval
YEARS	3.5		1	2	3		2.5	Total=12
Test Population	Laboratory and Animal Studies	FILE NDA	20 to 80 Healthy Volunteers	100 to 300 Patient Volunteers	1,000 to 3,000 Patient Volunteers	FILE NDA		Post-marketing safety monitoring
PURPOSE	Assess safety and biological activity.		Determine safety and dosage.	Evaluate effectiveness. Look for side effects.	Verify effectiveness, monitor adverse reactions from long-term use.		Review Process	Large-scale manufacturing
					Expedited Review: Phases II and III combined to shorten approval process on new medicines for serious & life-threatening diseases.			Distribution
								Education
% of all new drugs that pass			70% of INDs	33% of INDs	27% of INDs		20% of INDs	

Figure 7.A. The success rate of drugs for each phase of the development process.

studies also determine how a drug is absorbed, distributed, metabolized, and excreted and the duration of its action.

Clinical Trials, Phase II: In this phase, which takes about two years, controlled studies of approximately 100 to 300 volunteer patients (people with the disease) assess the drug's effectiveness.

Clinical Trials, Phase III: This phase lasts about three years and usually involves 1,000 to 3,000 patients in clinics and hospitals. Physicians monitor patients closely to determine efficacy and identify adverse reactions.

New Drug Application (NDA): Following the completion of all 3 phases of clinical trials, the company files an NDA with the FDA if the data successfully demonstrate safety and effectiveness. The NDA must contain all the scientific information that has been gathered. NDAs typically run 100,000 pages or more. By law, the FDA is allowed 6 months to review an NDA. In almost all cases, the period between the first submission of an NDA and the final FDA approval exceeds that limit; the average NDA review time for new molecular entities approved in 1991 was 30.3 months.

Expedited Process: Under a plan implemented by the FDA early in 1989, Phases II and III may be combined to shave 2 or 3 years from the development process for medicines that show sufficient promise in early testing and are targeted against serious and life-threatening diseases.

Approval: Once the FDA approves the NDA, the new medicine becomes available for physicians to prescribe. The company must continue to submit periodic reports to the FDA, including any cases of adverse reactions and appropriate quality-control records. For some medicines, the FDA requires additional studies to evaluate long-term effects.

The importance of this in the course of disease remains unclear. Although some researchers still think that the virus kills cells simply by reproducing in them, many hold that the deterioration of the immune system depends on subtler processes. Cells producing large amounts of HIV would be excellent targets for a *tat* inhibitor. At present, one such *tat* inhibitor, the drug Ro 24-7429, is under trial. If it proves effective, with acceptable side effects and toxicity, it may be well suited to combination therapy regimes with RT blockers. In any event, *tat* inhibitors as a class should not stand or fall on the basis of the first drug in the class to reach trials.

Drug companies and research laboratories in the United States and the United Kingdom are also developing protease inhibitors that act by blocking the viral enzyme that cuts other viral pre-proteins into the proteins needed for viral assembly. The structure of the enzyme has been worked out precisely through X-ray crystallography, allowing drugs to be tailored to its shape. Though not quite as conceptually neat as *tat* inhibitors, which just turn the virus off, they may be just as effective, particularly because there is a large body of knowledge regarding inhibitors of protease in other biological systems.

Even though few drugs that enter clinical trials are eventually approved for marketing, it is reasonable to assume that there will be more drugs against HIV available within the next few years for 3 reasons: there are more than 88 products already in clinical trials in the United States; there is a reasonably large market; and the costs of getting a treatment for HIV infection to market are probably comparatively low.* The U.S. FDA has recently moved through approval of some AIDS drugs with unprecedented speed (see Boxes 7.2 and 7.3).

---

*There is some debate about the actual cost of drug development and the size of the market. Determining the cost of drug development usually depends on whether the information comes from a drug company or one of its critics. In addition, the market for AIDS drugs is considerably smaller than that for other products, such as antihistamines. Many estimates of the cost of drug development fail to factor in research funding provided by the federal government, as in the case of the United States where the National Institutes of Health in Bethesda, Maryland is the most significant funder of research into drugs for AIDS and other diseases.

However, the best time for using such drugs has yet to be demonstrated to the satisfaction of all. In 1989, a trial in the United States showed some advantage, over a relatively brief follow up of 13 months, to treatment with AZT of HIV-infected individuals without the symptoms of AIDS or HIV infection. A longer-term Anglo-French study, called Concorde, is still underway to assess the advantages of early AZT use over a number of years. The issue is still open to question, though early AZT use has become standard in some places. It is possible that patients receiving benefits from early AZT will receive less benefit later.[6]

Box 7.3: AIDS Activism and Drug Development

Mark Harrington, AIDS Coalition to Unleash Power (ACT-UP), New York, New York

ACT-UP, the AIDS Coalition to Unleash Power, was founded in New York City during March 1987 after activist and playwright Larry Kramer delivered a speech excoriating the pace of research on new treatments for AIDS. Starting from a base in New York's Greenwich Village, ACT-UP rapidly spread around the country and abroad. Five years later, there are ACT-UP chapters in Canada, Australia, the United Kingdom, France, Germany, and Italy.

ACT-UP is a participatory democratic organization that stages direct action, including civil disobedience, to target institutions that impede AIDS research, limit access to new treatments, or discriminate against people with HIV. In the United States, ACT-UP has been a pivotal force for changing the system under which new drugs are tested and approved.

The original focus of ACT-UP's direct action was the U.S. Food and Drug Administration (FDA), which oversees drug development and which must approve new drugs before they can be sold. Between 1981 and 1987, the FDA had approved just one drug to fight AIDS—the antiviral AZT, which was priced at $10,000 a year by its maker, Burroughs-Wellcome. The FDA also restricted access to new experimental drugs, denying potentially life-saving therapies to thousands of people with AIDS.

In October 1988, ACT-UP staged a massive demonstration at the FDA headquarters in Rockville, Maryland. Nationwide media coverage led to rapid changes in FDA policy. Beginning in 1989, the FDA granted activists the unprecedented ability to negotiate research policy. The agency sped up the pace of drug approvals and developed new expanded access mechanisms—sometimes called *Parallel Track*—to provide people with AIDS with experimental drugs outside of research protocols while clinical trials were still ongoing. ACT-UP and other groups developed considerable expertise in clinical trial design and applied this expertise to negotiations with drug companies, the National Institutes of Health (NIH), and the FDA.

Since ACT-UP's intervention, and under activist pressure, the FDA rapidly approved aerosolized pentamidine for PCP prophylaxis,

Although the question of offering early AZT therapy is not yet completely closed, experience with the drug supports a general tendency to early treatment. Anti-HIV drugs with few side-effect profiles may be used in such a way at some point. The same is true of prophylaxis or treatment for the opportunistic infections (OIs) that strike people with AIDS. Treatments for these infections can greatly improve the expectations and the quality of life of people with AIDS who have access to them (see Table 7.2).

---

ganciclovir for CMV retinitis, EOP for AIDS-associated anemia, fluconazole for cryptococcal meningitis, foscarnet for CMV retinitis, AZT for children with AIDS, and ddl for people with advanced HIV disease who are intolerant to or failing AZT therapy. ACT-UP also spurred the FDA to lower the dose of AZT by 50 percent after clinical trials showed the lower dose was safer and just as effective. After a year-long campaign led by ACT-UP, Burroughs-Wellcome lowered the price of AZT to $3,200 a year.

ACT-UP also worked with Bristol-Meyers Squibb to develop a Parallel Track program for ddl that provided the drug to 23,000 people with AIDS while ddl's clinical trials were ongoing. Similar expanded access programs have been developed for other AIDS drugs, including ddC.

After a May 1990 demonstration at the NIH, ACT-UP and other activist organizations won policy-making roles within the NIH AIDS Clinical Trials Group (ACTG), which designs and conducts most federally funded major clinical trials of new AIDS treatments.

ACT-UP's major victories in transforming clinical research were

won by an unusual combination of tactics, which included inside negotiation and outside agitation, massive demonstrations, targeted "zaps" or small strikes against selected targets, letter-writing campaigns, and use of the mass media. None of these efforts would have been effective had not AIDS activists learned the jargon of the medical establishment and turned it toward their own aims.

There remain many significant obstacles to the goals of AIDS treatment activists. Most people who need new AIDS drugs lack adequate health care, and even those with access to treatment lack information about their therapeutic options. The peer-reviewed medical journals publish important results many months or even years after they are available to AIDS insiders. Drug companies are uncomfortable sharing preliminary information about experimental therapies, and resent AIDS activists' hard-won influence on the development process. NIH research remains a bureaucratic labyrinth, and is threatened by cuts in federal AIDS research funding levels. The FDA's reforms speeding drug approvals

Therapy and Prophylaxis for Opportunistic Infections

The most notable success to date is prophylaxis for pneumocystis carinii pneumonia (PCP). Aerosolized pentamidine, and more recently the much cheaper drug Bactrim®, have been shown to ward off this form of pneumonia in people infected with HIV. These drugs may have done something to put off the later stages of the disease in many cases; they have also reduced hospitalization. As yet, primary prophylaxis (prophylaxis given before the first occurrence of an OI) is available only for PCP. Trials are presently going on to show whether some

---

remain under attack from members of Congress intent on preserving the agency's consumer protection role. Defects in understanding of the detailed pathogenesis of HIV-induced immune suppression limit the efficacy of existing anti-HIV drugs. Finally, AIDS treatment activism itself is threatened by burnout, attrition from disease and death, and political fragmentation within the AIDS activist movement.

Most AIDS treatments remain inaccessible to most people around the world who are living with AIDS. Moreover, until the United States develops a health care system which delivers treatment to all its inhabitants, the gains won by ACT-UP and other AIDS activists remain accessible only to a fraction of the 1 million or more HIV-infected people in the country.

The process of democratizing research and making it more accessible to its constituents—the people with serious and life-threatening diseases—remains incomplete. After five years of AIDS treatment activism, a cure is still nowhere in sight. Yet ACT-UP's accomplishments, however imperfect, have provided life-extending and sometimes life-saving treatment

options to thousands of people with AIDS, and have irrevocably transformed the drug development system in America.

A logical outcome of the successes of AIDS activism in the industrialized world (as exemplified in this profile by ACT-UP), will be to connect issues and struggles in the developing and industrialized countries. Thus, while access to AZT was reduced by high prices in the industrialized world, suitable trials and access to AZT, other antiretroviral agents and drugs to treat opportunistic infections are all extremely limited or totally absent in the developing world. A history of AIDS activism would also include many courageous and creative efforts in communities and countries around the world. Women refusing to continue subservient sexual roles, community groups working for human rights and dignity, groups working to permit sex education in schools, and people with HIV infection and AIDS fighting discrimination—all are activists. Their collective story needs to be documented and told. It is a global story which is making global history.

—The Editors

Table 7.2: Approved AIDS medicines as of January 1, 1992

Drug name	Manufacturer	Indication
Bactrim™+ trimethoprim and sulfamethoxazole	Hoffmann–La Roche (Nutley, N.J.)	PCP treatment
Cytovene® ganciclovir (IV)	Syntex (Palo Alto, Calif.)	CMV retinitis
Daraprim®+ pyrimethamine	Burroughs Wellcome (Research Triangle Park, N.C.)	Toxoplasmosis treatment
Diflucan® fluconazole	Pfizer (New York, N.Y.)	Cryptococcal meningitis, candidiasis
Foscavir® foscarnet sodium	Astra Pharmaceutical (Westborough, Mass.)	CMV retinitis
Intron® A+ interferon alfa-2b (recombinant)	Schering-Plough (Madison, N.J.)	Kaposi's sarcoma
NebuPent® aerosol pentamidine isethionate	Fujisawa Pharmaceutical (Deerfield, Ill.)	PCP prophylaxis
Pentam® 300 IM&IV pentamidine isethionate	Fujisawa Pharmaceutical	PCP treatment
PROCRIT®+ epoetin alfa	Ortho Biotech (Raritan, N.J.)	Anemia in Retrovir®-treated HIV-infected patients
Retrovir® zidovudine (AZT)	Burroughs Wellcome	HIV-positive asymptomatic and symptomatic (ARC, AIDS), pediatric and adult
Roferon®-A+interferon alfa-2a, recombinant/ Roche	Hoffmann–La Roche	Kaposi's sarcoma
Septra®+ trimethoprim and sulfamethoxazole	Burroughs Wellcome	PCP treatment
VIDEX® didanosine (ddI)	Bristol-Myers Squibb (New York, N.Y.)	Treatment of adult and pediatric patients (over 6 months of age) with advanced HIV infection, who are intolerant or who have demonstrated significant clinical or immunologic deterioration during Retrovir® therapy
Zovirax® acyclovir	Burroughs Wellcome	Herpes zoster/simplex

Source: Pharmaceutical Manufacturers Association, Washington, D.C. (1991).

of the treatments for other OIs or HIV-associated infections might also be used prophylactically. There are also trials aimed at proving the efficacy of new treatments for these OIs. Cytomegalovirus infections of the retina, for example, can presently be treated with two drugs, ganciclovir and the recently approved Foscavir®. The latter has side effects that are different from those of AZT, and the effects of ganciclovir and AZT can exacerbate each other. An oral form of either drug might be a good prophylactic. A new PCP drug, 566, developed by

---

Box 7.4: Alternative AIDS Treatments

Jon M. Greenberg is the founder of Treatment Alternatives Research Project (TARP), a project of the PWA Health Group, New York. TARP is dedicated to seeing controlled clinical studies of commonly used alternative treatments.

Since the beginning of the AIDS pandemic, numerous alternative treatments have been used, often in combination with conventional medical treatment. Approaches as varied as herbal compounds, nutritional supplements, Traditional Chinese Medicine, special diets, physical manipulation, and spiritual and psychotherapeutic techniques have all been grouped together under the heading of alternative treatments. Although many of these approaches have suggested some degree of effectiveness—in laboratory studies or anecdotal reports—very little is actually known about them. The confusing array of possibly effective but largely untested treatments and techniques makes truly informed decisions about how to spend precious treatment dollars nearly impossible. Available information, while often based on empirical evidence from other disease studies, has not been adequately confirmed by controlled studies with HIV-infected persons.

Although alternative treatment practitioners are often ill-prepared to conduct the type of studies needed on the treatments they prescribe, many conventional medical researchers have been ignorant of the possibilities and principles of use of such treatments. AIDS researchers usually learn of a possible therapeutic agent when a pharmaceutical company presents and promotes the potential therapy as a candidate for clinical trial. By that time, much of the preclinical work has already been done at the company's expense. Without such advocacy and promotion, potential therapies without pharmaceutical sponsors are rarely brought to the attention of most AIDS researchers. Consequently, researchers and, by extension, clinicians and people with AIDS are missing potentially valuable therapeutic agents and techniques.

The economics of drug development also work against the need for research on alternative treatments. Unless a pharmaceutical company stands to profit from a drug for which they hold the patent and that they can produce and market, there is little reason for them to invest time and money in developing the agent. Many alternative treatments for AIDS fall outside of the traditional profit-making scheme of drug development.

Burroughs Wellcome, may improve treatment when prophylaxis fails. Various antibiotics and antivirals are in use or in trials against other opportunistic infections. The increased perception of the importance of these drugs can be seen from the trend in the number of drugs in development. In the four years from 1988 to 1991, the number of anti-infectives in development and use rose from 6 to 23 (see Table 7.1).

To date, the fate of drugs aimed at improving the body's response,

---

It is often argued that the real problem lies within the institutionalized bureaucracy that requires prohibitively expensive studies. Although this may be partially true, major changes in the system cannot be expected to happen quickly enough to help people who need effective treatments and reliable information now. It is also important to emphasize that while biases against nonpharmaceutical treatments may be built into the system, the criteria used to judge conventional treatments are equally applicable to alternative treatments. The type of information ultimately required by the approving authorities is the same information needed by people with AIDS to make informed decisions: how much to take, how often to take, and what possible side effects can be expected. Historical and anecdotal evidence on a particular treatment, perhaps sufficient to get a rough estimate of these factors, can only be used confidently when there is a long history of use. Thus, for now, we must rely on methods developed within the established scientific community, which, if nothing else, should be able to produce information through a limited number of laboratory trials or dose-escalation studies. Unfortunately, without sufficient funds, even these tests remain prohibitively expensive for most alternative treatment practitioners and would-be researchers.

Given the lack of incentive in the private sector, research and development will need to come from the public sphere, with government and AIDS foundations funding research on treatments and care strategies that do not have pharmaceutical backing. But getting a share of the ever-tightening AIDS research budget is an uphill battle. Information is needed on both promising alternative treatments and not-so-promising treatments on which people with AIDS may be wasting vital resources. Promising alternative treatments, as with drugs developed by pharmaceutical companies, will need to be moved quickly and efficiently through the developmental and clinical process. The dogmas, biases, and economic disincentives must be put aside, allowing alternative and conventional medical communities to collaborate and share their respective areas of expertise in a joint investigative venture.

as opposed to fighting the virus and its associated infections, has proved disappointing. As yet, no immunomodulator is used as an approved therapy, and research into these compounds is not widely seen as hopeful—though that does not mean it is worthless. Separate from the immunomodulators are the cytokines, products of the body's immune system mimicked and mass produced by genetic engineering. Interferon 1 is a recognized treatment for people with Kaposi's sarcoma. Other cytokines, aimed to boost the immune system, are under

---

Box 7.5: Alternative Therapies

Compiled with assistance from Jason Heyman, *AIDS Treatment News,* and Jon M. Greenberg, ACT-UP/New York and founder of Treatment Alternatives Research Project (TARP)

Alternative therapies are used by a significant proportion of people with HIV, often to complement approved medical treatments. Alternative treatments have been investigated in laboratory settings and observational studies, and a few have undergone controlled clinical trials. Others are being used without having undergone any studies. For various reasons, usually lack of pharmaceutical sponsorship, many alternative agents have yet to be considered seriously as candidates for controlled clinical trials. Because so little is known about many of these therapies, categorizing or defining their use is a difficult and sometimes arbitrary process. An alternative therapy may be used for treatment of opportunistic infections, antiviral and/or immunomodulatory purposes, and for multiple conditions. Even where it may seem beneficial under certain circumstances, debate continues over why or how it works. Although often touted as nontoxic, some herbs or nutritional supplements can have significant toxicities if used improperly. More research is required to evaluate the efficacy and safety of many alternative therapies.

The following is a partial list of alternative agents and techniques illustrating the variety of approaches being used:

Plants and Plant Extracts

Derived from natural products or medicinal herbs, these are used for their possible antiviral properties and antibacterial and antifungal activity in the treatment of opportunistic infections. X = Investigated in single agent, controlled clinical trials; O = Observational study.

Treatment	Status
Acemannan (*Aloe vera* extract)	X (Canada)
Astragalus	
Bitter melon (*momordica charantia*)	O
Blue-green algae (Cyanobacteria)	
Burdock (*Arctium lappa*)	
Garlic extract	O
Glycyrrhizin (licorice)	X (Japan)
Hypericin (St. John's wort extract)	X (U.S.)
Iscador (European Mistletoe extract)	O
Maitake mushroom	
Mulberry roots and seeds	
Pine cone extracts	

trial—though some have powerful side effects. Other drugs, aimed either at offsetting the side effects of primary treatments (e.g., erythropoeitin, which mitigates anemia) or dealing with other symptoms, such as anorexia, are also in use or in trial.

There seems little doubt that, for people with access to the latest medications, the prospects will improve little by little over the next few years. This is not necessarily because there will be better treatments, though that does seem possible. It is also because as clinical

---

Red marine algae
  (*Schizemenia pacifica*)
Shiitake mushrooms   X (U.S. dose-
  (Lentinan)   finding study)
Siberian ginseng
  (Eleutherococcus)
Traditional medicinal herbs   O
Trichosanthin (Chinese
  cucumber root, GL,
  Q223, Compound Q)   X (U.S.)
Woundwart (*Prunella
  vulgaris*)

Numerous traditional Chinese medicinal herbs have been found to have anti-HIV properties.[a] Many other herbs and herbal compounds are used to alleviate drug side effects and treat various infections. For more details on use of medicinal herbs in HIV-infected patients and potential adverse effects of herbal use, see Kassler et al.[b]

Nutritional Supplements

Nutritional supplements are used to restore natural levels, to enhance resistance to opportunistic infections, and, when taken in high doses, to treat various HIV/AIDS-related conditions.

Treatment	Status
Vitamins and minerals	
Betacarotene	X (U.S.)

Calcium
Folic acid
Iron
Vitamin B6   X (U.S.)
Vitamin B12   X (U.S.)
Vitamin C (ascorbate)
Vitamin E
Other products
Acidophilus
Colostrum (bovine)   X (U.S.,
                       Denmark)
Co-enzyme Q10
  (amino acid)
L-lysine
N-acetylcysteine (NAC)
  (glutathione precursor) X (U.S.)
Selenium

Dietary Management

Dietary management is used to maintain or improve general health; special regimens can be used as a prophylaxis or treatment (such as eliminating refined sugar and yeast-containing products to prevent or treat fungal infections). (Observational studies are currently underway.)

Physical Therapy

Physical techniques are used to treat certain conditions, relieve physical symptoms, and improve comfort and

experience is gained, clinicians will become better at dealing with the complex mixtures of medication that they have to administer.

AIDS research has brought many changes in how clinical trials are conducted. One such innovation is clinical trials based in community settings, which will provide ever greater amounts of information about the practical efficacy of various combinations of treatments. Meanwhile, more rigorously controlled trials will test new drugs, and alternative therapies are being examined as AIDS treatments (see Boxes 7.4 and 7.5).

---

the quality of life. They are an option that can be combined with other regimens without interactions with other medications.

Treatment	Status
Acupuncture	X (U.S.)
Chiropractic manipulation	
Hydrotherapy	
Massage	

Spiritual/Psychological Approaches

These approaches seek to provide a holistic balance to complement other treatment strategies for HIV/AIDS. Although benefits are highly individual and subjective, they can contribute to an overall state of health.

Treatment	Status
Hypnotherapy	
Meditation	
Psychotherapy	
Spiritual healing	
Stress reduction	
Visualization	

Other Treatments

Treatment	Status
Aspirin	
Colonics	
DHEA (hormone)	X (U.S.)
DNCB (Dinitrichlor-obenzene), topical	(observational study)
Ozone therapy (super-oxygenation)	
Passive immunotherapy	X (U.S., France)
Shark cartilage powder	
Shark liver oil (Squaline)	
Snake venom (Soluteine)	
Thymus extracts	

a. WHO/GPA, Traditional Medicine Programme, *Report of a WHO informal consultation on traditional medicine and AIDS: in vitro screening for anti-HIV activity. Geneva: February 6–8, 1989* (WHO/GPA/BRA/89.5); WHO/Traditional Medicine Programme, *Report of a WHO consultation on traditional medicine and AIDS: Clinical evaluation of traditional medicines and natural products. Geneva: September 26–28, 1990* (WHO/TRM/GPA/90.2).

b. W. J. Kassler, P. Blanc, and R. Greenblatt, "The use of medicinal herbs by human immunodeficiency virus–infected patients," *Archives of Internal Medicine* 151 (November 1991):2281–88.

Vaccine Development

Although mass vaccination campaigns have previously focused on individuals yet to be infected with viral disease such as smallpox, polio, and the other childhood diseases subjected to immunization, current HIV/AIDS research has taken a novel approach, investigating not only the prophylactic vaccine, but also therapeutic vaccines for infected people—primarily intended to slow or halt the progressive damage to the immune system—and vaccines to stop perinatal transmission.

It is generally hoped that science will develop safe and effective vaccines during this decade.[7] At the end of 1991, 12 HIV-1 vaccine candidates were in phase I/II (safety/immunogenicity) trials (see Table 7.3). Major difficulties exist in the design of HIV vaccine clinical trials, involving ethical, behavioral, and scientific concerns, not the least of which are the questions of how to choose the most meritorious candidate vaccines and in what populations to test them. The continuing progress toward development of a vaccine against HIV infection has focused increasing attention on the question of its equitable distribution in both developed and developing countries. Whereas in industrialized countries, it may be the case that HIV/AIDS could be transformed into chronic manageable illnesses responsive to a range of therapies, development of a usable vaccine appears to be the only bright spot in the future for developing or poor countries of the world. In 1991, four developing countries (Brazil, Rwanda, Thailand, and Uganda) were approached by the World Health Organization (WHO) as possible sites for future clinical trials of vaccines, in order to facilitate the eventual participation of developing countries in large-scale studies when they begin.

The possibility of a vaccine has been much debated since a viral cause was first suggested for AIDS. Prospects have ranged from being deemed nonexistent to bright and beckoning. At present, optimism prevails for three reasons: the belief, by many people, that a vaccine is possible, on the basis of animal tests; the lack of side effects (at least in the short term) from use of preparations so far tested in people; and the fact that the search for a vaccine is seen as essential, even if the prospects of finding one have sometimes looked bleak. There is an imperative perceived in vaccine development that cannot wait on

Table 7.3: Candidate vaccines in development

Candidate vaccine	Manufacturer	Indication[a]	Phase of development
Recombinant gp160/ baculovirus system	MicroGeneSys (U.S.)	HIV+/–	II
Recombinant gp160/mammalian cells	Immuno-AG/NIH (Austria and U.S.)	HIV+/–	I
Recombinant gp120/env-2, 3/yeast	CIBA-GEIGY, Ltd./ Chiron/Biocine (Switzerland and U.S.)	HIV+	I
Recombinant gp120 IIIB	Genentech, Inc. (U.S.)	HIV+/–	I–II
Recombinant gp120 MN	Genentech, Inc. (U.S.)	HIV+/–	I–II
Recombinant gp120/mammalian cells	CIBA-GEIGY, Ltd./ Chiron/Biocine	HIV+/–	I
Synthetic p17 (HGP-30)	Viral Technologies, Inc. (U.K. and U.S.)	HIV- HIV+ (planned)	I
Gamma-irradiated HIV (gp120 depleted)	Immune Response Corp./Rhone-Poulanc Rorer, Inc. (U.S.)	HIV+	II–III
Vaccinia expressing env plus autologous vaccinia - env infected cells plus recombinant gp160	Pierre et Marie Curie University (France and Zaire)	HIV+/–	II–III
Recombinant p24/yeast system (Ty-gag)	British Bio-technology Limited (U.K.)	Phase I/II	I in HIV– volunteers II in HIV+ volunteers (planned)
Recombinant p24/baculovirus system	MicroGeneSys (U.S.)	HIV+	I
HIVIG (vaccine/IGG)	Abbott Laboratories (U.S.)	HIV+[b]	Clinical trials by NIH Heart and Lung Disease Group

Sources: Pharmaceutical Manufacturers Association, Washington, D.C., and survey by *AIDS in the World* (March 1992).

a. HIV+ is therapeutic; HIV– is to prevent infection.

b. To interrupt vertical transmission.

the technicalities of vaccine design. That is why groundwork for vaccine trials is now under way, while the question of which vaccine candidates to try is still being debated. It is likely that a vaccine may be discovered through enlightened empiricism before one can be designed based on immunological theory.*

At present, investigations are focusing on three different approaches to vaccination: *prophylactic, therapeutic,* and *perinatal.* The aim of prophylactic vaccination is to equip the immune system with the information it requires to defeat HIV when it attacks the body for the first time. The aim of therapeutic vaccination is to reinvigorate the already infected immune system, allowing it to combat more effectively the HIV-induced damage to the immune system. Perinatal vaccination has the limited aim of blocking the transmission of the virus from mother to child during pregnancy, during childbirth, and soon afterwards.

Most attention is focused on the first approach, both because it has huge potential benefits and because it follows the traditional aim of vaccination programs. Therapeutic vaccination would, if successful, herald a new era in the treatment of HIV and possibly of other diseases. Perinatal vaccination would have the advantage of being the easiest to test, but there is evidence that it may be of only limited use, even if successful intervention proves possible and difficult ethical problems could be overcome.

The evidence that a vaccine is possible comes principally from work done with primates, notably chimpanzees and rhesus monkeys. Rhesus monkeys, when infected with a virus (known as SIV-MAC) similar to HIV and originally found in mangabey monkeys, develop symptoms that are broadly similar to AIDS and that lead to death. Various strains of SIV-MAC have been isolated that cause disease of differing degrees of severity. At least one strain produces a notably un-AIDS-like acute disease, invariably fatal within days. Researchers who work with rhesus monkeys believe that the infection of monkeys with SIV provides a particulary good model for the infection of human

---

*The National Institutes of Health in the United States has stated the goal of undertaking vaccine efficacy trials by December 1993 at sites within the United States and by 1994 outside the United States (communication from NIH Office of AIDS Research, 1992).

beings with AIDS. They have found that vaccination with whole inactivated virus can, under some circumstances, lead to an immune response that protects the monkey when it is later exposed to live virus. The inference is that the immune system can, if forewarned, develop responses that neutralize the virus.

These experiments are encouraging but have their drawbacks. Many use fairly complicated immunization procedures (repeated vaccinations and booster shots) administered shortly before exposure to an infective virus; the inactivated virus in the vaccine is often the same strain as the live virus later used to determine whether there is any protection conferred. Also, the exposure to infective virus is often artificial, with the virus being given in a purified form instead of in the form of infected cells, which is how most people are probably infected. So far, most researchers have given the infective virus directly into the bloodstream by injection, rather than giving the virus across the mucous membranes, as actually happens in sexual infec-

---

Box 7.6: The Manhattan Project: Fact or Fantasy?

There is increasing talk about a so-called vaccine Manhattan Project among AIDS researchers. To evaluate it, consider the circumstances of the real Manhattan Project. There was a clearly defined problem—using a nuclear chain reaction in a weapon of war. There was strong incentive to participate, which meant that almost every nuclear physicist in the Allied countries was involved, including almost all the stars; there were practically unlimited funds available; there was a heavy emphasis on novel industrial processes, the production of plutonium (previously seen only in microgram amounts), and weapons-grade uranium; and there was an extremely powerful and centralized management structure. By the end of the World War II, the Manhattan Project made up a modest but appreciable fraction of the whole U.S. economy, occupying the time and talents of many thousands of workers.

The qualities of the Manhattan Project that might be transferred into vaccine research are these: strong goal orientation within a single program; unlimited resources; vast investment in new manufacturing technologies; and a powerful, authoritarian management structure. Even though its political likelihood seems low, the idea does have its attractions.

It clearly could have advantages at the technical end—many things now difficult might become possible. Research into sequencing and analyzing viral strains from around the world would be a priority, well suited to a centralized system (in fact, the database that would be built on is already, by a quirk of fate, sitting in

tion. This may have important implications for vaccine design. These tests do not show that long-term protection is possible, or that protection against all strains of the virus is possible. In 1991 a British group at the National Institute of Biological Standards found that they were protecting the control monkeys in their experiments simply by injecting them with uninfected human T cells. These cells are used to make most of the SIV vaccines, but no one until then had thought of doing the control experiment of giving the monkeys the cells alone. The implications of this finding are not yet clear, but it could mean that much of the protection in macaques comes about due to an immune response against cellular proteins as well as, or instead of, viral proteins.

Other evidence for the possibility of vaccination comes from chimpanzees. Unlike rhesus monkeys, chimpanzees can be infected by HIV. Unlike people, they appear to be able to live with this infection without being harmed. Experiments with chimpanzees are ex-

---

Los Alamos, New Mexico). So would ways to mass produce human proteins in human cells, which will be necessary for some of the subunit vaccine strategies. This would bring the program into direct competition with small biotechnology companies and have a large impact on that industry worldwide. The Manhattan Project did not put people out of work. A successful AIDS vaccine program along these lines might—and it would definitely have considerable effects on some companies.

However, the whole premise of such a program would be that the private sector was not equipped to do the job as well—a proposition for which there is some evidence. Large drug companies do not generally concentrate on vaccine research. Industry might even benefit if spin-off technologies developed in such a program were licensed out; new

innovations would follow abundantly. No sensible planner, however, counts on spin off to justify a program.

Whether the centralized approach would work at the level of scientific development, as opposed to facilitating technology, is less clear. Scientists do not take kindly to an imposed research agenda, even those who work in industry, where academic freedom is far from unlimited. Imposing those limitations on a large group, which must include the most able people in the field and ideally attract similarly able people from beyond the field, will not be easy. To some extent, of course, scientists will go where there is money for work, even if it means forsaking their favored field. Thus, money would clearly be an inducement. However, redirecting money toward HIV vaccines and away from other fields might have an unpopular air of coercion.

tremely costly and thus done sparingly. However, various possible vaccines have been tried on a few chimpanzees and found effective. Evidence that a human antibody directed against part of the virus's outer coat can stop the virus from infecting chimps is encouraging, but it is based on data from only a very few animals. And the vaccines that work on chimps are not of the same type as those that work on macaques: they are viral-coat-protein vaccines, not whole inactivated virus particles. Moreover, the model is always open to question because the chimpanzee's immune system, although similar enough on a molecular level to allow HIV to recognize and enter the chimps' immune helper cells, is sufficiently different that it stops the virus from doing any harm once there.

Taken together this evidence provides a sketchy—though far from conclusive—case for the possibility of a protective vaccine. But vaccine development is never based on the certainty of success. There is no way of finding out whether people can be protected from HIV

Goal-oriented projects have a tendency to narrow down options at an early stage. Such was not the case with the Manhattan Project, however, because of the high priority put on it at a national level. With unlimited money, it was possible to support two different technologies with two different designs and two different production facilities until the bitter end. That was, in some ways, wasteful. Any similar program, by keeping open all options, will also be wasteful in its undaunted exploration of a large number of blind alleys.

However, in this field particularly, options must be kept open. There is little theory firm enough to rule out approaches before they are tried. And there is also a tendency towards closure. People outside the community of AIDS researchers often perceive a reluctance to depart from orthodoxy, an unwillingness to move from a set of common assumptions. Though that perception is probably exaggerated, the situation would surely be worse within a monolithic research effort than it is at present. The advantage of uncoordinated research is diversity. In general, vaccines have come from small development programs followed by strongly designed, massive distribution programs.

The biggest question about such a program then becomes, Who pays? The sums involved, necessarily running into billions of dollars, mean that only the developed world could afford to pay. But will it? The benefits accrued from an effective vaccine would be enormous. The problem is that no developed country views such a vaccine as a matter of national survival, and only on issues of national survival have such programs previously been seen as justified.

except by a series of large scale trials. Before going on to consider the practicalities of such trials—a topic that has, in the past year, risen more or less to the top of the agenda in AIDS policy worldwide—it is worth studying progress in the other two development programs for a perinatal vaccine and a therapeutic vaccine.

A perinatal vaccine could be of great benefit in saving lives and resources. It is, in a way, the simplest form of vaccination. It has to stop the virus from doing one specific thing—transmitting itself across the placenta—and it has to do that only for a limited period of time. However, it is not proven that HIV is transmitted solely during pregnancy by crossing the placenta. A study on twins born to HIV-infected mothers has shown that the first-born has a significantly higher risk of infection than does the second-born. There may be HIV transmission during birth, in which case the role of a protective vaccine might be less. In addition, drugs that reduce the load of virus in the mother's blood might be a valid alternative or complement to a vaccine.

Therapeutic vaccination, if developed, will be a novel technqiue. The idea is that if the immune system is regularly reminded of what the enemy looks like, it can be kept in a state of constant alert and can provide a fuller immune response at all times, with a better prognosis. Various HIV vaccines are being studied in this way, including an inactivated whole virus. Animal trials based on the same procedure have not been effective. There have been some partly encouraging interim results published on human studies, but little more can be said until blinded trials have been finished. If those results are favorable, then therapeutic vaccines would look set to become important adjuncts to drug therapy.

If a prophylactic vaccine is to be shown to work, it must be tested in a population at risk of infection. That will require large-scale clinical trials. Planning for such trials is already in progress. In addition to the four developing countries already designated for preliminary groundwork necessary before a trial, other trials are likely. Trials are also probable in the United States. A great deal of epidemiological, behavioral, logistical, and virological work, as well as training and infrastructure support, will be needed to characterize the trial sites, which is why they must be chosen before the vaccine. Trials pose complex ethical problems. For example, how do researchers define informed consent where a population may be largely illiterate? How can poor countries in which the vaccine is tested ensure that they will have access to a vaccine proven effective once the trial is over, regardless of its cost?

The trial populations will differ from site to site, a logical necessity to avoid testing the vaccines in the same conditions everywhere. Counseling of subjects will be difficult. Vaccines may also differ from site to site, perhaps involving products resembling the strain or strains of the virus dominant in a given region. That is why virological groundwork needs to be done before trials can start. Whatever strain is chosen, the vaccine may include more of the virus than just its coat. Vaccines based on genetically engineered organisms make this approach easier. There are doubts about putting the first of these vaccines, those that use vaccinia, into people whose immune reac-

---

Box 7.7: What Can We Expect from an Effective HIV Vaccine?

June E. Osborn, M.D., Dean, School of Public Health, University of Michigan, Ann Arbor, Michigan

The development of a safe, effective vaccine to prevent HIV infection is and must continue to be a high priority goal for biomedical science. In some parts of the world, especially where seroprevalence has reached double-digit levels, such a weapon will be a merciful addition to present efforts to damp the waves of further HIV spread among young, sexually active men and women. Even a modestly protective vaccine (achieving, say, 70 to 80% efficacy) would be very useful, especially if it were made available to populations most in need, often those least likely to be able to afford it.

It is important to realize, however, that a good HIV vaccine will not be a panacea. Too often, the advent of an AIDS vaccine is depicted as the definitive solution to epidemic trouble—but it would not be, and we must not delude ourselves into believing that a vaccine breakthrough could abruptly end the crisis. Regardless of vaccine, the hard work of prevention through education and risk reduction will need to continue, as will efforts to provide care for the millions already infected.

To illustrate why its usefulness is likely to be limited, suppose that we had in hand an HIV vaccine as good as any viral vaccine yet created. Although it would almost surely require more than one dose (thus far only live virus vaccines have achieved full protection with a single administration), one could hopefully presume that it would be easily delivered, that problems of antigenic variation had been solved, and that it would be protective against exposure to HIV for at least a few years. How much could be expected of it?

First, it certainly would not be perfect in protecting the whole population. Even the very best of viral vaccines (measles vaccine is a good example) are less than 100 percent

tions might be extreme (e.g., people already HIV positive), but those doubts might be overcome if there was strong evidence that it would work. Other live vectors might be more acceptable.

The question of measuring the success of a trial is not clear-cut and involves the question of what end points to measure. The ideal vaccine would prevent 100 percent of infections. However, if vaccinated people get infected at a lower but still appreciable rate, the public health implications become more complex. The effect of such a vaccine on transmission of HIV would require careful computer modeling and raise very complex counseling and ethical problems in considering how to use it. An additional complication would arise if those vaccinated became infected, but, because of some improvement to their immune systems, did not go on to develop AIDS. To deter-

---

effective. In any large population of vaccine recipients, at least 1 to 2 percent, but often 5 percent or more, will turn out to be nonresponders, due to variation in human biology rather than to some inherent flaw in the vaccine. Repeated immunization can solve some but not all of that problem; invariably a group of susceptibles persists, providing an important part of the fuel for future epidemic fires should that particular virus be reintroduced after incomplete eradication. Those phenomena have been illustrated with painful clarity in recent recrudescences of measles, even in highly immunized populations.

That brings up a second important point: widespread use of virtually all efficacious viral vaccines results in a dramatic decrease in circulating "wild" virus in a population. Thus, not only does individual immune response protect most vaccine recipients directly, but also community (or herd) immunity makes re-exposure much less likely among remaining

susceptibles. Part of the reason this happens is that immunity to those short-incubation-period viral infections (whether invoked by natural infection or by vaccine) tends to be strong and durable.

But HIV is different from those other viruses in several crucial ways. Unlike measles or yellow fever viruses, once HIV infection is established, the virus remains potentially transmissible (through sex, injection of blood-contaminated materials, ingestion of breast milk or birth to an infected mother) for many years. That long interval of silent infection is usually unrecognizable without specific laboratory testing and is unassociated with symptomatic ill health. Unless general efforts at education and risk reduction are diligently maintained, infected people go about their normal lives unaware of either their status or the risk they may pose to others through sexual or injection risk behavior.

Furthermore, as a sexually

mine this would require a very long follow-up period, whereas most trials are designed to be reasonably short. Again, there is a question about health policy in such a situation. If these people are healthy, but still infectious, viral spread may continue unabated, or even intensify.

Overshadowing all these uncertainties is one of political will and power. If a protective vaccine is found, it would have its greatest effect in the developing countries. However, it is likely to be developed and produced, at least initially, in the industrialized world. If it is genetically engineered, it may be particularly expensive. Will the poor nations be able to afford it? The answer is probably no, unless specific steps are taken to provide them with access to the vaccine. This problem is seen as particularly acute for countries that will host the

---

transmitted virus, HIV is likely to pose a very different set of challenges for a would-be vaccine strategy. Constant circulation of virus in the community will create a steady likelihood of re-exposure if risky behavior continues, so that its protective effect would need to be sustained throughout the active sexual life of an individual, unless other risk-reduction measures are maintained. It is probably no accident that we do not yet have vaccines for sexually transmitted diseases, for the dynamics of spread are very different from the brisk, self-limited epidemics characteristic of childhood diseases and their effective vaccines.

Finally, any vaccine strategy presupposes delivery of the vaccine. One matter of greatest concern in the AIDS epidemic is the fragility of public health infrastructure in many areas where need is greatest. Already the cruel choice sometimes looms between childhood immunization programs (such as WHO's Expanded Program on Immunization) and HIV prevention activities. Adding a costly, multiple-dose HIV vaccine in such a stressed health care setting may even bring down the system, or it might inappropriately out-compete other critical public health activities because of public fear of HIV.

These sobering thoughts are not intended to discourage or disparage efforts in HIV vaccine research. As noted at the outset, an HIV vaccine will play a crucial role in global efforts to bring the pandemic under control. Rather, it is hoped that awareness of the limitations of such a vaccine strategy will inhibit hyperbole and prevent the abandonment of the useful prevention efforts that must be sustained no matter what. We must not succumb to the false hope that it will all be over when the vaccine comes.

trials, but it is general in the developing world. However, assuring access will require a massive centralized buying and distribution program supported by a large number of governments. The framework for such a program is not yet remotely in place. If it is not in place when evidence of effectiveness becomes available, the vaccine effort runs the risk of failing at its moment of triumph.

■■■■■■■■■   · · ·

EPIDEMIOLOGICAL RESEARCH

Like other forms of research, epidemiological research has expanded rapidly since the start of the AIDS pandemic. By the end of 1991, cohort studies on HIV infection and the evolution to AIDS were underway in more than 20 countries. Notably, most data from cohort studies came from industrialized rather than developing countries: a Medline search conducted by *AIDS in the World* found 8 times more studies in the United States than the total of *all* studies listed by Medline as being conducted in seven developing countries (Kenya, Zaire, Peru, Djibouti, Thailand, Singapore, Rwanda) from which it showed data. The *AIDS in the World* study found the following breakdown for 251 cohort studies analyzed: of 162 AIDS cohort studies for which the country was clearly specified, 94 percent were conducted in an industrialized country and 9, or 6 percent, in a developing country; of 66 such HIV cohort studies, 60, or 91 percent, were conducted in the industrialized world and 6, or 9 percent, in developing countries.

Among these studies, a wide variety of features and gaps are apparent. Most of the so-called natural history data available today is derived from studies in Western Europe and North America; very few natural history data are from the developing world.

A great gap exists regarding the study of HIV/AIDS and women. Although the majority concerned the general population, the largest single group studied was men having sex with men. Only one of the cohort studies was listed specifically for women infected with HIV. Thus, in spite of the number of women affected by AIDS, there is a dearth of data on progression of HIV infection in women.

Women have been relatively neglected in HIV/AIDS research programs. Women, until recently, had been grossly underrepresented among study subjects in the U.S. AIDS Clinical Trials Group (ACTG) network, as were injection drug users, minorities, and poor people. Women's participation in federally funded clinical trials may also be restricted on the basis of their reproductive status, with some agencies, such as the U.S. FDA, issuing guidelines stating that premenopausal females capable of becoming pregnant should be excluded from the earliest dose-ranging studies, except in cases of life-threatening illness.[8]

The health of women has rarely received as much research attention as has the health of men. As noted in *Searching for Women: A Literature Review on Women, HIV and AIDS in the United States:* "Even for illnesses and conditions to which men and women are equally vulnerable, researchers have favored men as study subjects and have assumed, often with little search for evidence to the contrary, that the male experience could be neatly extrapolated to women's experiences. . . . The long-standing belief that, except for gender-specific illnesses such as cervical cancer, disease manifestations will tend to be the same in the two sexes resulted in a reluctance to duplicate research in both men and women."[9] Where the prediction

---

Box 7.8: HIV/AIDS Literature Review: A Medline Search of Studies Conducted

Since the beginning of the HIV/AIDS epidemic, many research studies have been conducted. Despite the volume of studies, certain subjects have been underrepresented in this research effort. To investigate these gaps, a Medline search was conducted for the period 1989 through 1991.[a] Some of the findings are presented below:

Study type conducted	Number of studies	Percentage of total
AIDS cohort	179	71.3
HIV cohort	72	28.7
Total	251	100.0

Research topics	Cohort
General population	118
Men who have sex with men	76
Blood transfusion/ Hemophilia	28
Injection drug users	17
Vertical transmission	9
Associated with other diseases	7
Commercial sex workers	6
Other (nonspecific topics)	2
Women with HIV	1
Sex with HIV partner	1
Total (10 studies appeared twice)	261

Most of the research studies have been conducted by industrialized countries. This table reflects a line listing of countries and the number of studies conducted by each country:

proved false, medical care for women suffered as the state of women-specific knowledge lagged behind that for men. Recent efforts have begun to address these gaps.

◼━━━━━━━   •   •   •

BEHAVIORAL RESEARCH

Social and behavioral research has received relatively little attention and support in the past. In many respects, the stronger interest in biomedical research also indicates the continuing hope for and belief in a treatment and vaccine for AIDS. Table 7.4 shows that social and behavioral research accounts for only about 10 percent of the abstracts/papers indexed by Medline in 1988–1990.

Ten years into the epidemic, it is unfortunate that the potential of social and behavioral research has yet to be fulfilled. The vast number of HIV-infected people acquire their infections from sexual contact, and many of the remainder from the use of drugs: these two groups make up the prime subjects of behavioral research. Experts in behavioral research agree that traditional medical attitudes about information and behavior change are inaccurate, for the idea that people

Country	AIDS cohorts	HIV cohorts	Country	AIDS cohorts	HIV cohorts
United States	95	40	Djibouti	1	0
Netherlands	13	7	Norway	1	0
France	10	3	Thailand	1	0
United Kingdom	9	2	Singapore	1	0
Canada	7	1	Rwanda	0	1
Italy	4	1	Others	17	6
Austria	3	2	Total	179	72
Sweden	3	2			
Kenya	3	2			
Zaire	2	2			
Spain	2	0			
Denmark	2	0			
Germany	1	1			
Peru	1	1			
Switzerland	1	1			
Australia	1	0			
Belgium	1	0			

a. In searching Medline, the key words used were *HIV/AIDS cohort, longitudinal,* and *prospective studies*. This search yielded a total of 783 studies related to HIV/AIDS. However, to avoid possible duplication of citations, we are presenting data only for HIV/AIDS cohort studies. General population exposure groups for HIV include pregnant women, blood donors (nonpaid), HIV-infected persons, and serosurvey (when for a nonspecific group).

Table 7.4: Social and behavioral studies, 1988–1990[a]

Subject	Number of abstracts
Health behavior and HIV/AIDS	115
Sexual behavior	766
Commercial sex workers and HIV/AIDS	156
Homosexual(ity) and AIDS	835
Substance abuse and AIDS	427
Total abstracts	2,299
Total AIDS papers indexed, 1988–90	20,023

Source: MedLine search by *AIDS in the World* (March 1992).

a. *AIDS in the World* gathered data on behavioral research by conducting a MedLine search using the terms *AIDS* and *HIV* for the period 1988–1990. Both searches were unrestricted; therefore, the terms could be found in both the abstract and the title of the articles in the database. No language restriction was placed on the terms. On the resulting data, *AIDS in the World* refined the search using the following headings: health behavior, sexual behavior, prostitution, homsexual(ity), and substance abuse. After these headings were located, each key term was combined with AIDS and HIV individually to specify which studies to examine. For example, health behavior and AIDS were combined to determine the complex data set for this subject.

will change their behavior if informed about AIDS is clearly inadequate. There is obviously potential for behavioral intervention based on careful research. *AIDS in the World* will seek to study these research imbalances more closely in the 1993 edition.

. . .

WHO PAYS FOR AIDS RESEARCH?

The amount of public funding for HIV/AIDS research has expanded rapidly during the past decade. Based on a survey carried out by *AIDS in the World*, research spending by the 10 major industrialized countries and the European community (EC)* reached an estimated cumu-

*The survey by *AIDS in the World* of 10 major industrialized countries and the European Community was conducted between November 1991 and April 1992. In addition to the EC, *AIDS in the World* contacted officials in Australia, Canada,

lative total of $5.45 billion at the end of 1991. Only the United States reported spending on AIDS research before 1985. Although many countries have reported significant, steady increases in funding for AIDS research, the case of the United States is most pronounced, as the research commitment rose from $4 million in 1982 to $1.28 billion in 1991. U.S. resources for research in 1991 exceeded the entire amount of government-sponsored HIV/AIDS research spending by the other industrialized nations included in the survey. For the countries surveyed, 97 percent of total research expenditure involved research conducted within their own borders (see Table 7.5).*

The survey results of funding for international HIV/AIDS research activities—or research outside their own borders (i.e., developing countries)—provided by the development agencies of the 10 countries and the EC are shown in Tables 7.6 and 7.7. Although annual spending increased from zero before 1985 to a total of approximately $65 million by 1991, the cumulative total by the 10 countries amounted to just $179 million between 1985 and 1991, or nearly $28 million less than the amount spent for research in the United States alone in 1986. Again, the United States spent the most on international research, providing $130 million, or 73 percent of the total. France was second, with a total allocation of approximately $23 million. Among the rest of the countries surveyed, the amount spent internationally on research was small. Most of this funding was designated for Africa; among Asian countries, Thailand was the near exclusive beneficiary of international AIDS research funding, according to *AIDS in the World* survey results.

France, Germany, Italy, Japan, Sweden, Switzerland, the United Kingdom, and the United States. The same list of countries was contacted for international research spending.

*Attempts were made to determine the amount of research funding provided by private pharmaceuticals for AIDS research, but no single source could be found. The Pharmaceutical Manufacturers Association in Washington, DC, estimates that in 1992, U.S. pharmaceutical firms will spend about $10.9 billion total in all research and development of drugs, but it could not provide an estimate of the percentage of that figure devoted to AIDS or AIDS-related drug development and research. Likewise, global figures were unobtainable for private and corporate foundation spending. According to The Foundation Center in New York City, total private and corporate foundation grants for AIDS research between 1983 and 1990 totaled in excess of $16 million.

Table 7.5: National research funding for AIDS for selected countries: 1982–1991 (millions $U.S.)

Country	1982–84	1985	1986	1987	1988	1989	1990	1991	Total
Australia[a]		0	0.35	0.09	1.10	1.89	5.00	7.42	15.85
Canada[b]		0.82	2.07	4.37	7.63	7.34	7.51	6.41	36.15
France[c]		2.86	6.11	27.32	19.10	64.21	84.24	85.41	289.25
Germany[d]		0.34	1.48	4.23	9.02	10.66	14.24	15.61	55.58
Italy[e]		0	0	0	4.60	11.57	24.01	31.40	71.58
Japan[f]		0.02	0.53	1.09	6.61	9.48	8.88	9.69	36.30
Sweden[g]		0.02	0.11	0.70	0.82	1.18	1.12	N/A	3.95
Switzerland[h]		0	0	1.06	2.04	1.83	6.39	6.48	17.80
U.K.[i]		N/A	3.62	14.83	20.55	23.13	33.41	38.91	134.45
U.S.[j]	75.00	85.00	193.00	344.00	659.00	981.00	1,164.00	1,282.00	4,783.00
EC[k]		0	0	0.60	4.21	2.62	0.39	3.04	10.86
Year total	75.00	89.06	207.27	398.29	734.68	1,114.91	1,349.19	1,486.37	5,454.77

Detail of U.S. funding 1981–1984

	1982	1983	1984	Total
United States	4.00	24.00	47.00	75.00

Source: *AIDS in the World* survey.

Note: Budgets for Canada, Sweden, the United Kingdom, and the United States are based on a fiscal year (FY); thus figures for, say, 1985 are based on the budget for FY 1985–86.

a. Department of Community Services & Health. Budget leveling off, program being evaluated in 1991–1992.

b. Health & Welfare Department's National Health Research and Development Programme (NHRDP) and Medical Research Council. Breakdown for 1991–92: NHRDP $5.21 million; MRC $1.2 million.

c. Agence Nationale de Recherches sur le SIDA (ANRS); Centre Nationale de la Recherche Scientifique (CNRS); Office de Recherche Scientifique dans les Territoires d'Outre-mer (ORSTOM), which funds some domestic research as well; Institut Pasteur; Institut National pour la Recherche Médicale (INSERM); Institut National de la Recherche Agronomique (INRA). Breakdown for 1991:ANRS $33.71 million; CNRS $17.72 million; INSERM $16.1 million; Pasteur $16.2 million; ORSTOM and INRA $0.84 million each.

d. German Federal Ministry for Research & Health (BMFT).

e. Istituto Superiore di Sanità, Virology Department.

f. Ministry of Health and Welfare, Health Services Bureau, Infectious Diseases Control Office.

g. Swedish Council for Medical Research; Swedish Agency for Research Cooperation with Developing Countries (SAREC).

h. Swiss Federal Office of Public Health, AIDS Unit.

i. Department of Health, Research Development Division.

j. Public Health Services Agencies, Budget Division (includes all federal agencies), *Federal Government Spending for HIV/AIDS* (Washington, D.C., 1992).

k. Medical and Health Research Program.

Table 7.6: Annual official U.S. assistance allocated to support AIDS research outside the United States, 1985–1991 (millions $U.S.)

Source	1985	1986	1987	1988	1989	1990	1991	Total
USAID[a]	N/A	N/A	N/A	N/A	3.60	5.40	11.40	20.40
DOD	N/A	0.91	1.33	1.57	2.33	2.90	3.20	12.24
CDC	0.23	0.25	0.75	2.10	3.50	5.25	6.00	18.08
NIH	N/A	N/A	N/A	N/A	21.59	26.77	31.43	79.79
Total	0.23	1.16	2.08	3.67	31.02	40.32	52.03	130.51

Sources: *AIDS in the World* survey. USAID estimates based on research-related percentages of total spending on international AIDS programs.

a. For the years 1989, 1990, and 1991, research-related expenditures were 14.7%, 17.5%, and 19.5%, respectively, of the total international AIDS budget. DOD information from International Subcommittee of the Federal Coordinating Committee (FCCIS) database in consultation with DOD. Information on total NIH AIDS International Efforts/Collaboration based on communication of April 1, 1992; percentage provided by FCCIS in consultation with NIH communication of April 1, 1992.

Note: USAID = U.S. Agency for International Development; DOD = U.S. Department of Defense; CDC = U.S. Centers for Disease Control; NIH = National Institutes of Health; N/A = not available.

Between 1982 and 1991, approximately $5.63 billion were spent on AIDS research worldwide. Funds allocated to domestic research grew steadily between 1985 and 1991, during which period they nearly doubled each year. However, the rate of increase declined in 1991 for the first time since the beginning of the pandemic (see Figure 7.1). In 1991, approximately $1.55 billion were allocated to domestic and international research, compared with $1.40 billion in research funding allocated for 1990, or a mere 10 percent increase that hardly matched inflation. The $179 million in internationally funded research represents a small fraction (3 percent) of the world resources spent on research (see Figure 7.2).

Thus, the dichotomy of national versus international AIDS research spending by governments involves a difference of immense proportions: roughly 3 percent of the total research allocation was for international research funding ($179 million vs. $5.5 billion).* It can

---

*"A total of 559 AIDS-related research projects were identified in 1989 in 35 sub-Saharan African countries (range 1 to 82 projects per country). Of the 559 studies, 248 (44%) were reported to WHO through national AIDS committees,

be argued that scientific research conducted in the industrialized world will benefit all people, no matter where they live. Yet what is the power of the developing world to determine the course or direction of research? It has already been shown that the bulk of the HIV cohort studies involve people in industrialized countries. There is the need for a transfer of technology and resources from industrialized to developing countries. Would a person with AIDS in San Francisco, a woman with AIDS or HIV infection in New York or London, a clinician treating people with AIDS in Sydney or anywhere else in the industrialized world find such a scenario acceptable if the situation were reversed?

FUTURE DIRECTIONS: CAN THE PACE CONTINUE?

What is the prognosis for AIDS research for the remainder of the decade? Does the will exist to provide the resources—financial and intellectual—to dominate the epidemic? Based on an analysis of two indicators—the amount of spending on research and the number of research papers being published—it appears that by the beginning of 1992, the pace with which the industrialized countries had responded to AIDS had reached a plateau.

Projections of research spending for 1992, both nationally and internationally, suggest that the amount of funding allocated to re-

---

and 311 (56%), unknown to national AIDS committes, were identified through other sources, including lists of abstracts from international meetings and word of mouth. The research projects address the following topics: HIV-1 and HIV-2 seroprevalence among general populations and populations thought to be at risk of infection (62% of projects); knowledge, attitudes, and behavior in response to the AIDS epidemic (11%); perinatal transmission (11%); the association between HIV and other sexually transmitted disease (9%); the natural history of HIV infection (8%); the association between HIV and tuberculosis (8%), and rapid field diagnosis of HIV infection (4%). Other topics less frequently studied include possible prevention interventions (2%), evaluation methods (1%), and the cost of interventions for HIV/AIDS prevention and/or control (1%). Support for 47% of the projects are from national resources alone; 53% are collaborative projects with 87 external donors."[5-10] (Letter from D. L. Heymann, P. Bres, M. Karam, R. Biritwum, B. Nkowane, A. Sow, P. Kenya, E. G. Beausoleil, R. Widdus, and J. M. Mann, WHO/GPA, Geneva, and WHO, Regional Office for Africa, Brazzaville, Congo, "AIDS-related research in sub-Saharan Africa," *AIDS* [May 1990]:469-70.)

Table 7.7: Annual official assistance allocated to support AIDS research outside the country, 1985–1991 (millions $U.S.)

Country	1985	1986	1987	1988	1989	1990	1991	Cumulative total
Australia[a]	0	0	0	0	0	0	0.02	0.02
Canada[b]	0	0.38	0.06	1.46	0.35	0.78	1.16	4.19
France[c]	0.05	1.51	2.79	3.19	4.14	5.29	6.31	23.28
Germany[d]	N/A	N/A	N/A	N/A	N/A	N/A	N/A	3.18
Italy[e]	0	0	0	0	0	0	0	0
Japan[f]	0	0	0	0.43	0.40	0.38	0.41	1.62
Sweden[g]	0	0.21	0.41	1.11	0.67	1.61	1.81	5.82
Switzerland[h]	0	0	0	0	0	0	0	0
United Kingdom[i]	0	0	0.40	1.34	2.18	2.96	2.96	9.84
European Community[j]	0	0	0	0.38	0.05	0.05	0	0.48
Total[k]	0.05	2.1	3.66	7.91	7.79	11.07	12.67	48.43
Total + U.S.[l]	0.28	3.26	5.74	11.58	38.81	51.39	64.70	178.94

Source: AIDS in the World survey.

Note: N/A = not available.

a. Australian International Development Assistance Bureau.

b. International Development Research Centre.

c. Ministry of Cooperation and Development (MCD); ANRS; Pasteur Institutes (Bangui and Dakar); ORSTOM. No figures were available for INSERM, which has a small budget for international research inseparable from its domestic component. Breakdown for 1991: MCD $3.75 million; ANRS $1.5 million; Pasteur Institutes $0.33 million; ORSTOM $0.73 million.

d. Federal Ministry for Economic Cooperation, Division of Health, Population and Nutrition. In 1986 Germany began funding mostly intervention-linked efforts in 17 developing nations, totaling about $19.36 million through 1991. About $3.18 million was allocated to HIV-related research. No annual breakdown is available.

e. Istituto Superiore di Sanità, Virology Department.

f. Ministry of Health and Welfare, Health Services Bureau, Infectious Diseases Control Office.

g. Swedish Agency for Research Cooperation with Developing Countries.

h. Swiss Federal Office of Public Health.

i. Overseas Development Administration (ODA); Medical Research Council (MRC). International portion of MRC's budget was subtracted from the domestic portion. Breakdown for 1991: MCR $1.66 million; ODA $1.3 million.

j. EC Commission AIDS Programme.

k. Totals from 1985 to 1991 exclude German spending, which could not be broken down by year.

l. See Table 7.6.

$US (millions)

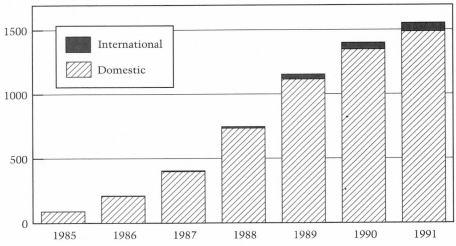

Figure 7.1. AIDS research funding, 1985-1991.
Source: AIDS in the World, 1992.

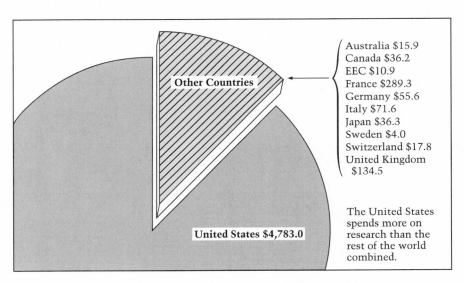

Other Countries

Australia $15.9
Canada $36.2
EEC $10.9
France $289.3
Germany $55.6
Italy $71.6
Japan $36.3
Sweden $4.0
Switzerland $17.8
United Kingdom
  $134.5

The United States
spends more on
research than the
rest of the world
combined.

United States $4,783.0

Figure 7.2. Research spending, 1981-1991 (in millions of U.S. dollars).
Source: AIDS in the World, 1992.

search on HIV/AIDS may be leveling off. The rate of increase in U.S. national spending on AIDS research began to level off before 1990. For 1993, projected budgetary increases by the U.S. government are 3.8 percent, whereas increases in research for non-AIDS projects is almost triple that level.[10] In 1993, the U.S. National Institutes of Health and Centers for Disease Control plan to allocate $34.1 million to international research activites. Of the $263 million to be spent on AIDS over the next five years by the U.S. Agency for International Development (USAID), about 17 percent will be for AIDS research outside the United States. Is it enough?

Another indicator is the number of papers on AIDS indexed by Medline. Following a meteoric rise between 1982 and 1989, the number of scientific papers on AIDS indexed by the U.S. National Library of Medicine has begun to level off as well, reaching an annual rate of increase of 5.4 percent, roughly comparable to the annual rate of increase exhibited in all other scientific disciplines (see Box 7.9). Yet the question remains whether the critical mass of energy and resources is being achieved and sustained to ensure growth and advancement of all the diverse scientific elements the world needs to confront a pandemic that shows no signs of reaching its own plateau.

Virus variability and natural history are current critical issues which raise challenges in terms of diagnostic treatment and vaccine development. To conclude this chapter, the variability of HIV and the epidemiology and natural history of HIV-2 will be addressed.

HIV VIRUS VARIABILITY

ançoise Barré-Sinoussi
titut Pasteur, Paris,
ance

The human immunodeficiency virus (HIV) is a cytopathogenic virus that causes AIDS. Two types of viruses have been identified: HIV-1, found worldwide, and HIV-2, found mainly in West Africa. Within each type, genetic variations occur, the implications of which are highlighted here.

The Genetic Structure of HIV

Retroviral genomes are composed of at least three genes named *gag*, *pol*, and *env*. These genes provide genetic information for the HIV nucleocapside antigens, reverse transcriptase, and surface proteins, respectively.

A similar DNA sequence of varying length (LTR or long terminal repeat) can be found at each end of the proviral DNA. This sequence contains elements that can promote proviral gene integration in the host cell's genome and expression of these genes.

The situation is more complex with regard to the HIV genome. It contains two additional sequences of genes located between *pol* and *env*, and next to *env*. These two sequences are made of at least six additional viral genes: *tat, rev, vif, vpr, vpu,* and *nef*. These genes regulate expression of viral DNA and are, therefore, involved in HIV replication. They can also modify the expression of certain host cell genes, thereby altering the normal biological processes of infected cells. The direct and indirect consequences of these alterations must be taken into account when considering the physiopathology of HIV infection. This is particularly true for the *tat* and *nef* regulator proteins, which may play an important role in the disease's progression in subjects exposed to HIV. This complex genetic structure is a specific characteristic of the lentivirus subgroup.

Box 7.9: AIDS Research 1982–1991: Do Research Papers Tell the Story?

Adapted from J. Elford, R. Bor, and P. Summers, "Research into HIV and AIDS between 1981 and 1990: The epidemic curve," *AIDS* 5 (1991):1515–19 (published by Current Science, Ltd.)

Just how rapidly has research into HIV and AIDS grown in the last 10 years? What have been its major areas of concentration? Where has the research been conducted? How accessible are the research findings? One measure of the volume and nature of research into HIV and AIDS comes from examining scientific papers published between 1982 and 1991. In fact, not all research findings are submitted or accepted for publication. Of those that are, there is always a lag between the funding and execution of the research and the publication of the results. A Medline search showed a meteoric rise in the number of papers indexed as HIV/AIDS, from 24 in 1982 to 6,552 in 1990. However, the most recent survey by *AIDS in the World* shows a leveling off in 1990 and 1991.

A two-page entry in the Centers for Disease Control's *Morbidity and Mortality Weekly Report* just over 10 years ago marked the dawn of a new age in research.[a] Since then, more than 30,000 papers on HIV/AIDS have been indexed by Medline. This figure would be remarkable in and of itself. The fact that none of the thousands of papers and posters at the seven international conferences on AIDS (unless otherwise published) or specialist journals, such as *AIDS Care, AIDS Education and Prevention,* and *AIDS Patient Care,* are indexed by Medline makes it even more so (see Figure 7.B).

Although the increase has been spectacular, the distribution of

Genetic Variability of HIV

The genetic structures of HIV-1 and HIV-2 are similar. However, in HIV-2, the *vpu* gene is absent and another gene, called *vpx*, is present. Precise comparative analysis of each genetic element of HIV-1 and HIV-2 revealed important differences between these two HIV viruses, especially for the *env* gene.

Genetic diversity is one characteristic of this family of viruses. Thus, differences in genetic sequence can be observed between variants of a same type of HIV found in different patients. Furthermore, several variants of HIV-1 (or HIV-2) may be found in a given patient. Recent data have shown that these strain variations occur in a patient during the course of HIV infection, as early as five days after infection and several months after exposure. HIV is submitted to selection by the host's immune system as it fights infection. This phenomenon may be the way the virus avoids destruction by the host's immune defenses. Persistent infections observed in patients may be a conse-

---

research, as reflected in the type and origin of the papers, has been uneven. The number of social/behavioral research papers indexed was low, perhaps reflecting the fact that some journals were excluded. In addition, only 3 percent of the papers discuss AIDS in sub-Saharan Africa, the source of a quarter of all AIDS reported cases.[b] Recently, the number of papers about, and by researchers from, Africa has increased, but not in parallel with the expansion of the epidemic.

A review of all HIV/AIDS entries indexed by Medline reveals the shifting areas of major interest in HIV/AIDS research. Although finding the cause of AIDS was a priority in the early 1980s, between 1983 and 1990 the proportion of papers concerned with the etiology of AIDS dropped from

25 percent to 3 percent. In that same period the percentage of papers concerned with the virus increased from 2 to 37 percent. The proportion of papers dealing with prevention and control reached a peak of 18 percent in 1988 but declined to 12 percent by 1990. Drug therapy and psychological aspects of HIV/AIDS accounted for an increasing, though still relatively small, proportion of indexed papers throughout the decade. The number of papers addressing the epidemiology of HIV/AIDS has remained constant at around 10 percent.

Medline also showed the predominance of English as the lingua franca of medical science, including HIV/AIDS (although selection bias may have slightly exaggerated its dominant position). This raises important questions about the accessibility of

quence of this viral escape mechanism.

This variability is not a property of the entire genome. *Gag, pol, vif,* and *vpr* genes are usually genetically stable. *Tat* and *rev* genes vary, but to a lesser degree than do *nef* and *env* genes. The *env* gene encodes for a glycosylated protein precursor, gp160. This precursor is then cleaved into an external gycoprotein (gp110/120) and a trans-membrane protein (gp41) by the host cell's enzymes.

Several domains can be distinguished from one another in these highly glycosylated proteins. The constant domains are called C domains; those that vary are V domains. We are beginning to familiarize ourselves with the biological roles played by these domains. For instance, domain C3 of gp110/120 is where the viral envelope protein attaches itself to the target cell membrane's CD4 molecule. This viral protein's degree of glycosylation seems to be an important factor in its affinity for the CD4 molecule.

The gp110/CD4 interaction allows for a change in the envelope protein's structure to take place. This change causes other protein domains to be exposed, namely, the V3 and C4 domains. The V3

published research for the countries most affected by HIV/AIDS. Interestingly, Russian assumed second place as the overall language of medical science, yet fell toward the bottom for HIV/AIDS research, alongside Chinese. (Both the USSR and China reported relatively few cases of HIV and AIDS in the 1980s.)

The overall rate of increase in published papers on HIV/AIDS certainly reflects an increase in the amount of AIDS research since 1982. However, there appears to be little doubt that the rate of growth of HIV/AIDS research publications is leveling off, corresponding—at least at one level—to a plateau in the rate of increase of AIDS research funding. Still, such activity remains high, representing an important percentage of overall medical research.

In conclusion, medical history has never seen so much attention paid to a particular issue in so short a time. It remains to be seen how HIV/AIDS may stimulate research on other issues. Certainly, the increase in the number of papers on HIV/AIDS will be less dramatic in the 1990s. The survey suggests that priorities should be given to prevention and to further development of drug therapies. Finally, countries and continents neglected by research in the 1980s must be granted increased priority in the decade to come, for this is where the burden of the disease will undoubtedly fall.

a. Centers for Disease Control, "Pneumocystis pneumonia—Los Angeles," *Morbidity and Mortality Weekly Report* 30 (1981):250–52.
b. World Health Organization Global AIDS Statistics. *AIDS Care* 3 (1991):349–52.

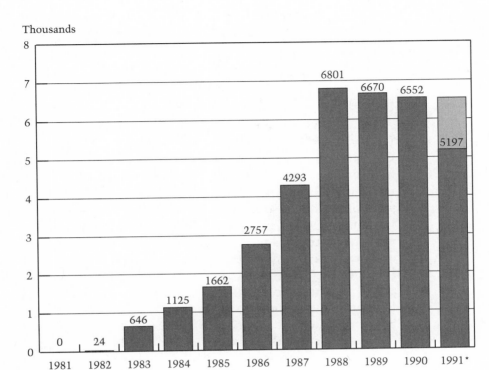

Thousands

*1991 data incomplete; total for 1991 is estimated on basis of previous year's experience.

Figure 7.B. A 10-year retrospective search: papers on HIV/AIDS indexed by Medline, 1981-91.
Source: Medline search by AIDS in the World.

domain is a major neutralizing epitope and plays a major part in the HIV virus's tropism for target cells. It is involved in the penetration of HIV into the host cell. The hydrophobic C4 domain of the gp41 transmembrane protein can anchor itself into the host cell's membrane, thereby facilitating fusion between the cell and the HIV virus. Other HIV viral envelope domains, such as V1 and V4, seem to be essential determining factors in HIV's pathogenic effect on the host cell.

Consequences of HIV Genetic Variability

HIV viruses' envelope proteins have many biological and immunological roles. The envelope's genetic variability therefore leads to differences between HIV variants in terms of biology as well as immunology. These differences affect:

- The physiopathology of HIV infection.
- The development of efficacious drugs and vaccines.
- The diagnosis of HIV infection.

Consequences for Biological Properties of HIV

Cells that carry a CD4 molecule on their surface are the main targets of HIV infection. These CD4 molecules have been identified as receptors for HIV. Target cells include the T lymphocyte CD4+ "helper" subgroup. They also include monocytes/macrophages or cells of similar lineage, such as dendritic cells, microglial cells in the central nervous system, Langerhans cells in the skin, Küpfer cells in the liver, and others. HIV is also capable of infecting certain epithelial cells, B lymphocytes after they have been altered by the Epstein-Barr virus (EBV), or cytotoxic CD8+ lymphocytes that have been altered by the Human T-Lymphotropic Virus (HTLV-1). Several CD4 cells, such as bone marrow precursors, human fibroblasts, and certain intestinal, neuronal, or endothelial cells, are vulnerable to HIV infection.

It must be stressed that differences are observed in different areas of viral activity according to the genetic variant studied. These areas are viral tropism for target cells, speed of replication, and rate of viral replication in the host cell. Several HIV variants with tropism strictly limited to macrophages have been described. These differences seem to result from mutations occurring in functional variable regions of the viral envelope, such as the protein's V3 domain.

The viral envelope's affinity for the CD4 molecule also seems to vary according to the genetic variant of HIV. This phenomenon can probably be explained by alterations in the secondary and/or tertiary structures of this C domain, which is located between two variable regions of the *env* gene.

Consequences for the Physiopathology of HIV Infection

Many factors seem to play a role in the slow progression of HIV infection to AIDS. Among these factors, phenomena attributable to virus/host and virus/cell interactions seem essential.

When viruses spread throughout the organism, highly virulent

HIV variants seem to undergo selection. These variants are capable of escaping the host organism's immune defenses and may be responsible for progressive reduction of T lymphocyte counts as infection progresses towards disease. One main biological characteristic of these variants is their highly cytopathogenic effect on CD4+ lymphocyte cultures in vitro.

This cytopathogenic effect is a result of the interaction between the CD4 molecule and the viral envelope. It leads, among other things, to the fusion of normal CD4+ lymphocytes and infected CD4+ lymphocytes that express the virus's surface antigens. This fusion results in the creation of nonviable giant multinucleate cells (syncytia).

However, this in vitro effect alone cannot explain the magnitude of the immune system disorder and the progressive but complete destruction of the CD4+ T lymphocytes. Some authors have suggested other mechanisms involving the viral envelope and immune responses aimed at this envelope. For instance, the expression of viral antigens on the surface of infected lymphocytes or the binding of free envelope proteins on the CD4+ lymphocytes' surface could lead to the lymphocytes' destruction. This destruction could involve cytotoxic T lymphocytes (CTL) or antibody-dependent cell-mediated cytotoxicity (ADCC), which could be directed against the viral envelope.

The presence of expressed viral envelope proteins on the surface of normal or infected CD4+ T lymphocytes could inhibit normal lymphocyte/macrophage interactions. These interactions are essential in any T lymphocyte-dependent immune response.

Consequences for Drug and Vaccine Development

Viral escape phenomena have been described in therapeutic trials. These trials were conducted on antiretroviral drugs, such as AZT or ddI.

HIV variants have appeared during long-term treatments by such reverse transcriptase inhibitors as AZT or ddI. The genetic changes seemed to be most pronounced in the *pol* gene.

This phenomenon supports the hypothesis that complex specific treatments can be developed using combinations of molecules. These combinations could inhibit the viral replication cycle in the host cell at the same stage or at different stages.

Most of the data found in literature seem to converge when it comes to the field of anti-HIV vaccine development. Research data stress the need for neutralizing humoral immune responses directed against the main neutralization epitope, called the *V3 loop*, in order to achieve protection against this infection.

Domains located on either side of the tip of this V3 loop differ in the envelopes of HIV variants. The conformation of this structure and, therefore, the antibody response directed against this epitope may vary from one variant to another. This variance leads to further delay in the development of the universal prophylactic vaccine to come.

Consequences for the Diagnosis of HIV Infection

Diagnostic tests for HIV infection rely on the detection of anti-HIV antibodies or viral genetic sequences. The reliability of the tests is determined by viral reagents used. HIV genetic diversity may lead to falsely negative results when testing for a particular type of virus. Furthermore, diagnosis of HIV-1 and/or HIV-2 infection creates an additional difficulty, because an HIV-1 test may not diagnose an infection by HIV-2, and vice versa.

One must be wary of anti-HIV antibody detection tests that have been developed using peptides synthesized from amino acid sequences corresponding to a perfectly well-known and characterized HIV variant. In a patient infected with a genetically unknown HIV variant, the use of such a diagnostic test may yield a false negative result. Infected patients may carry antibodies that are directed specifically against their own viral variants, which therefore, may not react to the peptides used as antigens in these diagnostic tests.

Diagnostic and/or confirmation tests using an entire purified virus or recombinant proteins as antigens are the only reliable tests available at present. Recombinant proteins used are mainly the *env* proteins, in association with synthesized peptides or not. Similar problems occur in the diagnosis of HIV infection through detection of viral genetic sequences after amplification using a polymerase chain reaction (PCR). This technique is appealing, as it is very sensitive to HIV. However, PCR use DNA primers that have been selected and synthesized according to our present knowledge of HIV genetic sequences. The genetic sequences used are those that seem to be common to the genome of all known HIV variants. One cannot be sure that these sequences will be present in all future HIV variants of an HIV-infected person.

This method must therefore be used rigorously and carefully. One must also be careful as to the test's reliability when used for initial HIV diagnosis. Thus, PCR is not often used for diagnosis of HIV infections, except in research laboratories and HIV infection in newborns. In this case, PCR is used along with other tests (antigenemia, IgA anti-HIV antibody titers, etc.) that confirm initial results obtained by PCR.

Conclusion

In the coming years as the HIV/AIDS pandemic continues to grow, the emergence of many variants of HIV should be expected. The diagnostic and therapeutic problems created will become increasingly complex. The efficacy of vaccines will depend on their capacity to cover an increasingly broad spectrum of variants.

But the very strength of the virus, which resides in its genetic variability, may make it more vulnerable to scientific discovery. As it takes on multiple aspects and acquires changing biological and pathogenic features, the virus exposes itself to a better understanding, on the part of research, of the mechanisms that regulate and signal these variations and of the constant characteristics that are central to its power. Therein lies some hope of understanding more deeply and with increasing precision the behavior of the elusive virus and of developing diagnostic methods, therapies, and vaccines that will contribute to its domination.

▬▬▬▬   .   .   .

THE EPIDEMIOLOGY OF HIV-2 INFECTION

n M. De Cock,
tor of Project
RO-CI in Abidjan,
d'Ivoire, and
çoise Brun-Vezinet,
f, Virology Laboratory
e Hôpital
at-Claude Bernard,
, France

The existence of HIV-2 was first suggested in 1985 following the demonstration in commercial sex workers in Senegal of serologic reactivity to antigens of simian immunodeficiency virus (SIVmac).[11] In 1986, researchers isolated the virus in persons with AIDS from Guinea-Bissau and Cape Verde.[12] Since then, the highest rates of HIV-2 infection have been reported in West Africa, with Guinea-Bissau the most heavily affected.[13,14] HIV-2 infection also exists in Angola and Mozambique, and sporadic cases have been reported from the Americas, India, and most European countries—particularly Portugal and France.

Routes of transmission[15,16] and risk factors[17,18] for HIV-1 and HIV-2 are similar. However, while the comparative efficacy of transmission of HIV-1 and HIV-2 has not been thoroughly studied, there is growing evidence that HIV-1 is transmitted more efficiently through heterosexual contact than HIV-2, at least early in the course of infection. This may explain why HIV-1 has spread more rapidly in West Africa than HIV-2, despite the fact that HIV-2 may have been present longer in many countries. Nevertheless, a study in Côte d'Ivoire showed a similar rate of infection in sexual partners of hospitalized medical patients infected with either HIV-1 or HIV-2, suggesting that HIV-2 infectivity increases over time as the infection progresses to disease.

HIV-2 seems less easily transmitted than HIV-1 from an infected mother to her fetus/infant as reflected in the higher rate of serological concordance between HIV-1–infected mothers and their living children. Furthermore, children born to HIV-2–infected mothers have a greater chance of survival than those born to women infected with HIV-1.[19,20] Precise transmission rates remain to be determined.

Disease Associations and Natural History

Epidemiological studies have shown similar disease manifestations associated with HIV-2 as with HIV-1 infection, including AIDS, tuberculosis, and other AIDS-related features such as oral candidiasis, hairy leukoplakia, pruriginous dermatitis, and varicella zoster.[21,22] In cross-sectional studies, similar types of immunologic abnormalities have been described in HIV-2- as in HIV-1-positive persons, including reduced CD4 cell counts, increased CD8 cell counts, and reduced CD4/CD8 cell ratios.[23] However, in asymptomatic persons these immunologic abnormalities have tended to be less marked than in HIV-1-infected persons.[24] As in persons with HIV-1 infection, mortality levels have been shown to be increased in HIV-2-positive persons followed prospectively.

HIV-2 seems to have a longer latency period than HIV-1. Evidence for this includes reports of HIV-2-infected persons with long survival;[25] an increasing age-specific prevalence of HIV-2 infection in certain populations;[26] the less marked immunologic aberrations in HIV-2- compared with HIV-1-infected persons in cross-sectional studies;[27] and the results of prospective cohort studies of HIV-2-infected persons. In Senegal, studies of female commercial sex workers have shown a greater incidence of AIDS in women who are infected with HIV-1.[28] Autopsy studies in Côte d'Ivoire showed that persons infected with HIV-2 had a greater frequency of certain lesions characteristic of long-standing immunodeficiency, including giant cell encephalitis and severe cytomegalovirus disease than persons infected with HIV-1.[29]

Diagnosis and Clinical Virology

Numerous tests are now available to detect HIV-1 and HIV-2 antibodies. Second generation assays most used currently incorporate recombinant and/or synthetic peptide antigens. Tests based on synthetic peptides corresponding to the N-terminal part of the viral transmembrane glycoproteins are the most specific for distinguishing between HIV-1 and HIV-2. Even with these tests, however, dual serologic reactivity may remain a problem in West African countries where HIV-1 and HIV-2 are spreading; the differentiation between dual infection and serologic cross reactivity in such cases is problematic.

First results of measurements of virus load in HIV-2-infected persons showed a lower rate of virus isolation and detection by polymerase chain reaction (PCR) in persons with higher CD4 cell counts than in those with advanced immunodeficiency.

Conclusions

HIV-2 is a pathogenic virus causing AIDS and associated conditions, whose routes of transmission are similar as those of HIV-1. Firm conclusions on natural history of HIV-2 require more prospective work, but a longer latency period is likely. Early in the course of infection, sexual and perinatal modes of transmission seem less efficient for HIV-2 than for HIV-1. Because the routes of transmission of HIV-1 and HIV-2 are the same, the same public health interventions should apply to these two virus infections.

CHAPTER EIGHT

. . . .

National AIDS Programs

National AIDS programs (NAPs) are made of people, structures, and resources. National AIDS programs are the combination of collective actions that take place within the boundaries of a nation and have an overall plan, a management and coordination structure, a budget, and a monitoring and evaluation capacity. These actions may involve governmental institutions and agencies, nongovernmental organizations (NGOs), and the private sector. The role of national AIDS programs is to ensure that people who are affected and those who are at risk acquire and are assured of the means for their own protection and well-being. Thus, there is a critical interaction between the individual, society, and the program: programs should be capable of promoting and supporting changes in individual behavior and health, as well as changes in dysfunctional social structures. Conversely, the programs should be capable of changing in response to societal or individual demands and pressures.

A diverse array of AIDS-related policies and programs has emerged during the first decade of response to the pandemic. Even in industrialized democracies, which share certain historical, cultural, societal, and economic characteristics, the response has varied widely (Box 8.1). This chapter examines the evolution of national AIDS programs and identifies some of the most important features, achievements, and current challenges. The next four chapters describe and analyze trends worldwide in implementing prevention and care strategies, the cost of these programs, and the level of international support for AIDS prevention and care.

Box 8.1: AIDS in the Industrialized Democracies

The Pandemic's Challenge to Industrialized Democracies

David L. Kirp, School of Public Policy, University of California, Berkeley; and Ronald Bayer, Division of Sociomedical Science, Columbia University School of Public Health. (Adapted from David L. Kirp and Ronald Bayer, eds., *AIDS in the Industrialized Democracies: Passions, Politics, and Policies* [New Brunswick, N.J.: Rutgers University Press, 1992].)

Although the HIV/AIDS pandemic has placed the heaviest burden on the world's poorer nations, it also presents economically advanced nations with a challenge many had come to believe would never be seen again. Yet despite their similarities, industrialized democracies have not all responded alike. HIV is a single virus, but it occurs in distinctive societies at distinct moments in their history and has thus led to public policy unique to each nation, its politics, and culture.

National Traditions Have Shaped Diverse Responses

The political coloration of individual governments has proved less significant in shaping the overall response to AIDS than have long-established traditions for dealing with matters of sexuality, drug use, privacy, the rights of vulnerable minorities, and perceived threats to the public health. These preexisting patterns of public policy are primarily responsible for the diversity of responses. And there is indeed diversity: public health officials in New York City and San Francisco chose to close or regulate the bathhouses, whereas authorities in Australia, the Netherlands, and Denmark let them stay open. Needle exchange programs have been accepted in the Netherlands but have caused bitter debate in Germany; the United States.

Britain, Sweden, and Australia decided to stress the fear of death in their AIDS information campaigns; the Netherlands, France, Spain, and Denmark selected a more benign approach. Only in the United States and Spain was there significant public outcry on the subject of schoolchildren with AIDS.

Investigating the Differences: Issues to Consider

Much of the comparative analysis of AIDS policy to date has involved extracting a single strand of policy from its context: needle exchange, for example, or the treatment of HIV-infected prisoners. We sought, quite differently, to locate the development of AIDS policy within the broader framework of social policy formation. To do this, we looked at how the industrialized democracies dealt with a number of selected issues: public health, drug abuse, homosexuality, sex education, confidentiality and discrimination, health and social security, and the policymaking process. We asked many specific questions about each area of concern. What, for example, is the country's tradition of reliance on the imposition of restraints on those deemed a threat to public health? What is the role of criminal law in drug abuse control? How well is the homosexual community organized? Do moralistic concerns shape the content of sex education? What is the scope of health insurance protection? Are interest-group constituencies involved in formulating and implementing health and social policy?

The Poles of Public Health Strategy: Contain-and-Control versus Cooperation-and-Inclusion

The mix of policy decisions on AIDS adopted by any country is not reducible to a single, simple formulation. Rather, it falls somewhere between two poles: the *contain-and-control strategy* and the *cooperation-and-inclusion strategy*. Contain-and-control relies on compulsion to identify those with HIV and isolate them as a way of preventing transmission of the virus. It derives from the historical tradition of public health codified around a century ago in the context of virulent epidemics. Rarely applied in recent decades, the philosophy nevertheless continues to characterize elements of the response to sexually transmitted diseases, particularly the emphasis on compulsory identification through screening.

Cooperation-and-inclusion reflects a newer tradition. It attempts to engage those most vulnerable to AIDS in education, voluntary testing, and counseling by protecting their privacy and social interests. This strategy is based on the effort to confront chronic noninfectious diseases that are linked to patterns of behavior (alcoholism, lung cancer, heart disease) and emphasizes the role of persuasion to modify life-styles linked to disease.

What Are the Lessons for the Future?

Each of the industrialized democracies had to decide a fundamental question: Which approach would be drawn on to prevent HIV spread? Thus far, the answers reflect the balance of political forces in each nation, the importance placed on privacy, the relative commitment to personal liberty, the value placed on voluntarism, and the changing epidemiology of HIV/AIDS.

In short, the politics of AIDS is the politics of democracy in the face of a critical challenge to communal well-being. The responses tell us a great deal not only about our recent past but also about how the next out-of-the-ordinary challenge to communal health is likely to be faced. If AIDS has taught us anything, it is that we can no longer believe that we are secure against such a threat.

Box 8.2: A Framework to Assess National AIDS Programs

The following criteria can be used to assess the quality and comprehensiveness of national AIDS programs.

Criterion 1. Voicing Commitment

Commitment is reflected by:

- Acknowledging AIDS at the highest executive level
- Creating programs
- Creating a multidisciplinary, multisectoral national AIDS advisory committee that reports to and interacts with the forum where policies are formulated and decisions are made
- Including HIV/AIDS prevention and control in the development plan, national budget, or organization's mandate

Criterion 2. Translating Commitment into Action

Ensuring consistency between policies and strategies endorsed in international arenas and domestic policies and activities for:

- Providing information and education
- Providing health and social services
- Creating and reinforcing a supportive social environment, with special attention to human rights
- Upholding international solidarity through the exchange of information, knowledge, skills, and resources and participating in international governmental and nongovernmental networks

Criterion 3. Coalition Building

Partnership between governmental and nongovernmental sectors in policy development and program implementation, as reflected in:

- A jointly stated policy and a mutually agreed on agenda delineating the respective roles and responsibilities of the governmental and nongovernmental partners
- A delegation of authority and resources by the governmental to nongovernmental programs and, in return, a commitment by the nongovernmental sector to adhere to mutually agreed on policies
- The participation of people affected by the pandemic in program development and implementation

Criterion 4. Planning and Coordinating

Establishment of a comprehensive plan:

- Stating objectives, targets, strategies, and evaluation criteria
- Focusing on the modes of HIV transmission relevant to the populations at risk and preparing a detailed plan of action
- Specifying population groups that would benefit from the program, and those who will not be reached
- Establishing functional links and ties with primary health care and social services
- Providing a mechanism for domestic and international coordination

Criterion 5. Managing

Strengthening program management through:

- Training and deployment of needed human resources

- Efficiently using existing structures and services
- Undertaking innovative and dynamic action

Criterion 6. Responding to Prevention Needs

Responding to individual and collective needs by:

- Providing information, supplies, equipment, prevention, and social services
- Prioritizing interventions according to risks and resources

Criterion 7. Responding to Care Needs

Responding to individual and collective needs for care by:

- Expanding coverage and increasing the quality of medical services
- Prioritizing interventions according to needs and resources

Criterion 8. Securing Financial Resources

Securing needed financial resources and accounting for their use by:

- Mobilizing resources nationally and internationally
- Developing and operating a reliable accounting system

Criterion 9. Sustaining the Effort

Ensuring the sustainability and self-reliance of effective programs by:

- Setting a course of action that reflects the needs and aspirations of the community served
- Concentrating on long-term activities that require minimal external support

Criterion 10. Evaluating Progress

Improving program efficiency by periodically:

- Monitoring and evaluating program's process and progress
- Applying evaluation findings in reorienting program direction

Criterion 11. Evaluating Impact

Improving policies and enhancing programs' cost effectiveness by:

- Conducting periodic evaluations of the program's impact on behavioral and epidemiological trends
- Applying evaluation findings to policy and program development

FRAMEWORK FOR ASSESSING NATIONAL AIDS PROGRAMS

AIDS in the World has developed a framework for assessing national AIDS programs (Box 8.2) in terms of policy basis, planning, management and implementation capacity, and resources and evaluation strategy. It particularly emphasizes the linkages among governmental, nongovernmental, and private sectors in the realization of a truly national AIDS program.

In order to collect information on national AIDS programs, *AIDS in the World* conducted a survey in 37 countries (Box 8.3). The characteristics of the countries surveyed are tabulated in Appendix 8.1. The survey findings are summarized for each country in Appendix 8.2 and are analyzed in more detail in relevant chapters.

Among the 37 countries surveyed, the Czech and Slovak republics

---

Box 8.3: *AIDS in the World* Family of Surveys

AIDS in the World (AIW) conducted a family of surveys from December 1991 through March 1992. The largest of these involved 38 countries and investigated national AIDS program policies, strategies, structures, functions, and financing patterns. Other surveys focused on specific elements of national AIDS programs, such as nongovernmental organizations (NGOs), blood transfusion services, program management issues, AZT costing issues, and injection drug use. (See Table 8.A.)

Because the main questionnaire on AIDS program structure and prevention services was sent to official national AIDS programs, the responses reflect the governments' account and perspective of their plans, services, and accomplishments. The nongovernmental organization survey provides a different perspective, focusing on the role NGOs have played in HIV/AIDS prevention and care. To develop a comprehensive picture, the following sections draw from the various surveys conducted by AIW, from documents and reports (both national and international), and from published literature.

Survey of 38 National AIDS Programs: Management, Financing, and Prevention Strategies

Countries were chosen from each of the 10 Geographic Areas of Affinity; within each area the variety of situations that are represented differ by the size of the national population, the type of government structure (federal versus centralized), the Human Development Index level, and the approach to AIDS prevention and control. Together, these countries included 74 percent of the world population and 82

Table 8.A: *AIDS in the World* family of surveys, December 1991–March 1992

Survey topic	No. of countries responding/invited to participate
HIV/AIDS program management, financing, and prevention strategies	38/44
Blood transfusion services	15/18
AZT availability and cost	15/15
NGOs	25/30
National program managers	14/15
Research spending	11/11
Injection drug use	22/30

percent of the cumulative number of AIDS cases reported since the beginning of the pandemic. (See Appendix 8.1.)

Prior to implementation, the survey questionnaire was pretested by three national AIDS program managers, revised, and then sent out to national AIDS programs in one of three languages (English, French, Spanish).

The response rate was very high, demonstrating the positive attitude of the programs surveyed toward international sharing of the information. Of the 44 countries that received a survey questionnaire, 38 (86 percent) responded, and most of them provided all the information requested. Gaps were filled in through follow-up communication with program managers or with alternative sources. Where they were available, AIW obtained copies of national AIDS plans and program evaluation reports issued by the countries or the WHO Global Programme on AIDS.

Appendix 8.1 summarizes selected indicators and characteristics that provide a general profile of each country's program. The results of this survey are discussed in the relevant chapters and are summarized in Appendix 8.2.

AIDS in the World expresses its gratitude to all respondents for their cooperation.

The participants, by Area of Affinity, were: (1) Canada, United States; (2) France, Germany, Italy, Netherlands, Norway, Sweden, Switzerland, United Kingdom; (3) Australia; (4) Argentina, Colombia, Mexico; (5) Cameroon, Congo, Côte d'Ivoire, Ethiopia, Nigeria, Rwanda, Senegal, Tanzania, Uganda, Zambia; (6) Haiti, St. Lucia, Trinidad and Tobago; (7) Czech Republic, Poland, Slovak Republic, Soviet Union; (8) Egypt, Morocco, Pakistan; (9) China, Japan; (10) India, Thailand.

responded separately. Both sets of responses are provided for questions covering events that followed the creation of the Czech and Slovak Federal Republic in March 1990. In such cases the number of respondents totals 38.

■■■■■   .   .   .

VOICING COMMITMENT

Do Heads of State Have the Right to Remain Silent?

National commitment to AIDS requires placing AIDS on the political agenda. Overall, political leaders have done so reluctantly, late, and with limited force. In 24 of the 37 countries surveyed by *AIDS in the World* in January–February 1992, the head of state had made a statement on HIV/AIDS.[1] In only four countries (Australia, Czechoslovakia, Mexico, and Tanzania) was this statement made before 1986, by which time the public had demanded information and collective action. To the credit of the 24 leaders who made statements, they publicly addressed the issue on several occasions. Repeat statements had been made in almost all of these countries within the twelve months prior to the survey. The content of these statements is analyzed in Chapter 9. Interestingly, many countries whose heads of state remained silent on HIV/AIDS rank lower on the Human Freedom Index of the United Nations Development Program (UNDP).[2] (See Table 8.1.)

Half of the heads of state who addressed the issue of HIV/AIDS did so only after 1988. In January of that year, a world summit on AIDS, organized jointly in London by WHO and the government of the United Kingdom, brought together delegates from 148 countries. One hundred ministers of health attended, more than had ever before assembled on a health issue. The summit resulted in a declaration that underscored the need for reinforced political commitment in the world's response to AIDS, for information, and for education. Following the summit, a number of governments apparently felt that it was time to address the issue of AIDS publicly. However, 13 heads of state included in the *AIDS in the World* survey took a year or more to express their concern about the situation publicly. To date, in 13 of the 37 countries surveyed, no public address has been made on AIDS by a head of state. (See Appendix 8.2 on program profile and Table 8.1.)

Table 8.1: First statement on AIDS by heads of state, 1981-1991, and Human Freedom Index (HFI)

First statement on AIDS by head of state	Ranking on HFI		Total
	Medium/low	High	
Before/in 1988	4	7	11
After 1988	9	4	13
Never	11	2	13
Total	24	13	37

Sources: Statements: *AIDS in the World, 1992.* Countries' ranking on Human Freedom Index: United Nations Development Program, *Human Development Report 1991.*

National AIDS Advisory Committees

National commitment also requires the creation of an advisory committee to guide policy and strategy design. Every country in the world has created such a committee. Initially, these committees were largely comprised of members of the scientific and medical professions and mainly provided technical advice. With a few exceptions, they were and still are responsible to the minister of health. As the need to involve other sectors and groups in national programs became clear, and pressure from other ministries and community-based organizations mounted, the composition of these committees changed to include more women, representatives from other government sectors and nongovernmental organizations, and people with HIV infection and AIDS. This change shifted the scope of the work of these committees increasingly to the social field, a task for which they were often unprepared in terms of their mandate or location within the government. In addition, as more governmental sectors began to participate in these committees, their focus shifted away from technical functions to coordination, a task they generally had no clear authority to perform. In particular, they exercised very little control over resource allocation. This prerogative was retained by the management team of the government program, in consultation with donor agencies in developing countries.

Gradually many national committees lost their focus and momentum. This evolution coincided with a shift of demand by policymakers and the public away from information on the nature of the pandemic and policy guidance and toward action. Other committees were set up by many countries with a coordinating mandate, creating a forum for discussing implementation issues and resource allocation. In many of these cases, national advisory committees were relegated back to their initially assigned technical functions, but they never fully regained their effectiveness.

Another common problem many of these advisory committees face is that their voice is often not heard, resulting in a loss of credibility. As a result, meetings are few and far between, public statements receive less attention, inadequate funding prevents committees from functioning efficiently, and, more important, committee advice exerts little influence on the political system. An added handicap is their place in the government hierarchy; in most countries, they report to the ministers of health, who, unlike ministers of planning, finance, or defense, are not among the most influential members of governments, even in times of health crisis. With an average tenure of office for ministers of health of one to two years, providing new officials with initial briefing is a regular task of national advisory committees and managers of AIDS programs. Often, this rapid turnover has resulted in ill-considered decisions motivated by the new minister's desire to act swiftly in a new political direction. When the committee is directly responsible to the head of state or the prime minister, as in Thailand, Uganda, or the United States, its work should have greater impact. Unfortunately, these expectations are not always met. In the United States, the action-oriented report of the National Commission on AIDS in 1991 did not trigger action by the executive office. In Uganda, the National Advisory Committee had great difficulty in securing a presidential endorsement to promote condoms.

Thus, the overall influence of national advisory committees has declined since their inception in the 1980s. Although the expansion of membership has created opportunities to debate policy issues more broadly, there are still too few examples of such policies being publicized, endorsed, and translated into action. An *AIDS in the World* survey of fourteen national AIDS program managers showed that since being established, all but two committees had been restructured. The reasons given for this restructuring included the need to involve more sectors, increase the representation of women, and heighten visibility

(Box 8.4). Clearly, there are two major needs: first, for a *think-tank* on AIDS removed from political pressures; and, second, for a coordinating committee, truly intersectoral and with the full participation of representatives of nongovernmental organizations and people with AIDS, to be powerful and effective participants in national policy and program development.

AIDS on the Development Agenda

Since the early years of the response to AIDS, policies and programs were guided by two motives misperceived by many people as antagonistic: a human rights/humanitarian approach and a public health

---

Box 8.4: A Mini-Survey of National AIDS Program Managers in 14 Countries

In February 1992, *AIDS in the World* carried out a mini-survey of 14 national AIDS program managers in the following countries:

Cameroon	Fiji	Papua New
Canada	Ireland	Guinea
Chile	Jamaica	Philippines
Congo	New Zealand	Tanzania
Ethiopia	Nigeria	Uganda

The purpose of this survey was to obtain NAP managers' views of the functions of their program, their evolution (for example, decentralization), relationship to NGOs and funding agencies, major achievements, and constraints. The programs were drawn from various regions and from both industrialized and developing countries. In view of its many large-scale programs, a heavier representation of countries from sub-Saharan Africa was deliberately chosen.

One manager interviewed requested feedback on this survey on the grounds that he had "responded to many global surveys before but never got any feedback on their results." *AIDS in the World* wishes to express its gratitude to this person and to other managers who took the time to participate in the survey and hopes that they will find useful information here.

The results of this survey are analyzed below. Responses are presented in Appendix 8.3 except for a few elements of information that are presented only in an aggregate form.

In the countries surveyed, public acknowledgment of AIDS as a national concern preceded the reporting of the first case of AIDS in one country, took place in the same year in 6 (42%), and followed it in the remaining 8 countries (58%) with a delay of 1 to 3 years. In 12 countries (85%), the initial governmental response was the creation of a task force; delayed response was reported from 3 countries, including 1 where information on the incidence of AIDS was suppressed.

Five countries created a national AIDS program during or before 1986

perspective. The economic argument was seldom raised. As noted in Chapter 6, efforts to evalute or project the economic impact of HIV/AIDS suffer from a lack of information. Thus, such evaluations are often based on a series of assumptions and alternate models using the approach of *scenario building.* In many countries, until recently, it did not seem necessary or politically advantageous to make the cost of AIDS a major public issue. It did not conform to the humanitarian agenda (cost is secondary to human rights) or to the public health perspective (the population must be protected at any cost). However, with the rising number of people and communities affected by the pandemic, the cost of prevention and care and the general economic

---

and the remaining 9 between 1987 and 1989. All programs are located within ministries of health, but in one instance, Fiji, the program is shared between ministries of health and education. Two-thirds of the programs are now into their fourth or later year of implementation.

All programs have a national advisory committee or an equivalent body. Eleven (78%) of these committees are answerable to the minister of health (in one instance, Chile, to his deputy), one to the prime minister (Tanzania), and one to the head of state (Uganda). The chairperson of these committees is a man in 11 (78 percent) of these countries, a woman in the remaining 3 (22 percent). As an average, these committees consist of 20 members (range from 9 in the Philippines to 50 in Jamaica). An average of 30 percent of this membership is made of women (range from 10% in Tanzania to 60% in Chile). Twelve committees (86%) include representatives of NGOs. Ten committees have met at least twice in the previous calendar year, one of them (Ethiopia) as many as 12 times.

Twelve Committees (86%) had been restructured since their inception. In all such instances, the involvement of sectors other than health, the integration of the program with other health initiatives, and the intention to gain more visibility were mentioned as reasons for restructuring. In 6 instances, it was also reported to be motivated by the desire to include more women as committee members.

The turnover of program managers has been high: since their creation, 10 (71%) of the 14 program managers initially appointed had been replaced, including 9 (64%) who had been replaced within the last 2 years. Death, studies abroad, promotion, and political and personal motives were stated as the reasons for the changes. However, there had been no significant staff change at a lower level of the program in the majority of these programs.

Six (43%) of the 14 programs were centralized; the remaining 8 (57%) had begun or completed their decentralization in the 4 years preceding the survey (in Jamaica, the program was decentralized since its

impact of AIDS have become topical issues, as is highlighted in ensuing sections on the financing of AIDS programs and the cost of AIDS. The section on financing summarizes the available information on the allocation of national resources in support of AIDS programs. The section on costing estimates and projects the cost of AIDS prevention and control. Later in this book, a section on the international transfer of resources shows that in 1991, these resources have declined for the first time since the beginning of the global mobilization against AIDS. It is clear that as the pandemic continues to worsen, AIDS programs will be forced to struggle with declining resources.

The economic perspective considers the impact of AIDS on de-

---

creation). Eight programs (57%) were reported as having experienced pressures from various sources that resulted in management changes. This pressure came from one or more sources: UN agencies including WHO (5 Programs), NGOs (4), donors (4), national advisory committees (3), ministry of health (3), other sectors (1), and the media (1).

Collaboration with NGOs was reported by all programs: in six (43%), collaboration had started before the creation of the national program. The other 5 established this collaboration an average of 3 years after the program was created.

Relations with NGOs were reported as very good (5, or 36%), or as good or fair (9, or 64%). All programs reported they provided funds to NGOs. The level of this funding represented an average of 15 percent of national program budgets (range from less than 5% in Cameroon to 50% in Chile).

In only one country did the source of major financing shift from one source to another (from WHO to the World Bank in Uganda).

The main achievements most frequently reported by program managers were, in descending order, creation of public awareness about AIDS, improvement of blood safety, promotion of condoms, and decentralization of the program. The participation of NGOs and the underrepresentation of women in national AIDS advisory committees were also common features across countries.

Among the constraints reported were the shortage of funds (10 programs, 71%), followed by difficulties in decentralizing management and implementation. The same constraints were stated as foreseeable in the forthcoming year.

This mini-survey provided insight into national program managers' concerns and reflected the transition that programs underwent in the late 1980s, a transition that is ongoing in many countries and raises questions about their long-term sustainability.

velopment in a decade that began in an environment of worldwide recession (Box 8.5). It has been proposed that in countries hard hit by HIV/AIDS, the impact on young, productive adults and their children will jeopardize national development. Placing AIDS on the development agenda is long overdue: this would stimulate the conduct of economic studies and the inclusion of HIV/AIDS related activities in national development plans, budgets, and international aid agreements. The World Bank has already taken steps in this direction (see

---

Box 8.5: AIDS and Development

Hans Moerkerk, Special Advisor, International Health Affairs, Ministry of Welfare, Health and Cultural Affairs, Netherlands

AIDS is much more than a health issue. Poverty, malnutrition, poor health care, lack of respect for human rights, illiteracy, inadequate housing, discrimination against women, and unresponsive political systems all exacerbate the impact of HIV on any given society. In a vicious circle, an HIV epidemic then undermines earlier progress and reinforces many of the worst facets of underdevelopment

The health care crisis in many developing countries was already acute before the impact of AIDS. Most of the developing world had made significant progress in the 1970s reducing infant mortality and increasing life expectancy. But some African countries spend less than 1 percent of their GNP on health! This continuing underinvestment in health care, together with an increasing economic crisis, had by 1980 led to increases in infectious diseases such as tuberculosis and STDs, rampant opportunistic infections, and endemic malnutrition in many parts of the world. This created an ideal context for the spread of HIV and made it almost impossible for most developing

country health care systems to launch an effective response.

We know that HIV/AIDS has an inordinate impact on the poorest countries, affecting economic, social, and political conditions. Unfortunately, for all the attention HIV/AIDS has received in the health sector over the last decade, it has been conspicuously ignored by politicians and by development technocrats. As such, we still lack concrete, detailed information about the real impact of the pandemic.

Although the overwhelming human costs of the pandemic are obvious, we now have at least some data on the direct developmental impact as well. The costs of caring for people with HIV are overwhelming even in middle-income countries like Brazil and Thailand, as outlined in this chapter. In Kenya, with an infected population of about 500,000 people, we can easily calculate that by the end of the decade alone, roughly 200,000 productive young adults will have burdened the health care system and died, denying the country of human resources in their prime. The Tourist Board of Kenya has indicated that fewer travellers are visiting the country because of AIDS, and that

Chapter 17), and the German International Cooperation Agency (GTZ) now includes AIDS systematically in its discussion with countries applying for aid.

These are positive steps, but they are accompanied by potential problems that require monitoring; economic development goals may overshadow human rights and basic humanitarian and public health principles. For example, investment in the training or higher education of HIV-infected persons or the allocation of resources to programs

---

there is an increasing AIDS-related shortage of workers.[a] In agricultural areas of east and central Africa, loss of life is undermining regular patterns of planting and harvesting, and causing expensive and inefficient transitions to less labor-intensive crops.[b] Even the costs of organizing funerals can be punitive, especially in areas of the world where such observances can involve 50 to 100 people over a several day period.[c]

The direct impact of AIDS on women in the developing world is particularly devastating. Not only does the disadvantaged position of women make it much more difficult for them to choose safer sex in their own lives, but a lack of prenatal care also makes it difficult for pregnant women with HIV to reduce the chances of infecting their children. Women bear a disproportionate burden of caring for the ill in the home. In many parts of the world, women whose husbands die of AIDS may be left with children but without access to inheritance. Areas with high AIDS-related mortality are seeing an erosion of the extended family structure that often provided such women with their only support.

In addition to all these direct costs, AIDS increases other infectious diseases, changes the process of human reproduction, and has the potential to affect migration patterns, political stability, and ecological balance.

Underdevelopment makes a response to AIDS more difficult, but ignoring broader social conditions around the epidemic will make effective programs impossible. The huge numbers of street children in many Third World cities are particularly affected by HIV—their seroprevalence rates in Manila and Rio de Janeiro are as high as 40 to 60 percent. But in trying to reduce new infections among street kids and care for those who already have HIV, it is completely ineffective to focus exclusively on a narrow behavioral type of health education. These children are unlikely to use injection drugs, but their sexual relations can be complex, including consensual, pleasure-oriented sex with their peers, formal or informal prostitution with adults, and high rates of sexual abuse and rape at the hands of both other street kids and establishment figures, including the police and the military. Children are living on the street and are vulnerable to HIV first and foremost because of poverty, but also because of the social

targeted at marginalized groups may be challenged by the assessment of costs versus projected economic returns.

■■■■■■ . . .

BEYOND WORDS: WHERE IS THE PROGRAM?

National AIDS programs are often perceived as government owned. Almost invariably overseen by ministries of health, they are generally implemented through government agencies and health services. Yet,

dislocation and cultural upheaval affecting many families in rapidly urbanizing societies, including families who could afford to keep their children at home if the children chose to stay. As challenging as it may be, HIV/AIDS programs for street kids have to affect all these factors—not just multiple sexual roles, the particular vulnerability of girls and young boys to rape, and pervasive poverty with its attendant epidemics of AIDS cofactors like poor nutrition and tuberculosis, but also the need to give entire communities the necessary resilience and flexibility to remain attractive and welcoming places for their own children. Indeed, we need a whole new conception of urban health.

What other policies would help us address the interlinked crises of AIDS and underdevelopment? There is a strong need to integrate health strat-egies into overall thinking on economic development and development cooperation. Development programs should give more concerted attention to strengthening families and strengthening local communities, both to prevent the spread of HIV and to help strengthen the response to the ill and the orphaned. The values inherent in early work on primary health care,

particularly the role of participatory health education, must be reasserted. Development strategies are necessary to support the fight against AIDS, but the stress should not be only on economic growth; political freedom to organize and respond and protection of human rights are also essential for success. Finally, given scarce resources and the accompanying pressure on governments to emphasize prevention instead of care, there is a strong argument that donors should earmark money for each purpose separately, even though the activities are interlinked.[d] Integrating these issues into both national development strategies and international development cooperation efforts requires the courage to consider new methods and concepts. Only such efforts will save the world from disaster.

a. AIDS documentary televised by the Kenya Broadcasting Corporation (July 1991).

b. David Norse, "Impact of AIDS on food production in East Africa," *AIDS Analysis Africa* (Nov/Dec 1991).

c. Robert Ainscow, "AIDS und die Entwicklungsländer," *Europa-Archiv* (Folge 14, 1991).

d. Malcolm Potts, Roy Anderson, and Marie Claude Boily, "Slowing the spread of HIV in developing countries," *Lancet* 388 (September 7, 1991).

the history of the mobilization against AIDS shows that although the involvement of ministries of health is necessary, it is not sufficient.

In industrialized countries, the response to AIDS began in the early 1980s as a community-based movement. Governments became active only when it was evident that the whole population—and not exclusively people who had been stigmatized even before the pandemic—could be affected by HIV and AIDS. Initially, governments reacted to the visible manifestations of AIDS, not to the silently spreading epidemic of HIV.

The emergence of national AIDS programs in industrialized countries resulted largely from the pressure exercised by community-based organizations. These early programs consisted of focused interventions intended to respond to groups and communities known to be affected by HIV/AIDS at that time: gay/bisexual men, recipients of blood and blood products, and, to a lesser extent, injection drug users. However, these first initiatives often lacked resources, coordination, and official legitimacy.

By the mid-1980s, governments in industrialized countries had created programs that emphasized mass media campaigns (discussed in Chapter 9), introduced HIV screening in blood transfusion centers, and collected epidemiological information to track the epidemic.

In federal states (Australia, Brazil, Canada, Germany, India, Nigeria, the United States, and many others), the national mobilization relied on a multilayered, multicentered system that involved different federal agencies and delegated responsibilities and awarded grants to appropriate institutions. In these nations, there are laws and institutions at the federal and state levels. The role of the federal program in these countries focused on providng technical support, monitoring epidemiological trends, and conducting research. Implementing and financing a large share of program activities was left to the initiative of each state. Given this decentralization, the survey conducted by *AIDS in the World* captured information on federal and state activities but was confronted with the difficult task of accessing information from individual states within federations. This information was often not available from federal agencies or ministries of health, illustrating the coordination problems that exist in many industrialized countries. The concept of program in these settings is wide and varied, ranging from a set of policies, federal laws, and budgets along with plans of activities and budgets formulated by each institution or group. Coordinating mechanisms and interaction exist: efficient in Australia where the interactions between federal and state levels are clearly presented in a newly formulated national program document; less so in the United States, where each federal agency competes with the others for a larger share of resources (with weak coordination), or in Brazil, India, and Nigeria, where much of the power rests with individual state governments.

Centralized states, such as France, Sweden, Norway, or the Netherlands, tended to create AIDS program structures that oversaw and financed program activities across the various disciplines, operating from a center located within the ministry of health or linked to it, and that played a more direct role in the implementation and monitoring of activities and in coordination with NGOs. In theory, a coordinated program would be easier to establish in these settings. In order to do this, certain countries (Norway, Sweden) initially created programs fully integrated with existing structures, allocating AIDS prevention responsibilities and resources to each of the existing departments. Others, France, for example, created a special national agency to oversee and coordinate multidisciplinary activities in relation to AIDS.

In developing countries, most programs were created in or after 1987, following the establishment of the WHO Global Programme on AIDS (GPA) and a resolution by the 167 WHO member states at the World Health Assembly in 1987 describing AIDS as a global emergency requiring an urgent and vigorous global mobilization.[3] The creation of and support for national AIDS programs was a high priority of GPA, which allocated more than half of its resources to this work. In the following years, several meetings brought together government representatives, creating a sense of global solidarity with an intensity not seen before in any disease control program. Indeed, unlike smallpox, tropical diseases, or even tuberculosis, AIDS had become a reality for both industrial and developing countries. (For tuberculosis, the combination of a declining level of interest, a feeling of complacency, a lack of global and long-term thinking, and a reduction in resources has led to a resurgent crisis as TB interfaces with HIV. The consequences are now being felt in both developed and developing countries.)

In 1987, WHO set forth criteria to define a National AIDS *Program*: (1) a National Advisory Committee on AIDS had to be appointed; (2) a focal point/program manager had to be identified; (3) a plan had to be formulated that was consistent with the global strategy approved by member states at the World Health Assembly[4] and included objectives, targets, and an implementation plan; and (4) the program had to have a budget allocation.[5]

After some initial hesitation, countries in sub-Saharan Africa began to mobilize earlier and in a somewhat more concerted manner than the rest of the developing world. By 1988, 144 of the 167 countries belonging to WHO had received support from GPA, and by the end of 1989, this number rose to 159; a global response was clearly underway.[6] By 1990, every country in the world had established a program, although they did not always fully conform to the WHO definition.

Figure 8.1 shows the year in which national AIDS programs were created in the 38 countries surveyed by *AIDS in the World*. The first programs were those in North America, Western Europe, and Oceania. Most programs in Eastern Europe and in developing countries were created in 1987–1988, as a result of the global mobilization against AIDS.

The program development process, while well established, continues to evolve as political realities change. The ongoing redefinition of the map of Eastern Europe, for example, has created a need for newly reconstituted states to create their own AIDS programs. This task must take place amid political tension, administrative chaos, and the increased risk of HIV transmission that accompanies disruptive social change and deepening economic crisis. As one program manager said in response to the *AIDS in the World* survey: "We still have an AIDS program but no longer a country. . . ."

Thus, the response has been universal if not always rapid. But what did these programs achieve?

EVALUATING PROGRAMS: WORDS OR ACHIEVEMENTS?

The success of a national AIDS program involves the extent to which it helps curb the course of the HIV epidemic and ensures quality care

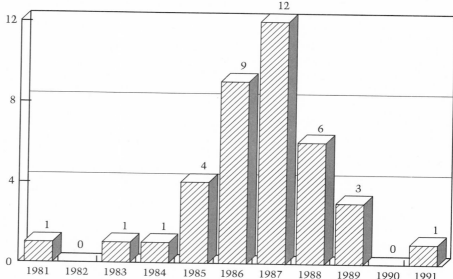

Figure 8.1. National AIDS program formation by year, 1986-1991.
Source: AIDS in the World, 1992.

to those already affected. On this basis, no program in the world can yet claim success. In addition, the monitoring systems created by these programs have generally not been sensitive enough to measure their own impact.

A second measure of success would be to document—and possibly quantify—behavioral changes that reduce the risk of exposure of the population to HIV infection. Apart from small community studies, which demonstrated that under certain conditions such changes *can* occur, such changes have either not occurred or not been convincingly documented.

To date, the achievements of national programs have, therefore, been measured by the degree to which they have raised awareness about AIDS and distributed such commodities as condoms, and more generally on the managerial efficiency with which activities are planned, implemented, and financed. Of the 38 countries surveyed by *AIDS in the World,* 24 reported having conducted some type of pro-

Table 8.2: National AIDS program evaluation in 38 industrialized and developing countries

	Program never evaluated	Program evaluated by national staff[a]	Program evaluated by national staff with international participation[a]	Total programs evaluated
Industrialized countries (n=16)	7	8	1	9
Developing countries (n=22)	7	4	11	15
Total	14	12	12	24

Source: AIDS in the World, 1992.
a. Program evaluated at least once.

gram evaluation. Of these, 12 were conducted by the staff of the program and/or by other staff within the ministry of health. International participation had been invited in the evaluation of 12 other programs, all but one of which were in developing countries. Seven of 16 programs (44%) in industrialized countries and 7 of 23 programs (30%) in developing countries had never been evaluated. (See Table 8.2.)

In general, the evaluation findings can be summarized as follows: Once created, programs became operational rapidly; they were successful in raising public awareness on AIDS issues, although they did not prevent (and at times they even generated) misperceptions among certain communities. The programs raised human rights issues and, in some instances, managed to prevent violations of these rights; and they exchanged information and, in some cases, resources at the international level. A common criticism, however, was a lack of focus and priority setting, weak management, and inability to involve other health programs, sectors, and NGOs more actively. By the end of the 1980s, pressure mounted on many programs to share responsibilities and resources with other governmental or nongovernmental groups. These pressures were exercised by ministries of health, other ministries, NGOs, and funding agencies, as revealed by the "mini-survey" of national program managers (see Box 8.4). The proposed changes involved structures, staff, and strategies.

∎ ∎ ∎   · · ·

EVOLVING PROGRAM STRUCTURES

Since the inception of national programs, much debate has focused on the issue of *vertical* versus *integrated* approaches to program management and implementation. This discussion became more animated as AIDS programs gained visibility and resources. Many of these programs rapidly outgrew their original structures. It was not unusual for a national AIDS program manager to achieve a more prominent public image than his or her supervisor, let alone others who had long struggled with mixed success to capture the attention of policy makers and the public on such health issues as primary health care (PHC), tuberculosis, or sexually transmitted diseases (STDs).

No AIDS program in the world was actually structured on a vertical model that, like malaria or leprosy, deployed specialized staff from a central management unit to the community level, dedicated to a single program and with a direct chain of command. Instead, AIDS programs created central management units that implemented activities through the existing structure, filtering through—but at times overwhelming—generally underfunded and understaffed health care systems.

Because AIDS programs had to operate through the several layers of health systems, the concept of integration was linked to decentralization, which necessitated the delegation of resources and authority to a level closer to or within the community.

National AIDS programs have had difficulties and have achieved varying degrees of success in the process of decentralization. Many have failed to support other governmental sectors and community-based organizations. National AIDS program managers have been reluctant to assign functions and resources to other entities in the health and social sectors, fearing a loss of control, resources, and accountability.

The linkage of HIV/AIDS and STD programs has become the central issue in restructuring HIV/AIDS programs (Box 8.6). In 34 of 38 countries surveyed by *AIDS in the World*, HIV/STD programs were reported as fully integrated in 14 countries (37%), partly integrated in

10 (26%), and separate in 10 (26%). Of the 14 countries that reported full integration, 6 had a separate program manager for each of the 2 programs, a sign that the concept of integration of services does not rule out retaining individual management entities at the center.[7]

Thus, at the beginning of this decade, most programs were undergoing a transition toward more decentralized and integrated programs. In many cases, this transition involved major staff changes.[8]

HIGH STAFF TURNOVER AND BURNOUT

National AIDS program managers and their key staff could be characterized as young, committed, overworked, and more likely than others to lose their jobs.

Box 8.6: AIDS and STDs

The evolving relationship between AIDS and the *other* sexually transmitted diseases (STDs) is a case study in scientific, medical, and public health politics. *In retrospect,* why did it take so long for AIDS programs and STD programs to work closely together, based on clear common interest and objectives? *In retrospect,* why did it take so long for health policy leaders to accept the reality of heterosexual HIV transmission? *In retrospect,* why did traditional STD programs give so little attention to sexual behavior—knowledge that, had it been available could have accelerated and dramatically improved the effectiveness of HIV prevention programs?

The Background

Prior to the 1960s, syphilis and gonorrhea were considered medical diseases, which required medical treatment. However, by the 1970s, a vastly increased number of sexually transmitted pathogens had been identified, cutting across the traditional disciplinary boundaries of infectious disease (bacteria, viruses, and parasites). Diagnosis, treatment and control of these diverse sexually transmitted pathogens were increasingly complex; a new group of experts, largely physicians, emerged to work on the STDs.

Whereas knowledge of clinical and microbiological aspects of STDs expanded rapidly, research into the behavioral aspects of STDs lagged far behind. Little attention was directed at the sexual behaviors themselves; constraints included longstanding problems with open discussion of sex, political constraints, and the strong medical orientation of many STD experts. The rapid progress of the STD specialty and ready access to effective therapy (including, with acyclovir, for a viral STD) contributed to making STDs, at least in the industrialized world, appear less threatening—causes of treatable morbidity but rarely associated with mortality.

As a new health issue, AIDS drew scores of young health and social workers to a field in which specific expertise was by and large nonexistent, and the established scientific, medical, or public health communities were often not eager to claim it. Furthermore, HIV/AIDS had to do with behaviors and practices that had not been the mainstay of preexisting programs or institutions: in the past, sexual behavior, injection drug use, and STDs received limited attention and resources and lacked trained staff. The emergence of AIDS created new demands. People were needed promptly to effect this change. Most of them were young; the average age of people attending national meetings and workshops on AIDS or the annual International Conferences on AIDS was in the thirties, even though the youngest AIDS

Meanwhile, in the developing world, few countries had developed comprehensive STD prevention and control programs. The combination of severe resource constraints, lack of a sound conceptual and strategic approach, and inattention from health policy makers contributed to the relative inattention and relatively low priority given to STDs. STD clinics were established, often linked with university hospitals in capital cities, and based essentially on a western medical model. Diagnosis and treatment of individuals with STD, rather than community approaches to STD control, were the norm. In 1986, as the HIV pandemic was breaking into international consciousness as a global problem, the entire STD program at World Health Organization headquarters in Geneva was operated by a single doctor.

In summary, by the early and mid-1980s, a strong scientific basis had been established for the diagnosis and treatment of STDs. In some industrialized countries, considerable progress had occurred in STD control, although the precise relationship between declining rates of syphilis and gonorrhea and specific STD programs was not always clear. However, in the developing world, the STD revolution in diagnosis and treatment lagged behind: family planning programs tended to avoid becoming involved in STD control, and specific STD programs were nearly always considered of low priority, understaffed, and underfunded. Finally, the gaps remained large, both in industrialized and developing countries, between medical and community approaches to STD control, as well as between medical and behavioral knowledge relevant to STDs.

The Arrival of AIDS

AIDS was discovered by infectious disease and cancer specialists, not by STD experts. Although the epidemiologists working on HIV/AIDS were often drawn initially from the ranks of STD experts, the specific features of AIDS epidemiology

workers were less likely than others to be able to afford to attend such meetings.

A unique feature of the group of AIDS workers who, over the years, succeeded in creating tight national and international networks is that the group included people with HIV/AIDS. Today, although the commitment and dedication of these people are as high as ever, the external pressures have increased, leading in many instances to loss of morale and burnout. From a functional standpoint, dilution of responsibilities and expeditious transfers were often hidden under the attire of study opportunity, promotion, or need for reorganization. Some of these staff, who were also people with HIV/AIDS, were more susceptible than others to exhaustion, sickness, and death.

(combining acute infectious and chronic disease approaches and methodology) brought many non-STD experts into the picture. Clinical expertise to manage opportunistic infections and cancers of people with AIDS was generally outside the scope of STD clinicians. The application of existing and new scientific tools for identification of the pathogen from lymph nodes and blood (not genital secretions) brought about a rapid influx of virologists and molecular biologists with prior backgrounds in cancer and non-STD infectious diseases.

In North America and Europe, the epidemic was initially thought to be a disease primarily of homosexuals and recipients of blood and blood products. Resistance to the idea of heterosexual transmission of HIV, which would have further supported the argument that HIV was "just another STD," helped keep the HIV/AIDS and STD worlds apart. Identification of the HIV epidemic among injection drug users

contributed further to a distancing of the HIV/AIDS problem from the world of traditional STDs. Finally, the urgency of AIDS and panics, such as occurred around the death of Rock Hudson (and many other prominent individuals in different societies around the world), had no modern precedent or counterpart among the STDs (the herpes scare was sharply limited in geographical terms and of relatively short duration).

In many respects, two different worlds emerged by the mid-to-late 1980s: the STD community, relatively underfunded and underappreciated by policy makers and the public; and the AIDS community, with funding and public interest at a level previously unimaginable for an STD.

Fortunately, several factors have led to an integration of HIV/AIDS and STD activities in many communities and most countries. First, epidemiological studies documented the strong interrelationships between HIV and STD transmission. Second, the lack of a medical solution to AIDS helped

By the end of the 1980s, there was a high staff turnover in most programs, at least at the management level. In clinical settings, professional and emotional stress required a frequent rotation of staff and the creation of coping schemes, which had not previously been customary.

Program staff had to learn new skills that were not traditionally taught in medical, nursing, or social sciences schools: how to deal with the media, convince administrators and politicians, raise funds, and respond to increasing and often uncoordinated demands from donor agencies. In short, they had to attend to immediate needs of their patients or their programs while communicating with and persuading policy and decision makers and the public at large. They had to be attentive to events occurring both within their professional world and on the public, administrative, and political fronts.

Furthermore, in order to respond to demands with the required degree of urgency, staff in many countries were often initially allowed

---

policy makers recognize that sexual behavior would be critical for the future of the pandemic. Third, individual STD and AIDS experts learned to bury the hatchet and sought increasingly to find ways of combining efforts. Thus, while some STD experts publicly proclaimed that the way to major funding for STD was through AIDS, and some AIDS experts deplored the idea of bringing AIDS work *down* to the level of worldwide STD efforts, the basic concept of integration is fundamental and has been increasingly widely accepted. Symbolic steps, such as the joining together of the VIII International Conference on AIDS and the III STD World Congress (July 19–24, 1992, in Amsterdam, the Netherlands), have been accompanied by real efforts to consider the optimal ways to join HIV and STD prevention, beyond rhetoric, at community and national levels.

Conclusion

The problem of establishing effective HIV/STD control programs presents a tremendous challenge. Yet the global morbidity and mortality from all STDs require that a joint effort go far beyond a simple application of the limited approaches that have characterized past STD efforts. It remains to be seen whether the leadership will emerge that will bring sexually transmitted diseases forward into a modern, global era in which sexual behavior will be seen as the fundamental issue, thereby unifying efforts to understand and prevent not only HIV/AIDS and STDs, but also sexual violence and problems of reproductive health. A new nomenclature is needed: the terminology *AIDS and other STDs* is divisive and awkward. Is a new concept of *sexual health* or *conditions associated with sexual behavior* ready to be born?

or encouraged to bypass hierarchical procedures or were awarded exceptional status and prerogatives, creating resentment and irritation among other program staffs.

Local, national, and international institutions do not like change. Many instititions worried about the rapid growth of AIDS programs. Thus, once national mobilization was well underway in the late 1980s, institutions began to reduce some of the exceptional attributes of programs and reclaim certain prerogatives of their staff. Some AIDS program managers feared a return to business-as-usual mentality in a society in which a sense of complacency toward AIDS was clearly increasing. Others, however, saw the routinization of programs as an opportunity to increase their capacity to deliver goods and services in a sustained manner.

In 46 countries that participated in at least one of the series of surveys conducted by *AIDS in the World*, it was found that 27 (59%) government AIDS programs had changed manager since their creation; 20 (43%) had done so during the last 2 years. Long-term program sustainability will require that changes be made creatively and innovatively. Well-trained personnel will be needed, and staff turnover will have to be held to a minimum.

While these changes continued to occur within the structures of government and institutions, NGOs were consolidating and expanding their work, not without difficulties of their own.

COALITION BUILDING: NGOs AT WORK

Nongovernmental organizations have been at the forefront of the response to AIDS in most countries of the world. Economists argue that NGOs focus on social needs that cannot be met otherwise due to *market failure*, that is, the inability of private firms to profitably provide necessary services at an affordable cost. Political scientists say NGOs exist to provide public goods (such as health services) to groups of people too small or marginalized to be served by the state.[9] Both agree that NGOs working in AIDS typically offer the advantages of being cost-effective and responsive to new needs and of having access to target communities.

For volunteers and activists involved in NGOs, the chief strength of the organizations would almost certainly be seen as their ability to represent effectively the needs and values of a particular constituency. Although they have recognized weaknesses, NGOs clearly serve certain functions well and can effectively complement and improve governmental response.

In most industrialized countries, the first significant nongovernmental response was from groups of volunteers and activists who formed their own organizations to provide care to their sick friends, educate their peers, and advocate for more attention and funds. These nonprofit, AIDS-specific NGOs are usually referred to as AIDS Service Organizations or ASOs (see "AIDS Service Organizations in Transition" in Chapter 17). ASOs now exist in most countries of the world, although in the developing world they usually emerged somewhat later in the epidemic, with the initial volunteer response to AIDS being organized by other, preexisting NGOs.

By 1991, WHO/GPA had identified more than 200 NGOs and ASOs working on AIDS issues in Africa; the Pan American Health Organization (PAHO) estimated that 500 NGOs and ASOs were fighting the pandemic in Latin America; and the National AIDS Information Clearinghouse in the United States listed about 16,000 organizations working on AIDS in the United States (although this includes some government agencies as well).

NGOs encompass a wide variety of organizational styles and missions, and their role in response to AIDS has varied accordingly. Some NGOs can be described as charities that seek to alleviate suffering directly, and their role in the pandemic has been to provide material or medical assistance, usually to a limited geographic area (often at a district level). This type of organization, often church based, is particularly active in Africa. Some charities evolve into development groups and help communities develop the necessary skills and resources to alleviate and/or avoid health problems. The community counseling approach of the Salvation Army in Chikankata, Zambia, is an example. In contrast, advocacy groups seek to influence the broader political and economic environment. As already established NGOs working on such issues as women's rights, access to essential drugs, and Third World debt have generally started collaborating only recently on AIDS, it has been left to the ASOs to initiate many AIDS-related advocacy campaigns. Finally, public service subcontractors play a role as nonprofit, privatized service delivery vehicles for the state, whose activities change with governmental priorities and investments. Several American public service contractors who have been awarded large contracts are particularly prominent in developing country activities, such as the social marketing of condoms.

Organizations can also be distinguished on the basis of their founders or the mix of their staff and volunteers. People's organizations or self-help groups are founded and controlled by a distinct community sharing a collective interest. Volunteer organizations bring together people (usually both unpaid volunteers and paid staff) with shared values and vision. International NGOs usually grow out of or support voluntary organizations that promote international financial and technical cooperation. Government- or donor-organized NGOs (GONGOs and DONGOs) are created to pursue specific objectives of government or donor policy, which for one reason or another cannot be directly addressed by the parent organization.[10]

The World Health Organization surveyed 406 NGOs working on AIDS in developing countries in 1990. The results give an indication of different NGO program priorities (more than one NGO is often involved in a particular project, so these data do not fully reflect the distribution of NGO projects.[11] (See Table 8.3.)

A review conducted by *AIDS in the World* illustrated trends in the response by nongovernmental organizations to AIDS. In Zimbabwe, NGOs dedicated to AIDS (ASOs) preceded the response of other NGOs to AIDS. By 1990, 30 NGOs/ASOs were working on AIDS in Zimbabwe, including 11 NGOs that had expanded their scope of work to address AIDS-related issues. (See Table 8.4.) In contrast, in Mexico, preexisting NGOs expanded their scope of work to encompass AIDS work. Concurrently, ASOs created their own program. The total number of NGOs/ASOs working in Zimbabwe, Australia, Canada, and Mexico increased from one in 1983 to 176 in 1992.

AIDS in the World also conducted an in-depth survey of 25 of the world's most prominent ASOs, including 12 in developing countries and 13 in the industrialized world. The majority of these ASOs in both industrialized and developing countries considered their priorities to be public policy and advocacy, followed by counseling and education. (See Table 8.5.)

As expected, a constant problem for NGOs is sustaining financing

Table 8.3: AIDS-related activities listed by 406 nongovernmental organizations (NGOs) in developing countries, 1990

Specific AIDS-related activity	% of NGOs
Provides education/information for specific groups	72.7
Provides education/information for the general public	55.2
Offers AIDS counseling	51.5
Is involved in community development	43.4
Provides primary health care	42.4
Conducts counselor training	33.0
Offers family planning service	26.1
Supervises home care for people with AIDS	25.6
Offers sexually transmitted disease programs	22.9
Conducts research	20.7
Performs blood testing for prevention or care	18.2
Offers drug abuse counseling	7.6

Source: WHO Global Programme on AIDS Inventory of NGOs working on AIDS that received development cooperation or assistance, WHO/GPA/DIR. 19.5-1990.5.

Table 8.4: Number of NGOs and ASOs newly responding to AIDS, by year, 1983–1991

Year	Zimbabwean NGOs	Zimbabwean NGOs and ASOs	Australian ASOs	Canadian ASOs	Mexican ASOs	Mexican NGOs and ASOs (excluding universities)
Pre-1983		1				1
1983			2	3	1	3
1984		1	1	1		
1985		2	9	10	1	5
1986		1	2	6	4	6
1987		4	2	9	8	8
1988	1	4		9	11	18
1989	4	8	2	7	10	19
1990	3	4	3	6	6	13
1991	3	5		1		
Total[a]	11	30	21	52	41	73

Source: AIDS in the World, 1992.
a. As of January 1992.

Table 8.5: Percentage of ASOs in industrialized and developing countries listing specific activity areas among their priorities, January 1992

Activity area	Industrialized countries (n = 13)	Developing countries (n = 12)
Public policy and advocacy	92	73
Counseling with testing	75	46
Counseling for people with HIV infection	67	55
Education for other NGOs	58	50
Education in schools	50	60
Education for heterosexuals	58	60
Education for sex workers	67	73
Education for sex workers' clients	58	55
Education for IDUs	67	50
Education for urban poor	58	50
Condom distribution	33	60
Promotion of sexual abstinence	0	9
Needle exchange	8	0
Drug rehabilitation	0	0
Human rights monitoring	25	27
Legal advocacy work	42	27
Blood transfusion and banking	0	0
Home care	33	10
Institutional care	8	0
Buddying services	42	0
Health promotion for people with HIV infection	75	45
Mass media campaigns	25	55

Source: AIDS in the World, 1992.

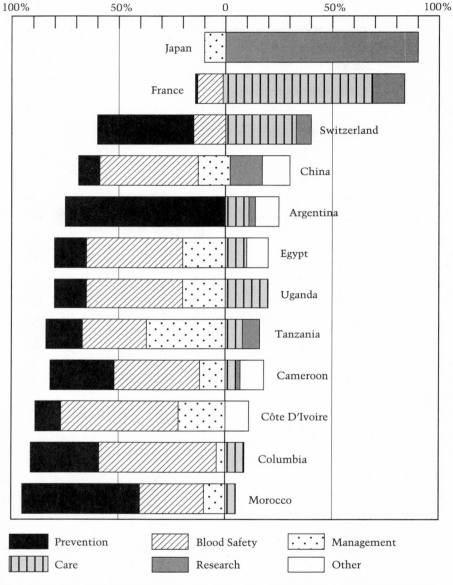

Figure 8.2. Proportional allocation of resources available to ministry of health national AIDS programs from national and international sources, for one year, 1990-91.
Source: AIDS in the World survey, 1992.

for their activities. The mini-survey of national program managers (Box 8.4) revealed that the government national AIDS programs allocated an average of 15 percent (range of 5 to 50 percent) of their budget to NGOs. Today, short- and long-term financial issues are a major concern of both governmental and nongovernmental programs.

FINANCING NATIONAL AIDS PROGRAMS

Funds made available to governments through their national programs came from national and, for developing countries, international sources. Figure 8.2 shows the proportional allocation of these funds to program elements, which have been regrouped in broad categories: management, blood safety, prevention, care, and research. In industrialized countries, NAP resources focus on care, research, and prevention. In developing countries, the larger share of these funds goes to prevention, blood safety, and the strengthening of program management. In countries in sub-Saharan Africa, where the needs for care are enormous, only small amounts of funds are allocated to care. Some of the care cost is covered by the governments through hospital and primary health care networks. Of course, such funds do not normally pass through national AIDS program management units.

In developing countries, program sustainability is vital. Can these countries finance their NAPs over time? Figure 8.3 shows financing trends for two countries, Ethiopia and Thailand, for the period 1989–1991.

Financing Prevention

Ethiopia's economy is in crisis. Years of civil war, drought, and political instability have left the country bankrupt and heavily dependent on external donors for financial support. Figure 8.3 shows that from 1989 to 1991 external funds decreased by 20 percent, from $2.0 million to $1.6 million. Because these funds comprise the majority of NAP budgets, the program is now suffering greatly. However, even in the face of overwhelming resource allocation problems, the central government has increased its share of funding for the NAP. In 1989, it provided almost $300,000, one-seventh of the NAP budget; in 1991,

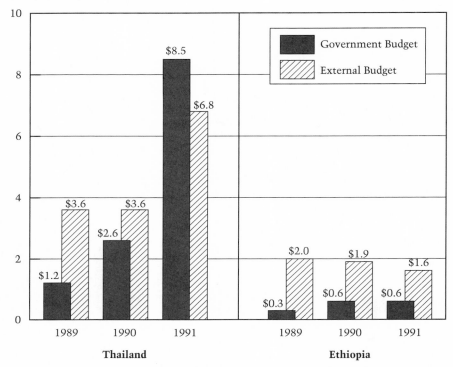

$US (millions)

Figure 8.3. National AIDS program budgets in Ethiopia and Thailand, 1989-1991 (in millions of U.S. dollars).
Source: AIDS in the World, 1992.

the government's contribution rose to more than $650,000, representing 29 percent of the NAP budget.[12]

Thailand has benefited from both a rapid and generous response from international donors and the government. Figure 8.3 shows that during the period 1989–1991 the NAP budget, including national and international funds, increased more than 300 percent, from $4.8 million to more than $15 million. During this time the Thai government's contribution to the AIDS budget increased more than 700 percent, from $1.2 million to $8.5 million. In 1989, the government provided about a quarter of the NAP budget; by 1991–92, this portion

Table 8.6: External financing of national AIDS program budgets, selected countries and years (millions $U.S.)

Country	Year	Bilateral	International organizations	NGO	Total
Cameroon	1990–1992	2.4	0.7	0.07	3.2
Côte d'Ivoire	1989–1991	2.3+	2.1	—	4.3
Tanzania	1988–1991	5.9	9.1	—	15.0
Morocco	1991	1.0	0.3	—	1.3
Pakistan	1990–1992	—	0.4	—	0.4
Trinidad	1991	—	0.3	—	0.3

Source: AIDS in the World, 1992.

had risen to over 50 percent. For the Thai government, as measured by both public statements and internal allocation of resources, HIV/AIDS has become a high priority.[13]

The *AIDS in the World* survey provided some insights into external financing sources for prevention programs. Table 8.6 shows external funding of NAP budgets as reported, for varying years, for 6 countries in Africa, Southeast Aisa, and the Caribbean. In many cases there is no amount reported for NGOs. This by no means implies that NGOs did not provide resources, but rather reflects an information gap between government program managers and NGOs. This information would be useful for ensuring more equitable distribution of services and better coordination of activities.

As expected, external financing varies widely across countries. In Cameroon and Morocco, bilateral aid represented at least 75 percent of external funds. In contrast, in Tanzania, Pakistan, and Trinidad, international organizations were the main source of external funds. Chapter 12 reviews trends in international transfer of resources from industrialized countries and international organizations in support of AIDS programs in developing countries.

Financing Care

In general, it is expected that medical, psychosocial, and social services would be financed for HIV/AIDS as for other diseases, through preexisting mechanisms. This typically involves a mix of insurance for workers, government funding, self-finance, community-based income generating schemes, and other means. The lack of health insurance in developing countries shifts much of the financial burden to the individuals, families, and governments.

The laboratory diagnosis of HIV infection requires reagents, laboratory equipment, and trained personnel. Eleven percent of the countries that responded to the *AIDS in the World* survey reported that voluntary testing was available on a fee-for-service basis but free testing was unavailable. This is likely to limit access to testing for persons in lower income strata in these countries. Over 40 percent of countries reported no charge to individuals, and 46 percent reported that tests were available to individuals either for a fee or at no charge. The cost of free tests was absorbed by the government, provided by external donors or manufacturers of the test kits, or covered by other sources.

In the area of medical management, a study in Rwanda indicated that 92 percent of both inpatient and outpatient costs for persons with AIDS were met through public funds. The remaining 8 percent was paid out-of-pocket.[14] Reports on 6 home care programs in sub-Saharan Africa, which provided a range of medical, psychological, and social support services, reported that the programs were highly dependent on external funding.[15] This dependence threatens the programs' long-term viability.

A study in Thailand noted that many of the people with AIDS are injection drug users and sex workers who have no health insurance. In the same country, only about 10 percent of the costs of delivering medical care were reportedly recovered from persons receiving treatment.[16]

The method of financing AIDS care determines who will have access to and receive different types of care. Some countries, such as Ethiopia and other sub-Saharan African countries, will continue to depend on external resources to finance their NAPs. The issue of who will pay for meeting the needs of people with AIDS is in question. Increased competition for scarce health care resources will likely exacerbate inequities in access, decrease quality of services and care, and further strain the fragile health care infrastructure in many developing countries.

With one exception, the United States, industrialized countries have a national health care system. Industrialized countries in Europe, in addition to Canada, Australia, New Zealand, and Japan, have some type of nationalized health systems ranging from national insurance with health services provided by both the public and the private sectors to systems where the government is the sole provider. The debate over AIDS care in these countries tends to focus more on the levels of care to provide, not on how to finance it. For example, in Switzerland it has been estimated that almost 98 percent of all citizens are covered by the health insurance system.[17] In France, 70 percent of patients are completely covered by social security, and 25 percent are covered at least partially.[18]

Though socialized health insurance and care systems address some financing and access problems, others are unresolved. For example, Switzerland's health insurance scheme is considered one of the best in the world. Virtually all Swiss nationals are covered, and for those who do not have insurance, their Canton of birth provides support. However, it is unclear what type of care is received by the marginalized citizens, such as injection drug users who tend to avoid the formal health care system. Despite the efficiency of the system, some fear that such persons do not receive medical care until their physical condition deteriorates badly.

France currently faces a fiscal and political crisis that could significantly affect health care service financing. Over the past decade, the portion of the national budget allocated for health services has risen dramatically. Hard decisions to adapt the social security system to existing economic realities will have to be made. In the United States, the lack of a national health care system makes finance a critical element in determining who receives care and what kind of care they receive. Figure 8.4 shows a summary of major funding sources for HIV/AIDS care, based on information provided by the insurance industry, the federal and state governments, and research studies. It was assumed that out-of-pocket costs total about 21 percent of all health care expenditures in the United States.[19] If this were applied to the 1989 funding figures, the amount attributable to the "other" category would be $527 million.

In 1989, approximately $2 billion was spent in the United States on care for HIV-infected persons and people with AIDS; excluding life

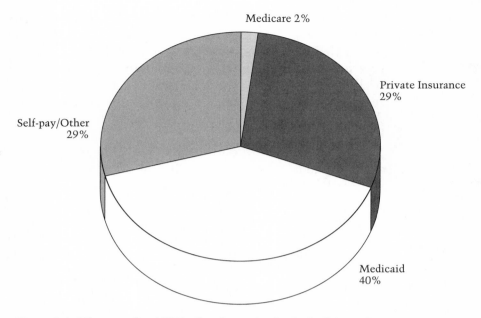

Medicare 2%

Private Insurance
29%

Self-pay/Other
29%

Medicaid
40%

Figure 8.4. Who pays for AIDS-related care in the United States?
Source: Report of the U.S. National Commission on AIDS, August, 1991.

insurance payments, approximately $1.5 billion was spent by the federal and state governments and insurance companies. Between 1986 and 1989, funding for HIV/AIDS care rose by over 340 percent.

With approximately 35 million uninsured persons in the United States, finance issues have already begun to dominate the national debate on AIDS patient care. Between 1984 and 1987, public financing of AIDS inpatient care rose from 25 to 41 percent. Privately funded inpatient care decreased from 49 to 43 percent in the same period.[20] It is unclear if this indicates a shift in insurance financing or a change in the composition of AIDS cases.

Currently, in the United States, many large urban area hospitals are absorbing the costs of treating people who have no resources. A 1987 nationwide survey of public hospitals reported that more than 60 percent of people with AIDS in public hospitals were injection drug users who had no insurance. The same survey found that, overall, about 31 percent of AIDS admissions to public hospitals had no private resources. Public hospitals had to absorb a deficit of $218 per day per AIDS patient.[21] Communities, charities, and other organizations that fund public hospitals are currently subsidizing care for people with AIDS. Alarmingly, it has been reported that private insurers are finding ways to exclude people with AIDS from receiving insurance.[22] The issue of how to finance the care of people with no insurance or resources will continue to be hotly debated in this decade.[23]

SHARING THE COST: THE NEED FOR SOLIDARITY

AIDS treatment would be unaffordable to most people with AIDS on an out-of-pocket basis. Meeting this need is both an individual and collective responsibility. Collective funding can help to ensure that this need is met and that persons and families affected are not financially crippled in the process. Figures 8.5, 8.6, and 8.7 present examples of individual and collective cost sharing for Rwanda, Thailand, and the United States. These countries represent different levels of costs and the collective ability to finance health care needs (Box 8.7).

Rwanda is a relatively poor sub-Saharan country with a $320 per capita GNP, and where HIV/AIDS has been prevalent for over a decade and the number of cases of AIDS is relatively high. Figure 8.5 shows that the annual cost for a person with AIDS is estimated at $358. This is more than double the per capita consumer spending, for all needs, of $166 per year. Typically, the annual spending per person for health care in this country averages $6.60. The cost of care for one person with AIDS would represent 216 percent of the total annual budget for consumer spending, or 54 times what the same person would typically spend for health care in this country.

Another approach to financing AIDS-related care is that it might be spread across the entire population, thereby reducing the risk and burden for any individual. Spreading risk is commonly done in both the private (insurance) systems and public (social welfare program) sectors. Figure 8.5 shows that about $4.98 per capita is spent by the government of Rwanda on public health. Calculating the total 1990 national cost of AIDS care and dividing it over the entire population result in a per capita cost of approximately $0.50: about 10 percent of the government budget for health. This is an important burden in a country where there is a dearth of resources to fund essential primary health care programs. This comparison, however, underscores the fact that even a minimal increase in the allocation of funds to the health sector would be collectively bearable and individually beneficial to people with HIV/AIDS. It would go a long way toward ensuring better care for people with AIDS and express a national solidarity.

In Thailand, a person with AIDS receiving hospital-based care could expect to pay between $658 and $1016 annually. Assuming a midpoint estimate of $837 dollars per year, this person would have to spend almost 35 times his or her annual personal spending for all health care.[24] (See Figure 8.6.) The national expenditure for health averaged $11.50 per capita in 1990. Calculating the national cost of AIDS care and dividing it over the entire population results in a cost of less than $0.01 per person, a small addition to the allocation of public funds to the health sector.

The United States has one of the most modern and extensive health care systems in the world. It is, however, available only to

---

Box 8.7: The Impact of AIDS: Can the National Health Care System Cope?

Lazare Kaptue, Inspector General, Ministry of Health, Yaounde, Cameroon

Before the AIDS pandemic, our health care system in Cameroon was already suffering severely from the scarce resources due to the unprecedented economic crisis. The AIDS pandemic has made things worse. Most local and foreign resources that could have helped us improve the functioning of our health care services are devoted to HIV/AIDS. The situation is such that the Ministry of Health has been accused by the public of concentrating on AIDS and neglecting other diseases, such as malaria. Since 1988, we have spent $13.3 million on HIV/AIDS. During the same period we have spent less than $1.9 million on other communicable disease control programs.

In the hematology department of the teaching hospital at Central Hospital in Yaoundé, more than 50 percent of the activities have shifted to HIV/AIDS. In Central Hospital, three-quarters of hematology beds are occupied by AIDS patients. Hospitals keep only those patients who are seriously ill. The others are seen in outpatient units or in the community. Before the AIDS pandemic, most of our activities were focused on sickle cell anemia. Since AIDS, however, sickle cell anemia patients unfortunately receive less attention.

AIDS has increased tremendously the need for training and personnel. In all of Cameroon, there are 90 HIV testing sites staffed by more than 250 technicians. Seminars have been organized for 60 doctors and 20 technicians on the appropriate use of blood. Some are planned on

those who can afford it. Figure 8.7 shows that a person with AIDS would have to spend approximately $32,000 per year for inpatient and outpatient care. Excluding AIDS, this represents about 17 times what a person would annually spend out-of-pocket on health care. By spreading the costs of AIDS care over the entire population, this expression of solidarity would cost approximately $12.00 per person annually.

> *The problem is not our resources but our priorities. In recent years we have witnessed the most military build-up in the history of the world. We went from spending under $160 billion on arms in 1981 to nearly $300 billion in 1987. The expenditures amounted to $1.6 trillion in just seven years, or $12,000 for every taxpayer in America. If we had spent a million dollars a day since the birth of Christ, the total expenditure would have been only half that for the weapons outlays of the past seven years.* (Dr. J. Larry Brown and H. F. Pizer, *Living Hungry in America*)[25]

---

nosocomial HIV transmission. The AIDS pandemic has created the need to train a new category of personnel, namely counselors, because the work load is so heavy that the doctors and nurses alone cannot cope with the situation. With the increase of HIV prevalence and the number of AIDS patients, we will need thousands of counselors to cover the whole country.

Can government health services alone cope with AIDS? The answer is definitely no. This is why we are developing community-based care. Our experience in this field is not yet as advanced as Uganda's, for example, but we are doing our best to develop these activities. A few national NGOs are operating, and we are encouraging the creation of others. With the increasing number of AIDS patients, they are going to play a major role in helping government health services cope with the pandemic.

Has the response to AIDS generated innovative action in the national health system? The answer is yes. In the field of blood transfusion, the AIDS pandemic has convinced health personnel of the necessity for appropriate use of blood. Now, blood transfusions have been reduced in many hospitals to a minimum, to only those that are absolutely necessary. Also, with the use of condoms and the reduction of sexual partners, the number of patients presenting with STDs has decreased in many health centers. An innovative program has also been introduced to educate sex workers. Innovations in counseling and community-based care benefit other health programs.

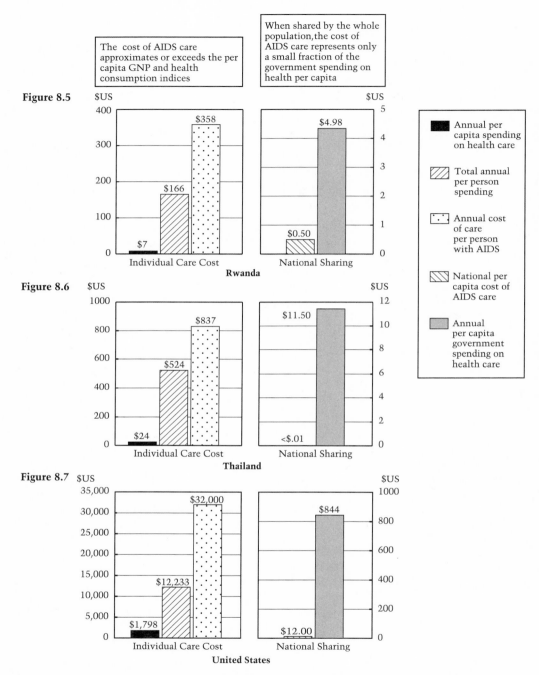

Figures 8.5, 8.6, 8.7. Individual per capita spending on health care, and the nation sharing the cost, 1990-1991.

Source: AIDS in the World, 1992.

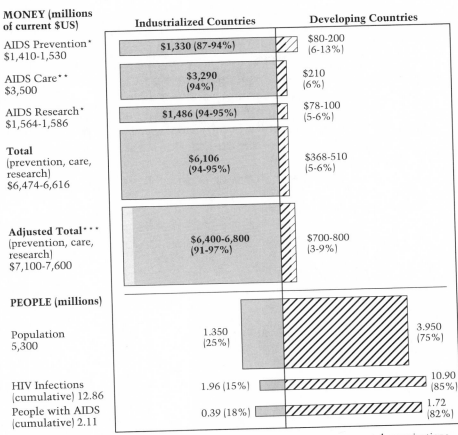

MONEY (millions of current $US)	Industrialized Countries	Developing Countries
AIDS Prevention* $1,410-1,530	$1,330 (87-94%)	$80-200 (6-13%)
AIDS Care** $3,500	$3,290 (94%)	$210 (6%)
AIDS Research* $1,564-1,586	$1,486 (94-95%)	$78-100 (5-6%)
Total (prevention, care, research) $6,474-6,616	$6,106 (94-95%)	$368-510 (5-6%)
Adjusted Total*** (prevention, care, research) $7,100-7,600	$6,400-6,800 (91-97%)	$700-800 (3-9%)

PEOPLE (millions)		
Population 5,300	1.350 (25%)	3.950 (75%)
HIV Infections (cumulative) 12.86	1.96 (15%)	10.90 (85%)
People with AIDS (cumulative) 2.11	0.39 (18%)	1.72 (82%)

*Includes only government resources, not the private sector or nongovernmental organizations.
**Care costs of adults AIDS only (not pre-AIDS HIV diseases).
***Adjusted for management cost, inflation, increased access to antivirals, underreporting of expenditures, and dollar value.

Figure 8.8. Estimated costs of AIDS prevention, care, and research in industrialized and developing countries, 1991-1992 (one year).
Source: AIDS in the World, 1992.

As the number of persons with AIDS increases, the unit cost might remain constant, but the total national cost would rise. At some point even spreading the cost over the entire population would involve difficult internal resource allocation decisions.

In a spirit of solidarity, foresight is needed on the part of governments and international bodies to plan for the future as projected in Chapter 2 on HIV. The transfer of financial resources both nationally and internationally is only one of many manifestations of solidarity. Chapter 12 examines international financing in support of AIDS prevention and care.

For a comparison of estimated global costs of AIDS prevention, care, and research, see Figure 8.8.

Box 8.8: The Danger of Complacency

Maureen Law, Senior Fellow, International Development Research Center, Ottawa, Canada

Despite the increasingly grim projections concerning the AIDS pandemic and its demographic, economic, and social impact, many people involved in the international AIDS effort believe the sense of urgency that marked the late 1980s has abated noticeably, at least in industrialized countries. This has been identified by the Global Commission on AIDS as one of the critical issues for the 1990s.

There appear to be a number of factors contributing to this phenomenon: unrealistic expectations that the problem will soon be solved by vaccines and drugs; a public view that the epidemic has levelled off or peaked and is declining in industrialized countries; the belief that heterosexual spread is not a serious problem in industrialized countries;

and fatigue about AIDS on the part of the media, politicians, and the public.

In some highly affected countries, this apparent complacency may actually represent denial, as the true dimensions of the disaster become apparent. In other countries, complacency may be the result of the mistaken belief that certain societies are virtually immune to HIV/AIDS because of cultural factors, including religious beliefs and practices.

Whatever its roots, complacency is extremely dangerous. It leads to the failure not only of individuals to protect themselves, but also of governments to sustain a high level of commitment and action, especially in regard to public education and other preventive efforts, such as condom distribution.

There is particular danger that public complacency in wealthy countries, combined with the economic recession that is affecting many countries at present, will result in

TROUBLE ON THE HORIZON

Confronted with weak national commitment, fragile and moving structures, declining resources, and a growing sense of complacency, national AIDS programs and the people they are intended to serve are in jeopardy (Box 8.8). As seen in the following chapters, where efforts are made by programs to provide a coordinated response to the growing crisis, there are clear signs of positive individual responses. Meanwhile, national programs are falling behind. Many governments, constrained by their lack of resources, continue to avoid the reality of the pandemic: more people become infected because they do not have sufficient access to information and services; more individuals require care they cannot afford; and more families and communities are affected by the impact of a pandemic that has only begun.

---

failure to increase the bilateral transfer of funds to poor countries or to sustain or increase contributions to multilateral and other international efforts against AIDS—at the very time when needs are increasing dramatically, especially for the care of the sick and orphaned. In less affluent countries, complacency may lead officials to ignore the need to shift priorities in national spending, perhaps from military and police to health and social services.

Because the mass media clearly have been the major source of information to the public on AIDS, they obviously have a critical role in combatting complacency. Although media coverage will likely continue to be extensive, it is important that the information people receive through the media be accurate and balanced so that it does not aggravate existing tendencies to ignore or deny the seriousness of the situation. For example, premature media enthusiasm for new drugs or vaccines may contribute to complacency in some places, whereas in others, the problem may be with unduly catastrophic reporting that generates hopelessness and denial.

Yet the media's primary role is to report news, not to educate the public. As a result, governments and nongovernmental organizations need to persevere in developing and promoting both general and targeted AIDS information in order to increase public knowledge and maintain public concern.

Advocacy must continue to be one of the cornerstones of the AIDS effort if the danger of complacency is to be overcome and AIDS is to remain high on the national and international agendas.

To compensate for the varying capability of government programs to expand or even sustain their actions, NGOs are expanding the scope of their work. But as later chapters show, they too are undergoing a transition involving a mix of opportunities and risks. Private sector involvement in the global effort is uneven, guided more by self-interest than social responsibility: research hinges on the profit motive; insurance companies silently build fences against people with HIV infection; the latex market, stimulated by skyrocketing individual demand for condoms, thrives.

What is the prognosis for the latter part of the twentieth century? For national programs, the prospects on the horizon are unclear, if not grim. It appears that governments and national and international institutions are facing mounting pressure to *lower* the profile of AIDS programs rather than *raise* the profiles of other health and social issues. Some may be forced to make difficult decisions regarding social and economic issues. Because of the lack of foresight and courage to address AIDS as a truly unprecedented health crisis, these changes are likely to be too little, too late. And in a worsening pandemic, they can have a severe and tragic impact on individuals and societies. Thus, as the collective response falters, individuals must continue to struggle for their own protection and survival. They will need to exercise increased pressure on national AIDS programs to obtain more meaningful responses to their demands and needs.

CHAPTER NINE

. . . .

Prevention

section was
pared in collaboration
Mitchell E. Cohen,
D., a consultant
cializing in HIV/AIDS
vention.

An analysis of prevention activities over the past decade shows that prevention can work. At the individual and community levels, there are many examples of successful HIV prevention, some of which are described in this chapter. However, to understand better both the successes and the failures, and to identify the challenges for the coming years, an analytic framework for HIV prevention is required. An analysis of prevention programs worldwide has identified three elements as essential to the success of HIV prevention:

- information and education
- health and social services
- a supportive social environment

The capacity to design, deliver, and improve this prevention package engages individuals and their partners, HIV prevention programs, and social systems. Whether they involve homosexual men, injection drug users, sex workers, or adolescents, the combination of these three elements in creative, innovative, and courageous ways have proven their ability to slow HIV transmission. Yet if any of the three elements are missing, it can be stated unequivocally that prevention is not being given a fair chance to succeed.

Information and education are the first requirement, and the details of this work are critical. Most important is the involvement of target groups—the people to be reached by program design and implementation. Examples abound of experts deciding what other

Table 9.1: Awareness knowledge of HIV/AIDS in selected countries[a]

Group/Study/Country	% knowledge AIDS (general)	% knowledge sexual transmission	% knowledge blood transfusion	% knowledge transmission and injection	% knowledge condoms as prevention	% knowledge perinatal transmission	% perception of personal susceptibility
Commercial sex workers							
Mhalu et al.[3]							
1988–89							
Dar es Salaam, Tanzania							
Public house workers							
Program participants	97	96	62	NR	71	NR	NR
New recruits	96	88	46	NR	32	NR	NR
Ngugi[4]							
1992							
Nairobi, Kenya	100						8
Hassig[5] (1992)[b]							
Cameroon							
Before intervention		79					
After intervention		96					
Tanzania							
Before intervention		97					
After intervention		100					
Mexico							
Before intervention		53					
After intervention		98					
Pleak, Meyer-Bahlburg[6]							
1988–89							
Manhattan, U.S.	86						

General population

Van de Walle[7]
(1990)[b]

United States	99	88	NR	97	NR	NR	NR
Nigeria	46	90	NR	85	NR	NR	NR
Gabon	90	42	NR	39	NR	NR	NR

Chikwem, Chikwem, Ola[8]
(1988)[b]

Nigeria	NR	79	57	55	13	18	NR

Wilson, Mehryar[9]
1984–1989

Central African Republic	84	93	NR	50	47	77	62
Chad	60	78	NR	NR	38	39	40
Côte D'Iviore	86	95	NR	56	42	89	27
Lesotho	94	95	NR	NR	77	85	23
Mauritius	92	93	NR	52	84	83	22
Rwanda	98	97	NR	40	NR	68	24
Sudan	69	89	NR	NR	NR	54	15
Togo	64	93	NR	76	39	80	52
Tanzania	87	82	NR	40	13	70	16

Drug users

Selwyn et al.[10]
1985
New York City, U.S.

Methadone clinic	NR	92	NR	97	52	90	NR
Detention center	NR	99	NR	97	63	83	NR

Kleinman et al.[11]
1986
United States

Drug users	NR	38	14	58	NR	NR	NR
Nonusers	NR	36	17	31	NR	NR	NR

a. References for this table, shown in superscript numbers, are in the Reference Notes for Chapter 9.
b. Parentheses indicate publication date.

Table 9.1 (cont.): Awareness knowledge of HIV/AIDS in selected countries[a]

Group/Study/Country	% knowledge AIDS (general)	% knowledge sexual transmission	% knowledge blood transfusion	% knowledge transmission and injection	% knowledge condoms as prevention	% knowledge perinatal transmission	% perception of personal susceptibility
Adolescents							
Weisman et al.[12] 1989 Baltimore, U.S.							22
Seltzer, Rabin, Benjamin[13] 1989 New York City, U.S. Females	98	100	57	81	NR	NR	NR
Rotheram-Borus, Koopman[14] 1991 New York City, U.S. Minority gay/bisexuals	82						
Lorenzetti et al.[15] 1990 Italy	NR	95	NR	98	92	NR	NR
Landefeld et al.[16] 1988 Cleveland, U.S.				79			
Carroll[17] 1988 Rhode Island, U.S.					89		
Thomas, Gilliam, Iwrey[18] 1989 United States Black college students	NR	96	97	96	90	90	NR
Gray, Saracino[19] 1990 United States	NR	99	99	NR	NR	90	NR
Abraham et al.[20] 1991 Scotland	23	NR	NR	NR	NR	NR	15

Romer, Homik[21]						
DeMoya, 1988, Santo Domingo, Dominican Republic	90					
Deniaud, 1988, France	70					
DiClemente, 1985, San Francisco, U.S.	80					
Kapila, 1988, United Kingdom	NR					
King, 1988, Canada	80					
Ouedraogo, 1989, Burkina Faso	90					
Pavri, 1988, Bombay/Pune, India	90					
Perucci, 1988, Rome, Italy	80					
Roscoe, 1987, Michigan, U.S.	90					
Sonenstein, 1988, United States	90					
Strunin, 1986, Massachusetts,U.S.	NR					
Wilson, 1988, Zimbabwe	70					
Zuegin, 1987, Switzerland	80					
Ibanga, Williams, Ibanga[22] (1985)[b]						
Nigeria	20	NR	83		85	
National Research Council[23]						
1987–88						
United States						
Females						
White		98		96	87	82
Black		94		91	86	87
Hispanic		91		87	68	90
Males						
White		96		92	90	80
Black		87		83	83	82
Hispanic		85		85	82	81
Hingson, Strunin, Berlin[24]						
Massachusetts, U.S.						
1986		91	93	91		
1988		99	89	99		
Sugerman et al.[25]						
1990						
United States						
Homeless youth	75	85		86	86	86

people need to know, and how to tell them about it. Information and education are necessary, but hardly sufficient.

The second key element of success involves *health and social services* linked to the information messages. For example, if the message is to use condoms—then obviously, condoms must be readily available, of good quality, and affordable. It is striking how often information campaigns have been launched without considering the specific concrete needs for local services which will result.

The third element is more complex, but just as important as the other two—a *supportive social environment*. This means that people are supported rather than coerced, and that active steps are taken to prevent discrimination and promote human rights.

When these three elements have been combined, as they have in innovative and creative ways in communities around the world, then HIV transmission is slowed. One example is provided by the experience of a group of Zairian sex workers: when provided with information, counseling, condoms, treatment of other sexually transmitted diseases, and social support, the rate of new HIV infections plummeted from 18 percent per year to just 2 percent per year.[1] Conversely, no program which fails to include each of these elements has been demonstrated to be effective. Therefore, the adoption and adaptation of each of these three elements to local circumstances, customs, and realities, appear critical in creating successful HIV prevention programs.

——————— · · ·

INFORMATION AND EDUCATION

For many, information was thought to be the key to behavior change.[2] Therefore, prevention programs usually focused on increasing awareness about modes of HIV transmission and information on how to avoid becoming infected. Examples abound of increased awareness following information campaigns (see Table 9.1).

Even so, experience over the past decade has shown that by itself information is insufficient to change behavior. For example, at one time it was commonly believed that the possibility of dying of AIDS would prompt individuals to change their behavior. Widely disseminated information about the risk of AIDS, however, has failed to achieve such a result. This failure of information to lead reliably, regularly, or predictably to behavior change has been documented repeatedly in varying cultures and contexts and underscores the need for a comprehensive approach to prevention, combining the three elements essential to its success.

Relying solely on information also has risks. Misperceptions and misunderstandings have been common in AIDS information programs and serve as barriers to adopting preventive behavior. Correcting such misperceptions has been a theme of HIV prevention programs in many settings (see Box 9.1). Unfortunately, even with complete and accurate information, adoption of prevention behavior is far from assured.

When a person sees AIDS as inevitable, there is little motivation to change behavior; people must have hope that preventive behavior will reduce their chances of infection. Prevention programs which provoke anxiety have been associated with adopting preventive behaviors, but extreme anxiety can lead to denial, avoidance or a sense of fatalism.[26]

The search for love and intimacy may also create an obstacle to adoption of safer sex practices. The belief that steady partners are "safer" than occasional partners is widespread and persistent.[27] Therefore, beyond information, the interaction between partners is an important factor in deciding to practice and maintain safer sexual behaviors.

Messages

Messages are more effective when they can be directed toward a specific target population. The language and the approach must be shaped to reflect specific needs and solutions that are appropriate for different communities.

An analysis of the information/education programs of 38 national AIDS programs revealed that in over 90 percent of both industrialized and developing countries, the main messages were caution about lifestyle and correcting misperceptions. About 80 percent of the countries surveyed have provided information about how to assess personal risk. Far fewer countries included messages countering discrimination, partner negotiation, and testing; partner negotiation and testing messages were more commonly reported from industrialized countries (see Figure 9.1).

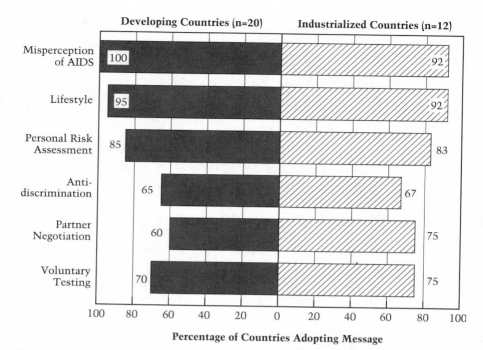

Developing Countries (n=20) **Industrialized Countries (n=12)**

Misperception of AIDS	100 / 92
Lifestyle	95 / 92
Personal Risk Assessment	85 / 83
Anti-discrimination	65 / 67
Partner Negotiation	60 / 75
Voluntary Testing	70 / 75

Percentage of Countries Adopting Message

Figure 9.1. Messages of HIV/AIDS information, education, and communication programs: Analysis of the content of 32 national AIDS programs, 1991-1992.
Source: AIDS in the World, 1992.

Box 9.1: Early Perceptions and Misperceptions about AIDS in Tanzania

Justin Nguma, Muhimbili College of Health Sciences, Dar es Salaam, Tanzania

In many countries around the world, the onset of the AIDS pandemic was met with varied perceptions both at the community and government levels. For example, in the late 1970s most Americans perceived AIDS to be a disease of homosexual men, injection drug users, and people of Haitian origin because they were the ones most affected by it. Thus, individuals who did not identify with these groups falsely believed that they were safe from AIDS. In Tanzania, AIDS took its first toll in the Kagera region on young men and women involved in illegal trade across the border with Zaire, Rwanda, and Burundi. The trade flourished on illegal buying and selling

of currency, minerals, alcohol, and basic commodities that were in short supply in Tanzania, especially after the border war with Uganda in the late 1970s.

One commodity that made history in this trade was colorful shirts, some of which had an eagle emblem on the back or the inscription "Juliana." The shirts became very popular among the youth and spread like fire around the country. As the death toll continued to rise among these traders, the Kagera communities started to perceive the disease as having something to do with the nature of the trade. In particular, they believed that witchcraft was the main cause of these deaths and that the dying were bewitched by their colleagues (as a result of cheating in their business deals) or by their competitors. The communities

Most countries surveyed reported that their main prevention themes aimed at reducing sexual transmission of HIV, include using condoms, reducing the number of partners, and preventing and treating sexually transmitted diseases (STDs). Each of these approaches was cited slightly more frequently in industrialized than developing countries, with the exception of prevention and treatment of STDs, which received more emphasis in developing countries. Fewer countries selected abstinence as a major theme; industrialized countries were about twice as likely to promote abstinence as developing countries (see Figure 9.2).

Message *content* is more effective when it is clear and unambiguous. Yet the past decade has revealed how cautious many HIV prevention messages have been when talking about sex, condoms, and drug injection. Prevention messages have been full of inferences to sexual practices which were as likely to confuse as to inform. For example, the warning against exchanging "bodily fluids" may have avoided offense, but it was interpreted incorrectly as including sweat, saliva, and tears, for which there is no evidence suggesting a possible role in HIV transmission.[28]

Ambiguous messages can result from lack of cultural sensitivity, self-censorship, and imposed censorship. Among adolescents and

---

named the disease Juliana, symbolizing a disease resulting from the trade on Juliana shirts. A majority of Tanzanians, therefore, perceived AIDS as a disease of illegal traders and smugglers. As in the case of homosexuals and injection drug users in the United States, those who did not identify themselves with this trade falsely believed that they were not susceptible to HIV infection. Because the majority of AIDS patients, particularly those suffering from diarrhea and fever, were noticed to lose a lot of weight, the communities later renamed the disease "Slim."

The new name, "Slim," came to serve as a community's visual criterion for determining who could be carrying the AIDS virus. Just as homosexuals, Haitians, and injection drug users were being discriminated against in the United States as possible carriers of the AIDS virus, slim people, especially when they happened to be strangers, were often discriminated against in casual sex situations based on this perception. People were more likely to have casual sex with strangers who were plump and overweight than with those who appeared extraordinarily slim. This misconception became the major target of the early IEC messages. It was critical to dispel this myth and alert the public that anyone could be carrying the AIDS virus irrespective of his or her physical appearance.

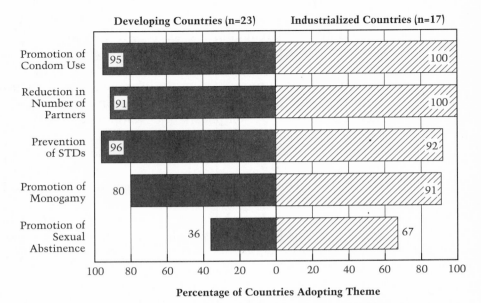

Developing Countries (n=23)   Industrialized Countries (n=17)

Promotion of Condom Use	95	100
Reduction in Number of Partners	91	100
Prevention of STDs	96	92
Promotion of Monogamy	80	91
Promotion of Sexual Abstinence	36	67

100 80 60 40 20 0 20 40 60 80 100

Percentage of Countries Adopting Theme

Figure 9.2. Themes of HIV prevention programs in 38 national AIDS programs, 1991-1992.
Source: AIDS in the World, 1992.

young adults who say they have adopted monogamy, further probing may reveal a pattern of serial monogamous relationships lasting from only a few weeks to several years.[29] In another instance, a campaign was conducted in the Netherlands to counter common misunderstandings about HIV. The format was purposefully ironic, and their research found that as much as 25 percent of the population failed to understand the irony.[30] As an example of censorship, the first brochures in England about safer sex were confiscated as obscene.[31] Indeed, nongovernmental organizations often produce more provocative messages and images than governments—sometimes in opposition to government policy and other times with its consent.[32,33] (See the *AIDS in the World* survey of nongovernmental organizations, Chapter 17, "AIDS Service Organizations in Transition.")

A further barrier to HIV prevention through information is the gap between the literacy level of the audience and the level at which a brochure or pamphlet has been written. A study in the United States reviewed 137 HIV-related brochures and found that between 2 and 16 percent of the target audience were at a reading level below that of the material. Two studies evaluated the readability of inserts in condom packages and concluded that all texts required a reading level above the education level of many people at risk for HIV.[34]

Material can be pretested with the intended audience for comprehension and impact. The audience can then provide feedback to the producers of the material, and necessary changes can be made to improve design. This type of research contributed greatly to the success of interventions such as the social marketing campaigns of condoms in Zaire,[35] the "Hot Rubber" campaign in Switzerland,[36] and in-school prevention material in the Congo.[37] Pretesting also has the advantage of obtaining the cooperation of key members of the target populations.

In the future, more emphasis needs to be given to messages emphasizing partner negotiation, as partner interaction is one of the most powerful influences on adoption of safer sexual behavior. In addition, an immense gap remains between the receipt of a message and subsequent behavior.

Channels

Developing clear and appropriate messages is an essential part of the information/education component of the HIV prevention process. Making sure they are heard is another. Few programs start with a formal analysis of their communications environment, and many fail to consider the best combination of channels for reaching a particular target audience: radio, newspapers or television; brochures or posters; counseling, theater or outreach and self-help groups. Instead, most programs start with a channel in mind because it is the predesignated choice or simply the channel already available to the program.

Reach and frequency must be considered when selecting and evaluating the effectiveness of a communications channel. Reach refers to the number of people who can potentially be exposed to the message. Frequency refers to the number of times the message is repeated. HIV prevention messages in the mass media are often published or broadcast as public service announcements, often at the discretion of television or newspaper managers. Little information has

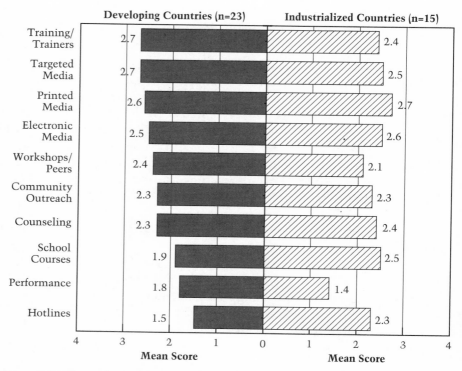

Figure 9.3. Channels used for information, education, communication on HIV/AIDS in 38 national AIDS programs.
Source: AIDS in the World, 1992.

been collected on the frequency with which they are shown; thus, one of the key variables for mass communication is often uncontrolled.

Data on the number of brochures printed are often used by programs as an indicator of activity. Less frequently, are there records of the quantities delivered to various distribution points. Stockpiles of brochures are sometimes found in warehouses and storerooms without any systematic plan for distribution. Most programs are constrained by the small number of counselors, teachers, and outreach workers that can be hired. Consequently, there is rarely an attempt to calculate the overall reach of the program.

There is consensus that mass media channels create awareness and set the agenda, while interpersonal channels are more likely to influence behavior.[38-40] In developing a media plan, the per contact cost and the overall budget for the program are key variables. Per contact, mass media costs significantly less than counseling or other types of personal contact, and when trying to reach the general population, the reach of the message may be greater than for other channels. Still, the absolute cost of producing the message and arranging or purchasing media time may be quite high.

Lower cost channels and specialized media may be more efficient, however, when programs target specific populations such as sex workers or gay men. Gay newspapers have clearly been effective in reaching gay men.[41-44] Newsletters have been created to reach commercial sex worker (CSW) groups, and workbooks have been created to reach students. In addition, the use of popular culture is particularly effective in increasing awareness; some of the more innovative channels used to reach populations have been performances and music.

The *AIDS in the World* survey indicated that in industrialized countries, print media are used most frequently, followed by targeted media, electronic media, and school courses (see Figure 9.3). Training of trainers is used most frequently by developing countries, followed by targeted media, printed media, and electronic media. School courses are used more frequently by industrialized countries, while performances are used more frequently by developing countries.

HEALTH AND SOCIAL SERVICES

Beyond increasing awareness and providing information, prevention projects have led to behavioral changes (see Table 9.2). A selection of studies from the published literature demonstrates increases in condom use, declines in the number of sex partners, changes in sexual venue, and modification of needle-using and sharing practices. In all these instances, information/education was complemented by supportive services.

There is a wide range of supportive services which may be required to help people translate information into behavior. Relevant health and social services include testing and counseling, treatment programs for injection drug users (IDUs), support groups and condoms.

The logic of information and education programs must be followed through at the local level to ensure that predictable health and social service needs are anticipated and met, and that emerging needs are detected. At the local level, the details of service, design, and accessibility will make the critical difference.

Supportive services include the provision of information, care, and commodities through governmental, nongovernmental, and private networks. Their efficiency increases as the individuals and communities for which they are intended participate in their design and implementation. HIV/AIDS prevention and care involves a wide range of services and channels, some of which serve multiple purposes (maternal and child health services, primary health care, STD clinics, for example), while others respond more specifically to needs created or revealed by the pandemic (IDU or CSW outreach programs). From another perspective, some services involve personnel dedicated to a specific task (laboratory technicians, condom quality controllers), while other services are delivered through a broad range of health and social workers who may be called upon to perform HIV/AIDS related tasks in the course of their work (counseling, health education).

The effectiveness of the response to HIV/AIDS depends on the extent to which services designed to meet community needs are geographically accessible, financially affordable, occur in a favorable environment (quality of interpersonal contact, confidentiality, tolerance, compassion), are delivered by skilled personnel, and are sustainable over time. Thus, health and social services will require the use of multiple channels, the participation of trained human resources, effective management and coordination, and the continued availability of funds.

How prevention needs have been met among certain target populations is explored in the following sections. The gaps between knowledge and misinformation, and empowerment and powerlessness, will repeatedly surface as consistent themes.

■■■■■■   .   .   .

SUPPORTIVE SOCIAL ENVIRONMENT

Regardless of the quality and reach of information/education and the quality and accessibility of health and social services, the broad social environment within which these activities take place will play a major role in determining the success of an HIV prevention program. Like the first two critical components of prevention—information/education and health and social services—a supportive social environment must be created, or at least promoted.

The term "empowerment" is useful to describe the process through which individuals assume for themselves the power to determine their behavior. An individual is not empowered by others; rather, a person must empower himself or herself. Therefore, the positive role of the social environment is to remove barriers to personal empowerment and to facilitate this process. The capacity of a social environment to promote individual empowerment will also be explored further in Chapter 14 on vulnerability.

Community Norms

AIDS pushes the frontiers of community norms, which reflect collective values, many of which are taboo topics of discussion. Understanding community norms and how to involve communities in the process of changing norms is an important part of HIV prevention.

Broadly, two positions on freedom of discussion about AIDS prevention can be distinguished. The first, *public health* viewpoint advocates providing information as completely and widely as possible, regarding all possible methods of HIV prevention. The second position, broadly characterized as *moralist,* takes the view that some information is harmful or otherwise unacceptable; thus, some options (e.g., abstinence, or saying "no" to drug use) are strongly, even exclusively favored.

Community norms surface in the language used to speak about AIDS. In a constrained societal climate, it is difficult to say certain things clearly. Thus, the warning to avoid exchanging "bodily fluids"—a term used in recommendations in the mid-1980s—probably avoided causing offense, but at the cost of clarity. In Uganda, the recommendation for "zero grazing" was a clever reference to monogamy, but the message was frequently misunderstood.[57]

Word selection is important because it is linked to the struggle between HIV/AIDS prevention and care efforts on the one hand and the status quo of the community's thinking on the other. Words carry

Table 9.2: Individual and partner behavior change over time in selected populations[a]

Population/Study	Behavior change: Condom use	Behavior change: Sex partners

General Population

Haussser et al.[45] Switzerland 1989-90, Age 17–30 [N = 1,182, 1,211, 1,213, 1,231, 1,227] Telephone survey

Use with casual sex partners

	Jan. 87	Oct. 87	Oct. 88	Oct. 89	Oct. 90
Always	8	18	28	48	48
Sometimes	25	44	59	19	15
Never	67	38	13	32	37

No.of partners

	9/86–4/87	5/87–12/87	1/88–12/88
Women			
>1 partner in past month	21	16	18
>1 partner in last 6 months	57	49	53

Van Haastrecht, van den Hoek, Coutinho[46] Amsterdam 1982–1989 STD clinics [N = 1,582]

Condom use

	9/86–4/87	5/87–12/87	1/88–12/88
Men			
Always	10	20	25
Never	60	58	45
Women			
Almost always	7	30	31

% Reporting casual partners in last 6 months

Jan. 87	Oct. 87	Oct. 88
18	14	15

Wellings[47] Dubois et al. Switzerland 1989 Age 17–30 [N = 1,182, 1,211, 1,213] Telephone survey

Use with casual partners in last 6 months

	Jan. 87	Oct. 87	Oct. 88	1989
Never	67	38	13	
Sometimes	25	45	58	
Always	8	17	29	

More than one partner in last month

	1986	1987	1988	1989
Sample	9	11	8	9
Singles	22	22	19	21

Brorsson Sweden 1989 General survey (N = 4000)

Use on last occasion of sex

Nov. 86	Dec. 87	1988	1989
14	23	30	31

2 or more partners in past year

Nov. 86	Dec. 87	1988	1989
19	24	23	23

United Kingdom 1986–1989 Age 18–24 [N = 111, 260, 1,156, 1,176] General survey

Netherlands 1987–1989 General survey [N = 137]

Use of a condom in last month

	April 87	Sept. 87	Oct. 88	Oct. 89
Sometimes	21	33	31	43
Always	9	28	46	40

Adolescents

Cochran, et al.[48]
California
1986-87
University students (N = 182)

Use by sexually active students

	Winter 86	Fall 87
Men	59	68
Women	31	55

Unprotected vaginal intercourse

	Winter 86	Fall 87
Men	89	94
Women	80	89

Gay/Bisexual

de Vroome, Sandfort, Tielman[49]
Netherlands
1986-1989
Mailed questionnaire (N = 329)

% adopting safer sex

1986	1987	1988
34	+10	+10

de Wit, et al.[50]
Netherlands
1985-1989
N = 976

% practicing unprotected anal sex

Receptive		Insertive	
Pre	Post	Pre	Post
65	26	79	33

Ekstrand, Coates[51]
San Francisco
1984-1988
Mostly white, single, well-educated
Telephone survey (N = 686)

% practicing unprotected anal sex

All receptive		All insertive	
84-85	87-88	84-85	87-88
64	19	69	19

Rec. w/ejac.		Ins. w/ejac.	
84-85	87-88	84-85	87-88
64	9	69	9

No. of sex partners

Multiple		Anonymous	
84-85	87-88	84-85	87-88
80	52	52	30

Pollak, Moatti[52]
France
1985-1988
General survey (N = 999, 1,200, 1,200, 1,500)

No. of partners

	1985	1986	1987
None	5	8	9
One	16	24	28
2-5	31	33	32
6-10	21	17	17
11-20	17	11	8
>20	10	7	6

Table 9.2 (cont.): Individual and partner behavior change over time in selected populations[a]

Population/Study	Behavior change: Condom use	Behavior change: Sex partners

Hessol et al.[53]
San Francisco
1988
City clinic (N = 310)

Mean no. of partners with receptive anal intercourse w/ ejaculation w/o condom

	1978	1980	1982	1984
	14	20	10	1

Ross, Freedman, Brew[54]
Australia
1988
Gay establishments (N = 172)

	1986	1988
Men who never used during anal sex		
Receptive	56	38
Insertive	56	41
Men who never used during sex		
Yes	129	159
No	42	11
Men who used in past 2 months		
Always	31	56
Never	41	22

Martin, Dean, et al.[55]
New York City
1985–88
Gay organizations (N = 624)

% of men who had unprotected anal sex

	1981	1985	1986	1987
Receptive	77	51	26	17
Insertive	85	57	30	23

% of men with certain nos. of partners

	1981	1985	1986	1987
None	3	3	5	7
One	8	14	16	19
2 or more	90	83	79	74

Commercial sex workers

Van Haastrecht, van den Hoek, Coutinho[56]
Amsterdam
1986–88
STD clinics (N = 32, 27, 37)

9/86–4/87	5/87–12/87	1/88–12/88
59	78	68

Medium no. of partners

	9/86–4/87	5/87–12/87	1/86–12/88
Past month	35	14	15
Past 6 months	165	130	50

a. References for this table, indicated by superscript numbers, are in the Reference Notes for Chapter 9.

many different meanings, or codes. Examples of the evolving language of AIDS include:

- Prostitutes—now widely referred to as commercial sex workers;
- AIDS patient/victim—people/person with AIDS;
- Drug addict—injection drug user;
- Hemophiliacs—people with hemophilia;
- Promiscuous person—person with multiple sex partners;
- Target group—target behavior.

Decisions about safer sexual practices are rarely made in isolation, yet most HIV prevention interventions are aimed at the individual. Studies have found that men who participated in the gay community and were responsive to community norms were also much more likely to adopt informed AIDS prevention behavior, while those who isolated themselves adopted fewer and less effective behavior changes.[58-60]

In summary, both HIV prevention programs and individuals in the society are strongly influenced by prevailing community norms of behavior and discourse.

Policy Support

The formal expression of community norms is found in the legislation and laws which affect HIV prevention policy. Laws may reflect tradition and societal mythology rather than social realities, as noted in the discussion about commercial sex workers (see Box 9.2). In addition, there is often a naive confidence in the ability of laws to influence human behavior (see Box 9.3).

At the policy level, the central conflict reflects the moralist/pragmatist dichotomy. Some policies can have a direct impact on prevention measures: obscenity laws and postal regulations can limit circulation of explicit HIV prevention materials; regulations on condoms can increase their cost or make them unavailable;[61] failure to halt discrimination in housing and unemployment can render testing and counseling programs ineffective; laws prohibiting possession of needles and syringes or limiting their distribution can actually increase needle sharing. Sometimes, policies have unexpected results. For example, the reduction in fire fighting services in the South Bronx of New York City led to further decay of the district, a surge in drug injection, the dispersement and disintegration of the community, and ultimately, the exposure of community members to higher risk of HIV infection[62] (see Box 9.4).

Policies which discriminate against certain groups work against HIV prevention. Nongovernmental organizations often played a critical role in representing those who found themselves outside the mainstream community values, and were ignored or discriminated against by government policy.

Empowerment

Self-efficacy and belief in the capacity to control one's environment are important factors in adopting and sustaining safer behavior. On

---

Box 9.2: Commercial Sex Workers: Police or Policies?

Cheryl Overs, Coordinator, Network of Sexwork Related HIV/AIDS Projects, Paris

In some countries, sex workers are screened for HIV, and those found to have the virus are detained in special facilities where they are supposed to be rehabilitated or retrained. In other places, people with HIV are prevented from working in the sex industry by imprisonment or detention in medical or quarantine facilities. Specific legal, or quasi-legal, actions are often taken to prevent HIV-infected sex workers from continuing to work. These include closing commercial sex venues, taking police action against sex workers suspected of carrying HIV, and screening photos of HIV-infected sex workers on television in the form of community service announcements.

There are few protests in either industrialized or developing countries against the idea that the removal of people with HIV from the sex industry is sound policy. In some regions, the media have contributed to this climate by portraying HIV-infected sex workers as vampirelike creatures stalking the streets to spread death. For obvious reasons, governments and health

authorities are quick to respond to public demand that an HIV-free pool of sex workers be maintained. Education campaigns remain relatively rare and are widely seen as an unreliable or soft option in the political climate around AIDS and prostitution.

There are several assumptions underlying these actions aimed at removing people with HIV from the sex industry. One is that it is possible to identify people with HIV. However, the nature of HIV with its long *window period* and the formidable logistics involved in repeatedly testing an often unwilling population mean that even if it were desirable, there is probably no way to accurately identify HIV-positive sex workers in most countries. Furthermore, actions for preventing those who are HIV positive and want to continue sex work from doing so, are also unlikely to succeed. They may even exacerbate the incidence of risk behavior by creating a second illegal or underground tier of the sex industry.

There is a widespread but largely unexamined assumption that HIV-positive sex workers will transmit the virus. Where safe sex practices are the norm in the sex industry, there is

the collective level, belief in the power to effect change was reflected in the early development of nongovernmental organizations (NGOs). Certainly, for many street kids, CSWs, and women with low levels of empowerment, this sense of low personal efficacy is a harsh reality. Interventions which help empower individuals have been shown to be effective.[63,64] These include inducing policy changes, establishing peer support groups where empowerment is gained through collective action, workshops that improve skills in condom use and partner negotiation, and outreach programs which focus on group empowerment. Several studies in Africa have shown that monogamous women married to men who have multiple sexual partners are becoming

---

evidence that this is not the case. On what basis could a particular act, which is promoted in official campaigns if it occurs in private, be regarded as an unacceptable risk if it is accompanied by the exchange of money?

One argument is that the greater the number of sexual partners a seropositive person has, the greater the risk of accidental transmission during protected sex. (Do sex workers necessarily have more partners than non-sex workers?) From this perspective, taking special measures to prevent a person infected with HIV from receiving payment for sex may be based on a notion that the client is entitled to a smaller chance of contracting HIV (as a result of a safe sex accident) than other people who are having protected sex with partners of unknown status. Even if unsafe services are provided, how can setting clients of sex workers aside as a group deserving special protection be justified—particularly when there is consensus among sex workers that where unsafe services are provided, it is always at the client's demand.

These attempts to ensure that men can have sex with seronegative sex workers reflect the idea that the small amount of money which exchanges hands absolves the client of responsibility for his own sexual health. A brothel owner who supports this consumer rights approach described HIV-positive sex workers as a *faulty product.*

Depending on one's view, it is appropriate, morally reprehensible, or criminal for people with HIV to participate knowingly in risky activities with uninformed partners. This view rests alongside the idea that each person is responsible for protecting him or herself from HIV. How these concepts are worked into policy responding to people with HIV who knowingly place others at risk will, of course, vary enormously from country to country. But it is clear that those decisions and policies should apply according to the behavior of individuals. The exchange of money bears no impact on the rights and responsibilities held by two individuals who have sexual intercourse, protected or otherwise, in the age of AIDS.

Box 9.3: HIL Revisited

Justice Michael Kirby,
Supreme Court, Australia

It came to me in a flash. There was a new virus running parallel to the devastation caused by HIV. Like its counterpart, it was virtually universal, spreading rapidly, causing a great deal of havoc and pain. I refer to HIL—the contagion of Highly Inefficient Laws. I revealed my discovery at a conference in Paris. Later, even President Mitterrand smiled. But this is no smiling matter.

HIL has continued to spread, and like HIV, it mutates. Different strains of HIL are seen in different parts of the world. So far, there have been three major manifestations of the same virus: HIL-1, HIL-2, and HIL-3. As manifestations of the same virus, they all attack the body politic.

HIL-1 is universal, mandatory HIV testing. So far, HIL-1 has only been found, for certain, in Cuba, although there were strong outbreaks at one time in Bulgaria and parts of the former Soviet Union. In most other parts of the world, HIL-1 has been stamped out. In a few states of the United States, premarital testing for HIV was mandated by legislation. In Illinois, which commenced such screening in 1988, only 23 of the 150,000 people tested in the first 11 months were found to be HIV positive (i.e., 1 in 6,500). The cost of the HIV test per person ranged from $25 to $125. Illinois officials estimated that the cost of finding each of the 23 infected people came to $228,000. Meanwhile, the number of couples seeking marriage licenses in the state decreased by 55 percent.

If universal testing had been adopted in the United States, HIL-1 would have revealed about 1,300 HIV infections in persons who would not otherwise have been identified as HIV positive—at a cost of $100,000,000 nationwide. Little wonder that HIL-1 has been readily contained. Yet in the early days of the HIV epidemic, HIL-1 appeared very dangerous indeed. It may yet spring up in small and relatively isolated communities with authoritarian cultures, sharing an exaggerated notion of the effectiveness of state control of public health crises.

HIL-2, on the other hand, continues to spread everywhere. This is the mandatory screening of particular vulnerable groups who are not in a strong position to protest or resist. This is an extremely virulent strain of HIL.

Sex workers and prisoners, together with drug-dependent persons and homosexuals, are the targets of compulsory systems of mass screening, directed at so-called high-risk groups. It is easy to mandate compulsory screening, but how effective is it? How often must it be repeated? Is it any more cost-effective than the Illinois experiment? Does it not merely pander to the prejudices of society, whilst providing little efficient protection? The alternative strategies are likely to be much more effective, but also much more controversial.

The third mutant HIL-3 involves the requirement for a certificate of HIV negativity at international frontiers. If one were really trying to make this strain of HIL effective, the first group to be targeted would surely be tourists. These swashbuckling merry-makers often leave behind them at home the inhibitions—sexual and otherwise—that restrain the spread of HIV. Dump them and their millions on tropical beaches or in crowded Asian resorts, and the risk of the unprotected spread of HIV increases. Yet tourists are the darlings of late twentieth-century economies. No one would target them with HIL-3. Instead, it is returning nationals, immigrants, refugees, foreign students, and applicants for long-term residence who are required to prove that they are HIV free. WHO, at least, realizes the inefficiency of such certificates. The window period. The need for constant testing. The false negatives. The cost involved. The basic rights of HIV-positive people to travel. HIL-3 is a very blunt instrument for containing the virus of HIV in a world constantly on the move.

Yet HIL-3 still has to be watched closely. If accurate instant tests for the presence of HIV were invented, they might be installed in the form of universal testing at international frontiers. Not only is the intrusive practice of checking one's biological baggage at customs questionable, but the restrictions that would certainly accompany such a watch-dog policy also promise to exacerbate discriminatory practices. Even worse, once HIL-3 takes root in a few countries, the dangers of replication and retaliation threaten to take a further toll on human rights.

The last decade has seen our societies tested. Tested by HIV, which has come upon us like a dark cloud out of nowhere—unexpected and threatening. But darker still can be the actions of humankind below the cloud. The history of epidemics, and of the legal responses to them, has been one of cruelty and gross inefficiency. It behooves an informed world to target the HIV pandemic with keen attention to basic human rights. That is why, in our strategies concerned with HIV, we should remain vigilant to the dangers of HIL. Out of the melancholic predicament of HIV may even come a better appreciation of the utility and the limitations of the law where human behavior and public health are the targets of the law's concern.

infected with HIV, their only risk factor being powerlessness to influence their husband's behavior. In such situations, reform of laws governing property distribution and divorce may be much more important in helping to prevent HIV infection than condom distribution.

■■■■■   .   .   .

INTERVENTION PROGRAMS

The *AIDS in the World* survey found that national AIDS programs universally included messages for the general population and the

---

Box 9.4: From Fire Service Cuts to AIDS

Dr. Rodrick Wallace, New York Psychiatric Institute

What factors determine the level of HIV infection within the heavily infected urban epicenters of the United States? Several recent studies document the connection between the hollowing out of inner-city communities and the role of these communities as epicenters of the AIDS pandemic.[a] Using New York's South Bronx as an example, they identify a new and disturbing paradigm for the spread of HIV/AIDS.

During the 1970s, as part of an official planned shrinkage policy, a series of cuts were made in New York City fire services, including major reductions in services to poor minority neighborhoods, such as the South Bronx. These cutbacks to already vulnerable communities led to a contagious—and continuing—cycle of housing loss, forced migration, social disruption, and spiraling social and public health problems. Between 1972 and 1976, the New York City Fire Department staff was reduced by 30 percent, and 50 firefighting units from the South Bronx and other areas with already high fire rates and high

population density were disbanded or removed. At the same time, the number of initial response companies—critical to containing a potentially devastating structural fire—was also reduced.

The loss in personnel, overburdening of remaining fire services, and increases in uncontrolled fire and building abandonment spread destruction in ever-widening circles. Neighboring buildings were infected by spreading fire or by increased susceptibility to fire from overcrowding, undermaintenance by absentee landlords, and vandalism centered around already abandoned structures. Adjacent neighborhoods, overcrowded and overstressed by the absorption of displaced people and increased social problems, soon fell victim to the same ills. By 1980, between 50 and 80 percent of housing units in heavily affected communities were lost—a figure unprecedented in an industrialized nation not involved in total war. Where communities once lived, hulks of burned and abandoned buildings and vacant lots remained. Both the devastated zones and nearby communities receiving displaced

military. Beyond these two groups, the emphasis of target populations varied substantially between industrialized and developing countries (see Figure 9.4).

Over 90 percent of the industrialized countries surveyed by *AIDS in the World* reported targeting IDUs, homosexual and bisexual men, HIV-infected people and people with AIDS, and prisoners. The next tier of targeted populations in industrialized countries were health care workers and CSWs. Fewer industrialized countries targeted religious leaders, community leaders and migrant populations. In developing countries, programs were directed toward opinion and religious

---

persons experienced rising rates of homicide, suicide, drug and alcohol abuse, HIV infection and AIDS.

Several factors explain the impact of the burnout of the South Bronx on the spread of HIV/AIDS. Forced migration expanded injection drug use from a tightly clustered region of the South-Central Bronx to a more geographically extended community, exposing a larger population to interaction with injection drug users. The disruption of personal, domestic, and community social networks intensified existing problems of violence, substance abuse, and prostitution, which are associated with increased levels of HIV transmission. The loss of social structures also limited community ability to disseminate information and reinforce social norms regarding behaviors that help prevent HIV/AIDS. Displacement, as well as increased poverty, reduced access to health care among an already underserved population.

The fate of the South Bronx reflects the vulnerability to HIV infection created by processes of urban decay already widespread in many U.S. cities, including Detroit, Newark,

Philadelphia, Chicago, Wilmington and Miami, as well as New York City. The scattershot of individually oriented interventions, such as public education and condom and sterile needle distribution, have proven insufficient to stem the HIV epidemic. Disease control strategies must address the social context in which HIV is transmitted. A broad approach to prevention is needed, including the social and physical restoration of affected communities, in order to reverse the conditions that increase individual and community vulnerability to HIV transmission.

---

a. R. Wallace, "A synergism of plagues: 'Planned shrinkage', contagious housing destruction and AIDS in the Bronx," *Environmental Research* 47(1)(1988):1–33; "Urban desertification, public health and public order: Planned shrinkage, violent death, substance abuse and AIDS in the Bronx," *Social Science and Medicine* 31(7)(1990):801–13; "Social disintegration and the spread of AIDS: Thresholds for propagation along with sociogeographic networks," *Social Science and Medicine* 33(1991):1155–63; R. Wallace and M. Fullilove, "AIDS deaths in the Bronx 1983–1988: Spatiotemporal analysis from a sociogeographic perspective," *Environmental Planning A* 23(1991):1701–23.

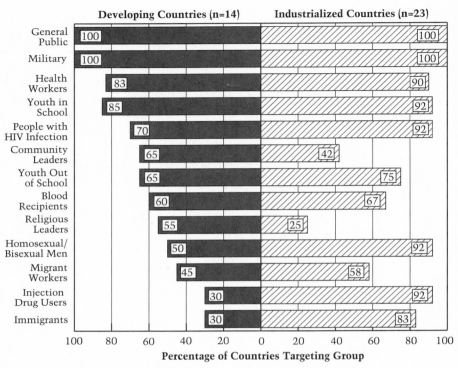

Figure 9.4. Target groups by developed and developing countries.
Source: AIDS in the World, 1992.

leaders, indicating a greater reliance on existing networks. For both industrialized and developing countries, there was a gap in information efforts targeting out of school youths and migrant workers. In the following section, interventions directed toward certain of these target populations are profiled in greater detail.

Targeting the General Population

Prevention programs that target the general population attempt to reach the vast majority of people, often through the use of mass media: billboards, newspapers, television, and popular music. The impact of the media has been well documented. Although some countries continue to report low levels of knowledge about safer sex techniques,[65] in the past decade, awareness about AIDS has increased dramatically in the general population. Individuals aware of HIV and AIDS often report some behavior change, usually a reduction in the number of sexual partners and greater care in choosing partners. Unfortunately, whether this has an important impact in communities with a high prevalence of HIV has yet to be established.[66]

HIV prevention needs of the general population differ depending on the country and community. In communities with high HIV prevalence, a campaign whose objective is raising awareness about risk and promoting safer sexual behavior would be appropriate. In low prevalence countries, raising undue fear may be counterproductive. In Australia[67] and the United Kingdom,[68] fear campaigns resulted in many persons at no or little risk seeking access to counseling and testing services. The long-term negative impact may be a credibility gap between the initial message of high risk and the reality of low current risk for many communities. The Netherlands, for example, made a conscious decision not to have a general population campaign until 1987 because it feared that the alarm to the public would serve no useful preventive purpose. In Switzerland, an early decision was made against using fear tactics.

In several sub-Saharan Africa countries, the general population is considerably more at risk than the general population of North America, Western Europe, and Oceania. In some countries, such as the Congo, general population campaigns were started as the magnitude of the AIDS problem became known. Others waited, apparently reasoning that since nothing could be done, why alarm the public—a fatalism that may be linked to political motives or a collective sense of powerlessness.

As shown in Figure 9.5, three-quarters of the countries in the *AIDS in the World* survey stated that one of their top three themes to the general population was use of condoms. Over two-thirds of the developing countries had messages to counter misperceptions and to modify risky lifestyle. Few countries mentioned increasing fear of AIDS as a major theme of their programs.

Only 17 percent of the developing countries and 21 percent of the industrialized countries mentioned testing as a major theme for the general population. More discouraging was the finding that only 26 percent of the developing countries and 43 percent of the industrial-

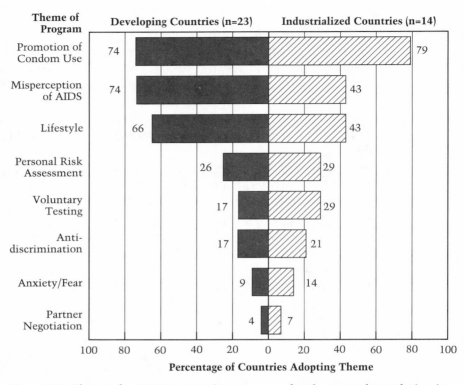

Theme of Program	Developing Countries (n=23)	Industrialized Countries (n=14)
Promotion of Condom Use	74	79
Misperception of AIDS	74	43
Lifestyle	66	43
Personal Risk Assessment	26	29
Voluntary Testing	17	29
Anti-discrimination	17	21
Anxiety/Fear	9	14
Partner Negotiation	4	7

Percentage of Countries Adopting Theme

Figure 9.5. Themes for AIDS prevention programs for the general population in selected developing and industrialized countries.
Source: AIDS in the World, 1992.

ized countries included messages designed to help people to assess their own risk. General population campaigns to reduce discrimination have generally been neglected. This is a major omission, since fear of discrimination often discourages individuals from seeking prevention and care services.

Adolescents

The increasing incidence of AIDS among young men and women in their early and mid-20's lends urgency to the need for effective HIV prevention programs targeted at youth. Adolescents may not yet have established their sexual habits, and if safer behaviors can become their norm, then there is an opportunity to limit infection in the next generation.

HIV/AIDS prevention programs have targeted two categories of young people: in-school and out-of-school youth. A further breakdown may include urban and rural youth, orphans and street kids, and youth in institutions. Within these strata, men and women often have substantially different needs. In many cultures, young women are partially protected by religious and cultural tradition from early sexual intercourse and are thus at lower risk for HIV infection. In other cultures, young women are at considerable risk for early sexual activity, as evidenced by high numbers of teenage pregnancies. Particularly in parts of East Africa and Latin America,[69] rising fertility rates suggest that young women are at additional direct risk for HIV infection through possible complications with births and abortions, and indirect risk because early pregnancies generally interfere with efforts to educate women, provide them with work qualifications, and improve their status.

Generally, urban youth are more at risk than rural youth because they tend to begin intercourse earlier and because the prevalence of HIV is higher in the cities.[70-72] Those most vulnerable to HIV infection are adolescents living on the streets, who often engage in commercial sex work and are more likely than those living at home to start intercourse early.[73-76]

In areas where injection drug use is common, teenagers are at an even higher risk. Among some adolescents, use of alcohol or non-injection drugs may be part of a pattern of risk behaviors which includes unsafe sex. The reasons for HIV risk are complex and include disinhibition and potential interaction with peers who are also engaging in high risk practices.[77-85]

Awareness of HIV among adolescents is generally high. But in poorer communities, where the literacy rate is low, alternative material is often not available. Among adolescents, personal perception of risk is usually low and misperceptions continue about transmission modes and the efficacy of prevention measures. As in other populations, there is also a negative attitude among youth toward condoms.[86-88] For some, the search for love may sometimes represent a far more immediate reward than the adoption of safe sex.[89] Young people also tend to feel invulnerable, and research has shown that low

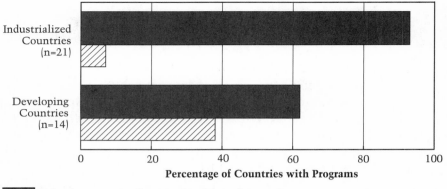

Percentage of Countries with Programs

School program implemented widely or frequently

School program rarely implemented

Figure 9.6. In-school HIV/AIDS prevention programs and level of implementation.
Source: AIDS in the World, 1992.

Percentage of Countries with Programs Widely or Sometimes Available

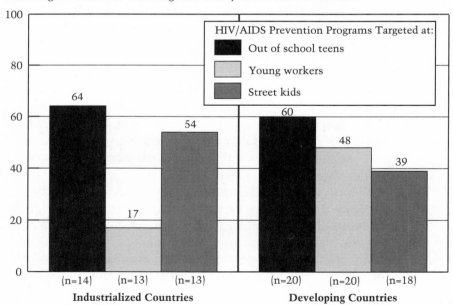

Figure 9.7. Availability of HIV/AIDS prevention programs for out-of-school youth in selected industrialized and developing countries.
Source: AIDS in the World, 1992.

risk perception is associated with higher risk activities.[90–92] The need, then, is for outreach and organization among adolescents which provides the skills and social support to help them practice safer behavior.

Adolescents are in the process of defining their independence and searching for role models: peers, athletes, rock and movie stars may all have a strong influence on adolescent behavior.[93] For HIV prevention, this suggests that there is a need to have role models who openly discuss and advocate safer behaviors.

Changing social patterns worldwide compound adolescent vulnerability to HIV infection. Among the changes accompanying a breakdown of extended, stable family networks is a redefinition of traditional role models for adolescents. Adolescents are initiated into both heterosexual and homosexual activity at earlier ages, yet they often marry later; this may lead to a higher number of sexual partners and greater risk of HIV infection.[94,95] In some areas of high HIV prevalence, younger women are increasingly under pressure from older men seeking sexual partners.

Prevention Programs: In-school programs for HIV education exist in about three-fourths of the industrialized countries in the *AIDS in the World* survey, with just over 60 percent targeting out-of-school youth (see Figure 9.6). In many countries, sex education is controversial in secondary schools,[96] with the unsupported fear that sex education leads to earlier initiation of sexual activity and a deterioration in moral values.[97] Outside the school environment, family planning clinics provide HIV/AIDS prevention information, but in developing countries in particular, these efforts target adult women, not sexually active adolescents.

In industrialized countries, programs for out-of-school youth were reported to be less frequent than in-school programs (92 percent vs. 64 percent); approximately 60 percent of developing countries reported both in- and out-of-school programs. Both industrialized and developing countries target out-of-school teens more than they target young workers or street kids, although young workers are a target population that could also be reached through programs in the workplace (see Figure 9.7).

As reported by *AIDS in the World* survey countries, themes differ between in- and out-of-school programs, and between industrialized

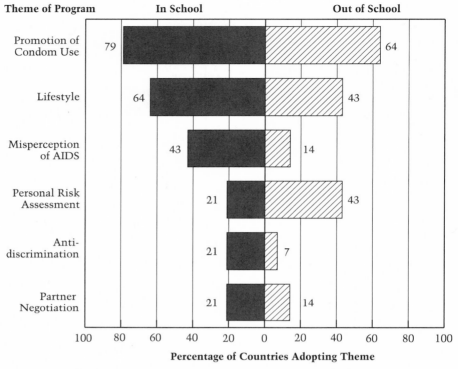

Theme of Program	In School		Out of School
Promotion of Condom Use	79		64
Lifestyle	64		43
Misperception of AIDS	43		14
Personal Risk Assessment	21		43
Anti-discrimination	21		7
Partner Negotiation	21		14

100 80 60 40 20 0 20 40 60 80 100

Percentage of Countries Adopting Theme

Figure 9.8. Themes for AIDS prevention programs for youth in 14 selected industrialized countries.
Source: AIDS in the World, 1992.

and developing countries (see Figures 9.8 and 9.9). Condom use is the most common theme for out-of-school youth. Half of the developing countries and 60 to 80 percent of programs in industrialized countries promote condoms for all youth. Few if any of the countries advocate HIV testing or use fear messages for either type of program.

While condoms were recommended, three-quarters of the countries surveyed reported that they were not widely available. Developing countries were more likely to report that condoms were unavailable. None of the industrialized countries reported that condoms were generally available in schools, but about half said they were sometimes available. As shown in Figure 9.10, condoms were more likely to be available in discos and other places where youths gather than in schools.

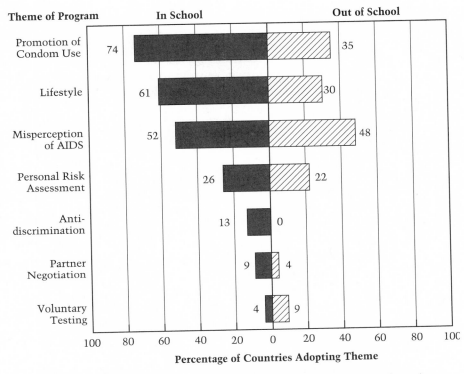

Figure 9.9. Themes for AIDS prevention programs for youth in 23 selected developing countries.
Source: AIDS in the World, 1992.

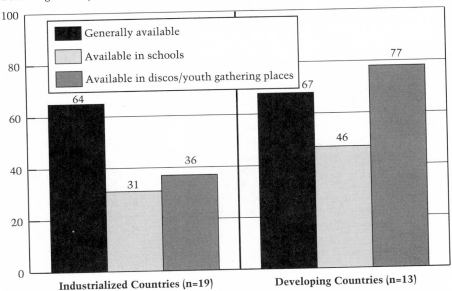

Figure 9.10. Condom availability for youth as reported by the AIW survey.
Source: AIDS in the World, 1992.

In addition to the government supported programs for adolescents, a large number of programs has been initiated by NGOs. The largest international NGOs conducting AIDS education programs have networks directly reaching millions of young people. The most important of these groups are the member societies of the International Federation of Red Cross and Red Crescent Societies (see Box 9.5), the Young Men and Women's Christan Association (YMCA/YWCA) movement and its affiliates, and the world scouting movement. All of these networks have simultaneously stimulated AIDS education efforts at the grassroots level and by leaders in national and international offices. The educational approach has been to balance traditional emphases on building youth self-esteem, encouraging positive peer pressure, and reinforcing indigenous cultural values with technical information on such issues as STD symptoms and condom use. The YMCA and the Red Cross movement place a significant emphasis on non-discrimination and care for people with HIV. The

---

Box 9.5: Preventing AIDS: A Continuing Challenge for Youth

Anne Petitgirard and Diane Widdus, International Federation of Red Cross and Red Crescent Societies

With 90 million youth members, the International Federation of Red Cross and Red Crescent Societies recognized the crucial need to reach out to young people as a primary part of its AIDS response. Together with the World Organization of the Scout Movement (WOSM), the Action for Youth project was born in 1989.

The long term objectives of the project are:

1. To provide young persons with the skills to increase their awareness of AIDS and to contribute to their communities' fight against AIDS.

2. To give youth leaders skills to incorporate ideas and methods for integrating AIDS-related activities and other health issues into their current programs for youth.

3. To strengthen the cooperation between the World Organization of the Scout Movement, the Red Cross and Red Crescent Societies, and other nongovernmental youth organizations, particularly at the national level.

To reach these objectives, a *training of trainers* approach was developed with a major role played by the target youth. This strategy included writing and distributing a training manual for youth leaders and the mobilization of young people through regional workshops and follow-up support.

Lessons Learned

Follow-up and evaluation missions have been completed in four countries selected from among those involved in the regional workshops. Several lessons already learned can help in our future plans.

world scouting movement is currently in the midst of an international controversy over its official policies of discrimination against homosexuals.

"Anti-AIDS clubs," a different type of nongovernmental AIDS education program organized by adults for young people, are becoming quite widespread in anglophone Africa and are growing in importance in Latin America and parts of the United States. They were first formed in Zambia, organized mostly by missionaries and by teachers in religious schools to discourage discriminatory attitudes to people with HIV and encourage community services on AIDS issues. Their prevention strategy consists of asking young people to take a membership pledge vowing sexual abstinence until marriage and monogamy thereafter. While these clubs have been very successful in attracting large numbers of teens, there has been to date no evaluation of their effectiveness in delaying the age of first sexual intercourse, use of protective barriers, or frequency of intercourse.

---

1. Long-term support is essential when a program is being developed worldwide that is based on peer education.

2. Pretesting and using participatory methods take time and money but improve the possibility that the final product will be used. To involve young people from the beginning has ensured that the manual was understandable, useful, practical, easy to read, and adaptable.

3. Participatory methods used during the workshops increase the confidence, competence, and motivation of participants in all aspects of their youth work.

4. A shift in policy toward the integration of AIDS awareness and health promotion into ongoing youth programs has occurred. AIDS awareness and prevention have also been more fully integrated into youth camps and regularly scheduled youth-leaders' seminars using, for example, focus groups, and plays.

5. With the Action for Youth project, we have learned more about the power of international NGO solidarity.

6. Evaluation and monitoring progress allow us to adjust the content from one workshop to another. Experience from one country forms the basis for the approach in the next. Further evaluation will explore whether there have been ripple effects on the communities studied during the previous evaluation missions.

7. The participatory process activates and sensitizes youth to issues surrounding AIDS and people living with AIDS.

More recently, self-organized youth programs have begun to emerge, both for young people with HIV to provide mutual support and education to their peers, and for young people in general. Two of the first significant efforts in this area were in Mexico and in Ghana, where "Youth for Population Information and Communication" has initiated both peer education and outreach to adults. Self-organized groups of young people have been significant in pressing school authorities for expansion of sexuality education programs and distribution of condoms in schools, as well as in making use of popular cultural vehicles such as rap music and street theater to help build a *safer sex* culture.

Street children, who are among the most at-risk adolescent populations, are difficult to reach. NGOs have initiated several efforts to reach these kids. Two such projects using different approaches are presented as examples in Boxes 9.6 and 9.7. In the first, Street Kids International produced a video and comic book for educating street

---

Box 9.6: Karate Kids: AIDS Education as Empowerment

Street Kids International

Karate Kids is an AIDS prevention education package including a 22-minute karate adventure cartoon video, training book for educators, and Karate Kids pocket comic book. The material was created in 1989 to provide simple, explicit AIDS health education for street youth in the developing world. It is now translated into 14 languages and used by educators in more than 100 countries.

The first challenge was to develop a video that could be used in several different countries. Through research, risk behaviors and values shared by street kids were identified:

- Street children engage in unprotected sex with multiple partners out of economic necessity or for comfort with their peers. Sexual abuse was fairly common.

- Injection drug use is a luxury and generally not affordable (although the situation may be changing in some Asian and Latin American cities). The most common substances abused were glue, gasoline, alcohol, and marijuana.
- Few street kids have access to education or health care; most are illiterate or semiliterate.
- Most survive by informal work as street vendors, scavengers, sex workers, beggars, and thieves.
- The most popular heroes among street kids everywhere are the vigilante movie stars.
- For protection and friendship street kids form youth gangs that have basic values of friendship, survival, and ingenuity.
- There is a basic mistrust of authorities.

Similarities in street culture were incorporated into the script: the

children about HIV and AIDS, its modes of transmission, and use of condoms. The second project conducted by the Brazilian Center for Children and Adolescents describes a program directed toward street girls in Recife, Brazil. Such outreach programs can be effective in encouraging self-esteem and empowerment, and offer education and employment opportunities to their participants.

Future Needs: An extensive review of the HIV/AIDS literature found information about 197 HIV prevention programs for adolescents (see Table 9.3). The most common program goal was raising awareness; the least common was peer support, which is among the most effective approaches to raising awareness and initiating behavior change. Approximately half of the programs reviewed were in North America or in Western Europe, and this is likely to reflect the bias of published and available unpublished reports.

There is still a considerable need to develop programs to reach

---

storyline is about a gang of kids in a market place who learn self-defense from a street leader named Karate, loosely based on the late actor Bruce Lee. One of the boys has unprotected sex with a Smiling Man, and eventually, the boy dies of AIDS. Karate and his girlfriend Rosa teach the kids that AIDS can come from sex and show them how to use a condom. In the context of the adventure story, the cartoon teaches what HIV/AIDS is, how it is sexually transmitted, and how infection can be prevented. The central message is "Protect yourself, protect your friends."

The video was pretested with health experts and street children in Nairobi, Colombo, Manila, Rio de Janeiro, New York City, and Toronto. Health experts identified factual problems, such as the time between infection and AIDS. The street kids were quick to point out inconsistencies in their life-style— children in the cartoon should be

barefoot because street kids don't have shoes. The kids were frustrated that the villain did not die, and they wanted more information about condoms. In response to the question Where does the cartoon take place?, most children said the market place in their own country, thus indicating the viability of the cross-cultural approach.

Systematic outcome evaluation about behavior change is underway but not yet completed. Feedback thus far indicates that the material is most useful in the hands of educators who are comfortable with the subject matter. They are able to stimulate lively discussions of sexual health, street life, and AIDS. The cartoon provokes strong criticism from authorities who do not accept the need for explicit sex education for youth.

Box 9.7: Working with Street Girls in Brazil: A Model for Prevention Education

Compiled from articles by Ana Vasconcelos, Brazilian Center for Children and Adolescents

Brazil is home to an estimated 17 million working and 7 million abandoned street children and youth. Perhaps 30 percent of the street children, many of them African Brazilians, are girls whose lives are characterized by poverty, violence, rape, and exploitation of their labor as domestics or prostitutes. They do not go to school. They are everyday at risk for HIV. And they are especially hard to reach with prevention education.

The Brazilian Center for Children and Adolescents is a nonprofit, nongovernmental organization in Recife, one of Brazil's poorest cities. Its purpose is to defend the individual and social rights of girls—especially those in the streets, brothels, and slums. We have developed two successful, interrelated projects that have made it possible to reach these girls with educational programs both directly and indirectly related to HIV prevention. Halfway House I teaches the girls about their sexuality and their role in society and works to empower them to take control of their lives. The Preventive Program trains teenage girls to work as health agents who reach out to educate and organize their peers.

Halfway House I: Empowerment through Self-Esteem and Behavior Change

Halfway House I is an open educational space available to girls ages 7 to 17. They receive schooling, psychological support, and food and are also referred for health and maternity care. The staff began the program by going into the streets to get in touch with the girls and to experience their reality. We did not go to judge, but to be educated, to understand, and to work out a program policy together. It was not always easy. The girls were suspicious and frightened, and many brought their street ways with them to Halfway House I. The project also came under fire from segments of society that found it hard to accept that we supported the street girls, left them free, and did not subject them to moralizing. We were going against the grain, for Brazil's customary treatment of abandoned children has been to design government policies to protect society against the so-called danger they represent.

It took several attempts to find a way we could all work together. Before they could think about new strategies for survival, the girls had to be given time to recall and then talk about their lives. We had to listen to and respect each girl's story, for only then could she begin to believe in herself. We learned that it was essential for each girl to build self-esteem and assert her self-worth before going on to work on other issues such as sex education.

The atmosphere at Halfway House I is open and nonjudgmental and allows the girls to act outside the passive/submissive role our paternalistic culture has always forced on them. Rules are discussed, decided on, and observed by everyone. The girls discuss their rights and obligations and begin to develop a critical awareness of their society and their role in it. They see that to make changes, they have to act and that when acting, they are no longer passive victims. Such changes are not easy, and confrontations are sometimes dramatic and difficult. Girls leave and return, caught up in self-doubt, until a time comes when they feel able to exercise their basic options.

The Preventive Program: A Model for Health Education in the Streets and Neighborhoods

Graduates of Halfway House I can join other Center programs and work toward generating income and acquiring professional skills. One of these, the Preventive Program, trains them to bring health and sex education to other girls. Its purpose is to avoid that absence of information that, together with sexual abuse and violence, continues to push girls toward the streets and brothels. Sexual abuse and violence within the family are common and often begin a cycle of pregnancy, poverty, attempts at abortion, and perhaps, prostitution. This usually happens against a background of total ignorance, on the part of the girls, of their bodies and

their own sexuality. Caught in the same web, their mothers can provide them with little of the information they so desperately need.

The first program trained 35 girls to provide information on health and sexuality in general and on AIDS and STDs specifically. Despite initial problems and delays, the program has become a model, and UNICEF is documenting its progress. Participants take part in research projects, talk to girls seeking help for specific emotional and health problems, and discuss with their peers such formerly taboo subjects as sexuality, pregnancy, and sexual abuse.

Lots of Talk: Making the Link between Self-Esteem and Health Issues

In both programs, girls spend a lot of time simply talking about their own realities. As they do so, they begin to realize that health depends on how one lives, awareness of rights, housing conditions, opportunities, education, and information. The girls go through a process by which they come to understand both that they are able to transform the reality in which they live and that it is a difficult process. They have learned, and they teach, that they have a right to health.

Table 9.3: Review of 197 HIV/AIDS prevention programs targeted to youth[a]

Item	No. of programs	% of programs
Region		
North America	53	
Western Europe	39	
Africa	53	
Asia	15	
Latin America	20	
Oceania	5	
Other	12	
Total	197	
Age targeted		
Under 18	155	78.7
Over 18	111	56.3
Where targeted		
In school	103	52.3
Out of school	114	57.9
Channels of intervention		
Media	95	48.2
Interpersonal/Peer	55	27.9
Outreach	119	60.4
Goal of intervention		
Awareness	137	69.5
Behavior change	82	41.6
Training of trainers	59	29.9
Peer support	30	15.2
Information for survey	66	33.5

Source: AIDS in the World, 1992.
a. Because of overlap in geographic areas covered and other program features, percentages do not add to 100.

young CSWs (both male and female), street children, and adolescent gay men. While there are a growing number of out-of-school programs, these tend to be pilot or small projects and reach only a small number of street children and out-of-school adolescents. Opportunities exist to reach youth in schools, in the workplace, at STD clinics and prenatal/maternal and child health clinics, and in the street.

Poverty, discrimination, and poor health care have to be addressed if countries are to stem the epidemic in the upcoming generation of adults. Yet discrimination is conspicuously absent as a theme in HIV/AIDS programs for adolescents in government-sponsored programs. The underlying social factors that increase the vulnerability of adolescents to HIV infection should be addressed. Rural development programs that would slow the flow of migration to cities by offering economic opportunity and improved health care may also be an effective HIV prevention strategy. Young people often believe they are not at risk because they associate risk with belonging to a group rather than practicing certain behaviors.

HIV/AIDS and Reproductive Health

The interactions between HIV infection and contraceptive methods, pregnancy, breast feeding, and reproductive tract infections, and between these proximate factors and their socio-cultural determinants (e.g., gender relations, sexuality, and fertility goals) have just begun to be explored. These relationships are central both to country-specific approaches to AIDS prevention and to the achievement of reproductive health goals such as healthy fertility regulation, safe childbearing, and child survival. In many countries, existing reproductive health infrastructures offer one of the most appropriate frameworks for AIDS prevention and research. By sharing expertise and resources, AIDS, family planning, maternal and child health, and other reproductive health initiatives can complement and strengthen each other (see Box 9.8).

The life cycle is marked by key reproductive events—conception, pregnancy, birth, child growth and development, and adolescent and adult sexuality (see Table 9.4).[98] With regard to human reproduction, the predominant routes of HIV transmission are sexual and perinatal. The sexual transmission of HIV and its prevention have been addressed in Chapter 2. Chapter 15 will include a review and analysis of the epidemiological, individual, and societal issues associated with HIV transmission from mother to fetus/infant.

During the past decade, two broad problems have emerged in the interaction between HIV/AIDS and reproductive health programs.

First, it has often been difficult to integrate services for prevention of HIV with existing reproductive health and related services, particularly in family planning and maternal/child health. These difficulties have many sources, including earlier reluctance of some family planning organizations and services to be identified with AIDS. At another level, the need for HIV prevention to deal explicitly with sexuality has created difficulties, as family planning (and STD) programs often worked less, or less successfully, with sexual behavior issues. The difference between pregnancy prevention needs and STD prevention and control objectives also created confusion and occasional conflict: should condoms (known to be relatively less useful than other available methods for pregnancy prevention) be recommended *in addition* to oral or injectable contraceptives? Questions were also raised about the safety of use of different contraceptive technologies by HIV-infected women.

Second, the conceptual framework within which reproductive health services were established also needed to be broadened. For

---

Box 9.8: The AIDS and Reproductive Health Network

Founded in 1988, the AIDS and Reproductive Health Network is a growing multi-disciplinary group of scientists in Africa, the Americas, Asia, and Europe conducting research on AIDS in the context of reproductive health. Through co-equal collaborative exchange, investigators from diverse disciplines and countries seek to strengthen their own and other members' research capacities and products, and to increase the utility of their research for the prevention of AIDS and the promotion of reproductive health.

The network was initiated through the generous support of the John Merck Fund. The Ford Foundation also made a contribution toward the network's capacity-strengthening activities in Africa. The Rockefeller Foundation, the Ford Foundation, the International Development Research Centre (IDRC) of Canada, Family Health International and the American Foundation for AIDS Research, and the John D. and Catherine T. MacArthur Foundation are providing support for research projects conducted through the network. The network's secretariat is located at tne International AIDS Center, Harvard AIDS Institute, Boston, Massachusetts.

Table 9.4: Major life-cycle events, reproductive health, and AIDS problems, and interventions

| Life-cycle event | Problems | | Reproductive health/ AIDS intervention |
	Reproductive health	HIV/AIDS	
Conception	Infertility	Transmission	Family planning Perinatal care
Pregnancy	Malnutrition Anemia		Abortion
Birth	Birth practices Breast feeding	Perinatal transmission	Obstetrics Breast feeding
Childhood	Infections Malnutrition	Transfusion	Child health care
Adolescence	Sexuality STDs	Sexual transmission	Sex education STD control
Adulthood		AIDS infection sarcoma social economic emotional	AIDS response infection control oncology counseling/care
Death			Medical care

Source: L. C. Chen, J. Sepúlveda Amor, and S. J. Segal eds., *AIDS and Women's Reproductive Health* (New York: Plenum, 1992).

example, family planning services were not usually linked with STD control; sexual violence and child sexual abuse were often managed separately from maternal and child health services. A broader framework was clearly required, capable of incorporating STDs (including HIV/AIDS), reproduction (including sterility), sexual violence, and other health problems linked with human sexuality. In turn, the experience with HIV/AIDS prevention and care highlighted once again the critical importance of societal roles and status, particularly those of women. Issues of reproductive rights and access to abortion were central to discussions about AIDS and reproductive health. Finally, the need for this broader framework re-emphasized the fundamental

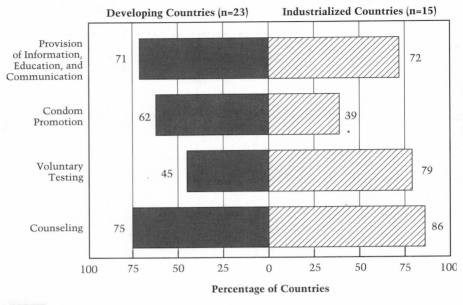

Developing Countries (n=23)   Industrialized Countries (n=15)

Provision of Information, Education, and Communication   71   72

Condom Promotion   62   39.

Voluntary Testing   45   79

Counseling   75   86

100   75   50   25   0   25   50   75   100

Percentage of Countries

Service available in all or all MCH clinics.*

Service rarely or not available in MCH clinics.

Figure 9.11. Prevention services at maternal and child health clinics in 38 countries surveyed.
Source: AIDS in the World, 1992.
*The survey provided an indication of service availability but does not provide a measure of the completeness or quality of services when provided.

lack of knowledge about human sexuality or consensus about public health strategies regarding sexual behavior.

Persons of reproductive age who are confronted with HIV infection need information, education, and counseling in addition to access to voluntary HIV testing, optional pregnancy termination, contraception, and care for women who give birth and for their potentially infected newborns. In populations that are more severely affected by the HIV/AIDS pandemic, maternal and child services are often deficient. In addition, the *AIDS in the World* survey revealed that the integration of HIV prevention in maternal and child health clinics remains minimal (see Figure 9.11). In only about one third of the

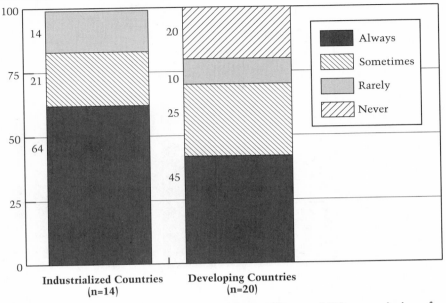

Percentage of Countries with Programs

Figure 9.12. HIV prevention programs about mother-to-child transmission of HIV targeted at teenagers in 34 countries surveyed.
Source: AIDS in the World, 1992.

countries surveyed—both developing and industrialized—was information/education on HIV/AIDS available in maternal and child health clinics. Other approaches, such as condom promotion, voluntary HIV testing, and counseling were available in less than half of the industrialized and developing countries surveyed. Of particular significance was that only 36 percent of industrialized countries reported offering voluntary testing to pregnant women, while an even lower proportion (14 percent) offered pre/post-test counseling on a regular basis. Prevention programs based on information/education and targeted at teenagers were reportedly available in about half of the countries surveyed. In 16 percent of the industrialized countries and 30 percent of the developing ones, these services were rarely, if at all, available (see Figure 9.12).

Upon learning of her infection with HIV, a woman and/or her

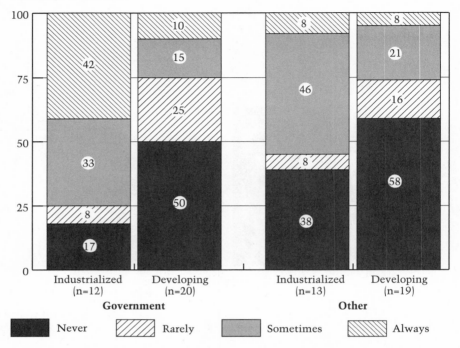

Figure 9.13. Access to abortion in government and other facilities.
Source: AIDS in the World survey, 1992.

partner may be motivated to avoid pregnancy. However, one study based in New York City indicated that when female IDUs in methadone maintenance programs were told they were HIV positive, they were just as likely to conceive as those told they were not HIV infected.[99] Similar results have been reported in other parts of the world. For example, a study in Kinshasa, Zaire, showed that knowledge of serostatus among mothers did not significantly affect the probability of future conceptions.[100]

Women who would wish to terminate their pregnancy are still confronted with societal and legal barriers. The *AIDS in the World* survey showed that abortions were never or seldom offered in government facilities in over three-quarters of the developing countries (see Figure 9.13). In more than one-half of the developing countries sur-

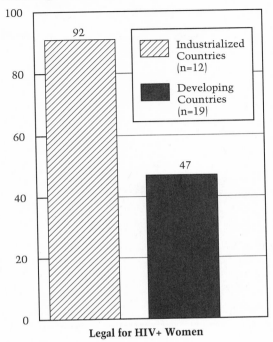

Percentage of Countries

Figure 9.14. Access to legal abortion for women with HIV infection.
Source: AIDS in the World survey, 1992.

veyed, abortion was illegal with no exception in the case of maternal HIV infection (see Figure 9.14). In addition lacking access to abortion services, the level of contraceptive use is lowest in regions with the highest rates of heterosexual transmission of HIV: Africa, Latin America, and Asia (see Table 9.5).

Prevention activities related to HIV and reproductive health should by no means be focused on women alone. Such efforts should also involve men, using the most appropriate communication channels. In certain social and cultural contexts, these channels may rely partly on older members of the community who also require information and education.

The challenges for AIDS and reproductive health involve both efforts to integrate services and strategies on an operational level, as

Table 9.5: World regions according to 1990 population, crude rates of births and deaths, contraceptive prevalence, and HIV-1 infections among adults

Region	Population (millions)	Crude rates per 1,000		Contraceptive prevalence (%)	HIV infections	
		Births	Deaths		No. (thousands)	Rate per 100,000 population
World	5,272	25.7	9.3	45	8,040	152
Industrialized countries	1,210	13.8	9.6	68	1,510	125
Developing countries	4,062	29.2	9.2	38	6,530	161
Africa	653	42.6	12.9	3–40	5,030	770
Asia	3,085	26.0	8.7	15–65	500	16
Latin America	442	26.4	6.8	25–30	1,000	226
North America	279	13.6	8.8	65	1,000	358
Europe	787	14.1	10.2	60–65	480	61
Oceania	26	19.0	8.3	—	30	115

Sources: L. C. Chen, J. Sepúlveda Amor, and S. J. Segal, eds., *AIDS and Women's Reproductive Health* (New York: Plenum, 1992). Population and crude rates: K. C. Zachariah and M. T. Vu, *World Population Projections, Short- and Long-term Estimates* (Washington, D.C.: World Bank, 1988). Contraceptive prevalence: W. P. Mauldin and S. J. Segal, "Prevalence of Contraceptive Use: Trends and Issues," *Studies in Family Planning* 19 (6) (1988):335–53. HIV infections: WHO Global Programme on AIDS, 1988.

well as to confront serious issues of common concern, including the quality and safety of reproductive health services; the lack of innovative sexual behavior research; the lack of women-controlled intravaginal agents which could prevent HIV transmission yet permit pregnancy, if desired; difficulties in discussing sexuality in "traditional" reproductive health settings; and perhaps most critically, reproductive rights and the role and status of women (see Box 9.9).

Commercial Sex Workers

The fact that commercial sex workers (CSWs) have multiple partners has led to the assumption that they would play a major role in the spread of HIV infection to the general population.[101] This simplistic view of CSWs as vectors of disease promotes stereotypes of dangerous women preying on naive clients. Sex work generally responds to client demand; if clients demanded safer sex, then it would become the norm, yet the importance of client education is rarely recognized.

In the *AIDS in the World* survey, less than one third of the 38 national AIDS programs provided estimates of the number of CSWs in their country, and the figures provided appeared rather conservative (see Table 9.6). Despite lack of information on the size of the CSW population, the promotion of condom use for CSWs is now included in almost all country programs. Nevertheless, at the first level of prevention, the challenge remains to develop a demand for safer sex and a consistent and affordable supply of condoms.

For CSWs, like others, the major risk is unprotected sexual intercourse, and this varies widely among CSWs. Yet as a group, CSWs are

---

Box 9.9: Women, AIDS, and Reproductive Issues

Mellous M. Mhloyi,
Population Studies Program,
Department of Sociology,
University of Zimbabwe,
Harare

Five years or even 2 years ago, the idea that AIDS would become an epidemic of women and children would have been met with considerable skepticism. But the epidemiology of the disease is changing. The distribution of infection has shifted heavily toward the developing world and is accompanied by a shift in mode of transmission to heterosexual and vertical. Increasingly, women and children are becoming infected. Awareness is also growing that women are more vulnerable to HIV infection than are men. In part, this is because the direction of sexual spread favors male-to-female transmission. Yet a much more important cause of vulnerability for women are the socioeconomic and cultural contexts in which women live. Without equal status, they have no decision-making power on issues that determine their health and welfare, the welfare of their children, and the relationships in which they are sexual partners.

The Context of Vulnerability: Sexuality and Socialization

The disadvantages that impoverish women socially and economically and put them at increased risk starting in early childhood are an inextricable part of the socialization process. Especially in developing countries, societies foster and nurture an inferiority complex in women. Discrimination begins in infancy in those Asian countries where son preference is most pronounced. In Latin America and Africa, where son preference also exists, discrimination begins when schooling starts. Having little or no education means that women participate in the labor force at

much more likely to use condoms than women in the general population.[102]

Commercial sex workers have a high level of awareness of AIDS (see Table 9.1). Given the transient nature of commercial sex work in most communities, however, there is a constant need for information about modes of transmission and safer sex. Street workers and those in brothels form friendships, and there have been some instances where these groups have provided the peer support and "house rules" to assure safer sexual behavior. This is less likely to happen among outcalls and escort services where the CSW acts more independently and in an isolated environment.

In general, commercial sex work is a direct result of economic pressures. Studies comparing other low skill vocations with commercial sex work have generally found that the pay is often much higher for the latter.[103] When CSWs rely on the client for money to pay for food, housing, or drugs, they are not in a position to be adamant about

---

low levels. Coupled with their lack of property rights, this makes them economically dependent on men, further undermining their power to make decisions about their lives and health.

How women are socialized about their sexuality also increases their vulnerability to HIV. Generally, women are socialized to please men sexually, but not to express their own sexuality overtly. They are also expected to link sex with fertility. All of this nurtures a silent norm regarding sexuality issues; breaking the silence involves risks because it means challenging the social constructs that give men control. For most women, breaking the silence in an attempt to initiate safer sex may result in rejection.

Yet most men do not want to use the condom. Even for parents who know that they are HIV infected, many factors combine to reduce the

likelihood of contraception use in limiting vertical transmission: the high value placed on children; social and religious attitudes; son preference in Asia, and desire for large families in much of Africa and to some extent, in Latin America. The option of abortion is not only a difficult choice to make, but also rarely available.

The Circumstances of Vertical Transmission: Asking the Questions that Need to be Asked

Increasingly, prevention strategies will need to take into account central issues around reproduction—an area where a great deal of research still needs to be done. Given the context of vulnerability in which women and children live, what issues need to be investigated in order to facilitate change?

In the long run, we need to look toward empowering women and girls

demanding safe sex.[104] In some countries such as the United States or Australia, drug use is often associated with commercial sex work.[105] In those communities where commercial sex work and drug use overlap, there exists an additional risk of HIV transmission (see Box 9.10).

Thus far, the male sex worker has not been targeted extensively for HIV prevention. There may be an assumption that male sex workers are members of the gay community, but research indicates that, as in female sex work, there are many subcultures within male sex work. Those who are more isolated from the gay community and more in need of money, are at greater risk of HIV infection.

Interventions with sex workers have led to increased knowledge and behavior changes including safer sex, mostly the adoption of condom use. As shown earlier in Table 9.1, the level of information is generally high among CSWs despite the highly transient nature of many CSW populations.[106]

Figure 9.15 indicates that two approaches to HIV prevention among CSWs—condom use and periodic voluntary visits to STD clin-

---

so that they have more control over their own lives. This begins with asking what strategies can be used to educate about the importance of treating children of both sexes equally. In the shorter term, the question is how, given their low status, can women prevent infection? We need to understand more about women's actual sexual practices and patterns within their cultures. How motivated are they to actually practice safe sex? How often and under what circumstances do they demand condom use, and what is their partner's reaction? How, most basically, can open communication on sexuality be fostered between partners?

We also need to know more about how HIV-seropositive women relate to childbearing. Are they willing to forego having children? Will they be able to exercise that choice? In some countries, 10 to 20 percent of pregnant women are HIV infected, yet how many knew their status before conceiving? To what extent are they willing to abort? Are facilities readily available to them? If not, how can governments be convinced of this urgent need?

Restructuring the Social System

Despite the many unanswered questions, it is clear that if their situation is to improve, women need social and economic empowerment. If behavioral changes are to be effected and sustained, the socioeconomic and cultural contexts must change so that they support the choices individuals make. Because the objective is to reorder social systems, men—who are in control of such systems—also need empowerment.

Table 9.6: Female-male commercial sex workers (CSWs), estimated by government AIDS programs

Geographic Area of Affinity/Country	Estimated no.	Proportion	
		Women	Men
North America	NA	NA	NA
Western Europe			
Netherlands	20,000	95	5
France	17,500	90	10
Sweden	700	99	1
Oceania	NA	NA	NA
Latin America			
Colombia	NA	90	10
Sub-Saharan Africa			
Ethiopia	NA	100	0
Uganda	NA	100	0
Tanzania	20,000	100	0
Nigeria	NA	95	5
Zambia	NA	100	0
Cameroon	NA	100	0
Congo	2,000	100	0
Senegal	80,000	95	5
Caribbean			
Trinidad/Tobago	600	99	1
Haiti	700[a]	NA	NA
Eastern Europe			
Czech Republic	75,000	85	15
South East Mediterranean			
Egypt	500[a]	95	5
North East Asia			
China	NA	100	0
Southeast Asia			
Thailand	150,000	95	5
India	1,000,000	NA	NA

Source: AIDS in the World survey, 1992.
a. Significant underestimation assumed.

Box 9.10: Trading Sex for Drugs

dy Fullilove, HIV Center, York

In the early 1980s, drug dealers in the United States developed a new method for processing and consuming cocaine. Crack—which refers to the sound that is made as the drug is being "cooked"—is a short-acting, highly addictive, smokeable form of cocaine. Crack produces an intense high that lasts for approximately twenty minutes. The crash from this high is so painful that users will go to extreme lengths in order to maintain the state of euphoria and avoid the crash. This cycle of getting high, crashing, and then getting high again can easily degenerate into a binge that can last for many days. The end typically comes when the user cannot obtain more crack or when exhaustion sets in.

Efforts to market the new product began in a few U.S. cities and spread across the country during the latter part of the 1980s. The marketing and distribution of crack have been remarkable. Initially, the drug was targeted to women as the ultimate feel-good drug and targeted to men as a potent aphrodisiac. Because it is rapidly addictive, many casual consumers became steady customers. The combination of crack's addictive properties coupled with efforts to market the drug as a sexual aid provided the perfect stage for a new form of prostitution. Many crack-addicted women discovered that as long as they were willing to offer sex in exchange for crack, there would be more than enough male customers.

This sex-for-drugs barter, which has become a standard part of the crack scene in places like New York City, involves performing some sexual act for either crack or money. The specific act and the amount of drug/cash involved in the transaction are both negotiable. Because the addict is often desperate, however, a very unfavorable exchange—both in terms

of money and safety/desirability of the sexual act—may take place. Consequently, even when money is offered in the exchange, it is typically only enough to permit the user to step to that next high.

Interestingly enough, this barter economy is extremely sensitive to the user's need to obtain the wherewithal to purchase the next hit. Observers have reported that a shrewd negotiator will pay only enough money to buy a prospective partner's next vial. In the grip of so powerful an addiction, the ability to set limits or to say no is rapidly lost.

Women in the sex industry who are paid for their services, and who are able to work in stable, protective environments, appear to have the best chance for protecting their health and personal safety. Women engaged in sex-for-drugs exchanges, by contrast, may get as little as one high per sexual contact. Because a crack binge is composed of many highs, women on a binge may repeatedly engage in the sex-for-drugs exchange without regard to personal safety.

Sex-for-drugs exchanges place both partners at high risk for sexually transmitted disease. Increases in syphilis and gonorrhea have accompanied the crack epidemic throughout the United States. Crack use has also begun to emerge as a risk factor for HIV infection through the practice of exchanging sex-for-drugs. Because the risk behavior is closely linked to addiction, the treatment of the addictive disorder must be the primary focus of prevention efforts. Yet treatment for crack addiction must remain cognizant of the sexual trauma that some women have undergone as a result of their addiction. Treatment strategies must link recovery from addiction with recovery from past trauma as well as to the establishment of safer sexual practices.

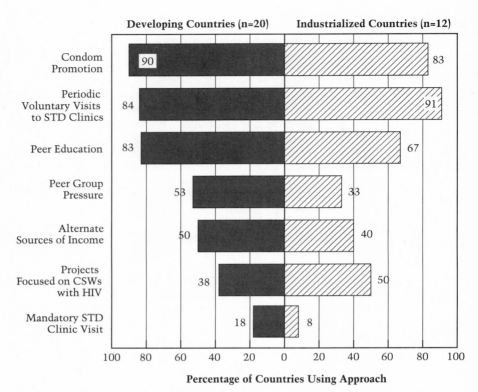

Developing Countries (n=20)　　　**Industrialized Countries (n=12)**

Condom Promotion: 90 | 83
Periodic Voluntary Visits to STD Clinics: 84 | 91
Peer Education: 83 | 67
Peer Group Pressure: 53 | 33
Alternate Sources of Income: 50 | 40
Projects Focused on CSWs with HIV: 38 | 50
Mandatory STD Clinic Visit: 18 | 8

100 80 60 40 20 0 20 40 60 80 100

Percentage of Countries Using Approach

Figure 9.15. Approaches used for HIV/AIDS prevention among commercial sex workers, 1992.
Source: AIDS in the World, 1992.

ics—are used by over 80 percent and 90 percent in both industrialized and developing countries in the *AIDS in the World* survey. Condom use is a major message to CSWs in all countries in the survey (see Figure 9.16). Testing was emphasized twice as much in industrialized countries compared with developing countries. Programs to help find alternative sources of income were more commonly reported in developing countries.

Focusing on CSWs without educating their clients overlooks the unequal balance of power, as clients who demand unsafe sex also control the marketplace. One indicator of the lack of success in edu-

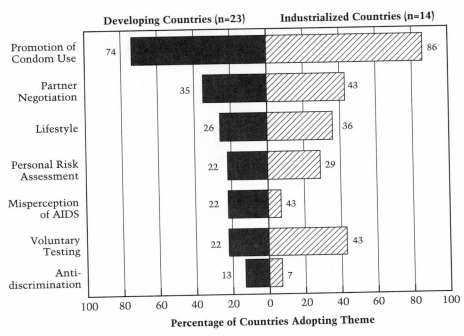

Figure 9.16. Themes of prevention targeted to commercial sex workers, 37 countries, 1992.
Source: AIDS in the World, 1992.

cating clients is that in many countries, clients are willing to pay more for unprotected sex.[107] In a recent review conducted by WHO, between a fifth and a third of CSW programs targeted both the sex worker and their clients, yet few targeted male sex workers and even fewer programs targeted sex workers' business managers, despite the important role they play in defining the sexual practices of commercial sex workers (see Table 9.7).

Box 9.11 highlights a program in the Cross River State of Nigeria, illustrating how an integrated approach can increase awareness of risk and use of condoms among female CSWs.

Future Needs: The world of commercial sex work is highly diverse, which directly impacts the design and implementation of HIV prevention programs.

Table 9.7: A review of programs targeted at commecial sex workers (CSWs) and/or clients[a]

Program	Region		
	Africa	*Americas*	*Asia*
Target audiences			
Female sex workers	31	23	18
Male sex workers	1	6	4
Female and male sex workers	1	4	3
Sex workers only	19	20	11
Sex workers and clients	12	5	6
Clients only	5	—	—
Sex workers, clients, and business managers	5	2	3
Project characteristics			
Projects using peer education	11	11	8
Average number of peer educators	104 (7)[b]	45 (3)	845 (2)
Projects providing STD services	5	3	4
Projected reach			
Under 2,000 sex workers	14 (18)	13 (15)	3 (5)
2,000–10,000 sex workers	4 (18)	2 (15)	2 (5)
Under 2,000 clients	2 (8)	—	1 (1)
2,000–10,000 clients	6 (8)	2 (2)	—

Source: WHO Global Programme on AIDS.

a. The number of countries and number of projects identified per region are as follows: Africa 20 countries/36 projects; the Americas, 12 countries/26 projects; Asia, 6 countries/ 21 projects.

b. Parentheses indicate number of projects reporting data.

The challenge is to understand these diverse systems and work within them to support HIV prevention by using peer support, persuading owners and managers of establishments to support safer sex, and educating clients. Misperceptions that continue in any community should be actively identified and addressed, such as the frequently mentioned misperception that "regular" partners are safer than clients.

Most programs addressing CSWs are actually projects (often pilot projects) and are small in size, reaching relatively few CSWs. As a result, there are now useful prototypes of many types of programs, but these have yet to be widely implemented. Despite growing consensus that peers make more credible educators than outsiders, CSWs are still not involved widely enough in design and implementation of prevention programs.

Although condoms are the most frequently recommended prevention measure, demand exceeds supply in many areas. Assuring a consistent supply of condoms must be a high priority. Furthermore, the acceptability of testing and counseling in prevention is highly contingent on the assured anonymity and/or confidentiality of testing results, plus the availability of counseling and care for infected persons. Without appropriate prevention services and alternative employment for HIV-infected CSWs, testing services will have little impact, while mandatory testing programs will be counterproductive.

The development of sustainable programs to prevent HIV infection among CSWs requires an understanding of the subculture and involvement of CSWs in the design and implementation of the program. Ultimately, issues of commercial sex work in the context of AIDS will best be addressed by dealing with the larger issues of gender discrimination and inequality.

Homosexual Practices

Much of the information reported about the behavior change related to HIV originates from studies done in gay communities. The decline in HIV incidence among cohorts of gay men in the United States and Europe has often been cited as one of the most rapid and extensive changes in human behavior ever observed.[108] Ample evidence indicates that prevention efforts slowed the progression of HIV in gay communities and that many men adopted safer sex practices to avoid HIV infection.

There is some evidence of risk of transmission among women practicing unprotected woman-to-woman sex.[109] However, as most of the available data on same-sex behavior concentrates on male-to-male behavior, this section highlights findings from this group.

To date, most data on the incidence of HIV among gay men involves well-established urban gay communities in North America, Western and Northern Europe, and to a lesser extent, in Mexico and Brazil. Important cohort studies of gay men over the past ten years have provided a unique historical view of the epidemic. In many urban gay communities, there has been a dramatic decline in HIV incidence as documented in Chapter 2. Less information exists about HIV sero-

---

Box 9.11: Implementation of an AIDS Prevention Program among Prostitutes in the Cross River State of Nigeria

Eka Esu-Williams, Society for Women and AIDS in Africa (SWAA)

The Cross River State of Nigeria (estimated population 3,000,000) borders the Republic of Cameroon. HIV infection was first identified in the state in 1987, with the first AIDS patients seen in 1989. Data from 1985 to 1989 indicate an HIV seroprevalence of 0.2 percent in the general population. There was a reported 1 percent seroprevalence among women practicing prostitution tested in 1989 and 1.5 percent in male clients and partners of prostitutes tested in the same year.[a] This project initiated a targeted intervention program to serve 19 sites in the sea port of Calabar, and 5 sites in the border town of Ikom. Activities included peer-based health education, condom promotion/distribution, and a sexually transmitted disease (STD) treatment clinic.

Preprogram studies in Cross River State revealed a community of full-time prostitutes who live and work in highly structured hotel and housing settings where the proprietor/owners and hotel managers have substantial influence. Each setting has a prostitute leadership structure consisting of a chairlady who sets rules, a deputy chairlady who relays the rules to the prostitutes, and a policing agent who enforces the rules. The chairladies and deputy chairladies were trained and given the designation of peer leaders; they looked after the logistics of condom availability and related information on the importance of condom use.

During the one-year period between September 1989 and September 1990, more than 1,000 clients and other sex partners and 450 prostitutes were reached in the 19 Calabar sites. In Ikom, 700 full-time prostitutes and more than 1,500 clients and other sex partners were reached. The number of condoms distributed to all sites during this one year period ranged from

prevalence among bisexual men. However, a number of studies among STD clinic patients show lower HIV prevalence among bisexual than self-identified homosexual men.

Large-scale behavior change occurred first in 1981 in San Francisco and New York City, and by 1984, reached Western Europe. The different patterns of HIV incidence rise and decline suggest different levels of adopting and maintaining safer sex. For example, countries like the Netherlands and France had an early decline in incidence and then a plateau, suggesting both a continued level of unprotected anal intercourse and, probably, a relatively open sexual network. In all cities, studies confirm that safer sex is far from universal, with a large variation among groups in the same country, across geographic boundaries and in different cultural settings.

4,000 to 58,000 monthly. While condom acceptance was high, supply difficulties accounted for a substantial range in condoms distributed. Among 102 prostitutes surveyed, 66.7 percent stated they had used a condom during their most recent sexual intercourse; 99.5 percent of those using condoms took the initiative in suggesting their use, and 100 percent of the prostitutes using condoms supplied the condoms to their clients/partners.

While program flexibility allowed for a pragmatic approach to peer education which was effective in reaching full-time prostitutes and their partners, a similar structure does not exist among part-time prostitutes and their clients. Video showings and condom and leaflet distribution have been supported by trained hotel proprietors/owners and managers. This wider exposure may have an impact on part-time prostitutes: it has been suggested that those with discretionary control in bar, night club, and hotel settings may play a pivotal role in health interventions in areas of Africa where there is little discernible organization or leadership among prostitutes.

This program has taken a proactive position of serving as an advocate to prostitutes in situations of harassment. This has been helpful in building trust with the target population. Concurrently, official support for program activities was solicited and received from the Cross River State Ministry of Health and the Cross River State AIDS Committee. In addition to the implied message of concern this relays to the target community, such official approval may stifle harassment from the police and others.

---

a. E. Williams, N. Hearst, O. Udofia, et al. HIV infection and prostitutes in Nigeria. Presented at the VI International Conference on AIDS and Associated Cancers in Africa, Marseille, France, October 1989; E. Williams, N. Hearst, and O. Udofia. Sexual practices and HIV infection of female prostitutes in Nigeria. Presented at the V International Conference on AIDS, Montreal, Canada, June 1989.

In gay communities in which HIV incidence declined, behavior changes included reduction of the number of partners, condom use, refraining from anal sex, and abstinence. Bisexuals in North America and Europe may also have adopted safer sex practices,[110] but changes among gay men have been more extensive and more consistent.[111,112] Among all groups, unsafe sex is practiced most often with regular partners, and for bisexuals, several studies show that unprotected sex is more likely with female partners than male partners.[113]

A troubling observation is the recent increase in HIV incidence indicating a tendency to return to unsafe sex; this appears to reflect the difficulty for those who have changed to safer sex of maintaining their safe behavior. A further explanation is the less frequent adoption and maintenance of safer sex among young gay men, some of whom mistakenly believe that the AIDS epidemic is no longer a threat to the gay community.[114]

Recent studies among homosexual men in Thailand suggest that established gay communities have begun to adopt safer sex practices.[115] Nevertheless, the observed *success stories* may not be widely generalized. In countries like India and those in Eastern Europe,[116,117] where the epidemic is in the early stages, and in countries where there are few resources for prevention and services, such as in Latin America or North Africa, HIV incidence among men who practice homosexual behavior is most likely increasing. The ability of these gay communities to take a proactive stance is low as they usually have few funds, little organization, and no formal recognition.

Prevention Activities: The rapid spread of HIV and subsequent drop in infection rates in certain gay communities can best be explained by the fairly closed sexual network within these communities. This enabled the infection to spread rapidly, but at the same time, to be recognized early, and for the communities to utilize established channels in its response. Building on the growing movement to prevent the epidemic of STDs, the gay community sent out early warnings about AIDS through existing newspapers and newly formed organizations; in San Francisco, the first AIDS brochure was distributed in 1981.

In almost every instance, prevention programs in gay communities started before official government programs. In many communities, the threat of HIV was recognized by a small group of men, who then started or expanded small NGOs that have, in many instances, been transformed subsequently into the major nongovernmental HIV/AIDS prevention and care organizations. Among these are the Swiss AIDS Foundation, the Terrence Higgins Trust in England, the Bobby Goldsmith foundation in Australia, the Gay Men's Health Crisis in New York City, the San Francisco AIDS Foundation, and COC in the Netherlands.[118] In England and the United States, these groups designed and circulated early brochures and supplied condoms; gay newspapers provided a constant flow of medical and prevention information to the communities.

Approaches differed early in the epidemic. For example, condoms became the central focus of the Swiss group, including design, manufacture and distribution of their own brand of condoms. Information was the main focus of the Dutch group which targeted many visitors and distributed information in venues such as saunas, bars, and theaters. Some gay communities, however, feared stigmatization and discrimination, which inhibited targeted prevention. Gay organizations in France, for example, felt that specific programs targeted toward gay men would be stigmatizing and that the overall impact would be negative.[119]

In most communities, the first response to those promoting behavior change was to see them as naive collaborators with an *enemy* who was using AIDS as an excuse to reverse hard-won sexual freedoms.[120–122] Denial was facilitated in the mid-1980s by the fact that only a few men were seriously ill or had died of AIDS. Through 1987, researchers were providing optimistic estimates that only a portion of those with the virus would progress to AIDS, and only some of those would die.

Even though the gay community was divided regarding the threat of HIV, many men did take precautions. As the risk factors became clearer, as AIDS became more visible, and as death rates climbed, more men changed to, and others maintained, safer sex. Some, however, did not, including many of those living in more rural areas and who were not part of a gay community.

In response to a perceived need for additional information, a wider network of information was developed to reach more isolated gay and bisexual men, using outreach at "beats," in parks, car parks, and public toilets.[123] Telephone hotlines were created to provide anonymous information to gay men, and as the epidemic progressed, to bisexuals, heterosexuals, and IDUs.

Health professionals and many gay men believed that knowledge of serostatus would lead to the adoption of safer sexual behaviors. Yet the effect of knowing one's HIV serostatus has been found to be inconsistent.

Given an unclear impact on prevention, combined with evidence that knowledge of seropositive status led to depression and a continued fear of discrimination in housing and employment, most gay communities did not recommend testing or remained neutral on the subject. Only in the past two years, as the possibilities for early treatment increased, have some gay groups in Europe and North America started to promote testing, usually in unlinked, anonymous systems.

As in other populations, awareness of modes of transmission and safer sexual practices was not sufficient motivation for behavior change among gay men. For example, while awareness about condoms was high, many gay men had negative attitudes about condom use and did not use them. Others held a variety of misperceptions that allowed them to rationalize lower HIV risk for themselves.[124] The creation of erotic material using condoms was a response to these negative attitudes; the idea being to make safer sex sexy.[125] Yet even with positive attitudes and correct information about risk, numerous studies have suggested that information reaches a level of saturation and that other emotional needs and situational factors may be more important.[126]

Recently, programs seeking to strengthen partner support and provide an opportunity to increase a sense of self-efficacy have helped many gay men to adopt safer practices. Skill enhancement exercises such as partner negotiation and safer sex workshops have been designed to provide skills and social support using small group discussions and role playing. Experience in the STOP AIDS project in San Francisco (which reached over one quarter of the gay men in San Francisco) and in the safer sex workshops in New York, Amsterdam, and Zurich has reinforced the value of these personalized approaches.[127–129]

Peer and community support has been essential for adopting and maintaining safer sex among gay men. One of the major achievements

Percentage of Countries Adopting Theme

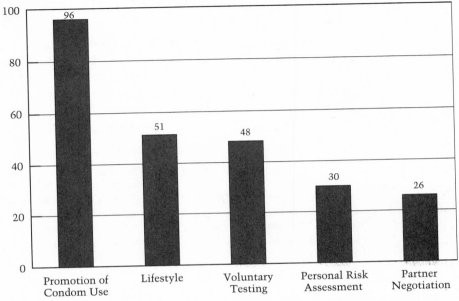

Figure 9.17. Themes of prevention targeted to homosexual/bisexual men in 27 selected countries, 1992.
Source: AIDS in the World, 1992.

of community-based and AIDS service organizations, in addition to providing services, was the creation of new social networks in which safer sexual activity became the norm.

Current Prevention Programs and Future Needs: The types of messages targeted to gay and bisexual men in the *AIDS in the World* survey countries were fairly consistent. Of 38 countries, 27 reported targeting prevention programs to homosexual/bisexual males, including all countries in North America, Western Europe, Latin America, and the Caribbean. All except Egypt said their main message to this population included use of condoms and practicing safer sex. As shown in Figure 9.17, about half of the countries promoted testing and being cautious, around 30 percent had messages about how to assess personal risk, and one quarter promoted partner negotiation.

Relatively few prevention activities have been evaluated. However, the overall success of prevention programs in gay communities has as much to do with broad coverage as with the effectiveness of any single campaign. Most communities have had a variety of targeted posters and brochures, videos, and broad-based coverage in the gay media. Those programs offering a wider variety of components for different gay and bisexual populations were more likely to succeed than those relying on a single approach.

The next challenges include the application of strategies in coun-

---

Box 9.12: Dehomosexualization

Dennis Altman, Australian Federation of AIDS Organizations

It is not an accident that AIDS was first recognized among U.S. gay men; while HIV-related illness almost certainly existed before 1981 in Central Africa and possibly among other groups in the United States, the perception and naming of the syndrome required access to the sophisticated medical technology of a developed medical system. This led in turn to the first term given to AIDS, that is, gay-related immune deficiency. For much of the 1980s, AIDS was defined, at least in Western countries, as a homosexual disease (or, as the headlines put it, "the gay plague").

As it became increasingly clear that this was inaccurate and that HIV was widely spread, both regionally and among diverse populations, there were moves from both the gay movement and the health profession to destigmatize AIDS by downplaying the gay link. Even though homosexual men were often the group most affected—in much of the developed world, but also in some areas of the developing world, such as parts of South America and Southeast Asia—there was great stress on the

idea that AIDS threatened everyone equally, and a corresponding reluctance to speak openly of the devastation being caused to the gay community. In many countries, this has meant insufficient resources available to provide education, support, and services to homosexual men.

With only a few exceptions, governments were unwilling to support AIDS organizations that were openly gay-identified, and WHO provided much less support for gay-related support and research than for other groups considered at risk. Despite its origins in the gay community, the Terrence Higgins Trust in Britain has for a long time been ambivalent about acknowledging the extent of its gay constituency, in part because of perceived pressures from the government. Often AIDS organizations themselves, even when their primary constituency was gay men, sought very hard to position themselves as representing the general community. Considerable political pressure was placed on a number of community organizations to de-emphasize their gay identity, even where homosexuals remained by far the largest group who were infected and in need of services.

tries where HIV is expanding among gay and bisexual men and where governments are still reluctant to acknowledge the existence of gay communities or their need for support and resources (see Box 9.12). In long-affected communities, there is a need to maintain safer sex for those who have changed and a need to inform younger gay men that they are vulnerable to HIV. For men who are difficult to reach, interpersonal programs are likely to be the most effective. Among partners, programs should be designed for those who are in steady relationships. Furthermore, strategies have to be developed that will

---

One consequence of this has been lack of recognition and support for gay communities in all but a few countries, even where they have provided the basis for AIDS organizing. Yet the AIDS epidemic has seen an upsurge of organizing among gay men—sometimes alongside lesbians—who have often taken the lead in developing wider programs for AIDS awareness, prevention, and care. This is true not only in Northern Europe, North America, and Australasia, but also in developing countries, such as Malaysia and Mexico. In others, such as Zimbabwe, local gay communities were among the major supporters of HIV organizations.

In the developed world, AIDS has contributed to the increasing militancy and visibility of the lesbian/gay movement; certainly, the spectacular rise of ACT-UP in the United States was in part fueled by anger at the denial of the special stake of the gay community in the epidemic. In many areas of the developing world, AIDS has provided the impetus and the urgency to develop a gay movement. Yet official reluctance to recognize this remains strong and has led to AIDS organizations in such countries as Canada and Australia having to restate very strongly the need for governments to recognize the implications of HIV epidemiology in their particular societies.

Although the great bulk of HIV infection is increasingly due to heterosexual spread in the developing world, it is important to remember that programs that ignore the existence of significant homosexual populations are less likely to succeed. The firsthand testimony of organizers and educators in countries, such as Brazil, Thailand, and India, attests to the fact that homosexual worlds exist, that they are by no means confined to the demands of Western sex tourists, and that official denial and prejudice contribute to the spread of HIV and to ugly discrimination against those infected and affected. The belief that all gay men are rich, white, and define themselves as members of gay communities is one of the more dangerous myths contributing to the growth of the epidemic.

allow minimum risk for unprotected sex within a long-term relationship. These strategies recognize a need for intimacy that is often given as a reason for unsafe sex with regular partners.

Providing condoms and information at venues where men have sex with men could be greatly improved. Owners and managers of commercial establishments such as massage parlors, saunas, bars, and other commercial establishments should be encouraged to provide affordable, high quality condoms and HIV prevention information. Where commercial sex work occurs, managers and sex workers could more forcefully insist on condom use.

Reaching bisexual men will remain difficult. Pilot projects for bisexual men who practice homosexual activities at venues such as parking areas along highways and parks have been targeted by outreach workers and could be expanded. New approaches to reaching bisexual men have to be created.

A major obstacle to HIV prevention is the negative legal status of homosexuality. The lack of legal recognition of gay rights inhibits the distribution of condoms and HIV prevention programs. If homosexual behavior between consenting adults continues to be a source of discrimination, substantial structural and psychological barriers will remain for prevention activities.

■■■■■ · · ·

CONDOMS

This chapter has until now examined elements of HIV prevention programs as they apply to various target populations. Among the strategies that cut across these programs and populations is the consistent use of quality condoms to prevent sexual transmission of HIV (see Table 9.8). As a widely implemented prevention strategy, condom use exemplifies the empowerment of individuals and interaction between people who want to protect themselves and others against HIV infection; the supportive or adversarial role played by the societal environment; and the effectiveness of programs designed to raise awareness, create demand, facilitate access to an affordable and sustained source of supplies, and ensure the availability of quality products.

There is a global trend of increased demand for condoms, the

Table 9.8: Effectiveness of condoms in AIDS prevention[a]

Country	Group studied	Seroconversion nonusers	Seroconversion condom users	Time (months)
Greece[130]	Sex workers	12/350 3.43%	2/270 0.74%	12
Kenya[131]	Sex workers	20/28 71.43%	23/50 46%	
Tanzania[132]	Public house workers	10%	22%	12
United States[133]	Homosexual/ bisexual men	97/4083 2.38%	7/977 0.72%	24
United States[134]	Discordant couples	12/14 85.71%	1/10 10%	12–36

a. References for this table, indicated in superscript numbers, are in the Reference Notes for Chapter 9.

development of an improved worldwide logistic system to assure delivery without lapses in supply, and the expansion of markets to CSWs, homosexual and bisexual men, sexually active adolescents, and married men and women. Almost never mentioned by health officials 10 years ago, today nearly all *AIDS in the World* survey countries include condoms as a part of their HIV prevention program. Although there are many variations, the basic message is that consistent condom use during vaginal or anal sex with partners of unknown or HIV-positive serostatus is necessary. However, condom use does not necessarily accompany increased awareness (see Table 9.9).

Factors Related to Condom Use

Many studies show that *attitudes* toward condoms are strongly related to use.[145–148] Condom use is also linked to *beliefs* about the efficacy of condoms as a barrier to HIV infection.[149,150] Those who misunderstand the latency between HIV infection and AIDS, and people who have had experiences with condoms of poor quality are more likely to believe that condoms are an ineffective barrier to HIV infection. The complexity of the interaction between attitudes and experience was shown in a village in northern Tanzania, where people

Table 9.9: Condom use pre- and post-intervention in selected countries[a]

Population/Study	Condom use			Intervention used

General population
deVries et al.[135]
Netherlands
1989
Telephone survey (N = 6,000)

Use in last 6 months

	Pre	Post
Study sample	20	31
Nonstable partners	30	83
Ages 15–25	10	50

Intention to use condoms in future

	Pre	Post
Study sample	23	33
Nonstable partners	65	79
Ages 15–25	34	54

Mass media campaign

Tipping[136]
Somarc, Morocco
1990
Males
General survey

Use after 1 year of campaign

Baseline 1988	Current use
5	24

Mass media, public relations, trade promotion

Hassig, AIDSTECH[137]
Africa, Latin America
Males

Reported condom use with follow-up

	Pre	Post
Cameroon	N = 200	N = 200
Ever used	55	75
Recent use	45	65
Zimbabwe	N = 75	N = 58
Recent use	39	47
Used always	21	36
Tanzania	N = 449	N = 198
Ever used	49	95
Used always	11	40

Peer education
Condom distribution

Adolescents
Rotheram-Borus et al.[138]
New York City, U.S.
1988 1990
Publicly funded shelters for runaways (N = 78, 67)

General knowledge about HIV/AIDS, coping skills, access to health care and other resources, and individual barriers to safer sex

Consistent use

	Nonintervention	Intervention
	22	25

By number of interventions

	3 mos.	6 mos.
0–2	33	11
3–9	3	18
10–14	40	20
15–30	57	63

Gay/Bisexual
Valdiserri et al.[139]
Pittsburgh, U.S.
1986–87
Pitt Men's Study (N = 265, 319)

I. Small group lecture only
II. Small group lecture and skills training

No. of sex partners per practice in past 6 months

Sexual practice	Baseline		First follow up		Second follow up	
	I	II	I	II	I	II
Insertive anal	1.8	1.4	1.4	1.3	0.9	1.0
Receptive anal	1.6	1.5	1.1	0.9	0.7	0.5
Condom w/insertive	0.8	0.5	0.6	0.9	0.5	0.8
Condom w/receptive	0.8	0.4	0.6	0.5	0.4	0.7
Mutual masturbation	4.1	4.2	3.0	3.5	2.9	3.6
Insertive oral	5.7	4.5	3.9	3.4	3.3	3.8
Receptive oral	6.3	4.8	4.2	3.3	3.8	3.3

Kelly et al.[140]
Mississippi/Louisiana
1989
Gay bars (N = 659)

Peer leaders employed to endorse change

No. of partners

	Intervention city		Comparison city	
	Pre	Post	Pre	Post
0	70	80	69	71
1	7	5	8	8
2	4	3	4	4
3	2	1	4	3
4	2	1	7	7
5	3	0.9	3	4

Table 9.9 (cont.): Condom use pre- and post-intervention in selected countries[a]

Population/Study	Condom use	Intervention used
Drug users	*Intended condom use*	Education sessions
Dengelegi, Weber, Torquato[141] New York City, U.S. 1988 Detoxification facility (N = 100)	Pre (N = 100) Post (N = 67) 21 51	
Friedman et al.[142] Brooklyn, New York 1990 A section of Brooklyn (N = 600)	*Reported condom use* Pre Post* 23 33 * 6 mo. follow-up	Former IDUs as outreach workers used to form community
Commercial sex workers Hassig, AIDSTECH[143] Africa, Latin America	*Reported condom use with follow-up*	Peer education, condom distribution

	Pre Post
	Cameroon N = 100 N = 100
	   Ever used 83 90
	   Recent use 63 90
	Zimbabwe N = 40 N = 50
	   Recent use 18 72
	Tanzania N = 311 N = 122
	   Ever used 52 77
	Mexico N = 195 N = 207
	   Recent use 68 91	

Fox, et al.[144] Honduras 1988 Clinic N = 130	*Reported condom use/10-week interval* Pre Post 19 31[b]	Lectures on STDs and AIDS information, condom distribution

Note: Pre = pre-intervention; Post = post-intervention.
a. References for the table, indicated in superscript number, are in the Reference Notes to Chapter 9.
b. Ninety percent of women used condoms when available free of charge.

who felt at risk of HIV infection were the first to use condoms. This self-selected group was also among the first to be diagnosed with AIDS—most resulting from infections which occurred long before they started using condoms—and some linked getting AIDS to their adoption of condoms.

Attitudes and beliefs are closely related: negative attitudes about condoms lead to the belief that they are not effective, and the belief that condoms are not effective leads to negative attitudes about their use. For example, in Bangladesh, breakage was cited as the most common problem in condom use, and women complained far more than men of burning sensations and allergic conditions. These complaints are likely to have been due to deterioration in the condoms because of poor storage,[151] and to lubrication which may irritate the vagina. But the overall effect was a dislike for condoms as well as a belief that they were not effective.

Strong psychological factors often compete with awareness of AIDS risk. For example, love was often given as a reason for not using condoms, as they were perceived to interfere with intimacy.[152] Some condom promotions have addressed this issue directly by suggesting that condom use is an expression of concern and love.

A strong sense of self-efficacy is another factor related to condom use. Where one partner does not feel he or she has any control in a sexual encounter, the desires of the other partner take precedence. Some people choose not to use condoms if they think their partners will disapprove, or if they believe that condom use implies infidelity. Condoms are less frequently used with regular partners than with occasional partners.[153] A main factor in the decision to use or not to use condoms is concern about the views of peers and adherence to social norms.

Condom Demand

The global need for condoms, according to the Center for Communication Programs at Johns Hopkins University (Baltimore, Maryland, USA), is about 13 billion annually, twice the number currently used.[154] The gap between need and use is not necessarily dictated by supply. To date, neither latex supplies nor manufacturing capacity appear to be limiting factors. In 1991, an estimated 6 billion condoms were used, while the global production capacity is about 8.5 billion condoms.

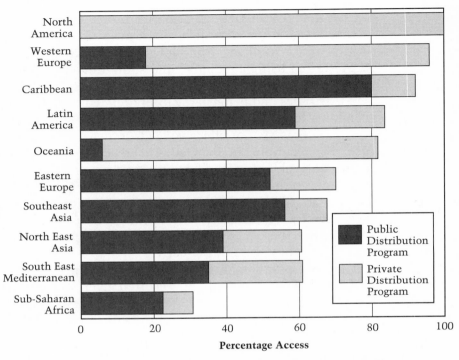

Figure 9.18. Access to affordable condoms by Geographic Area of Affinity.
Source: Population crisis committee, 1991.

Latex, the raw material for condoms, is widely available, and condoms are produced in several countries. Industry experts note that there is considerable capacity to expand if demand increases.[155] However, in a survey of six condom manufacturers who together supply about 20 percent of the world market, there was no consensus on future need.

About half of the countries surveyed by *AIDS in the World* indicated that supply met demand, two did not know, and seven did not respond. All industrialized and Southeast Asian countries in the survey, except for the former Soviet Union, said supply met demand. Despite the oft-heard comment that African men would never use condoms, programs in sub-Saharan Africa were the most likely to say that condom supply did not meet demand (see Figure 9.18).

The Logistics Link

Over the past five years, considerable progress has been made in assuring that quality condoms are available and affordable for HIV/AIDS prevention. Table 9.10 displays the many factors that are necessary to assure that sustainable supplies of quality condoms reach the user.

Over 90 percent of the *AIDS in the World*-surveyed countries report importing condoms, with many developing countries supported by international agencies. The number of condoms imported for AIDS prevention varies by country. The largest distributor of condoms to developing countries is the U.S. Agency for International Development, which distributed about one billion condoms in 1991 (see Table 9.11).

Targeting Condom Distribution

Before AIDS, condoms were typically distributed through primary health care facilities, family planning, and maternal/child health clinics. The primary target for condoms was married women. Unmarried women, men, and sexually active adolescents—the populations most often at risk for HIV infection—were largely excluded from these channels.[156] Distribution through the health care system tended to be based on a *push* system, where condoms were treated like medication coming into a country and would be proportionately allocated to clinics. Given a finite supply of condoms, this meant that a supply to high risk populations could not be sustained.

Over the past five years, there has been some movement to combine distribution of condoms for family planning with distribution of condoms for AIDS prevention. While there is little data to suggest the level of integration, groups such as the International Planned Parenthood Federation (IPPF) and their affiliates worldwide have started integrated programs. However, this requires training and the development of new outlets and distribution systems, including community-based distribution in some countries.

Today, targeting condoms to men, CSWs, adolescents, and sexually active singles has become part of most HIV/AIDS prevention programs. Those programs are more likely to have outlets in bars, hotels, and other areas where sexual transactions might be initiated.

Table 9.10: Elements of condom logistics

Phase	Primary questions	Key parties/accomplishments
Program planning and development	Who coordinates activities? What is the demand and supply? What is the cost? Who are the target populations?	National AIDS program, donor/funding agency, NGOs, ministry of health establish coordinated sustainable program with clear objectives.
Logistics management information system	What is the best management information system (MIS) for managing flow of condoms to assure sustainable supply with minimal stock?	Recipient and donor agency implement a demand-based MIS system.
Procurement	What are the specifications of condoms and methods to assure quality? How will condoms be purchased, and what will be standard for quality and testing?	National regulatory body and manufacturer to agree on quality. Purchaser links purchase to quality assurances.
Manufacturing	How is manufacturing quality assured?	Manufacturer adopts rigorous testing procedures.

Research has demonstrated that teenagers will effectively adopt condom use where sex education exists and condoms are available.[157] Yet in certain countries, condoms are illegal to sell to minors, or outlets do not provide them to adolescents.

Most surveys indicate that men purchase condoms in local markets and pharmacies,[158] where *AIDS in the World*–surveyed countries report them to be widely available. Prices and quality vary considerably. Although the market system is more responsive to demand, availability and affordability are often major barriers to use.

Contributions from international agencies will be difficult to sustain as agency priorities change; thus, there is a need to develop self-sustaining condom programs. Particularly in developing coun-

Table 9.10 (cont.): Elements of condom logistics

Phase	Primary questions	Key parties/accomplishments
Shipping and receipt	What is the shipping schedule to assure continuous supply? When do condoms arrive, and how are they stored (customs, warehouse, transport)?	Purchaser and recipient order a continuous supply of condoms and arrange for shipping, customs, and delivery. Recipient takes control of condoms.
Registration, condom management, and distribution	Who receives condoms at central facility? How are they stored and who controls inventory, inspections, and quality monitoring? Is repackaging for national activities required? Who processes orders and prepares shipments?	Recipient and affiliated programs receive condoms and assure that supply meets demand. Condoms are marketed and packaged to appeal to consumers.

Source: Prepared with the collaboration of Suzanne Thomas, John Snow, Inc., Arlington, Virginia.

tries, adopting and maintaining a demand-driven or pull-type management information system for condoms has been slow. Social marketing programs provide an alternative.

Innovative Marketing Approaches

Social marketing programs bridge the gap between public free distribution of condoms which often reaches only a fraction of the population at risk, and private market distribution which is often expensive and limited. Social marketing increases demand among target populations through advertising and public promotions. The sale, rather than the free distribution, of condoms has had three benefits: first, they have raised the value of condoms in the consumers' mind. There are several studies which indicate that as long as the price of condoms

Table 9.11: Condoms provided by supplier, African region (in thousands)

Supplier	1987	1988	1989	1990	Total[a]	% total[a]
WHO	0	0	0	61,834	61,834	12.5
International Planned Parenthood Federation	1,808	4,967	3,007	6,496	16,278	3.3
United Nations Population Fund	10,238	6,190	8,477	20,533	45,438	9.2
USAID	33,768	69,264	93,408	175,458	371,898	75.1
Total	45,814	80,421	104,892	264,321	495,448	100.1
% Total	9.2	16.2	21.2	53.3	99.9	

Source: WHO/GPA, Conference on AIDS in Africa, Dakar, Senegal, December 1991.
a. Because of rounding of numbers, percentages do not add to 100.

is affordable, they will be bought even when they can be obtained for free.[159,160] One study in Bangladesh showed that 70 to 80 percent of respondents to a survey paid for condoms that they could have obtained for free, citing reasons of time and convenience.[161] A second benefit of sale is that profit incentives have encouraged local merchants to stock and sell condoms, thus increasing distribution. Third, in theory, the profit from the transaction is used to make the condom program self-sustaining; however, evidence on the achievement of this goal is weak.

More than 30 countries have social marketing programs underway; these programs are subsidized by outside funds and have not, as yet, become self sustaining. Box 9.13 discusses the social marketing program initiated in Zaire which unfortunately has essentially been stopped as a result of civil unrest. While advertising condoms and creating a market among men has been important, perhaps the most critical success was the development of a distribution infrastructure. Yet even where a program is well conceived and executed, political instability can jeopardize its continued success.

In any condom promotion program, understanding the preferences of the target population is vital. For example, although condoms are often available in pharmacies, many people find this an inconvenient and often embarrassing place to purchase them. In France until 1987, the only legal distribution channel for condoms was through pharmacies. However, a French opinion survey revealed a high level of acceptance for condom vending machines and sales over the counter, in the open, or in bathrooms. More than 50 percent of people surveyed supported condom sales in outlets such as service stations, newspaper kiosks, restaurants, schools, streets, and public buildings. Based on the need to prevent AIDS, on public acceptance for a greater variety of outlets, and on a perceived demand, distribution of condoms in France has greatly expanded.

The Swiss "Hot Rubber" condom campaign stands as an example of how NGOs can develop a new market for condoms. They succeeded in developing a new condom market—gay men—and a new distribution system through mail order and commercial establishments catering to the gay community. The result was a high level of condom sales and revenues which funded other NGO activities.

Box 9.13: Social Marketing of Condoms in Zaire

ay Drosin and Banakpo gagele, Population Services nternational

The Zaire Contraceptive Social Marketing and AIDS Mass Media Project is proving that huge and needed increases in condom use are possible in areas where HIV prevalence is high and condom use has been practically nonexistent. Before the Zaire project began, fewer than 300,000 condoms were distributed per year in this country of 38 million people. The social marketing project began in 1988 and sold nearly and a million PRUDENCE brand condoms in its first year at a price equivalent to $0.01 per condom. In 1989, sales increased to 4 million; in 1990, to 8 million; and in 1991, to more than 18.3 million condoms.

The Zaire social marketing experience has become a powerful model in Africa's fight against AIDS. Its lesson is simple and straightforward: the systematic marketing of high-quality condoms sold at affordable prices and intensive use of available mass media channels can compel massive numbers of people to protect themselves from AIDS.

Population Services International (PSI) started the Zaire project in 1987 with support from a private foundation in the United States. In 1988, the United States Agency for International Development (USAID) and AIDSTECH, a USAID-supported project managed by Family Health International, joined the effort with funds adequate to expand the project nationally and to support the development and airing of AIDS prevention messages. PSI is now devoting substantial energy and endowment to replicating the Zaire project in ten more African countries. These projects delivered nearly 40 million condoms in 1991 in countries where, as recently as two years ago, the total number of condoms distributed was less than 5 million per year.

Condom and Lubricant—Past and Future

The past decade has not seen fundamental changes in condom design. The development of the female condom is discussed in Chapter 15. Although condoms come in two basic sizes, options include different colors, shapes, thickness of latex and lubricants. While most variations are used for marketing, they do affect the quality of the condom. All else being equal, thicker condoms are found to be more durable than thinner condoms. The tradeoff in thickness is sensitivity—both perceived and real.[162]

The lubricants used with condoms contribute to sensitivity and durability. During use, lubricants reduce friction and thus, the likelihood of breakage. Recently, especially for condoms directed toward homosexual populations, lubricants are offered in a separate sack along with the condoms. Packaging, brand recognition, color, and texture can be important marketing attributes for condoms. Though not necessarily criteria for reliability, they may be among the most important factors in developing sales and market visibility.

The efficacy of spermicides in preventing sexual transmission of HIV is still undetermined. Studies have shown that tiny concentrations of nonoxynol-9, 1/100th of that used on condoms, quickly inactivates HIV and decreases the viability of HIV-infected lymphocytes *in vitro*.[163] Unfortunately, spermicides may cause vaginal irritation in some women.[164] Additionally, allergic reactions to condoms have been reported, ranging from mild to anaphylactic, with some brands proving far worse than others.[165,166] Such factors could affect both continuation of use and increased risk of HIV transmission.

Plastic condoms are another innovation, and these may be available around the world in 1992. Their main advantage is that they may be stronger and have a longer shelf life. A comparison of the advantages and disadvantages of plastic and latex condoms is shown in Table 9.12.

Quality at the Factory and in the Warehouses

Condoms can break if they are designed or manufactured poorly, stored improperly, or used incorrectly. From the manufacturing viewpoint, the serious consequences of condom failure has placed added emphasis on condom quality. Yet despite the significant number of

Table 9.12: Comparison of plastic and latex condoms

Plastic	Latex
Reuse possible, though not recommended	Green (biodegradable)
Stronger than latex: less likely to break, thinner	Elastic
Potentially much longer shelf life: estimated shelf life of over 10 years	Could last much longer than 5 years with impermeable seals and high-quality packaging
Less likely to deteriorate in developing country settings	
Can be used with oil-based lubricants	

Sources: Robin Foldesy and Michael J. Free, personal communication.

condoms distributed for family planning during the past three decades, many agencies and countries have only recently adopted quality standards. Quality testing includes a test for holes based on water leakage or electronic testing, tensile strength based on stretching and inflation tests, and artificial aging procedures based on heating of condoms.

There is some dispute about whether laboratory tests are reliable measures of quality,[167,168] the principal question being the ability of *in vitro* tests to predict *in vivo* performance.[169] In addition to the relationship between *in vitro* tests and actual use, little is known about the relationship between the various marketing features, such as lubricated vs. unlubricated, reservoir tip vs. no tip, smooth vs. textured, and performance.[170]

Once condoms leave the manufacturer, they may weaken considerably due to problems of transportation, storage, and distribution; thus, it is necessary to provide periodic quality checks of condoms in storage. Many countries have become aware of issues of quality, and all of the *AIDS in the World*–surveyed industrialized countries and about half of the developing countries report some type of quality testing. WHO has contracted with Program for Applied Technology and Health (PATH) to establish laboratories in developing countries to test condoms that have been stored for long periods.

While manufacturers say that condoms may be good for up to five

Table 9.13: Recommendations for longer-lasting condoms

Opaque or foil wrapping

Standard thickness rather than ultra thin

Cool, well-ventilated storage

No direct sunlight, moisture, or pollutants

Proper handling or packaging to prevent tears

years, studies show that at two years, many condoms have deteriorated beyond acceptable standards due to poor conditions in transport or storage.[171] There are measures that can be taken at both the packaging and storage stages to prolong condom life. High-quality, impermeable and opaque packaging protects condoms better; and square packages are believed to be better than rectangular, because they place less stress on the latex. While ultra-thin condoms (0.04 mm) are advertised to provide greater sensitivity, they may deteriorate as much as one year faster than condoms of standard thickness.[172,173] Lubricants used in packaging condoms may also provide some protection against the elements, but the exact effect is yet to be studied.[174]

Humidity, sunlight, heat, and pollution all deteriorate latex. The ozone in smog has been shown to cause deterioration of unwrapped condoms, and nitrogen dioxide, which is also found in smog and has corrosive properties, can penetrate thick walls of plastic.[175] Consequently, warehouses should be kept under 40 degrees centigrade and well ventilated (see Table 9.13).

The Human Factor

Human error is a significant factor in condom breakage. Damaging condoms by using teeth or scissors to open a package, ripping the condom with fingernails, unrolling it before use, and using oil-based lubricants which significantly deteriorate the latex, are all frequent.[176,177]

Experience in condom use clearly makes a difference. A French study of 254 people revealed considerable differences in breakage rates among groups divided by sexual preference, profession (CSW or not), and degrees of experience, ranging from 0.6 percent breakage for CSWs to 9.8 percent among inexperienced homosexuals and bisexuals.[178]

For the inexperienced, most instructions inserted in or printed on the condom box are likely to be insufficient. A U.S. study of the directions on condom package inserts revealed that of fourteen sets of instructions, all required a reading level of the eighth grade or above.[179] An Australian evaluation of condom instructions found that a tenth or eleventh grade reading level was necessary to fully comprehend the instructions. By comparison, the author cites a sixth grade reading level when the test was applied to a lead article in a local newspaper.[180]

Several interventions have increased correct condom use by introducing skills training. Clearly, correct condom use can be learned and practiced, with the result being more condom use with less breakage.

Gaps

The largest gap is between current use and the level of use considered necessary to reduce the spread of HIV. Active government and, to a lesser degree, church opposition to condom distribution and promotion have been fading as condoms take on the less controversial image of disease prevention over that of birth control. The next challenge will be to convert this acceptance of condom promotion into effective programs.

This will require creating demand in new markets—among all sexually active individuals, including adolescents. Negative images of the condom have to be reversed, and messages with appropriate themes created. There is much to be learned about the appropriate mix of messages which appeal to different target groups.

Integrated public, semi-private and private sector distribution have to be established. There is little chance that a supply-oriented, clinic-based distribution will have a major impact on HIV transmission. While distribution at maternal/child health and family planning services should be enhanced, they reach primarily married women who are a small proportion of those at risk. At these facilities, there must also be new strategies developed for women who wish to conceive.

Social marketing may provide the best clues for achieving this integration, for it gives equal attention to high profile advertising and marketing techniques and the development of a suitable infrastructure. A goal of social marketing programs should be to make programs self-sustainable; a great danger in effective creation of demand through advertising is not having a consistent supply.

Condom logistics have made great strides over the past several years, and gains have been made in designing and implementing quality standards. Logistics training is a priority for many countries; developing simple, but effective management information systems will be necessary before demand-based condom systems can be implemented.

New products are long overdue. The female condom has taken too long to develop, test, and market. Little is known about the efficacy of spermicides and other possible chemical barriers. What other barrier products might be designed for use by women?

INJECTION DRUG USE

This section was prepared with the participation of Patricia Case, Director of the Center for Health Promotion, Department of Health and Social Behavior, Harvard School of Public Health, Boston, Massachusetts.

It has been known since early in the HIV/AIDS epidemic that injection drug users (IDUs) risk infection with HIV via contaminated injection equipment. The question has been how to reach and help a relatively hidden population commonly thought to be self-destructive and incapable of change. The reality is very different and was summed up by the United States National Research Council in 1989: "Prejudice and stigma have caused some people to believe that certain groups are incapable of changing their behavior, but data from surveys of injection drug users . . . do not support this notion. In general, it is important to point out that the groups at highest risk of infection in this epidemic also respond most favorably to the conditions under which all people respond best—that is, supportive economic, political and social conditions."[181]

Planning prevention strategies which target IDUs raises a number of difficult and often controversial issues concerning individual rights and social policy toward drug use. Should testing be voluntary or coerced? What is the role of law enforcement agencies? How can access be assured for treatment, sterile injecting equipment, education, and counseling? Does the country or society acknowledge the

Table 9.14: Main drugs used by injection drug users, reported by government AIDS programs

Country	Heroin	Amphetamines	Cocaine	Other
Argentina			+	
Australia	+	+		
Canada	+		+	+
China	+			
Czech and Slovak Federal Republics	+	+		
France	+		+	
Germany	+		+	
Haiti	+	+	+	
India	+	+		
Italy	+			
Japan		+		+
Mexico		+		+
Netherlands	+		+	+
Nigeria	+		+	
Norway	+	+		
Pakistan	+			+
Poland	+			
St. Lucia				+
Sweden	+	+		+
Switzerland	+	+	+	+
Tanzania	+			
Thailand	+			
United States	+	+	+	
USSR/CIS	+	+		

Source: AIDS in the World, 1992.

Box 9.14: How Many IDUs in the World?

AIDS in the World has estimated a midpoint of 3.4 million IDUs in a sample of countries that represents 61 percent of the world population. This amounts to an overall rate of 105 IDUs per 100,000 population. In extending this estimate to the world population, global numbers of IDUs could range as high as 5.5 million.

Table 9.15: Estimated numbers of injection drug users (IDUs) in selected countries

Geographic Area of Affinity/Country	Estimated no. IDUs	Mid-point (range) no. of IDUs per 100,000 population (1990)
North America		
Canada	90,000	339
United States	1.2–1.4 million	522 (481–562)
Western Europe		
France	70,000–100,000	151 (125–178)
Germany	50,000–80,000	84 (64–103)
Ireland	4,000	108
Italy	150,000	263
Netherlands	15,000	100
Norway	3,000–4,500	89 (71–107)
Sweden	8,000–10,000	107 (95–118)
Switzerland	25,000	378
United Kingdom	150,000	262
Oceania		
Australia	90,000–130,000	652 (533–770)
Latin America		
Argentina	900,000	2,785
Costa Rica	1,000	33
Sub-Saharan Africa		
Nigeria	50,000–100,000	69 (46–92)
Caribbean		
Bermuda	2,200–4,700	5,948 (3,793–8,103)
Puerto Rico	30,000–45,000	1,078 (862–1,293)
Eastern Europe		
Czechoslovakia	4,000–6,000	32 (25–38)
Poland	20,000–25,000	59 (52–65)

Table 9.15 (cont.): Estimated numbers of injection drug users (IDUs) in selected countries

Geographic Area of Affinity/Country	Estimated no. IDUs	Mid-point (range) no. of IDUs per 100,000 population (1990)
South East Mediterranean		
Israel	5,700–8,500	155 (124–185)
North East Asia		
China	90,000	8
Hong Kong	33,500	573
Japan	17,100	14
Southeast Asia		
India	50,000	6
Indonesia	700–800	<1
Malaysia	30,000–35,000	182 (168–196)
Philippines	400–500	<1
Thailand	50,000–100,000	135 (90–179)
Total	3,139,600–3,575,600	

Sources: Canada, United States, France, Germany, Italy, Netherlands, Norway, Sweden, Switzerland, United Kingdom, Australia, Argentina, Czechoslovakia, Poland, China, Japan, India, Thailand: *AIDS in the World* survey respondents; Ireland: national AIDS program, personal communication, 1992; Costa Rica: Asociacion de Lucha contra el SIDA, personal communication, 1992; Nigeria: Nigerian embassy, Washington, D.C., personal communication, 1992; Bermuda: W. Robert Lange, Addiction Research Center, U.S. National Institute on Drug Abuse, personal communication, 1992; Puerto Rico: H. M. Colon and M. A. Garcia, estimated extension of drug abuse in Puerto Rico, Department of Anti-Addiction Services, Commonwealth of Puerto Rico, 1987; Israel: Anti-Drug Authority, personal communication, 1992; Hong Kong: Narcotics Division, personal communication, 1992; Indonesia: Center for Communicable Disease, National Institute of Health Research and Development, personal communication, 1992; Malaysia: Health Services Division, Ministry of Health, personal communication, 1992; Philippines: National AIDS Prevention and Control Program, Department of Health, personal communication, 1992.

scope of the IDU/HIV problem or deny its existence? The answers to these and related questions will, to a large degree, determine the speed and extent of HIV's spread through a given IDU community.

Who Are the Injection Drug Users?

Although there are significant variations among countries, the main drug injected worldwide is heroin, followed by cocaine and amphetamines. Any injectable drug, legal or illegal, can be associated with HIV transmission (see Table 9.14). Despite the perception that only intravenous injection is dangerous, HIV can be transmitted through subcutaneous and intramuscular injection as well. Public health organizations have lately changed their terminology in order to reflect this, substituting the acronym IDU (injection drug user) for the earlier term IVDU (intravenous drug user).[182]

Yet the drug an IDU injects does have some bearing on the degree of risk for HIV infection. The physiological effects of drugs influence the pattern of use, and risk increases with the frequency of injection. Cocaine, for example, with its shorter duration of effect, may be injected many more times a day than heroin. There is also a link between certain drugs (e.g., crack cocaine) and increased sexual activity. If the sexual activity is unprotected, the risk of infection with HIV increases.

Injection drug use is a worldwide phenomenon, and there is evidence that the number of IDUs is growing. In addition, there have been reports that injection drug use is being adopted as a practice where other forms of drug ingestion were once more common. As drug supply routes shift worldwide, so, too, does the pattern of drug use along those routes. For example, smoking opium has long been a practice in Yunnan province in Southern China, but there has been a major increase in the flow of heroin through Yunnan. While heroin use increased substantially, injection equipment is scarce and often shared. As of July 1991, 96 percent of the known HIV-infected individuals in China were from Yunnan and nearly all of them were IDUs.[183] In Hong Kong, a transit point for the heroin from Yunnan, 80 percent of the IDUs are HIV infected.[184] In Brazil, the city of Santos—part of a cocaine supply corridor—has one of the highest per capita cumulative AIDS case rates in that country (111/100,000); nearly half are IDUs.[185]

Table 9.16: Perceived increase or decrease in injection drug use

Increasing		Stable	Decreasing
Australia	Nigeria	France	Argentina
Canada	Norway	Thailand	Haiti
China	Pakistan		Sweden
Czech and Slovak Federal Republics	Poland		United States
	Senegal		
Germany	Switzerland		
India	Tanzania		
Italy	USSR/CIS		
Japan			

Source: AIDS in the World, 1992.

Of 22 countries responding to the *AIDS in the World* country survey, 4 claimed that their IDU problem was decreasing, 16 felt it was increasing, and 2 considered the situation stable.

Wherever injection behavior has been adopted more recently, or the HIV epidemic has just reached the IDU population, evidence of HIV infection may not yet be apparent. Also, IDUs are often reluctant, for a variety of reasons, to be tested for HIV and are unlikely to be counted unless they are in treatment. Thus, at the VII International AIDS Conference in Florence, Italy, in 1991, only 38 of 122 abstracts dealing with IDUs involved individuals not in treatment and only 6 focused on developing countries.

The Needs of Individual IDUs

While the advent of the HIV/AIDS pandemic has not reduced drug use, IDUs have responded to the threat of HIV infection. In cities around the world—San Francisco, Bangkok, Edinburgh, Geneva—

needle sharing has declined and needle/syringe disinfection practices have improved. On the other hand, IDUs who may have changed their injecting behavior relatively quickly have not changed their sexual practices.[186]

Considerable experience now exists worldwide with intervention and education programs aimed at changing drug using and sexual behavior of IDUs. Some of these programs have succeeded, but it is difficult to determine which activities within a given program were most effective. It is clear, however, that the most successful strategies consider both the individual needs of the IDUs and the social/cultural context of injection drug use. Risk behaviors for IDUs are embedded in social relationships—between IDUs, within the drug culture and the society at large. Most prevention efforts, however, have focused primarily on individual behavior change rather than on the social context of injection drug use.

What are the components of successful prevention programs for IDUs? First, information and education can provide a basis for influencing behavior change, although alone they are inadequate. IDUs need detailed information about the risks associated with both drug use and sexual behavior. Education must do more than admonish ("Just say no," "Don't share needles"), it must speak specifically to an individual's interests and practices. Knowing the details of injection practice is critical for education; choice of drugs can influence risk (e.g., injecting cocaine means injecting more often) as could going to shooting galleries, or certain injecting practices like booting, in which blood is drawn into the syringe. Thus, it has been important to inform IDUs that sharing unsterile cookers (used to prepare heroin for injection) as well as needles can be dangerous.

Similarly, education about sexual behavior and HIV transmission

---

Box 9.15: Why Do People Share Syringes?

1. Lack of access to own syringe

- In withdrawal and unable to resist injecting drugs at the time
- Unable to buy syringes at night—pharmacies closed
- New injector or does not own syringe
- Cannot afford new syringe

2. Cultural practice to inject and share together

3. Inability to inject oneself and dependency on others to administer drugs

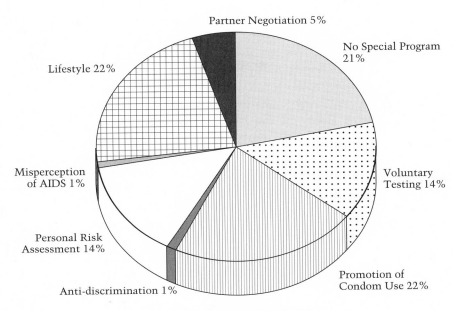

Partner Negotiation 5%

No Special Program
21%

Lifestyle 22%

Voluntary
Testing 14%

Misperception
of AIDS 1%

Personal Risk
Assessment 14%

Promotion of
Condom Use 22%

Anti-discrimination 1%

Percentage of Countries Adopting Message

**Figure 9.19. Most frequent HIV/AIDS prevention messages targeted at the
injection drug user population, 35 countries, 1992.**
Source: AIDS in the World, 1992.

should be designed with full understanding.[187] Intervention targeted
to gay-identified IDUs may miss heterosexually *identified* male injection drug users who engage in homosexual *behavior*. Heterosexual
transmission of HIV from IDUs to their non-injecting partners is an
important route of spread. Accordingly, several countries have targeted IDUs for condom promotion.

Behavior change among IDUs also needs the support of specific
health and social services. If an IDU is motivated by a prevention
education message and decides to seek treatment, that treatment
must be promptly available or the need for drugs may prevail. The
demand for drug treatment is increasing, but so, too, is the length of
the waiting lists at treatment centers. "Inadequate funding" is generally blamed for the shortage of treatment slots.

For IDUs who continue to inject, harm reduction programs that supply bleach and syringes can help reduce the spread of HIV, but only if supplies are readily and consistently available. Harm reduction programs which not only make supplies available but also bring the IDU into closer contact with the whole spectrum of social services often have considerable success. For example, an estimated 70 percent of IDUs in the Netherlands are in contact with the social service network, as compared to only 20 percent in the United States.

The third component of successful programs recognizes that injection drug use is part of a complex of social relations. Social and peer supports can be extremely influential in helping someone maintain safer practices, stop injecting or seek treatment.

The Social and Cultural Context of IDUs

The nature and effectiveness of prevention efforts are largely determined by the dynamic context of injection drug use. Ideally, education and support services for IDUs would be backed up by public support and by a social environment that would encourage every successful program. Unfortunately, this is rarely the case when IDUs are the target population. Often perceived as both outlaws and outcasts, enslaved by their addiction and lacking the power of individually motivated change, IDUs are frequently the target of societal anger and enforced behavior change. Wherever drug use is criminalized, users become the target of policies and laws which impede rather than help prevention efforts.

This problem is well illustrated by the example of testing. When deciding whether to volunteer for HIV testing, an IDU may understand the value of early treatment, but he or she also knows that access to such treatment will be very limited. In addition, there is the lack of social services and of immediate access to drug treatment to be considered, as well as the stigma and the potential legal consequences of testing positive for HIV. Despite all these problems, programs that have encouraged testing for IDUs (both in and out of treatment) have had some success.[188] Compulsory testing, on the other hand, neither motivates behavior change nor encourages prevention and serves only to drive target populations underground (see Table 9.17).

Another area in which social context has significant impact on

Table 9.17: Mandatory and voluntary HIV testing for injection drug users reported by national AIDS programs, 1992

Country	Voluntary testing recommended	Price charged for tests	% of those tested who receive counseling	HIV negative counseled?
Australia	Yes	Free	76–100	Sometimes
Canada	No	Free	51–75	Sometimes
Czech Republic	Yes	Free	76–100	Sometimes
France	Yes	Free	Unknown	Sometimes
Germany	Yes	Free or at cost	76–100	Always
India	Yes	Free	0–25	Never
Italy	Yes	Free	76–100	Sometimes
Mexico	Yes	At cost	76–100	Always
Netherlands	No	Free or at cost	76–100	Always
Nigeria	Yes	Free	0–25	Sometimes
Pakistan	Yes	Free	100	Always
Slovak Republic	Yes	Free	100 HIV+	Never
Sweden	Yes	Free	0–25	Sometimes
United Kingdom	Yes	Free	76–100	Always

Source: AIDS in the World, 1992.

prevention efforts is access to needles and syringes. Access may be legally restricted; possession of needles may be illegal; or the cost of a syringe, either through a legitimate outlet or on the street, may be high. In some countries, not enough syringes may be available. Legal restriction or criminalization of syringe possession is a compelling reason users may share syringes. In the United States, for example, 11 states and the District of Columbia outlaw simple possession of a syringe—and also have the highest rate of HIV infection among IDUs in the United States.

Legalizing the possession of syringes, increasing over-the-counter sales and needle exchange programs are all efforts targeting prevention

Table 9.18: Access to syringes in 14 selected countries, 1992

Country	Over-the-counter syringe sales	Syringe exchange programs	Paraphernalia laws
Australia	+	+	No
Brazil	+	–	Yes
Canada	N/A	+	No
France	+	–	No
Germany	+	+	No
India	+	+[b]	No
Mexico	+	–	No
Netherlands	+	+	No
Nigeria	+	–	No
Sweden	–	+ (Malmö)	Yes
Switzerland[a]	+	–	N/A
Thailand	+	–	Yes
United Kingdom	+	+	No
United States[a]	+	+	Yes (48 states)

Source: AIDS in the World Survey, 1992.
a. Varies widely by state or canton.
b. Being implemented.

to the IDU population. Of 24 countries responding to the *AIDS in the World* survey, 12 allowed over-the-counter sales of syringes, 8 had exchange programs, and only 4 had laws criminalizing possession of injecting paraphernalia (see Table 9.18).

Yet within a given country, the situation can vary widely. For example, only 2 cities in Sweden (Lund and Malmö) had a needle exchange program, and in the United States, even states which allow over-the-counter sale of syringes may have laws criminalizing possession of injecting paraphernalia.

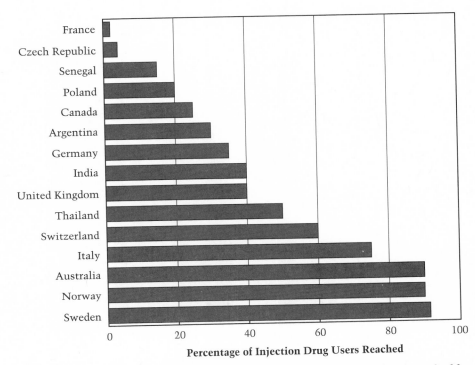

Figure 9.20. Proportion of injection drug users estimated to have been reached by various HIV/AIDS prevention programs, 16 countries, 1992.
Source: AIDS in the World, 1992.

Programs and Policies

Given the reported increase in injection drug use worldwide and its clear association with the spread of HIV, it would seem to be extremely important for national AIDS programs to not only target the IDU population, but also to ensure that they are using the most effective messages and approaches. At this stage in the epidemic, however, the success in reaching IDUs with prevention information varies considerably from country to country (see Figure 9.20). For example, in response to *AIDS in the World*'s survey, France, with an estimated 151 IDUs per 100,000 population and the Czech Republic (32 IDUs/100,000) reported reaching only a very small (under 5 percent) proportion of their IDU population with prevention efforts. Swe-

Percentage of Countries Using Theme

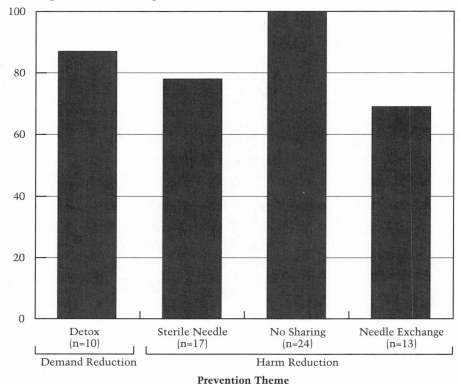

Figure 9.21. Main themes in HIV/AIDS prevention programs for injection drug users, 35 countries, 1992.
Source: AIDS in the World survey, 1992.

den (107 IDUs/100,000) and Australia (652 IDUs/100,000), on the other hand, claimed to have reached over 90 percent of IDUs. Voluntary testing (usually free of charge) is recommended for IDUs in 78 percent of 32 countries in the survey, and most provide counseling for IDUs infected with HIV.

Two main prevention message approaches to IDUs are in general use today. The first focuses on demand reduction: "Don't use drugs." The second recommends harm reduction: "Don't inject drugs; if injecting, inject safely." Countries surveyed by *AIDS in the World* report using these approaches with various messages to reach IDUs (see Figure 9.21).

Some prevention programs that have incorporated the message "don't inject drugs" often focus on drug substitution with methadone. Methadone, a heroin substitute, which is taken orally, can eliminate the risk associated with heroin injection. Methadone programs are limited in scope and apply exclusively to heroin injectors. IDUs who inject other drugs remain at risk, even if they are on methadone.

There is growing evidence that oral opiate substitution programs can be effective in reducing the risk of acquisition of HIV infection among IDUs. This risk reduction is mediated by the decrease of injection drug use and needle sharing practices. However, methadone availability alone is not sufficient. The concurrent provision of health education and counseling in a supportive environment is necessary to reduce the risk of HIV infection in IDUs and possibly achieve eventual abstinence.[189]

Harm reduction messages and programs focusing on safe injecting have emphasized not sharing needles, disinfection, syringe exchange, deregulating syringes, outreach and counseling. These campaigns have had considerable success. A 1988 study of a bleach disinfection program for IDUs in San Francisco reported a 22 percent decline in needle sharing over two years.[190] Declines in needle sharing have also been reported among syringe exchange clients in the United Kingdom,[191] Geneva,[192] Edinburgh,[193] and many other cities.

Gaps in Programs Targeting IDUs

While some attention has been paid to studying why IDUs have reduced risky behavior, it is not clear which elements or combinations of factors of existing programs and approaches are most successful in promoting change. An even greater gap looms in understanding and responding to the social construction of addiction, drug use, and needle sharing. Programs are not targeting poverty and social inequality, strong predictors of HIV infection. As long as prevention efforts focus only on risk reduction for individual IDUs without addressing the larger question of addiction itself, their success will be limited.

With the exception of attempts at user self-organization, little effort has been made to intervene in the social relationships or networks of IDUs. Although needle sharing is considered high risk behavior, little is known about specific needle-sharing practices and the context of this behavior. For example, women have been reported to share syringes more frequently than men.[194,195] Understanding the reasons for gender-specific risks would improve prevention education.

Studies are needed of sexual behavior among IDUs, even though risk through sexual transmission may be important. Finally, testing for HIV is proposed to produce behavior change in IDUs, yet studies upon which this hypothesis were based included intensive pre- and post-test counseling. Which variable led to behavior change?

Tracking the Future: Denial and Vulnerability

Addressing these questions and others raised by the IDU/HIV constellation will require political will on the part of many countries. However, two forms of denial may interfere. First, when injection drug use is thought of as "not a problem," the issues which make IDUs vulnerable to HIV infection are ignored. In Nigeria, for example, there is substantial current and future vulnerability to an injection related HIV epidemic. Heroin supply routes are being developed around the capital, Lagos, and an injectable drug supply is therefore becoming increasingly available. Informal reports to *AIDS in the World* indicated that the city now has some 50–100,000 IDUs, yet there is no program targeting IDUs, and no funds currently allocated to develop such programs.

The situation is similar in the Czech republic. More than two-thirds of the heroin seized in Europe is coming through the so-called "Balkan route."[196] There are 4,000–6,000 IDUs in the country, a severe shortage of syringes, even for medical purposes,[197] and no funding to develop or expand the few existing programs. Rapid development of prevention programs in these and other countries where there has been a shift in heroin supply and where syringes are unavailable could save the lives of IDUs, their sexual partners and their children.

The second form of societal denial of IDUs, which is also critically important for preventing HIV transmission, involves the marginalization and stigmatization of IDUs. Once again, political will is the critical need—not just within a society or nation, but internationally. Policy makers need to move beyond a focus on individual practices and look to the social roots of injection drug use if they want to stop the spread of HIV among their IDU populations.

BLOOD SAFETY AND BLOOD PRODUCTS

section was
pared with the
ticipation of Dr. Robert
l, former Head of the
od Programme of the
rnational Federation of
Cross and Red
scent Societies (IFRC)
Geneva, and currently
Medical Director of
Red Cross Blood
tre in Australia; other
tributors included: Dr.
ony F. H. Britten,
er Head, Blood
gramme, IFRC, and
essor Ian Gust,
earch and
elopment Director,
., Ltd., Victoria,
tralia.

A decade ago, in mid-to-late 1982, the U.S. Centers for Disease Control reported cases of AIDS among people with hemophilia and in at least one child who had received multiple blood transfusions. The reality of blood-borne HIV transmission was widely recognized by early 1983.

Yet in 1992, HIV transmission through blood is still a tragic—and preventable—reality in many developing countries. The history of control of HIV transmission through blood and blood products is filled with conflict and drama, and illustrates with stark clarity the gap in HIV prevention between rich and poor countries.

Blood, Blood Products, and Blood Transfusion

The first blood transfusion was reported in 1667, involving blood from a lamb given to a man. Apparently, a second transfusion followed the first, with nearly fatal results from an acute hemolytic reaction—making the point from the very beginning that blood is a potentially dangerous, as well as life-saving, product.

The modern era of blood transfusion started during World War II, when battlefield medicine developed and became expert in use of blood and plasma. Today, blood transfusion is a highly complex field, combining the latest knowledge of immunology and physiology with practical management of a wide range of services.

There are two major types of blood products. The first group is obtained from whole blood itself, and includes both cells in the blood (red blood cells, platelets, and buffy coat elements) and plasma. The second group is derived from separating the plasma into different components (fractionation) such as albumin, immune serum globulin, and factor VIII (anti-hemophilia factor).

From Blood Bank to Integrated Blood Transfusion Service

The key concept in modern transfusion medicine is the *integrated blood transfusion service*. The integrated system seeks to ensure a timely supply of adequate amounts of safe blood and blood products, where needed and at an affordable cost. The integrated system must consider donor recruitment, collection, testing, storage of blood, preparation of appropriate blood products, appropriate use of the different products, and complex record-keeping and logistical tasks. In many developing countries, in the major hospitals, blood obtained from a donor is subjected (or not) to simple tests of compatibility and safety, then infused into the recipient. The global reality is stark: while the integrated system is a reality in industrialized countries (albeit with residual problems), the people of the developing world rarely receive the full benefits—and often suffer the risks—of blood transfusion.

How Much Blood Is Collected and How Much Is Needed?

In 1986, the International Federation (formerly the League) of Red Cross and Red Crescent Societies *(Red Cross)* estimated that 80 million units of blood are collected each year.[198] However, the geographical distribution is markedly unequal: 33 million of the units are collected in Europe, 23 million in Asia/Pacific (of which 9 million are from Japan alone), and 19 million in the Americas, with only 2 million units collected annually in Africa (of which fully half were collected in the Republic of South Africa) and 2 million in the North Africa/Middle East region.[199]

The Red Cross estimated that to achieve self-sufficiency, countries would need to collect, each year, approximately 10 units of blood per hospital bed. However, tabulating units of blood collected per population reduces the built-in inequity of using hospital beds as a part of the standard. The geographical differences are striking: in the industrialized world, approximately 50 units are collected per 1,000 population each year; in *middle income* countries this rate drops to 10; while for the developing countries, an aggregate average of 1 unit is collected annually per 1,000 population.[200]

Blood is generally prescribed by a medical authority, and nearly always by a physician. Unfortunately, practices such as single unit transfusions (almost never necessary), giving a unit of blood before surgery as a prophylactic measure, or simply providing blood when it is not needed, remain important problems. In 1984, WHO estimated that in industrialized countries, 20 to 25 percent of red blood cell transfusions and up to 90 percent of (expensive) albumin administrations were not strictly necessary.[201] In Africa, when strict indications for blood were followed, an approximately 60 percent decline in blood transfusions has been documented. The patterns of prescription of blood vary from industrialized to developing countries: in the latter, a much larger proportion of blood is used for women and children (see Figure 9.22).

What Is the Reality of Blood Transfusion Services Worldwide?

In 1984, as the impact of the HIV/AIDS pandemic on blood services was just starting to be realized, WHO conducted a global survey of blood transfusion service organizations.[202] The results were shocking—as can be read in the direct language used in the final WHO report. Actual blood transfusion services in the developing world were the exception, while hospital-based blood services were the rule. The situation involving trained personnel and training programs was char-

---

Box 9.16: International Blood Transfusion: Size of the Problem

thony F. H. Britten, rmer Head, Blood ogramme, International deration of the Red oss and Red Crescent cieties

Many efforts have been made to strengthen blood transfusion services in developing countries, thus far, with only limited progress. This may be due to the fact that the problem is significantly larger than the resources which have been applied to its solution. No serious effort has been made to assess or to provide the financial resources necessary to strengthen blood transfusion services worldwide. However, a logical application of what little is known may make a useful start.

The cost of providing a modern blood service is approximately US$100 per blood donation in industrialized countries (this figure is close to reality in the United States). Currently, developing countries spend approximately $20 per donation. Each year, 80 million blood donations are made worldwide. An increase in blood collection levels in developing countries to 50 million donations per year, with an increase to $50 in expenditures per donation, would require total resources of $2.5 billion.

Where will this money come from? Will it come from international assistance? This seems unlikely, since present expenditures on international blood transfusion services assistance is about $50 million—just 2.5 percent of what is needed. Should we look for a huge increase in international funding? Or should we seek to optimize what can be done with the limited resources now available? Or are technological breakthroughs needed? Progress will require a definition of priorities, understanding of what types of assistance are useful, and improved coordination of the efforts of the many concerned organizations.

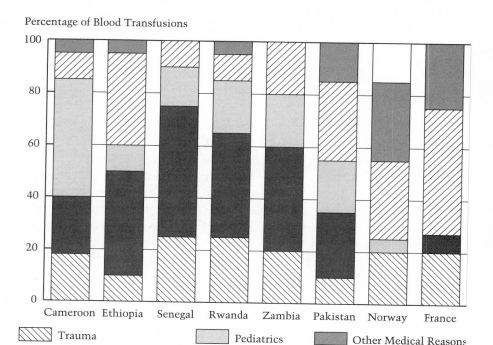

Percentage of Blood Transfusions

Figure 9.22. Distribution of blood transfusions by medical and surgical indications, 8 countries, 1991.
Source: AIDS in the World, 1992.

acterized by "gross inadequacy," and inspection and quality control programs were considered "abysmally poor." To illustrate these severe evaluations, WHO pointed out that of the twenty-two African countries responding to the survey, only one had any legislation on blood transfusion, only four had any official training or certification activities for blood service personnel, and only one had instituted a national quality control system. Similarly, in the Americas, only five of sixteen countries surveyed had quality control programs, along with only two of seven Southeast Asian countries responding to the survey.

Who Is Responsible for Blood Transfusion Services?

Many different systems exist worldwide, reflecting a combination of history, politics, and economics.[203] The United Kingdom has a government-operated service; in Canada, Finland, and Australia, the national Red Cross agency provides the blood (overall, through its over 140 national societies, the Red Cross provides 25 to 33 percent of the world's blood); in Denmark, it is hospital-based; the United States has a mixed system; in Zimbabwe, the blood system is private; and in Syria, the blood system is operated by the military. In Finland, the blood service is centralized at the national level; in France, it was divided along regional lines. In the developing world, the dominant pattern is a patchwork of hospital-based, private, semi-official, and sometimes official systems.[204]

What Is the Cost of Blood?

While it is costly to establish the infrastructure for a blood transfusion service, the major costs are operational.[205] Thus, a blood service in a developing country can be well housed, but literally paralyzed by a shortage or absence of critical laboratory reagents, supplies, or sterile blood collection bags. In the United States, the American Red Cross supplies about 6 million units (50 percent of the domestic demand for blood) at a total cost of $500 million annually.[206] Thus, in the United States, the total cost per unit of blood has been estimated at $70 to $100. In Zimbabwe, Zambia, Pakistan, Ethiopia, Côte d'Ivoire, and Senegal, the cost of a single unit of blood was estimated at $30 to $50. In sum, for developing countries, the cost of a single unit of blood may well exceed the total annual per capita health budget. But the cost of blood substitutes is equally unaffordable in developing countries (see Table 9.19).

What Are the Dangers of Blood?

In addition to immediate transfusion reactions (hemolytic, febrile, allergic) and risks of bacterial contamination and infection, several delayed reactions may be associated with blood transfusion. These include hemolytic reactions and the risk of transmitting infectious agents such as malaria, Chagas' disease, syphilis, hepatitis B, hepatitis C, HTLV-I, and HIV-1 and HIV-2. The risk of infection transmitted through different blood components is shown in Table 9.20.

Blood as an International Commodity

Blood and blood products are exchanged and sold through a major international network. For example, as the Swiss tend to collect more

Table 9.19: Average cost of blood and blood substitutes charged to health care facilities in selected countries, 1991 ($U.S.)

Country	Whole blood (per unit)	Plasma (minimum 200 ml)	Crystalloids		Colloids	
			0.9% Saline (per liter)	Ringer lactate (per liter)	Dextran or equivalent (per liter)	Hydrox starch (per liter)
Australia	8	—	1.50	1.50	26	no license
Cameroon	20	10	6	6	14	rare
Côte d'Ivoire	10–38	10–38	3.2–6.1	2.8–7.9	13.3	—
England/Wales	47	26	2.6	4.8	16.8	—
Ethiopia	17–25[a]	—	6	6	6	6
Finland	(53)[b]	68	4.8	6.6	—	22.4
France	77	16	1.2	1.7	14	18
Mexico	—	—	4.8	10.8	33.4	no license
Norway	142	152[c]	1.5	—	15	15
Pakistan	35	25	—	30–40	—	—
United States	60	17	1.1	1.5	25	—
Zimbabwe	—[d]	—	1.3	1.3	—	—

Source: AIDS in the World, 1992.
a. Provided to hospitals free of charge.
b. Red cell concentrate.
c. Per kilogram.
d. A report of the EEC AIDS Task Force concluded that the cost per collected unit amounted to $32 in Zimbabwe, $38.7 in Uganda, and $51 in Rwanda: R. W. Beal, W. Brunger, E. Delaporte, et al., *Safe Blood in Developing Countries: A Report of the EEC's Expert Meeting* (European Economic Community AIDS Task Force, 1992.)

red blood cells than required for national needs, Swiss blood was sold to shortage areas such as New York City, Greece, and Saudi Arabia.[207] Even under the best conditions, red blood cells have a short shelf-life. However, the major commercial interest is in plasma, and the commercial plasma industry is well developed, particularly in the United States. As plasma fractionation is not performed in about 80 percent of countries,[208] most blood services need plasma; the United States is the world's major plasma exporter, accounting for 60 percent of plasma world trade.[209] The commercial plasma industry has been

Table 9.20: Transfusion-transmitted infection through blood components, and relative risks[a]

Risk	Blood component
Zero	Plasma protein solution Albumin solution Immunoglobulin
Unit	Whole blood Red cell concentrate Fresh frozen plasma Platelet concentrate
Pool	Cryoprecipitate Anti-hemophilic factor Factor IX concentrate Anti-Thrombin III

Source: R. W. Beal and J. P. Isbister, *Blood Component Therapy in Clinical Practice* (Cambridge, Mass.: Blackwell Scientific Publications, 1985), p. 203.

a. The size of the pool may range from 5–10 units (cryoprecipitate) up to 50,000 individual units in large-scale industrial processes.

strongly criticized in the past, particularly for its practice of obtaining plasma in developing countries.[210] Plasmapheresis, the process of obtaining plasma, involves removal of blood and separation and retention of the liquid plasma, followed by reinjection back into the same person of their red blood cells. The image and reality of obtaining plasma from poor donors (at a cost one-tenth of the cost in industrialized countries)[211] for the benefit of rich countries was considered morally abhorrent and has been somewhat reduced or even eliminated in recent years. The lack of a universal labelling or enforced marketing code for blood also works to increase potential for abuses. The major organizations active in efforts to improve global blood supply are the Red Cross, WHO, and the International Society of Blood Transfusion.

Paid, Family-Replacement, and Voluntary Donors

The focus on voluntary (non-renumerated) rather than paid donors is a keystone of international efforts to improve the safety of blood and blood products.[212] Voluntary non-renumerated blood donation is safer

Table 9.21: Infective markers and blood donation

Disease sought and location	Ratio of prevalence in paid/unpaid donors	Reference
Hepatitis B (U.S.)	3:1	*Lancet* 1 (1975):838–41 M. Goldfield in T. J. Greenwalt and G. A. Jamieson, *Transmissible Disease and Blood Transfusion* (1975), 141–51
Non-A, non-B hepatitis	2.5:1	*Gastroenterology* 72 (1977):111–21
Hepatitis "carrier" rate	11.9:1	Prince et al. in Greenwalt and Jamieson 129–40
Hepatitis C (U.S.)	280:1	*J. Clin. Microbiology* 29 (1991):551–56
Hepatitis C (several countries)	8:1 to 55:1	Abbott slide data
HIV (U.S.)	7.4:1	*JAMA* 263 (1990):2194–97
HIV (Mexico)	70:1	*Bull. PAHO* 23 (1989):108–14
HTLV-1 (U.S.)	10:1	*Transfusion* 30 (1990): 780–82

Box 9.17: Prevention of HIV Transmission in Blood Products: Four Methods

Decreasing the transmission of HIV through blood and blood products remains an issue of prevention. Four key methods have been identified:

Donor Selection: When relying on the general population for blood donations, no screening method will ever be totally fail-safe. However, appropriate education, counseling, and well-designed questionnaires are all emphasized. In addition, voluntary blood donation has proven to be much safer than paid or otherwise renumerated donation.

Laboratory Testing: All donations should be tested for HIV. In practice, however, this is thwarted by lack of structures, services, funding, and coordination. When HIV prevalence is especially low in the general donor population, other approaches may be considered—such as pooling samples of blood for testing.

Appropriate Usage: Guidelines should be strictly followed to ensure that blood and blood products are not used unless absolutely necessary. In many countries, for example, transfusions are prescribed in situations where blood substitutes such as volume expanders could be used, but these are not always available or affordable.

Viral Inactivation: The production of certain blood products, including plasma can ensure viral inactivation through heat processing.

All four of these modes are interdependent; one cannot be ignored without reducing the efficacy of the others, thus the need of comprehensive, coordinated blood transfusion services.

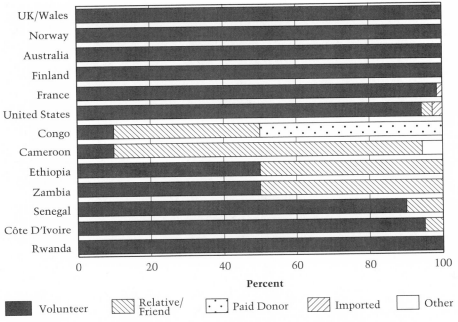

Figure 9.23. Percent blood donations by type of donors in selected countries, 1991.
Source: AIDS in the World, 1992.

than paid or replacement donation (see Table 9.21). Whenever a new, or newly recognized disease is identified as a potential transfusion-transmitted infection, the level of positive markers in the paid donor population has exceeded the level among voluntary donors. Again, the general pattern reflects differences between industrialized and developing countries. In industrialized countries, unpaid volunteers are the rule, but in developing countries, they are often the exception.

There are several known viruses that can be transmitted through blood and blood products. The screening of blood donations with commonly available reagents will not reduce the risk of transmission of most of these viruses (see Table 9.22). The stricter application of prescription criteria by health personnel, the prevention and control of infectious diseases, particularly in tropical areas, and a more effective approach to maternal and child health will help reduce the risk of transmission of blood borne viral agents (see Figure 9.23).

Table 9.22: Viruses that can be transmitted through blood and untreated blood products

Virus	Classification and description	Identification/ Reference[a]	Diseases	Modes (and rates) of transmission	Diagnostic markers	Blood antigen concentration	Vaccines
Cytomegalovirus (CMV)	Family: Herpesviridae enveloped DNA virus	1956: Independently by Smith, Rowe, and Weller[213,214,215]	•Often asymptomatic •Mononucleosis in young adults •Generalized infection in the young and immunosuppressed	•In utero (1%) •Perinatal (8–60%) •Oral and respiratory •Venereal •Organ transfer and blood transfusion	Virus isolation and detection of IgM antibodies to the virus	Cell associated	•Live attenuated vaccine, Towne strain, developed by Stanley Plotkin •Phase III trials
Human T-cell leukemia virus type 1 (HTLV-I)	Family: Retroviridae enveloped RNA virus	1980, Polesz et al. and, independently, Hinuma et al., 1981[216,217]	Adult T-Cell leukemia	•Breastfeeding •Venereal (male to female much more common than reverse) •Blood transfusion	•Antibodies to purified virus •NA hybridization of malignant cells	Cell associated	Experimental vaccines •Subunit envelope proteins •Live recombinant, vaccinia-expressing envelope proteins
Human T-cell leukemia virus type II (HTLV-II)	Family: Retroviridae enveloped RNA virus	1982, Kalyanar-aman et al.[218]	Associated with T-cell variant of hairy cell leukemia	Not fully defined	Can be distinguished serologically from HTLV-I	Cell associated	None
Human immun-odeficiency virus I (HIV-I)	Family: Retroviridae enveloped RNA virus	1983, Barré-Sinoussi et al.[219]	AIDS	•Prenatal (20–50%) •Venereal (0.1–1.0%) •Blood or blood products (95–100%)	•Antibodies to core and envelope proteins •Major core protein P24	Cell associated	None
Human immun-odeficiency virus II (HIV-II)	Family: Retroviridae enveloped RNA virus	1986, Kanki et al. and Clavel et al.[220,221]	Not fully defined	Not yet defined, assumed to be similar to HIV-I	Serologically distinct from HIV-I, but cross reacts	Cell associated	None

Virus	Classification and description	Identification/Reference[a]	Diseases	Modes (and rates) of transmission	Diagnostic markers	Blood antigen concentration	Vaccines
Hepatitis B virus (HBV)	Family: Hepadnaviridae enveloped RNA virus	1965, Blumberg et al. discovered viral surface antigen.[222] 1968, Prince showed antigen specific marker of Hepatitis B. 1970, Dane et al.[223] identified complete viral particle.[224]	• Hepatitis • Chronic infection associated with cirrhosis and primary hepatocellular carcinoma	• In utero (5–90%) • Perinatal (10–50%) • Venereal • Blood transfusion and inoculation of blood or blood products (95–100%)	Viral antigens HBsAg, HBcAg, HBeAg, and antibodies to these antigens	Up to 10^8/ml	• First-generation vaccines, derived from plasma of infected individuals and chemically inactivated, licensed in 1981 (MSD) • Second generation HBsAg expressed in yeast, 1986 (MSD & SB) • Experimental third generation includes other antigens (PreS) and live vector systems
Hepatitis C virus (HCV)	Family: Flaviviridae enveloped RNA virus	1989, Choo et al.[225]	• Hepatitis • Chronic infection associated with chronic liver disease, possibly carcinoma	• Venereal (probable) • Blood transfusion and inoculation of blood or blood products	Antibodies to non-structural protein of the virus	Often only 10^2/ml	Experimental vaccines under evaluation in animal models
Hepatitis delta virus (HDV)	Not classified, viroidlike incomplete virus requiring concomitant HBV infection	1977, Rizzetto et al.[226]	• Hepatitis • Chronic infection associated with liver disease	Not fully defined	Antibodies to whole virus	10^2–10^8/ml	Preventable by HBV vaccine

Source: I. Gust, Research and Development Director, GSC Ltd., Victoria, Australia.

a. References, indicated by superscript numbers, are in the Reference Notes for Chapter 9.

In summary, blood is a complex, lifesaving product. Worldwide deficiencies in blood collection, distribution and use existed before the HIV pandemic; HIV has served to highlight—yet again—the tremendous gap in safety and availability of precious resources in the industrialized and developing countries.

HIV, Blood, and Blood Products

HIV was able to take full advantage of the existing blood and blood product "system" worldwide. HIV infection through blood and blood products has accounted for approximately 5 percent of the global burden of HIV infection. This burden would have been multiplied many-fold if in addition to Factors VIII and IX (for people with hemophilia), the much more common and widely used "immune serum globulin" had been HIV-contaminated. This potential catastrophe was averted because the method of preparation involved physical and chemical processes which—unknowingly but extremely fortunately—completely inactivated HIV.

Blood transfusion is the most efficient, and also, at least in theory, the most easily preventable mode of HIV transmission. Receipt of an HIV-contaminated unit of blood is associated with a 95 percent or higher probability of becoming HIV infected, due both to the large volume of HIV transfused and the intravenous route of exposure.

Prevention of HIV transmission through blood followed immediately upon the establishment of an epidemiological linkage with blood transfusions and blood products. In 1983, donor deferral programs were instituted in the United States and many industrialized countries. In the United States, for example, the prevalence of HIV antibodies among first time donors declined from 0.08 percent in 1985 to 0.02 percent as a result of pre-donation counseling and the creation of alternate testing sites (see Figure 9.24). Following licensure of the HIV antibody test in early 1985, industrialized countries established systems to ensure universal HIV screening of blood. In the industrialized countries, the largest single component of added cost involved personnel to provide pre- and post-HIV test counseling. Following initiation of screening, the residual risk of HIV infection from a blood transfusion was essentially limited to the so-called *window period* of (usually) several weeks between HIV infection in a blood donor and

HIV Seroprevalence (percent)

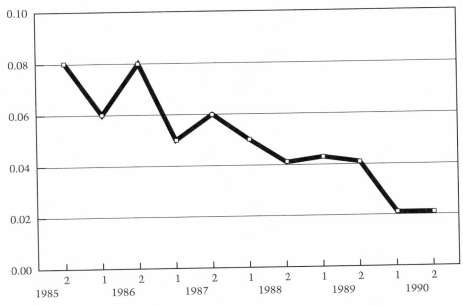

Figure 9.24. Prevalence of HIV in first time male blood donors in the USA, 1985-1990.

the time of appearance of anti-HIV antibodies (and therefore of a positive HIV test).

In the developing world, the advent of HIV had a tremendous impact on blood transfusion, unveiling once again the major, pre-existing deficiencies in blood collection and use. The additional costs included: testing equipment, reagents and other supplies, training and quality assurance systems, along with systems for record-keeping and counseling. Thus, in April 1986, a WHO survey found that 56 percent of African countries reported at least some HIV screening of blood for transfusion; nearly all involved a few, often university-based, hospital settings.[227] More shocking was the study in Kinshasa, Zaire, in February 1990.[228] At that time, of 733 medical institutions surveyed, 62 offered blood transfusions. Of these, half had refrigerators, only 10 percent were able to perform the basic cross-match to determine donor-recipient compatibility, and bacterial contamination of blood was considered "common." Of the 62 facilities providing blood transfusions, only 72 percent screened for HIV; thus, of all the units of blood transfused in Kinshasa in February 1990, over one-fourth were not tested for HIV. At about this same time, HIV seroprevalence among blood donors at Mama Yemo Hospital in Kinshasa was about 5 percent—or 1 in 20. In 1991, WHO conducted a survey of the percent of donated blood which was screened for HIV. In most of the devel-

---

Box 9.18: HIV Testing in Developing Countries

Dr. Debrework Zewdie, Steering Committee Member, Global AIDS Policy Coalition

Since 1987, testing for HIV has been a major component of AIDS control programs in developing countries. Testing has been used mainly for screening of blood and blood products for transfusion purposes, and for studying the prevalence and incidence of HIV infection in different areas and population groups. Yet the cost has been high. In Ethiopia, the cost of laboratory testing for HIV in 1990 was $700,000. As the pandemic progresses, what are the major obstacles faced by blood testing programs in developing countries?

Developing countries have responded to AIDS with great improvements in the general standard of their laboratories, particularly in laboratory safety and quality control. Yet many testing programs still suffer from poor—or absent—quality control and supervision, mainly due to a shortage of trained personnel. While early screening programs depended on the use of existing in-country personnel or on expatriates, donors took few steps to train them. Even today, refresher training courses are rare and, when they do occur, insufficient. Training and retraining of

testing personnel are essential to maintain self-sufficiency and good diagnostic standards.

HIV screening assays used in developing countries must have three important attributes: speed, manual performance, and visual reading. The most frequently used products to detect HIV-specific antibodies are the enzyme-linked immunosorbent assay (ELISA) kits. Particle agglutination and immunodot tests are also widely available for routine screening, require no instrumentation, and can be performed in some instances in less than ten minutes. Though highly sensitive and reproducible, these simple and rapid assays are, unfortunately, not highly specific: there are false positive results. Confirming or supplemental tests, such as Western blot (immunoblot), indirect immunofluorescence assays (IFA), and radioimmuno-precipitation assay (RIPA), are technically demanding and expensive. Some laboratories in Ethiopia have solved this problem by combining screening assays—there are some highly sensitive and specific ones—and limiting supplemental assays to anomalous results. This approach cut testing costs by up to 90 percent in some laboratories.

The inability to maintain equipment

oping countries and in some selected countries in eastern Europe, the proportion of blood donations which had been screened ranged between 50 and 99 percent.

The International Response

While support for HIV screening in existing blood transfusion systems was considered to be justified as an emergency measure, it was clear that only the creation or strengthening of blood services in the devel-

---

has been the bane of testing programs in developing countries, including Ethiopia. When testing for HIV first began in Ethiopia, equipment such as ELISA readers, water distillers and PH meters, were shipped to countries, often without any consultation with the recipients, nearly always without accompanying training. Within a short time, most of the equipment was out of order. No one knew how to repair even a minor problem. It was cheaper to replace the item rather than to bring someone in from abroad for repairs. No developing country uses standardized equipment which would permit different laboratories to share parts and facilitate the training of an individual—or the establishment of an office—to oversee the care of all equipment.

Problems associated with supplies of reagents used in AIDS screening can also create logistical nightmares and squander resources. Though they must be refrigerated, reagents may end up sitting in the sun waiting for customs clearance while laboratory supplies run out, and blood for transfusion is given unscreened. Large supplies are often threatened by power supply failures with no backup generator. The WHO/GPA, which buys and distributes reagents in developing

countries, may send reagents with a two-month shelf life to a country where they will not be used for six months (as with equipment, it is often easier in this case to replace these reagents rather than return them). Finally, reagents may possess weak positive control or cutoff values that are either too high or too low, but laboratories in developing countries lack access to company representatives for negotiating appropriate changes. Better coordination between international organizations and participating countries, and clearer agreements with companies producing the reagents, will go far toward alleviating these problems.

Access to new technology remains an important consideration for the future of blood testing in developing countries, particularly with new assays for the determination of T4/T8 ratios and for common opportunistic infections. However, rather than insisting on more advanced and expensive technologies, such as PCR and the Facs scan, the present priority in blood testing programs in developing countries must be to maintain and strengthen already functioning laboratories and to establish a better system of quality control and supervision.

oping world could provide medium- or long-term protection against continuing HIV transmission through blood. A survey of blood collection and blood screening practices among 7 industrialized and 8 developing countries in 1991 illustrates the variability of practices and policies for preventing transmission of HIV, as well as syphilis and hepatitis B virus, through blood (see Table 9.23).

In 1988, the Global Blood Safety Initiative (GBSI) was launched through collaboration among WHO's Global Programme on AIDS, the International Society of Blood Transfusion (ISBT), the Red Cross, the World Federation of Hemophilia, and the United Nations Development Program (UNDP). The explicit objective was to use the urgent concern about HIV safety and blood to mobilize the global commitment needed to make serious progress towards establishing integrated blood transfusion systems in all countries (see Box 9.19).

Box 9.19: The Global Blood Safety Initiative (GBSI)

The Global Blood Safety Initiative is a collaborative endeavor launched in 1988 by the Global Programme on AIDS (GPA) and the Unit of Health Laboratory Technology and Blood Safety (LBS) of WHO, the League of Red Cross and Red Crescent Societies (LCRCS), the United Nations Development Program (UNDP), the International Society of Blood Transfusion (ISBT), and the World Federation of Hemophilia (WFH), and is also supported by governments and other nongovernmental organizations.

The Objective is to ensure adequate and safe blood supplies, which are accessible to all and are appropriately used in all countries.

The Strategy is based on the conviction that this objective can only be achieved by well organized integrated blood transfusion services that are strengthened by a sustained cooperative world wide effort.

The Main Activities are

- promotion of recruitment and retention of safe blood donors improvement in processing and storage of blood improvement in exclusion of transfusion transmissible infectious agents
- encouragement of appropriate use of blood and blood products
- support and facilitation of relevant research

Table 9.23: Blood collection and HIV screening: Selected data for 15 countries, 1991

Country	No. of blood units received, 1991	Rate of blood units received per 1,000 population	% blood units received in urban and rural areas		Year HIV screening introduced	% blood units reported screened in 1991 for			Do donors who test HIV+ have access to results?	Do HIV+ donors receive counseling?
			Urban	Rural		Hepatitis B	Syphilis	HIV		
Argentina	—	—	—	—	1989	83	100	—	Yes	Frequently
Australia	1,000,000	57.19	—	—	1985	100	100	100	Yes	Yes
Cameroon	60,000	4.92	90	10	1986	45	45	90	Yes	Frequently
Congo	25,000	10.68	95	5	1986	50	20	100	No	No
Côte d'Ivoire	40,000	3.22	99	1	1987	100	90	100	Yes	Yes
England/Wales	2,200,000	38.35	—	—	1985	—	—	—	Yes	Yes
Ethiopia	30,000	0.59	50	50	1986	50	50	100	No	No
Finland	297,768	59.66	—	—	1985	100	100	100	Yes	Yes
France	3,903,600	69.30	—	—	1985	100	100	100	Yes	Yes
Norway	190,000	44.96	—	—	1985	100	80	100	Yes	Yes
Pakistan	225,000	1.78	75	25	1987	25	25	—	Frequently	Rarely
Rwanda	21,000	2.87	10	90	1985	100	100	100	Sometimes	Frequently
Senegal	20,000	2.66	95	5	1986	70	95	100	Yes	Usually
United States	13,000,000	51.75	—	—	1985	100	100	100	Yes	Yes
Zambia	49,000	5.61	46	54	1986	50	100	100	Yes	Yes

Source: AIDS in the World survey, 1992.
a. Reports include only blood units processed through national blood transfusion services, not those processed locally in some countries by peripheral health care facilities.

HEMOPHILIA AND HIV

HIV Incidence and Prevalence among People with Hemophilia

This section was prepared by Declan Murphy, S.T.L., M.A. in Ph., Executive Director, World Federation of Hemophilia; and Shelby L. Dietrich, M.D., FAAP, Medical Secretary, World Federation of Hemophilia, and Co-Director, Huntington Hospital Hemophilia Center.

Throughout the world, HIV has directly or indirectly affected the lives of people with hemophilia,* especially those living in the developed world. Of all high-risk groups, the hemophilia community is proportionately the most affected. Having learned from birth to live with one chronic and sometimes fatal disorder, many are now adjusting to living with a second disease with lethal implications.

The first cases of AIDS in people with hemophilia were reported by the U.S. Centers for Disease Control (CDC) in 1982. Since that time, AIDS has had a devastating impact. In the United States, as of January 1, 1992, CDC data on this group indicated a total of 1,876 AIDS cases in people with hemophilia; the overall case fatality rate is 64 percent, so it is presumed that almost 1,200 Americans with hemophilia have died of AIDS in the country. Approximately 50 percent of all persons with hereditary clotting disorders in the United States have been infected with HIV. Data from the Seroconversion Surveillance Project, a collaborative study by the U.S. Food and Drug Administration, the National Hemophilia Foundation, and the CDC indicate that people with severe hemophilia A were the worst affected (70 to 80 percent are HIV-antibody positive).

Background

In July, 1983, the World Federation of Hemophilia (WFH) established the World Hemophilia AIDS Center (WHAC) during its International Congress in Stockholm to facilitate collection of data on HIV/AIDS and to disseminate information. The Medical Advisory Board of WFH at the Congress received reports of 21 cases of AIDS in people with

---

*The authors of this section refer consistently to "people with hemophilia" and avoid the term "hemophiliacs." This choice of words is important: "people with hemophilia," like "people with AIDS," emphasizes the person first, the condition second, and avoids equating the condition with the person. For further understanding of this issue, consider the stigmatizing quality of (fortunately unused) terms like "cardiacs" or "cancerac."—*The Editors*

hemophilia. The first WHAC survey was conducted in 1984; subsequently, three surveys were conducted on an alternate-year basis.

In 1990, WHAC distributed a questionnaire to an international list of 500 physicians and hospitals previously identified as treaters of hemophilia; 114 physicians in 43 countries who treat 25,000 persons with congenital coagulation disorders responded. Two-thirds of the respondents knew the HIV status of their patients. The HIV prevalence rates of these patients varied widely by region. Few responses were received from Africa and the Eastern Mediterranean. Data for most of the countries in the Americas, however, were relatively complete: an overall HIV prevalence of 44 percent was found in this region. In Europe, the HIV prevalence was 24 percent. A low rate was found in Southeast Asia, but in the Western Pacific, including Japan, Australia, and New Zealand, it reached 28 percent.

AIDS cases in people with hemophilia increased dramatically over the 5 years covered by these surveys. In the Americas, the cumulative incidence of AIDS in people with hemophilia increased from 1 to 9 percent in the 1989 survey, and Europe has shown a similar increase from 0.9 to 9 percent. Australia, which initially had no cases, reported 8 cases in 1985, 21 in 1987, and 76 in 1989.

The data on the prevalence of HIV (Table 9.24) support several overall impressions:

- HIV prevalence rates are highest in those countries using pooled concentrates.
- HIV testing and reporting is low to nonexistent in those countries with poorly developed hemophilia diagnosis and treatment programs.
- The cumulative incidence of AIDS in people with hemophilia has increased ten-fold from 1984 to 1990.
- People with hemophilia in countries with volunteer blood donor programs have a lower rate of HIV prevalence, but have not been completely spared from HIV infection.
- HIV is being transmitted heterosexually from infected males with hemophilia to spouses/sexual partners in what is termed the "second wave" of infection, and on to children born to infected couples.

Although counseling, including risk reduction and safe sex practices, and emotional support were available for patients and families

Table 9.24: HIV testing by Geographic Area of Affinity

GAA	Country (no. of responses)	No. of people with hemophilia	No. tested for HIV antibodies	No. (%) HIV seropositive
North America	Canada (4)	486	395	186 (47)
	United States (18)	3,878	2,633	1,237 (47)
	Subtotal	4,364	3,028	1,423 (47)
Western Europe	Belgium (3)	428	250	16 (6)
	Denmark[a]	483	332	99 (30)
	Finland[a]	235	206	2 (1)
	France (12)	1,456	999	451 (45)
	Germany (East)	232	173	0
	Germany (West)	354	251	85 (34)
	Greece (85%)[b]	613	527	181 (34)
	Ireland (1)	430	—	—
	Italy[a]	2,254	1,924	543 (28)
	Netherlands (1)	58	32	0 (0)
	Norway[a]	—	318	21 (7)
	Portugal[a]	570	468	129 (28)
	Spain (4)	1,023	975	478 (49)
	Sweden (2)	363	363	88 (24)
	Switzerland (2)	417	340	68 (20)
	Subtotal	8,916	7,158	2,161 (30)
Oceania	Australia (11)	1,155	929	215 (23)
	New Zealand (2)	313	107	14 (13)
	Subtotal	1,468	1,036	229 (22)
Latin America	Argentina[a]	1,128	467	163 (35)
	Brazil (4)	1,764	1,167	642 (55)
	Colombia (1)	20	4	0
	Costa Rica[a]	152	136	55 (40)
	Ecuador (1)	7	7	0
	Mexico (1)	84	84	18 (21)
	Paraguay[a]	129	109	5 (5)
	Venezuela[a]	782	349	70 (20)
	Subtotal	4,066	2,323	953 (41)
Sub-Saharan Africa	Cameroon[a]	30	23	0
	Nigeria[a]	70	15	1 (7)
	South Africa (3)	130	87	1 (1)
	Subtotal	230	125	2 (2)
Eastern Europe	Bulgaria (1)	426	413	9 (2)
	Czechoslovakia (67%)[b]	738	600	17 (3)
	Poland[a]	1,551	1,205	15 (1)
	Yugoslavia (1)	484	204	73 (36)
	Subtotal	3,199	2,422	114 (5)

Table 9.24 (cont.): HIV testing by Geographic Area of Affinity

GAA	Country (no. of responses)	No. of people with hemophilia	No. tested for HIV antibodies	No. (%) HIV seropositive
South East Mediterranean	Egypt	1,549	40	1 (3)
North East Asia	Japan (4)	579	506	203 (40)
	Korea[a]	—	313	2 (1)
	Subtotal	579	819	205 (24)
Southeast Asia	India (1)	22	22	0
	Indonesia (1)	9	6	1 (17)
	Malaysia (1)	431	323	13 (4)
	Nepal (1)	26	—	0
	Thailand (1)	150	62	2 (3)
	Vietnam (1)	25	25	0
	Subtotal	663	438	16 (4)

Source: World Hemophilia AIDS Center, Los Angeles, Calif., October 1990.
a. Entire country.
b. Proportion of country covered.

Table 9.25: Global demography of estimated number of newborns with hemophilia

Continent/Area	Population (x 10^6)	No. of births per annum (x 10^6)	Expected no. of newborns with hemophilia
Africa	645	29.7	1,500–3,000
Asia	3,047	82.5	4,100–8,200
Australia/New Zealand	20	0.6	30–60
Europe	499	7.0	350–700
North America	275	4.4	220–440
South America	299	9.3	465–930
USSR/CIS	291	5.5	225–550
Total	5,076	139.0	6,890–13,880

Source: Prevention and control of hemophilia: Memorandum from a joint WHO/WFH meeting, *WHO Bulletin* 69(1)(1991):17.

of 91 percent of the survey respondents, the number of patients and families reached and the degree of behavior change resulting in consistent safe sex practices is unknown. Twenty-five percent of the respondents reported that female sexual partners were unaware that the male partner was at risk of HIV infection because of use of blood products. Also noted as barriers to counseling were religious and cultural differences, financial and time barriers, lack of expertise and questions of confidentiality.

World Patterns of Documented Hemophilia

In the developed world, AIDS is now the leading cause of death in people with hemophilia and represents the major medical, therapeutic, psychosocial, and public health problem in hemophilia. Hemophilia is the most common hereditary bleeding disorder. It poses a heavy social and economic burden. The incidence of hemophilia—15–20 per 100,000 males born, as based on an estimate found in surveys in several parts of the world—indicates that the disease is equally frequent in all ethnic groups and geographical areas.

Box 9.20: What Is Hemophilia?

Hemophilia describes a group of inherited blood disorders in which there is a defect in the clotting mechanism of blood. The molecular defect is the absence of, decrease in, or deficient functioning of plasma coagulation factors VIII or IX which cause hemophilia A (Classic Hemophilia) or hemophilia B (Christmas Disease) respectively. Since the defective gene is present on the X chromosome and transmitted by the mother to sons, all persons with hemophilia A or B are male.

In the early 1970s clotting factor concentrates were introduced and made possible dramatic improvements in the lifestyle and life expectancy of persons with hemophilia. Because prophylactic and therapeutic treatment was so effective, people with hemophilia could live relatively normal lives. Factor VIII or IX concentrates are produced from plasma pools containing 2,000 to 30,000 donations per pool, hence theoretically each individual could be exposed to the plasma of 1.9 million people in a single year. In the United States, a significant number of people with hemophilia were infusing with blood clotting concentrates on an average of one to two times per week, or 40 to 60 times per year. Unfortunately, this great advance in treatment exacted a cost of frequent exposure to and transmission of blood and plasma borne viral diseases, primarily hepatitis B, hepatitis C, and the human immunodeficiency virus (HIV).

Comprehensive Care of the HIV-Infected Person with Hemophilia

The exposure of people with hemophilia to a second chronic illness—HIV infection—has had significant impact on all parts of the hemophilia community. People with hemophilia and their families have been affected, as well as medical and psychosocial staff, hospitals, and the producers and suppliers of therapeutic materials for hemophilia (volunteer blood donor agencies and the commercial fractionation industry).

Patients and families are faced with the reality of a protracted and eventually terminal illness with the attendant financial, legal, psychosocial, emotional, and medical consequences. Staff and patients may feel alienated by litigation and experience feelings of guilt and anger. Staff face continuing emotional and physical stress due to patient deaths, illnesses, time demands, feelings of futility, and the problem of occupational exposure from needle stick or other accidents. Some physicians (especially surgeons) are reluctant to perform invasive procedures on HIV-infected patients. The 1990 survey of the World Hemophilia AIDS Center (WHAC) reported that more than half of the treatment staffs at their centers had been exposed to hepatitis B and/or HIV through occupational accidents, but no HIV seroconversion was reported. A major problem throughout hemophilia treatment centers has been patient concern that physicians who treat hemophilia are not always able or willing to remain their primary physician when the results of HIV infection become the primary medical concern.

Treatment Products

Although heat-treated Factor VIII concentrates were available prior to the identification of HIV to reduce hepatitis risk, there is evidence that heat treatment inactivated HIV was not available in the United States until 1984. Heat-treated concentrates subsequently replaced untreated concentrates in the United States and the rest of the world. Today the "triple safety net"—donor (voluntary or mandatory) screening and exclusion; donor plasma serologic testing; and viral inactivation treatment methods for concentrates—appears to have reduced the danger of HIV transmission via pooled plasma products to an extremely low level. However, it should be emphasized that no system can be considered 100 percent safe, as errors or mishaps may occur at any point in this safety chain. Since current clotting factor products seem free of the risk of HIV transmission, a new generation of individuals with hemophilia born since 1986 has not been exposed to and may never know the threat of HIV from blood products. Factor VIII concentrates produced by recombinant DNA techniques are currently awaiting licenses and are expected to eliminate the problem of transmission of viruses via human plasma donors.

National and International Response

The response in this area has directly correlated with the country's socioeconomic status. In countries with social security or welfare programs, patients can get assistance for additional costs due to HIV infection/AIDS. There are national hemophilia societies in at least 70 countries, taking a leading role in educating the community and government about the problems facing persons with hemophilia, especially those who have also contracted HIV/AIDS. Some have lobbied the national governments on behalf of those infected with HIV in order to seek financial compensation for damages caused by contaminated blood products. Since the advent of AIDS, the World Federation of Hemophilia (WFH) has played a major role in initiating and supporting national programs both to educate people with regard to HIV infectivity and also to help prevent further transmission of the virus.

Governmental Response

Many governments have reacted positively toward patients with hemophilia who contracted HIV/AIDS through contaminated blood products imported into the country with the government's approval. Under terms such as "compensation," "catastrophe relief," and "financial assistance," they have offered financial support to people with hemophilia who had seroconverted (see Table 9.26).

The amounts vary from country to country, as do the stipulations and procedural steps. It should be noted that these initiatives never come from the governments themselves, but rather originate from national hemophilia societies or individuals.

In the United States, a national strategy for preventing AIDS in hemophilia families has been outlined in which components of government (CDC, the Bureau of Maternal and Child Health) and the

Table 9.26: Status of financial assistance to HIV-infected people with hemophilia as of January 1, 1992

Group 0: Countries in which activities are not known

China	Honduras	Nicaragua	Trinidad & Tobago
Colombia	Iceland	Nigeria	Turkey
Cuba	Indonesia	Pakistan	USSR/CIS
Cyprus	Iran	Philippines	Zimbabwe
Czechoslovakia	Korea	Singapore	
Dominican Republic	Mexico	Somalia	

Group 1: Countries in which no compensation is planned

Algeria	Finland	Panama	Tunisia
Argentina	Israel	Peru	United States
Chile	Kenya	Poland	Uruguay
Egypt	Kuwait	Portugal	Venezuela
El Salvador	Luxembourg	Thailand	Yugoslavia

Group 2: Countries in which compensation is not yet planned, although HIV infections in people with hemophilia are known

Jamaica   South Africa

Group 3: Countries in which considerable activities were developed by the National Member Organizations (NMOs) to attain compensation, without having reached final solutions

Belgium	Costa Rica	Italy	Malta
Brazil	Greece	Malaysia	Portugal

Group 4: Countries in which compensation payments through the government have already been attained

Canada   Denmark

Group 5: Countries in which legislation already existed to allow for compensation

Bulgaria	India	Norway
Fed. Rep. of Germany	New Zealand	Sweden

Group 6: Countries with foundations/funds from private or government sources

Australia	Ireland	Netherlands	Switzerland
Austria	Japan	Spain	United Kingdom
France			

Source: World Federation of Hemophilia HIV Financial Assistance Committee, Heidelberg, Germany, December 31, 1991.

National Hemophilia Foundation provide planning resources and information to establish a national program for risk reduction. This program includes education, outreach, information dissemination, data collection and evaluation, and technical assistance to providers and chapters who perform or deliver the outreach, education, counseling and management at the local level. An early evaluation shows that coordinated efforts are making an impact on the transmission of HIV infection to sexual partners. Adoption of safer sexual habits has increased within the hemophilia community. In 1991, the CDC initiated a five-year project to evaluate methods for preventing sexual and perinatal transmission for people with hemophilia attending treatment centers. For this project, 7 treatment sites have been funded to conduct research among adults with hemophilia, and 11 sites will participate in a study of adolescents with hemophilia.

The most current WHAC survey (1990) reported a cumulative total of 2,383 CDC-defined AIDS cases in people with hemophilia from a total of 34,128 patients covered by the survey, or a cumulative incidence rate of AIDS of 7 percent. Additionally, 34 spouses and 5 children perinatally infected with AIDS must be added to this total. The life expectancy of people with hemophilia has been cut down drastically by HIV infection, causing lost decades of social and personal productivity. Paradoxically, those countries with the least developed systems of diagnosis and treatment have the lowest incidence of HIV in the hemophilia population. They had limited access to the technologically more advanced factor concentrates, which became contaminated in the late 1970s and early 1980s.

Major steps have been taken in purification of the clotting factor concentrates and improved donor screening and testing for plasma, cryoprecipitates, and blood components. The consequences of widespread HIV transmission from 1978 through 1984 via plasma concentrates and blood components continue to dominate the hemophilia community. Working through its 70 national member organizations, WFH is addressing these problems in a Decade Plan for the 1990s and will continue to coordinate medical, educational, and informational activities on an international basis.

CONCLUSION

This chapter has analyzed prevention programs targeted at specific populations. It provides examples and—where data were available—a measure of gaps between needs identified in populations at risk, services which often cannot meet these needs, and impediments created by constraining social environments. The inadequacy of services aimed at providing safe blood and blood products in the developing world is a vivid example of a situation where, in spite of the availability of an effective prevention technology, it remains inaccessible to a large part of the world population.

The first decade of HIV prevention has produced a great measure of success at the community level. The next challenge is to move from pilot projects and small programs to broad-based national efforts capable of altering the course of the HIV epidemic.

The recognition of three common denominators in successful HIV prevention programs—education/information, health and social services, and a supportive social environment—should strengthen the ability of communities and nations to implement effective programs. Each of the three components must be carefully considered at the local level, adapted to local culture, and implemented with available resources. Yet if any program lacks one of these three elements, it will be very unlikely to succeed.

In this manner, effective *global learning* about prevention is already taking place: the lessons from each community can be used to strengthen our collective knowledge.

Thus, the global record on prevention is mixed. Innovative and creative community programs around the world, serving different populations, have clearly shown that prevention can work. The common denominators for prevention have been identified. Now, the enormous challenge remains to make these programs widely available, sustainable, and capable of improvement based on evolving local and global experience.

CHAPTER TEN

. . . .

Providing Care

chapter was
ared by Charles
eron, an international
h economist, with the
stance of Julia
bard, a management
sultant. Both are
ed in Boston,
sachusetts.

No disease in history has raised such complex issues, required such a wide range of responses, or so mercilessly unveiled the preexisting, serious imbalances, inadequacies, and inequities embedded in health and social systems around the world. Even if all new HIV infections could be prevented as of today, there would still be a continuing increase in the number of people with AIDS during the coming decade and beyond and the gap between needs and services—already large— would become ever wider.[1,2,3] More realistically, by the year 2000, an estimated 38 to 110 million adults will have been infected with HIV, and as many as 24 million adults will have developed AIDS.

Thus, the HIV/AIDS pandemic raises the specter of a rapidly worsening global crisis in health care and social services, challenging our ability to cope humanely with dramatically increased needs. This crisis has already weighed heavily on many societies and will become even more serious in the years ahead. The needs of affected individuals, their families, and communities are diverse and complicated; and the psychological, social, political, and economic impacts of HIV/AIDS require thoughtful, integrated societal responses.

Three categories of needs must be considered: medical, psychosocial, and social welfare (see Box 10.1). In most cases, these needs are similar to those encountered in the care of many other conditions. However, in the context of HIV/AIDS, new or less traditionally accepted or expressed needs have also been articulated. For example, to a much greater extent and in a far more explicit manner, respect for the individual is seen as fundamental, regardless of the specific action and details of the program involved. HIV-infected people and those who care for them increasingly demand to be treated with dignity.[4,5,6,7,8] Table 10.1 provides a generic framework for discussion of these needs and different locations in which they can be met.

THREE KINDS OF NEEDS

Medical Needs

Like the specific aspects of the epidemic, the range of medical needs resulting from AIDS varies widely among communities and from one part of the world to another. In industrialized countries, medical management includes diagnostic, prophylactic, treatment, and counseling services. Medical care is provided by physicians, nurses, and other health professionals. Meeting the medical needs of people with HIV/AIDS can both prolong life and improve its quality.

Medical interventions depend on the capabilities of existing health care delivery systems and the availability of resources. In the industrialized countries in North America and Europe, people with AIDS have until now been seen primarily on an in-patient basis. Many are fortunate enough to receive first-rate care including diagnostics, complex and expensive treatment procedures, and an increasingly effective range of drugs.[7,11,12] Many new drugs are in development, and people with AIDS increasingly have access to experimental therapies. Alternative therapies and nutritional approaches are also widely available. Nevertheless, great inequities remain: in some cities, and among some groups of people with HIV/AIDS, basic medical needs are still not being met.

In the developing countries—especially in Africa and Asia—the picture is radically different. Whereas both traditional and alternative types of medical care are available through formal and informal health care delivery systems,[13,14,15] most therapeutic procedures and drugs were already available before AIDS. Health care systems in some developing countries are severely strained by the additional needs of people with HIV/AIDS. Even testing for HIV is not assured; supplementary confirmatory tests like Western Blot[16] are often unavailable

Table 10.1: Examples of services needed at different levels of the health/social welfare system

Type of service	Hospital inpatient/outpatient	Other facility (clinic, hospice)	Community (workplace, church)	Home
Medical Diagnostics Procedures Drugs Physical support	Tertiary care: Complex diagnostic and other biomedical procedures Intensive care Periodic checkups Trained health personnel	Secondary care: Diagnosis Treatment of severe illnesses Trained health personnel	Primary health care: Treatment of opportunistic infections Community support Trained health personnel	Individual access to: Self treatment Home-based care/nursing Medical supplies/ equipment Essential drugs Physiotherapy Information Condoms
Counseling/ Psychosocial	Pre-/post-test counseling Counseling during treatment Periodic assessment of psychological needs Trained counselors	Pre-/post-test counseling Counseling during treatment Trained counselors	Social contacts Community awareness and support Spiritual support	Social contacts Housing Home visits by support groups/ persons Psychological support to people with AIDS and friends and families Spiritual support
Social/Welfare	Periodic assessment of social/welfare needs Trained social/welfare workers	Periodic assessment of needs Linkage between health and social services Social support at work place Trained social/welfare workers	Community-based organizations/ ASOs to periodically assess needs and quality of life of people with AIDS ASOs and social services to attend to those needs Support to orphans Income generation Trained social welfare workers	Housing Financial support Food, clothing Support to orphans Administrative support Transportation Income generation Trained home visitors

or too expensive for routine use. Newer, specific antiretroviral therapies like Zidovudine (AZT) or ddI are unavailable for most people.

Psychosocial Needs

In the HIV/AIDS pandemic, psychosocial needs have been identified for the first time as a priority that requires a systematic and sustained public health response. Providing psychological support to people with HIV/AIDS, maintaining them within society, and strengthening their integration within existing societal structures is now seen as essential both for optimal personal health and for protecting public health and societal interests. In addition, as the pandemic proceeds, a widening circle of people affected by HIV/AIDS—and needing psychosocial support—is being identified, including families, health care providers (including those suffering from burnout), and even national AIDS program staff.

The most common mechanism for providing psychosocial support is usually called *counseling*. The English word *counseling* has no direct counterpart in many other languages. As used here, counseling

---

Box 10.1: Defining Needs: Different Approaches

What are the needs engendered by AIDS? Needs are dynamic, changing over time with an individual's state of health and with the evolution of the pandemic.

Defining the needs of persons affected by HIV can involve a formal review process, as has recently been done in Malawi,[9] or it can reflect informal consensus among HIV-infected persons, persons with AIDS, care providers, and government officials.[1,2,5,6,10] Although there are a number of studies attempting to define needs of persons with HIV and AIDS in industrialized countries, relatively little work of this kind has been conducted in developing countries. Comparisons across studies is difficult, due to different methodologies and

assumptions and substantial variation in questions asked by researchers.

In 1989, WHO developed a broad conceptual definition of care as "a comprehensive, integrated process which recognizes the range of needs for well-being; it includes services and activities providing counseling and psychosocial support, nursing and medical care, legal, financial, and practical services."[2,6] However, practical application of such a definition is difficult because of its all-encompassing nature. Many organizations have focused on 1 principal type of care (e.g., clinical management), a specific group of people with AIDS (e.g., orphans, injection drug users), or a specific location for providing services (e.g., hospital inpatient, home care). Clearly, no single classification system is ideal for all purposes.

includes provision of information, support for identifying and resolving issues of integration, care, and social needs, and psychological support. Thus, counseling for people with HIV/AIDS has both a preventive and a supportive role. Prevention involves informing people about protective behaviors and helps them avoid behavior that can expose others to HIV. Supportive counseling helps improve the quality of life through better coping with physical, emotional, and social problems. This typically includes assistance in dealing with anxiety, grieving, and exclusion of all kinds. Counseling can be individual or group; it may even occur at a community level. It is provided as part of the health care system or by community-based groups, nongovernmental organizations (including religious and spiritual societies), and by official institutions.[3,4,5,7,17]

International guidelines on counseling emphasize the importance of defining objectives, assessing effectiveness, integrating services within the existing health care system, and addressing confidentiality issues.[18]

How psychosocial needs will be defined—and addressed—varies enormously by country and social setting. Every society has traditions and mechanisms for providing psychosocial support. Yet HIV/AIDS creates specific challenges to traditions in several ways. First, the willingness and ability of societies to provide support to its already stigmatized groups will be challenged even further by the needs of marginalized people (e.g., injection drug users, sex workers, street children) who are HIV infected. Second, not all societies have traditionally approached confidentiality about health in a manner best suited to protecting the interests of the infected person. Third, many health systems do not emphasize the *dialogue* between provider and client, yet this back-and-forth ability to discuss and explore needs and fears, to locate strengths and solutions, is critical to the counseling process. Finally, modern health care systems worldwide have generally emphasized medical diagnosis and treatment rather than psychosocial support. For example, following diagnosis and treatment for cancer, psychological adjustment of the individual, support to the family, and the challenges of reintegration into the community may not be considered a routine part—or responsibility of—the health care system.

The psychosocial needs of HIV-infected people and people with AIDS challenge the status quo of prevailing concepts and available services. The needs are great; meeting psychosocial needs, as defined through dialogue between counselors and affected people, providers and clients, will likely be much more time and person intensive than will be meeting the medical needs of people with HIV/AIDS.

Thus, the novel element in HIV/AIDS is the extent to which the importance of psychosocial needs has been validated; they are essential in personal and public health terms. A major effort is now underway to translate this concern into appropriate strategies, training activities, and programs.

Social Welfare Needs

Social welfare needs in the AIDS pandemic include food and clothing, shelter and housing, drug rehabilitation, employment, schooling, and even funeral arrangements. In many cases, the extended families bound by tradition and culture may provide welfare support. Other options include governmental economic support for HIV-infected people and their families, self-help groups for HIV-infected persons, and organizations that support children orphaned by AIDS.[4,5,7,17]

How Has the World Responded?

In general, although many individuals and communities have responded in remarkable and creative ways to the needs of persons with HIV/AIDS, the collective societal response has been inadequate. Even in the limited area of medical needs, only a few industrialized countries have been willing and able to provide comprehensive care for the growing numbers of HIV-infected people and people with AIDS. As for psychosocial and social welfare needs, no nation has yet been able to address these problems fully. Every society has its particularly vulnerable groups—orphans in Africa, injection drug users in Europe, the uninsured, impoverished, or homeless in the United States. There have been some successes at the local level. Yet in the context of an expanding global HIV/AIDS epidemic, the response of society thus far raises legitimate fears of a massive, global failure.

Location of Service Delivery

Where services are delivered can be as important as what is delivered. (See Table 10.1.) Location has important implications for type and acceptability of care, access, effectiveness, cost, and service sustainability.[2,14,17] A large number of different locations for service delivery have been used to meet the needs of HIV-infected people and those with HIV/AIDS.[1,2,3,7] In addition, AIDS has stimulated demand and provided an impetus for change, spurring development of new, innovative service delivery systems.

Although AIDS care in many industrialized countries is typically hospital-based, community-based organizations (e.g., AIDS service organizations) have developed an increasing capacity to care for people in homes, hospices, and other community settings designed to provide familiarity and comfort. In contrast, in Africa and much of Asia, primary medical care is typically delivered in the home or at the community level, and tertiary care is delivered at central hospitals. Severely ill persons are referred from local health centers and hospital facilities according to their medical care needs.[3,8]

CARE: A GLOBAL OVERVIEW

The following section illustrates the global response to HIV/AIDS by describing models of care in selected industrialized and developing countries. The developing countries section contains sub-Saharan Africa, Latin America and the Caribbean, and Southeast Asia. Little information about care for those with AIDS could be found for countries in Eastern Europe, the South East Mediterranean, or North East Asia, with the exception of Japan. Industrialized countries include the countries of North America and Europe, Australia, and Japan. These examples provide interesting insights into approaches to meeting individual needs and into specific issues raised by the AIDS pandemic.

DEVELOPING COUNTRY EXPERIENCE

Sub-Saharan Africa

Currently meeting the medical needs of those affected by HIV is a greater challenge in sub-Saharan Africa than elsewhere due to the large and rapidly growing demand and extremely severe resource constraints.[3] In most African countries, AIDS is another major disease that must be addressed by an already inadequate health care delivery system.[2]

Diagnosis of AIDS involves clinical criteria developed by WHO in Bangui, Central African Republic, in 1985[19] and supplemented, as available, by HIV serological testing. However, large numbers of people with HIV disease remain undiagnosed, yet require care. In many health clinics in East and Central Africa, staff examine a patient, review the clinical history, and prescribe therapy without even rudimentary laboratory diagnostic support.[20] In 1989, WHO developed standardized treatment guidelines for adults, based on medical algorithms that can be applied in all types of service delivery settings.

The Zimbabwean and Ugandan ministries of health have also developed national treatment guidelines for opportunistic infections; however, these have not yet been evaluated. Following the Ugandan guidelines, using such criteria as the applicability of drugs for multiple purposes, perceived effectiveness, and cost, nine drugs were identified as essential for the care of people with AIDS.[21]

In 1988, a list was developed of commonly used drugs for HIV-related care in African countries. Table 10.2 lists the drugs and estimated costs for three levels of treatment: basic, intermediate, and advanced.[22] The cost per treatment episode ranged from $0.05 to more than $600 for treatment of a life-threatening fungal infection.

The use in Africa of antiretroviral drugs, such as AZT and ddI, continues to be debated. Major impediments to use include the lack of clinical studies on efficacy in the African setting, monitoring requirements, and high costs.[19,22,23]

Published studies of psychosocial support and care for people with AIDS in sub-Saharan Africa are rare. In Uganda, The AIDS Support Organization (TASO) includes counseling as an integral part of care for people with AIDS and their families (Box 10.2). Counseling is provided both at the TASO centers and in home care.[24] In Tanzania, a World Bank study found, not surprisingly, that nurses were used extensively at all levels of health care delivery, ranging from hospitals to home visits. They were critical for counseling and psychosocial care as well as for medical treatment.[25]

Social support and welfare are an important part of care in Africa. Traditionally, the extended family has played a crucial role in maintaining the integrity of families and communities under stress from

Table 10.2: Costs of various treatments for HIV-related illness

Drug	Drug unit	Drug unit/treatment episode	Cost/drug unit ($U.S.)	Cost/treatment episode ($U.S.)
I. indomethacin	tab 25 mg	20	0.003	0.06
paracetamol	tab 500 mg	20	0.004	0.08
loperamide	tab 2 mg	20	0.005	0.10
ORS	sachet 1l	5	0.070	0.35
gentamicin inj	40 mg/ml, 2ml	4	0.100	0.40
co-trimoxazole	tab 400+80 mg	40	0.014	0.56
nystatin	tab 100.000 U	30	0.031	0.93
amoxycillin	cap 250 mg	40	0.033	1.32
morphine	ml syrup	50	0.050	2.50
II. TB standard course	(1)			4.11
TB reserved regimen	(2)			5.10
Ringer lactate	1,000 ml	5	1.050	5.25
TB short course	(3)			9.27
Ketoconazole	cap 200 mg	20	0.950	19.00
III. acyclovir	cap 200 mg	25	3.026	75.65
antineoplastics	(4)			144.14
amphotericin B	inj 50 mg	18	14.250	256.50
flucytosine	cap 250 mg	1,512	0.400	604.80

Source: Adapted from S. Foster, "Affordable clinical care for HIV related illness in developing countries," *Tropical Diseases Bulletin* 87 (11) (1990):121–29.

Note: (1) = 2 months streptomycin, 10 months thiazine (thioacetazone and isoniazid); (2) = ethambutol in combination with other TB drug regimens; (3) = 2 months streptomycin, rifampicin, pyrazinamide, thiazina; 6 months thiazina; (4) = 6 doses actinomycin D plus 6 doses vincristine.

illness and death. Although there are few published reports, there are indications that the extended family has taken on this role with regard to AIDS.[26] However, communitywide fear, discrimination, ignorance of clinical manifestations, inability to provide adequate personnel, and other factors create barriers to broad social support.[3,27]

In Uganda, TASO provides information, food, some clinical support, and income-generating opportunities for HIV-infected persons, persons with AIDS, and their families. In addition, TASO's home visit program provides drugs, counseling, and other types of support to people with AIDS and their families. However, TASO is critically dependent on foreign resources; if outside aid were to be reduced, the program would end. It is unlikely that other countries in sub-Saharan Africa could afford a TASO-like program without sustained availability of external resources.[24,28]

Efforts to meet the needs of those affected by HIV in sub-Saharan Africa raise a number of important issues. First, meeting medical needs may include treating or preventing other diseases associated with AIDS, such as tuberculosis and sexually transmitted diseases, that have a serious impact on public health. Prevention and treatment efforts for these conditions must be coordinated with AIDS activities. Second, as more research on costs and quality of care in hospital settings is conducted, home care programs and other alternatives to hospital care are increasingly being considered. Finally, as family

---

Box 10.2: The AIDS Support Organization, Uganda

Noerine Kaleeba is the founder of The AIDS Support Organization (TASO), Kampala, Uganda. (Adapted from "Community-Based Care in an LDC: The AIDS Support Organization," Noerine Kaleeba, 1989.)

Before TASO, when a young Ugandan man or woman was diagnosed HIV antibody positive, there was nowhere he or she could go to find out more, to get questions answered, to talk about the illness.

The AIDS Support Organization (TASO) was created to provide support for people with HIV infection or AIDS and their immediate families. We work largely in the urban areas of Kampala and Masaka, offering medical, emotional, and practical assistance to families affected by AIDS. Our main aim is to encourage the family unit to provide a nucleus of support for the AIDS patient. Caring for a sick relative is a traditional practice in Uganda; yet AIDS is a disease that often frightens relatives away. We found that when time is spent with family members to explain how the disease is caught and how to care for a person with AIDS, and to talk through their fears, they are better able to cope with caring for the sick relative.

TASO provides basic material and medical support including eggs and milk for protein, oral rehydration salts to alleviate the effects of chronic diarrhea, and home care kits containing soap, antiseptic cream, and protective rubber gloves. These kits help families care for patients and avoid cross-infection through careless handling of body fluids.

Counseling sessions and home visits are carried out by more than 36 trained volunteers, reaching all levels of society—particularly families who cannot read government posters and leaflets. Many of TASO's volunteers are, themselves, HIV antibody positive or have lost relatives with AIDS.

In Africa, many people come from miles away for treatment and counseling. Often, they have just found out about their infection and are still in shock. This puts considerable pressure on the counselor. There is too much information to give all at once,

structures are strained, the social and welfare costs of helping children affected by the pandemic increase. Programs are now being developed to assist survivors, including orphaned children and the aged.

Figure 10.1 shows the reported prevalence of AIDS-related conditions in Rwanda, Tanzania, and Zimbabwe. Between 25 and 40 percent of patients with AIDS had active tuberculosis. In some sub-Saharan African countries, half of all people with newly diagnosed cases of tuberculosis are also HIV infected. In Tanzania,[29] for example, an effective tuberculosis control program, supported through collaboration with the International Union against Tuberculosis and Lung Diseases, had reduced the incidence of tuberculosis prior to the HIV epidemic. The spread of HIV since 1983, however, has brought a significant increase in tuberculosis incidence. By 1989, it was esti-

---

but you don't know when you'll see the person again.

Counseling people with HIV/AIDS about their future sex life is not easy. In Uganda, condoms are unpopular, and safer sex is not considered to be proper sex. Many men and women are in polygamous marriages. We have to advise these persons either to use a condom or to "stay away" from further sexual relationships.

The most difficult counseling situation is when a client refuses to tell a partner about the nature of his or her illness, and yet there is still a possibility that the partner is not infected. Some women—in trying to avoid telling their partner—say, "I'll keep away from him (sexually)." But this is virtually impossible. In this country it is men who decide when they want to make love.

Ours is a male-dominated society. Often relatives will encourage a man who appears fit and well to leave his wife with AIDS and find another, not realizing that he may pass the infection on to another woman. Local people recognize the symptoms of the illness AIDS, but they do not understand how a healthy-looking infected person could infect a sexual partner. Some women, and men, hope to run away from AIDS—to start a new life in a new place with a new family. We try to explain to HIV-infected women the problems associated with having more children in their situation. In some cases, a woman's husband has died of AIDS, and she doesn't know whether she has been infected (in fact, we don't advise people to take tests unless knowing the answer will definitely help them). TASO is developing a widow's project that will enable women who have lost their husbands to become economically independent.

In many countries, when someone is diagnosed HIV antibody positive, that's usually the end of the story—nobody wants to help. Through TASO, we hope to promote compassion and hope for people with AIDS and their families.

Percent

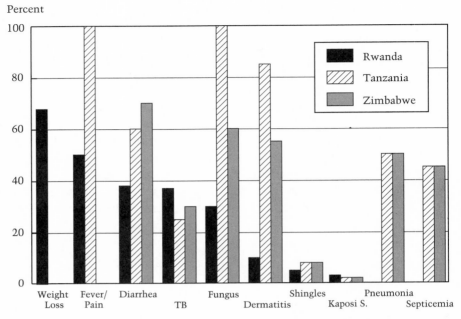

Figure 10.1. Prevalence of certain conditions in people with AIDS in three sub-Saharan countries, 1990-1991.
Source: *Tanzania AIDS assessment and planning study* (Washington D.C.: World Bank, 1992, forthcoming); D. Shepard and R. Bail, *Costs of care for persons with AIDS in Rwanda* (Geneva: WHO, 1991); Dr. Bent Jensen, personal communication (Zimbabwe, 1991).

mated that the number of new cases of tuberculosis was twice the number that would have been expected in the absence of HIV.[29]

The public health implications of combined TB/HIV are so serious that prophylactic treatment of tuberculosis deserves priority attention in countries where both are endemic. Studies in Kenya and Rwanda indicate that acute bacterial infections are also important causes of morbidity and mortality in HIV-infected persons. Studies are underway to determine if antibacterial interventions can reduce current and future morbidity and mortality.[19,30]

A second issue that has been given new urgency by the AIDS pandemic involves home care programs (Box 10.3). In developing countries, health care delivery systems, such as health centers and hospitals, have difficulty coping with the current and projected numbers of people with AIDS. Community- and home-based care programs increasingly are being considered for systematic expansion, as extensions of existing systems. Important considerations in developing such programs include selection of services, monitoring of quality control and patient satisfaction, availability of staff and financial resources, and effects on other health programs.

There is no standard model for home care. However, the basic idea in home care is to provide services—medical, psychosocial and welfare—to HIV-infected persons, people with AIDS, and their families through home visits. Some programs are connected to hospitals; others are entirely community-based.

A 1991 report on home care[17] analyzed 4 programs in Uganda and 2 programs in Zambia with respect to the resources needed to implement them and how they could be integrated into existing national AIDS programs. (See Tables 10.3 and 10.4.) All were administered by

---

Box 10.3: Home Care for Families with AIDS: New Role for Red Cross Volunteers

en Schietinger is a sultant in HIV policy and e for the AIDS Action uncil in the United States for Red Cross Societies rnationally.

In Rwanda, Red Cross volunteers have found a new role: teaching families how to care for people with AIDS and other chronic illnesses. The Rwanda Red Cross Home Care Project aims to prevent HIV transmission within the family and improve the quality of life for people with AIDS through better home care. Training is brief: after five days of preparation, including lessons in basic nursing skills and hygiene, the volunteers go back to their own communities throughout Rwanda.

Results are already being seen in the community. In one case, a volunteer noted that people were avoiding the house of a woman who was too sick to get out of bed. Wearing his Red Cross uniform to make a point, he helped the woman get out of bed, bathe, and dress in

fresh clothes. The impact on fearful neighbors was instantaneous. They began going to her house to help. Volunteers also provide education about AIDS. In the first 3 months of the program, 7 volunteers taught approximately 5,000 people about AIDS during meetings in schools, churches, and other public places.

The program is possible because of its low cost and its simplicity; because it does not require expensive medical supplies or foodstuffs, it can be implemented in a large area with a small budget. Two nurses in the central office provide ongoing supervision and guidance to the volunteers, who are teaching families in their own communities how to care for people with AIDS. The program demonstrates the effectiveness of using an existing infrastructure, such as the network of Red Cross volunteers throughout Rwanda.

Table 10.3: Elements of six selected home care programs, Uganda and Zambia, 1991

Services	Programs					
	CHIK	UTH	TASO-K	TASO-M	NSA	KIT
Administrative affiliation	NGO	Govt.-NGO[a]	NGO	NGO	NGO	NGO
Community initiated	No	No	Yes	Yes	No	No
Population served	Rural	Urban	Urban	Rural	Urban	Rural
Hospital or community based	Hospital	Hospital	Community	Community	Hospital	Hospital
Religious affiliation	Salvation Army	None	None	None	Catholic	Catholic

Source: Review of six HIV/AIDS home care programmes in Uganda and Zambia (Geneva: WHO/GPA, 1991).

Note: CHIK = Chikankata Program, Mazabuka, Zambia; UTH = University Teaching Hospital, Lusaka, Zambia; TASO-K = The AIDS Support Organization, Kampala, Uganda; TASO-M = The AIDS Service Organization, Mazaka, Uganda; NSA = Nsambya Mobile Home Care, Kampala, Uganda; KIT = Education Programme and Pastoral Care and Counselling Programme, Kitovu, Uganda.

Note: NGO = nongovernmental organization.

a. Program initiated in a government institution but now legally under the control of an NGO.

and dependent on nongovernmental organizations for materials and hospital-based support. All programs provided medical and nursing care, counseling, and material support. Four of the 6 had their own transport for use in home visits (four-wheel drive transport is essential for service delivery).

Typical medical supplies involved and material support provided in the 6 programs are listed in Table 10.5. There have been several unsuccessful attempts to develop essential drug lists. Four of 6 programs carried condoms, although the study showed that it is difficult to provide an adequate supply of condoms. None of the programs provided AZT. Material support included a number of items for physical comfort and nutritional needs, and even cash to initiate income-generating projects.

No formal studies have been reported on service quality or patient

Table 10.4: Components of six selected home care programs, Uganda and Zambia, 1991

	Programs					
Services	CHIK	UTH	TASO-K	TASO-M	NSA	KIT
Medical and nursing	X	X	X	X	X	X
Counseling	X	X	X	X		X
Pastoral	X		X[a]		X	X
Social support and welfare						
Transport		X	X		X	X
Income generation			X			X
Material support	X	X[a]	X	X	X	X
Relaxation class			X			
Social contact			X	X		X

Source: Review of Six HIV/AIDS Home Care Programmes in Uganda and Zambia (Geneva: WHO/GPA, 1991).

Note: CHIK = Chikankata Program, Mazabuka, Zambia; UTH = University Teaching Hospital, Lusaka, Zambia; TASO-K = The AIDS Support Organization, Kampala, Uganda; TASO-M = The AIDS Service Organization, Mazaka, Uganda; NSA = Nsambya Mobile Home Care, Kampala, Uganda; KIT = Education Programme and Pastoral Care and Counselling Programme, Kitovu, Uganda.

a. When available.

satisfaction.[17] However, the staff of the Chikankata program in Zambia reported that 95 percent of the 267 patients they visited over a two-year period preferred home visits to hospital care. In general, staff in all the home care programs indicated that patients and their families were satisfied with the programs.

A third serious issue in Africa is the increasing number of children of HIV-infected persons, many of whom are orphans, in need of assistance.[1,25,31] Although most are not infected with HIV, they nevertheless suffer from the impact of HIV. Their needs for clothing, guardians, education, freedom from discrimination, and health care make them particularly vulnerable.[31]

A report published in 1991 examined the needs of children in Rwanda, Uganda, Tanzania, and Zambia.[31] In most but not all cases studied, the extended family cared for orphaned children. To encourage this trend, a program in Rwanda was developed to help sensitize

Table 10.5: Medications, medical supplies, and material support typically provided in six selected home care programs, Uganda and Zambia, 1991

Medications	Medical supplies	Material support
Antibiotics	Medicine cups	Porridge (high energy)
Antifungals	Disposable syringes	Powdered milk
Antivirals	Disposable needles	Eggs
Antidiarrhoeals	Disinfectant for injuries	Soap for bathing and washing
Oral rehydration solution	Specimen bottles and cotton	Cocoa mix
Analgesics	Antiseptic solution for wound cleaning	Glucose drink
Antituberculosis drugs	Soap	Linen
Antimalarials	Bucket for water (for staff)	Rice
Multivitamins	Towels	Baby food
Herbal medicines	Bedding (sheets)	Baby formula
Iron	Disposable sheets	Soya bean
Cough syrup	Bedpans, urinals	Sugar
Antiemetics	Plastic sheets	Other donated foods
Antirheumatics	Dressings	Blankets
Antihistimines	Bandages	Clothing
Gentian violet paint	Gloves	School fees
Topical skin ointment	Aprons	Petty cash
Contraceptives	Condoms	Money for starting income-generating projects
Bronchodilators	Crutches	Labor charges
Sedatives		Bibles, rosaries

Source: Review of Six HIV/AIDS Home Care Programmes in Uganda and Zambia (Geneva: WHO/GPA, 1991).

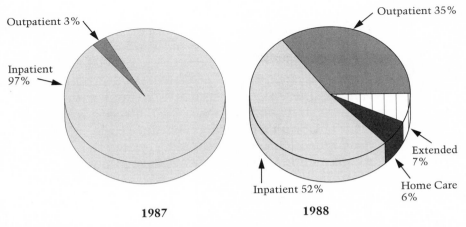

Outpatient 3%

Inpatient 97%

Outpatient 35%

Extended 7%

Home Care 6%

Inpatient 52%

1987   **1988**

Figure 10.2. Expenditure patterns on AIDS, San Juan, Puerto Rico.
Source: Y. Kouri, et al., "Improving the cost-effectiveness of AIDS health care in San Juan, Puerto Rico," *Lancet* 337 (1991): 1397-99

families to accept a child, either as part of the extended family or as a foster child.[31]

A study in Uganda by the United Nations Children's Fund (UNICEF) estimated that there were more than 600,000 orphans in the country by the end of 1989. This large number reflects the impact of war as well as AIDS and other diseases.

Central and South America

Central and South America present a complex mixture of more affluent and poorer communities.

A study of the costs associated with AIDS in Puerto Rico shows the potential impact of strategic changes for meeting medical needs.[32] The new plan emphasized outpatient, home care and hospice services, and creation of a rapid diagnostic laboratory. This approach shifted expenses dramatically between 1987 and 1988. In 1987, 97 percent of expenses were for inpatient care with no home-based care or hospice services available. By 1988, inpatient care had decreased to about half of total costs, while outpatient care increased from 3 percent of expenditures to 35 percent; 13 percent of expenditures were for home-based care and extended care. In addition, the average length of inpatient hospital stays decreased from 22.3 days in 1987 to 11.3 days in 1988. This led to a 75 percent decrease in inpatient costs per AIDS patient, freeing resources to fund additional outpatient services, education, research, and other activities. (See Figure 10.2.) This remarkable experience demonstrated that even with severe resource constraints, strategic planning of cost-effective services can improve the range of care for AIDS patients, reduce costs, and address AIDS patient management issues.[32] It should be noted, however, that Puerto Rico receives some assistance for AIDS care from the U.S. Federal Government, including limited amounts of AZT.

Southeast Asia

HIV is becoming a major issue for countries in Southeast Asia. Yet the recent onset of the pandemic and the current low number of AIDS cases provide the opportunity to prepare actively for meeting the care challenge with innovative programs.

As the large numbers of HIV-infected persons progress to AIDS, there will be an enormous increase in demand for health care services. For example, although Thailand had reported only about 150 cases of AIDS as of January 1, 1992, an estimated 400,000 Thais are now HIV infected. Even with the conservative assumption that only 20 percent of currently HIV-infected people will progress to AIDS within 5 years, this would result in a total of at least 80,000 new AIDS cases in Thailand between 1992 and 1996.

During 1990, the few people with AIDS were treated in special wards of infectious disease hospitals, such as Bamrasnaradura Hospital in Bangkok. No information was available about provision of care for persons with AIDS in other health care delivery settings. The Thai government planned to add AIDS wings—consisting of 50 to 60 beds per wing—to selected provincial hospitals in order to meet inpatient demand. Although this response was potentially viable in the short term, it was expensive and did not address serious resource issues that would arise in the future. Planning is now being undertaken to address the range of complex and longer-term issues associated with the projected increase in number of AIDS cases during the next decade. In India, the dramatic increase in the numbers of HIV-infected persons could also have a devastating impact on health care delivery systems.

INDUSTRIALIZED COUNTRY EXPERIENCE

Few studies have closely examined the types of care and locations of service delivery for people with AIDS in industrialized countries. In North America, Europe, Japan, and Australia a wide range of care is generally available[7,33] at a variety of locations accessible to groups or individuals in need.[7,12,34] However, access to care in industrialized countries is not uniform, and many persons with AIDS do not receive the full range of needed services. In the United States, for example, major problems exist with regard to access to health care for the large number of individuals with no health insurance.

Care in the United States is decentralized, with each state free to regulate health care delivery. There is no typical U.S. model of care. By contrast, France, Switzerland, the United Kingdom, and the Nordic countries have a more centralized, coordinated, and integrated approach to managing and delivering health care.

In Europe, people with AIDS often receive medical care in hospital wards, usually in internal medicine or infectious diseases departments. However, outpatient and community care, hospital-based outreach teams, and hospital-based extension services are becoming increasingly available.[5,6] Services are usually coordinated through social service organizations with significant involvement of private voluntary organizations and nongovernmental organizations. Outpatient and home visit services are widely used for delivery of drugs, counseling, and social welfare services.[35] Several trends in industrialized countries have been noted. First, there has been a decided shift away from inpatient hospital care to outpatient care. This trend is expected to continue. Outpatient care is generally less expensive and is becoming more feasible with increased ability to manage opportunistic infections in these settings. Earlier HIV diagnosis and the advent of such drugs as AZT and aerosolized pentamidine have prolonged and improved the quality of life for people with AIDS.

Outpatient care can raise awareness about the ongoing needs of people with AIDS. It can also reduce the cost per patient, as seen in France,[34] the United Kingdom,[34] and the United States.[12] Simultaneously, duration of inpatient stays is reportedly being reduced, thereby returning persons with AIDS to their homes and personal support systems.

In many industrialized countries, AIDS has provided a positive impetus for change in health care systems. The need for outpatient care, home care, and peer support has stimulated development of systems that benefit all persons with terminal diseases.[36] For example, AIDS has spurred development of hospices in the United Kingdom[6] and stimulated creation of NGOs and other voluntary organizations in Austria, the Netherlands, Spain, Sweden, the United Kingdom, and the United States. These organizations provide care primarily in the areas of psychological counseling and support, nursing, and long-term welfare support, including housing.[6,10]

Unlike developing countries, industrialized countries are generally able to provide comprehensive medical care for persons with HIV/AIDS. Currently, hospital bed capacity is not expected to be a major problem. However, AIDS must still compete for resources with other diseases and, more broadly, with other health programs and other national expenditures. Even in industrialized countries, important challenges remain. Psychosocial and welfare needs must be reviewed constantly to ensure that comprehensive and coordinated sup-

---

Box 10.4: Burnout among HIV/AIDS Health Care Providers

Adapted from statements by health care professionals in the United States, Brazil, Zambia, and Rwanda.

"Sometimes I feel while working with AIDS like the sons of Omulu-Obuluaie who forget their personal needs, limits and wounds to take care of others."—A Brazilian physician speaking of his eight years in the AIDS epidemic.[a]

As the number of people affected by AIDS continues to grow, the emotional, psychological, and physical toll on AIDS professional caregivers—physicians, nurses, counselors—must also increase. Increasingly, the individuals and institutions providing care to persons with HIV and AIDS are confronting what is commonly known as *burnout*. From São Paolo and San Francisco to Paris and Lusaka, AIDS health care professionals face the unique demands and stresses created by the pandemic. All must cope daily with the risk of accidental exposure, continuing social stigmas associated with the disease (and for those who care for it), inadequate resources, the lack of treatments and a cure, complex ethical and legal issues, and the devastating impact of watching young patients die. Some practitioners may also be dealing with the impact of AIDS in their own lives, through illness and death of friends, colleagues, and partners or because they themselves are infected or ill.

The effects of burnout are both personal and institutional. Burned out caregivers may experience difficulty functioning (professionally and personally), poor health, and

port is provided, to identify unmet needs, to monitor available services, and to ensure that all affected individuals and groups receive needed care. As HIV/AIDS evolves in industrialized countries, and as already marginalized groups are increasingly affected, the challenges of providing care will become more complex and difficult.

In summary, most countries have increasing difficulties in meeting some needs of people with HIV/AIDS. AIDS typically highlights the deficiencies in existing national health care systems.[37] The ability of those systems to respond must be strengthened today, as demand for the array of health care services and support will increase.

■■■■ . . .

IMPACTS AND CHALLENGES—GLOBAL VIEW

It is an enormous global challenge to meet the full range of needs of people with HIV/AIDS. As of early 1992, over 2.5 million AIDS cases were estimated to have occurred in adults. Of these adults, as many as 90 percent had died. Unfortunately, the medical, psychosocial, and social welfare needs of only a minority of these ill people were ade-

---

psychological distress. Where staff burnout is high, institutions suffer low morale, communication breakdown, increased staff conflict, decreased productivity, absenteeism, and higher turnover. Furthermore, when staff attempt to distance themselves emotionally, become cynical, or limit contact, AIDS patients and their families may also suffer.

Initial strategies to address burnout include creating formal and informal support groups, developing coping and stress management skills, and providing professional development opportunities. All help an individual bolster or renew his or her inner resources. Recently, there has been much discussion about institutional responses that can support both patients and staff. These changes may

not require the costly overhaul of established systems. Such institutional responses include: restructuring work distribution, benefits, and time schedules; improving communication at all levels; and acknowledging the difficulties facing staff.

Efforts to deal with burnout generally have been responsive rather than anticipatory. Few studies have examined the extent of the cost of burnout or evaluated the effectiveness of preventive measures. Health care systems must begin to prepare for the worsening of the pandemic and the resulting increase in burnout among caregivers.

---

a. Dr. Maria E. L. Fernandes, personal communication, March 23, 1992.

quately addressed. The vast majority in developing countries lacked access to adequate medical care; and paradoxically, some with medical care were without psychosocial care or attention to their social welfare needs. Societal systems, including health care and social service systems, were tested to the limit of their capacity and their ability to adapt and innovate in the face of expanded and new needs.

Yet by the year 2000, a tenfold increase in HIV infections and AIDS is anticipated: as many as 110 million adults will have become HIV infected, and more than 25 million new cases of AIDS in adults will have occurred. To prevent catastrophic gaps between needs and services, countries must prepare now. Lessons about cost reduction, effective and efficient service integration, and evaluation of needs and services must be applied to meet the future care challenge of the 1990s.

--- . . .

IMPACTS AND CHALLENGES OF HIV/AIDS IN INDUSTRIALIZED COUNTRIES

In quantitative terms, meeting the medical needs of people with AIDS will not have a major effect on the health care delivery systems of industrialized countries, at least in the foreseeable future. For example, in the United States, all HIV- and AIDS-related care accounted for less than 1 percent of health care expenditures in 1991.[12] In addition, the current oversupply of hospital beds in both Europe and North America and the trend toward outpatient treatment make it unlikely that these systems will be overwhelmed by the requirement of AIDS care. However, the need to optimize care for HIV-infected persons poses a qualitative challenge to all industrialized countries.

In Europe, social welfare and national insurance systems provide substantial coverage for AIDS care. The most important national issues to be resolved center on the types of services to be delivered and location of service delivery.[14]

In all countries there are unresolved national issues concerning vulnerable populations. For example, injection drug users may not have access to social networks that can provide support and care. Little work has been done to assess the needs of HIV-infected persons in prisons. Other issues for all countries include reducing discrimination, prejudice, and legal impediments. Many persons face housing and job discrimination, or health professionals reluctant to provide care.

Discussions with people with HIV/AIDS indicate that significant work remains to be done in meeting the medical, psychosocial, and social welfare needs of those who are infected. These needs include developing innovative medical interventions, improving the response of health care providers, and improving both quality of care and quality of life. Although medical needs are more tangible than psychosocial and social welfare concerns, the latter are equally pressing and may become the dominant questions of AIDS care in years to come. Furthermore, improving HIV/AIDS care may lead to broader reevaluation and strengthening of existing care systems for other chronic diseases and conditions.

· · ·

IMPACTS AND CHALLENGES OF HIV/AIDS IN DEVELOPING COUNTRIES

Whereas industrialized countries have the infrastructure, staff, and financial resources that are generally adequate to provide HIV/AIDS medical care (if equitably distributed), developing countries face a much less promising future. A 1990 study suggested that health care systems in some sub-Saharan African countries will not be able to provide significant amounts of medical care for future AIDS cases. Many countries will have to make painful choices between supporting AIDS care and care for persons with other diseases.[38]

AIDS patient care issues in the developing world can be summarized in two areas. First, AIDS care will require a complex set of responses from already overstressed economies and health care systems. AIDS strikes persons in their most productive economic years and requires medical, psychosocial, and social welfare support for patients and their families. These services may not exist in current systems. Human and financial resources allocated to AIDS care could lead to reduced food for family members, reduced income as those with jobs remain at home to care for AIDS patients, and reduced funds for school fees for children. As a result, children may leave school, become malnourished through neglect, or be abandoned.[14] (See Chapter 6 on the "Demographic, Economic, and Social Impact of AIDS.")

Second, human and financial resource constraints, lack of trained personnel, and limits in absorptive capacity of programs will limit the magnitude of response. In addition, the current economic uncertainties and problems in industrialized countries may eventually reduce the size of their contribution in support of health activities in developing countries. Economic issues include the global economic recession, shifts in resources to support conflicts such as the recent war in the Gulf, and the ongoing support for restructuring Eastern Europe and the former Soviet Union.

Developing countries and the communities, families, and individuals in those countries face an uphill struggle in their attempts to make more efficient use of existing resources. Even in the absence of formal planning at the national level, decisions will inevitably be made concerning resource allocation for AIDS and other diseases. However, crisis is not an excuse for a lack of planning. As shown in Puerto Rico, much can be done to obtain more from existing resources.

NEXT STEPS

Industrialized and developing countries can learn from each other to understand better the needs of HIV-infected people and to develop innovative solutions to meeting those needs. Although different levels of infrastructure development and amounts of resources exist, there are many global similarities.

In both industrialized and developing countries, resources are constrained, and choices must be made regarding which needs will be met and how they will be met. Inevitably, tradeoffs will be required.

All countries have both formal and informal or alternative systems for providing medical and other types of care. These informal systems draw on health care workers, traditional healers, families, loved ones, and others to meet the needs of persons affected by HIV. A sensible approach to the AIDS pandemic must integrate the needs of the affected and the potential offered by diverse groups of individuals, organizations, and institutions to meet those needs. Planning will be required at all administrative levels to assess needs, develop interventions, and provide adequate training, support, and infrastructure. A critical, and, in some ways, new dimension of HIV/AIDS care is the vital role of HIV-infected people and people with AIDS. They must be involved in defining the needs, developing innovative and responsive programs, and evaluating the efficiency and effectiveness of strategies and programs. The ability of a health and social system, of governments and society, to access and involve HIV-infected people and people with AIDS will be critical for optimal outcomes, regardless of the resources available. Resistance may be encountered among health and social service professionals to this kind of extensive and active involvement by "patients." Nevertheless, active leadership can help overcome this problem; people directly affected by the epidemic represent an extremely important resource and can contribute enormously to all phases of care.

STRENGTHENING ASSESSMENT TOOLS

In the future, a number of items can be monitored to (1) provide information to strengthen our collective ability to meet needs and (2) evaluate our progress. Such indicators are essential for determining the dimensions of the gap that exists between what is needed and what has been provided. Types of indicators include estimated numbers of persons with different types of needs, unit cost of meeting needs at different locations of service delivery, and national costs of meeting care needs.

Similarly, indicators are needed to assist both individual and collective efforts in measuring the quality of services provided and the quality of life of persons receiving services. Indexes, such as the Medical Outcome Study, must be developed and applied to ensure that the wide range of health needs are addressed.

Finally, because the needs of HIV-infected persons and persons with AIDS are likely to change over time, mechanisms are needed to assess these changes. It is important that health care delivery systems be sensitized and responsive as part of a long-term commitment.

BROADENING ACCESS TO CARE

One issue that consistently arises is the inequity of access to and use of services for segments of the HIV/AIDS-infected population. No community or country has yet succeeded in ensuring universal equity. Indicators are needed that are sensitive to specific populations, who may have limited or no access to services. For example, in the United States this could include tracking persons with HIV/AIDS to determine whether they have health insurance, what type of care they receive, and whether a definable relationship exists between the two.

Throughout the world, women bear an increasing individual and social burden of HIV/AIDS. Not only does gender bias lead to reduced access to care and support, but in most countries, women are also expected to nurture and care for AIDS-infected family members. This will likely reduce total family income as women are less able to spend time working outside the home.

Other vulnerable groups include the poor and socially marginalized groups. For example, in many countries HIV-infected injection drug users and poor persons with HIV and AIDS are likely to have no health insurance or social support networks, and few opportunities for employment. The result will be less access to all types of care and support.

Box 10.5: Quality of Care

To measure the impact of care on quality of life an evaluation scale must be available.[a] Most analyses focus on medical treatment and use scales that measure changes in various aspects of health status (e.g., individual comfort, mobility). Well-known scales include the *Karnofsky Index, Sickness Impact Profile, Symptom Distress Scale, Spitzer Quality of Life Index, McMaster Health Index,* and *Nottingham Health Profile*.[a,b] These and other indicators require information clarifying what types of care are covered (medical, psychological), how health status is measured (by patients or by care providers), and how different aspects of care are compared and weighted relative to each other.[b]

The *Medical Outcome Study* (MOS) has recently been proposed as a reliable quality of life measure for persons with HIV infection and AIDS. The MOS is a questionnaire in which patients rate their perception of 20 criteria, including physical functioning, role functioning, social functioning, mental functioning, health perceptions, and pain. The scale is especially sensitive to symptoms associated with HIV and AIDS.[a]

a. Wachtel et al., "Quality of life in persons with Human Immunodeficiency Virus infection: Measurement by the medical outcomes study instrument," *Annals of Internal Medicine* 16(2)(1992):129–37.
b. M. Drummond, "Output measurement for resource allocation decisions in health care," *Oxford Review of Economic Policy* 5(1)(1989):59–74.

PROMOTING INTERNATIONAL COOPERATION

In order to bolster individual and collective efforts it is vital to develop mechanisms that facilitate communication and exchange of knowledge and experience among nations and interested groups. For example, dialogue between health systems in Africa and Asia could provide an impetus for innovation and help nations build effective care systems, based on what has been learned from experience in these and other regions.

The few cost studies done to date indicate that the annual cost of medical care for a person with AIDS is about equal to the national per capita gross national product. Over the next decade, as the number of persons with AIDS grows, even the richest nations will face serious debate about which needs will be met and how they will be financed (see Chapter 11, "The Cost of AIDS Care and Prevention"). In many developing countries the magnitude of costs and impacts on health infrastructure, such as availability of hospital beds and drugs, has already reached dramatic levels. This could reverse advances made in health status in recent years.

A global response is needed to identify and help meet the challenges posed by the needs of people with HIV/AIDS. Support to developing countries that only covers prevention activities is not a humane or equitable response.

The world continues to wrestle with ways to respond to the pandemic. There are no ideal, yet practical solutions. The challenge is clear: What type of societies do we want? The AIDS pandemic is a complex, but ultimately manageable crisis that provides an opportunity to illuminate, both individually and collectively, the depth of our humanity.

CHAPTER ELEVEN

. . . .

The Cost of AIDS Care and Prevention

Is chapter was written
d researched by
arles Cameron, an
ernational health
onomist, with the
rticipation of Julia
epard, a management
nsultant. Both are
sed in Boston,
assachusetts.

Disease, disability, and death have always had a profound impact on individuals, families, and societies. Curbing the course of epidemic diseases and mitigating their impact have costs—both in human and economic terms. The cost of research into a vaccine or curative treatment has already been discussed. The question remains, how much has the AIDS epidemic cost in terms of care and prevention? Determining the cost of care and prevention is of growing importance to individuals and societies as the numbers of infections with HIV and cases of AIDS continue to increase in an uncertain global economic climate. Estimating the overall cost of care and prevention responses to AIDS has proved elusive so far, as only sporadic data from different countries and communities have been available. Yet such estimates are essential for decision makers and planners, who need this information to allocate resources now and in the future. Thus, assessing the cost of AIDS care and prevention is more than an exhaustive matter of global accounting. It is of vital importance in shaping the response to a global epidemic whose cost is increasing at a dramatic rate.

Why has estimating the global cost of AIDS care and prevention proved so difficult? The answer goes to the heart of the difficulties that AIDS presents to individuals, communities, and governments. AIDS funding is often integrated with that of other health and social programs, making it difficult to attribute expenditures specifically. Furthermore, the cost of AIDS today is born by a wide range of individuals, groups, and institutions. The needs of people with HIV/AIDS are diverse and changing: tracking a specific cost from each source to specific expenditures is difficult.

Costs associated with HIV/AIDS can be divided into four categories: *direct personal costs* to individuals, such as payments for medical treatment or insurance; *direct nonpersonal costs* associated with care and prevention activities for institutions, such as education and training programs; *indirect personal costs* that represent lost individual income or the cost of a person's time who is caring for a person who is ill; and, finally, *indirect nonpersonal costs* (or social opportunity costs) representing the loss of opportunities to treat other diseases in order to respond to AIDS.

The present analysis concentrates on the estimation of direct personal and direct nonpersonal costs, that is, on medical treatment and national prevention programs. What do these costs comprise?

■■■■■ . . .

THE COST OF PREVENTION: NONPERSONAL DIRECT COSTS

The cost of HIV/AIDS prevention varies widely around the world.* About 90 percent of the global resources mobilized for prevention are in North America and Western and Eastern Europe, areas that represent only 20 percent of the world's population and have 16 percent of the world's HIV-infected people (as of January 1, 1992). Expenditures in sub-Saharan Africa are a stark contrast: even though these countries contain about 10 percent of the world's population and 66 percent of the world's HIV-infected population, their proportion of global prevention spending is only 2.8 percent. In Southeast and North East Asian countries, the discrepancies are even more ominous: with more than half the world's population and a rapidly rising number of HIV-in-

---

*As part of the *AIDS in the World* survey of 38 countries, questions were asked about national AIDS program budgets, including the estimated budget for prevention activities. Using these figures, weighted per capita averages of prevention budgets were calculated for each of the 10 Geographic Areas of Affinity (GAAs) based on total budgets and total population. The per capita budget for prevention measure was useful for extrapolation of prevention budgets to the GAA level. Table 11.2 shows a summary of the prevention budgets for each GAA.

Table 11.1: Types of care costs

	Personal	*Nonpersonal*
Direct	Medical, counseling, and psychological care	Institutional costs for care and prevention
Indirect	Personal opportunity costs related to loss of income, the value of time associated with care provided by friends and family	Social opportunity costs of investing in AIDS versus other diseases

fected people, these countries spend less than 1 percent of the world's prevention resources (see Table 11.2).

The variation of per capita spending throughout the world is dramatic. For example, in the 7 European countries included in the *AIDS in the World* survey, prevention resources in 1991 ranged from less than $1 to over $3 per capita, with an average population-weighted resource value of $1.18. An enormous difference separates the industrialized from the developing world. Only in three geographic Areas of Affinity did 1991 per capita spending on HIV prevention exceed one U.S. dollar: North America, Western Europe, and Oceania. Less than $0.10 was spent per capita in Latin America, sub-Saharan Africa, Eastern Europe, the South East Mediterranean, and North East and Southeast Asia.

Prevention spending in North America exceeded the total amount spent for prevention in the rest of the world. In North America, approximately $2.70 was spent per capita in 1991 for prevention activities by the national AIDS programs. This figure represents only federal government spending and does not include that by lower levels of government, such as states and cities, nongovernmental organizations, the private sector, or individuals. Yet despite this relatively high level of spending, it still remains small when measured on a per capita basis. In the simplest of terms, annual federal spending per capita on prevention of North America in 1991 amounted to less than a month's supply of vitamins.

Such calculations can help us understand the magnitude of the social response to AIDS. Is the response equal to the need? Is there a

Table 11.2: Estimation of annual costs of prevention, 1991: Geographic Areas of Affinity and global totals

GAA/Country	1990 population (thousands)	Total NAP resources mobilized minus care and research (millions $U.S.)	Budget per capita ($U.S.)	Population weighted average by GAA ($U.S.)	Estimated 1990 population by GAA (thousands)	Total estimated cost by GAA (millions $U.S.)[a]	% of world population	% of world cost
1 North America				2.71	275,745	747.3	5.2	53.0
Canada	26,521	9.8	0.37					
United States	249,224	736.0	2.95					
2 Western Europe				1.18	435,312	513.7	8.2	36.4
France	56,138	75.9	1.35					
Germany	77,573	76.3	0.98					
Netherlands	14,951	20.3	1.36					
Norway	4,212	7.5	1.79					
Sweden	8,444	28.3	3.36					
Switzerland	6,609	8.9	1.35					
United Kingdom	57,237	113.6	1.99					
3 Oceania				2.23	26,199	58.4	0.5	4.2
Australia	16,873	37.6	2.23					
4 Latin America				0.03	414,207	12.4	7.8	0.7
Argentina	32,322	1.2	0.04					
Colombia	32,978	1.3	0.04					
Mexico	88,598	1.4	0.02					
5 Sub-Saharan Africa				0.07	526,745	36.9	10.0	2.8
Cameroon	11,833	2.5	0.21					
Congo	2,271	1.5	0.66					
Côte d'Ivoire	11,997	2.2	0.19					
Ethiopia	49,240	2.8	0.06					
Nigeria	108,542	0.1	0.00					
Rwanda	7,237	0.8	0.12					

Senegal	7,327	0.9	0.13					
Tanzania	27,317	1.0	0.04					
Uganda	18,794	1.2	0.06					
Zambia	8,452	5.5	0.65					
6 Caribbean				0.33	33,562	11.1	0.6	0.8
Trinidad and Tobago	1,281	0.3	0.23					
St. Lucia	150	0.1	0.60					
Haiti	6,513	2.2	0.35					
7 Eastern Europe				0.03	412,571	13.0	7.8	0.9
Czech and Slovak Republics	15,667	0.3	0.02					
Poland	38,423	4.8	0.12					
USSR	288,595	577.2	0.02					
8 South East Mediterranean				0.02	376,468	6.1	7.1	0.4
Egypt	52,426	2.5	0.10					
Morocco	25,061	0.7	0.01					
Pakistan	122,626							
9 North East Asia				>0.01	1,416,200	3.7	26.8	0.3
China	1,139,060	1.8	0.00					
Japan	123,460	1.5	0.01					
10 Southeast Asia				0.001	1,370,952	8.7	25.9	0.6
India	853,094	1.8	0.00					
Thailand	55,702	3.9	0.07					
Total[b]	3,703,809	1,472.5			5,289,951	1,780.8	100.0	100.0

Sources: 1990 population: World Bank, *World Development Report* (1991); 1991 national AIDS program (NAP) resources mobilized from *AIDS in the World* survey questions; 38 countries' NAP populations: *The sex and age distribution of population* (New York: United Nations Department of International Economics and Social Affairs, 1991).

Note: NAP = National AIDS program.

a. Based on weighted average costs x population.
b. Because of rounding, some totals may not match the actual sum of figures in the column.

right amount? What can reasonably be expected from prevention efforts? The results of the *AIDS in the World* survey suggest that around the world today, the level of spending on prevention remains far below the basic needs of societies and individuals. Annual amounts of resources allocated to prevention per person in 1991 ranged from $3.36 in Sweden to less than $0.01 in Nigeria. Even adjusting for the fact that a large segment of the population may not be targeted for prevention, these figures are very low. What results can be expected from such small investments?

Evaluating the effectiveness of this spending remains difficult because of the multifaceted and volatile features of HIV prevention. Determining the cost-effectiveness of prevention requires complex evaluation. This process is made even more difficult by the paucity of data on the impact of prevention activities carried out by national AIDS programs. Nevertheless, approximating the value of resources mobilized for prevention is one way of estimating the global response.

The *AIDS in the World* survey provided some indication of how 25 countries allocated resources for prevention and care in 1991 (see Table 11.3). Of 8 program areas, 4 related to prevention: sexual transmission, injection drug use (IDU), blood safety, and mother-to-child transmission. Generally, relatively more was allocated for the areas of prevention of sexual transmission and blood services. Very few or no funds were reported to have been allocated to the prevention of transmission of HIV from mother to infant and through injection drug use. The process of allocating and tracking resources, and reporting on their use, is in need of further refinement in both developing and industrialized countries.

THE COST OF CARE: PERSONAL DIRECT COST

The needs of people with AIDS are extensive and diverse, including medical, psychosocial, and social support services. These services must often be delivered in a variety of circumstances to changing groups of people. Care for people with HIV/AIDS is usually provided through existing health and social services. Programs have also been established in most countries to provide care in newly created facilities. Halfway homes in Thailand, nursing homes in California, sup-

Table 11.3: Allocation of resources by national AIDS programs to various prevention and care strategies in selected countries, 1990–91 (%)

Country[a]	Source[b]	Sexual transmission	Injection drug use	Blood safety	Mother to child	AIDS care	Total, prevention and care strategies
Latin America							
Mexico	R	37	0	46	5	12	100
Colombia	R	34	0	60	1	5	100
Average		35.3	0	52.7	3.2	8.9	
Sub-Saharan Africa							
Côte d'Ivoire	R	82	0	18	0	0	100
Cameroon	E	53	0	40	0	7	100
Tanzania	E	55	0	31	0	15	100[c]
Ethiopia	E	40	0	60	0	0	100[c]
Nigeria	E	51	0	24	0	24	100
Average		70.2	0	43.4	0	11.4	
South East Mediterranean							
Egypt	R	64	0	21	0	14	100[c]
Morocco	E	33	0	61	0	6	100
Pakistan	R	66	0	34	0	0	100
Average		54.6	0	38.8	0	6.6	
Other Areas							
Thailand	R	17	0	79	0	4	100
Australia	R	28	11	8	0	53	100
Sweden	R	75	14	0	0	11	100

a. These countries were selected on the basis of completeness of data from 38 countries surveyed by *AIDS in the World.*

b. Percentages of resource allocation to strategies were communicated by national AIDS program managers, based on reports (R) or, in the absence of reports, on program managers' best estimates (E). As figures were provided in combination with financial information and other program elements (including management and research), rates were indexed to a denominator that included only prevention and care strategies.

c. Because of rounding, numbers do not sum to 100%.

Table 11.4: Comparative cost of AIDS inpatient care in selected countries

GAA/Country	Year of study	Direct[a] medical cost/year ($U.S.)	Per capita GNP 1986–1988 ($U.S.)	Cost/per capita GNP	Study references
1 United States	1991	32,000	19,840	161%	Ref. 20
Canada	1983	33,900	16,960	200%	Ref. 6
2 Switzerland	1989	57,000	27,500	207%	Ref. 43
United Kingdom	1987–89	25,000–30,000	12,810	195–234%	Re.f 48, 50
France	1987	40,416	16,090	251%	Ref. 48, 54
Germany	1987	25,900	18,480	140%	Ref. 6
(Federal Rep.)		22,100		120%	Ref. 6
Greece	1988	38,482	4,800	802%	Ref. 48
3 Australia	1986	26,400	12,340	214%	Ref. 6
4 Brazil	1987	18,100[b]	2,160	838%	Ref. 6
Mexico	1990	1,430	1,990	72%	Ref. 14
		7,350	1,990	369%	
5 Rwanda	1990	358	320	112%	Ref. 2
Tanzania	1990	290	160	181%	Ref. 55
Zaire	1988	132–1,585	170	78–932%	Ref. 56
Zambia	1991	374	390	96%	Ref. 8
6 Barbados	1990	4,550	6,370	71%	Ref. 15
Puerto Rico[c]	1988	3,869	6,010	64%	Ref. 13
9 Japan	1987	161,945	21,020	770%	Ref. 58
10 Thailand	1990	1,312	1,230	107%	Ref. 9
	1991	658–1,016	1,230	54–83%	Ref. 57

Source: AIDS in the World, 1992. GNP derived from United Nations Development Program, *Human Development Report, 1991;* and World Bank, *World Development Report, (1991).*

a. Principally medical care, but in some cases also includes psychosocial care.

b. Mean lifetime costs.

c. The Commonwealth of Puerto Rico was studied separately from the United States.

port centers in privately rented apartments in Paris, and decentralized community-based care in Zambia and Uganda have all been created at the initiative of AIDS services organizations. Such initiatives, however, reach only a small number of people in need. The cost of providing care is analyzed below in two broad contexts, that of developing and industrialized countries. In developing countries, health care systems are commonly unable to meet the demand, and often critically short of financial and human resources and structures. In industrialized countries, the availability of services is generally greater, although access to services is not universal.

DEVELOPING COUNTRIES

Most cost studies in developing countries have focused on medical care alone, rather than including psychosocial or social welfare costs. Therefore, costs used in this analysis, by reflecting medical care, underestimate the total cost of meeting care needs. Overall, annual direct medical care costs ranged from 60 to 80 percent of per capita gross national product (GNP) in Mexico, Barbados, Puerto Rico, and low estimates for Zaire, to several times per capita GNP in some developing countries (Brazil, high estimates for Zaire). (See Table 11.4.) It should be noted that in almost all cases it is difficult to evaluate cost studies because of differences in methodologies, quality of data collected, currency values, and level of analysis.

Sub-Saharan Africa

In most countries, the costs of medical treatment vary according to the location of service delivery. This situation is particularly evident in sub-Saharan Africa. Costs of nursing care in Tanzania, for example, can range over six levels.[1] Generally, the more remote the location from central facilities, the lower the cost of care. Care at a reference hospital in major cities can cost more than 20 times as much as care provided at a dispensary and 50 times as much as home-based care provided in villages. However, it is difficult to determine which services are being provided, differences in quality or how well needs are being met among the different locations (see Figure 11.1).

Inpatient care is a relatively expensive way to deliver care for

Cost in Tanzanian Shillings (1$US=200Tsh [1990])

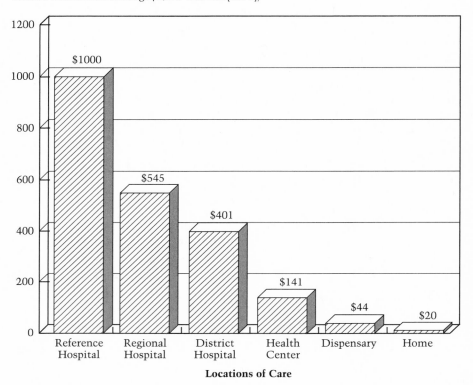

Figure 11.1. Average daily AIDS care costs,* by location of care, Tanzania, 1990.
*Average daily costs exclude drug costs.
Source: K. Pallangyo and R. Laing, *Background study on alternative approaches to managing the opportunistic illnesses* (Washington, DC: World Bank, 1990).

treatment of most diseases, including AIDS. In 1991, a study examined the types and costs of inpatient care for Rwanda.[2] The study showed that for the reference hospital examined, only five percent of costs were attributable to drugs and 18 percent for medical personnel. The remaining 77 percent represented indirect staff and general costs including overhead. In the university hospital studied, about 33 percent of costs were for drugs and personnel; two-thirds of costs were for indirect support. Neither location provided antiretroviral drugs.

Thus, specific clinical procedures and amounts of drugs given did not significantly affect total costs.

In Rwanda, the same study found that the cost per hospitalization for AIDS in 1990 ranged between $92 and $397. Assuming 1.7 hospitalizations per year, annual costs for a person with AIDS ranged from $156 to $675. Over 90 percent of total costs were for inpatient care, and public funds accounted for about 92 percent of lifetime costs. As the 1990 per capita GNP for Rwanda was $320, the cost of inpatient care ranged from 48 percent to 206 percent of per capita GNP.[3] A review of other studies indicated lifetime inpatient costs of people with AIDS in many African countries at about $325 and outpatient costs at approximately $33, for a total of $358 per patient.[4] Inpatient costs were approximately equal to per capita GNP.[5]

An attempt was made to estimate the hospital costs for projected AIDS cases in Rwanda. Assuming that about 30 percent of AIDS patients receive hospital-based care and that each case costs an average of $197 per admission, a significant increase in demand for hospital-based care is anticipated during the next few years. In 1988, AIDS patients accounted for only about two percent of Rwanda's hospital budget. However, by 1994, this will jump to over 11 percent of the nation's projected hospital budget (see Figure 11.2).

Several important policy implications emerged from this study. Overall, the cost of AIDS-related care is probably much higher, due to under-reporting of AIDS cases, the cost of outpatient care, and care for people who are infected with HIV but who do not have AIDS. The amounts spent on drugs, although substantial, were relatively small compared with other hospital costs. A reduction in costs per patient might be realized if treatment were more decentralized to district health centers where personnel and overhead are likely to be lower than in urban hospitals. For example, decentralization of tuberculosis treatment could reduce the length of inpatient stay, which represents the major component of treatment costs for AIDS patients. Although ambulatory and home care were not the primary focus of the study, patients reported that they would prefer non-hospital-based care. The main reason for accepting hospitalization was a perception that it was necessary in order to receive needed drugs. The question remains, can decentralized facilities and methods provide adequate quality care?

In sub-Saharan Africa, lifetime costs are assumed to equal annual

Percentage of National Hospital Budget

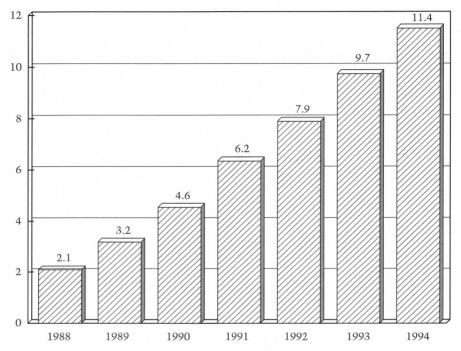

Figure 11.2. Cost of hospital-based AIDS care as percentage of national AIDS budget, Rwanda.
Source: D. Shepard and R. Bail, *Cost of care for persons with AIDS in Rwanda*, Consultant's Report, Global Programme on AIDS, WHO, Geneva (1991).

costs because of the short time between AIDS diagnosis and death. In addition, since annual per capita GNP approximates annual care costs, as indicated by studies in Africa, annual per capita GNP is a reasonable surrogate for expected inpatient hospitalization costs for each AIDS patient in this region.[6,7] On average, in sub-Saharan African countries, costs are estimated at $393 per year per person based on cost studies for countries where these have been conducted, and on per capita GNP as a surrogate for costs in other countries.

Home Care Costs: The Chikankata Hospital in Zambia provides an interesting example of a successful home-based care program. A 1992 study[8] reported on both the costs and the numbers of people receiving in-patient and home care for the periods 1988–89 and 1990–91, providing data to examine trends.

In 1988–89, 504 persons with AIDS received in-patient care at a unit cost of approximately $174—about 80 percent of the per capita GNP. Concurrently, 545 persons received care through the home-based program at a unit cost of about $85—half of the cost of in-patient care. By 1990–91, the unit cost of in-patient care had dropped to approximately $73 for the 372 people served. However, the number of people cared for through the home-based program grew by a third, yet unit costs dropped to $28. Figure 11.3 shows some of the products of home and in-patient care and their costs.

The trend appears to be increased use of home-based care. In addition, as Chikankata has gained experience in caring for persons with AIDS, the unit costs for both in-patient and home-based care have dropped, the latter remaining significantly less expensive than the former. The Chikankata study is a solid first step in better understanding what is being provided through home-based care programs, the resources needed, and their cost.

Another study examined the costs of home-based care for a district hospital in Zambia.[9] Costs were relatively high when capital costs and transport were included. Depreciation for vehicles represented about 38 percent of total program costs. The study reported that the costs of the entire home-based care program were about equal to 33 hospital days. As more experience is gained through similar costing studies for other home-based care programs, the cost effectiveness of home-care can be determined and used to allocate national and international resources.

Southeast Asia

Because HIV infection did not begin to spread in parts of Southeast Asia until the mid-1980s, the current number of AIDS cases is relatively small and few analyses of costs have been reported. In 1990, a small-scale study of treatment costs for AIDS patients was conducted at a reference hospital in Bangkok.[10] The average annual direct cost of diagnostic procedures and drug treatments was $1,312, of which 80 percent was for drugs. The antiviral drug zidovudine (AZT) accounted for two-thirds of total drug costs. In contrast, whereas antituberculosis treatment was included in 44 percent of all hospitalizations, it was relatively inexpensive, accounting for only 3 percent of drug costs.

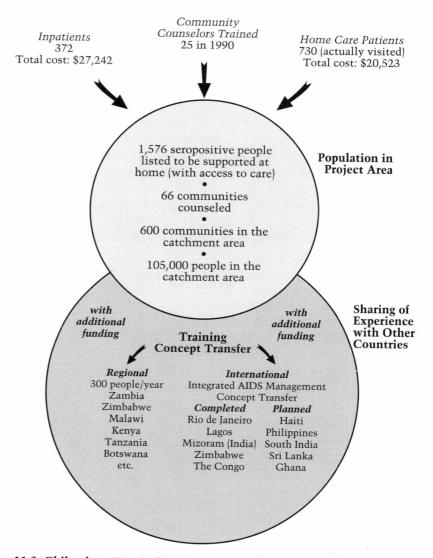

Figure 11.3. Chikankata Hospital AIDS care and prevention, 'products' of home and hospital care, October 1990–September 1991.
Source: I. Campbell, Medical Adviser, The Salvation Army International Headquarters, London. Presentation to the Congressional Forum on HIV/AIDS, Washington, DC, June 1992.

Table 11.5: Per person AIDS care expenditures in Thailand, 1991

	Range of costs:	
Location of care	Low	High
Inpatient		
Costs per day (material and labor)	$18	$22
Capital costs per day[a]	$1.4	$1.8
Patient days per episode	20	25
Drug cost per episode	$40	$60
Episodes per year	1.5	1.5
Percentage receiving treatment	20–60%	30–70%
Total annual cost	$642	$984
Outpatient		
Total cost per visit	$5.20	$6.40
Visit per year	3	5
Percentage receiving treatment	30–60%	40–70%
Total annual cost	$15.60	$32.00
Total inpatient and outpatient costs	$658	$1,016

Source: M. Viravaidya, S. Obremskey, and C. Myers, "The economic impact of AIDS on Thailand," Harvard School of Public Health, Department of Population and International Health, Working Paper no. 4 (March, 1992).
a. Value of resources lasting more than one year (building, beds, equipment, etc.).

However, it should be noted that the number of patient records reviewed was small and charges were used in calculations when cost data were not available.

The average length of stay for AIDS patients was 20 days, or 3.7 times that of non-AIDS patients in the same hospital. Because of the more intensive care required, AIDS patients incurred costs of $7.14 per day in the hospital, almost 40 percent more than non-AIDS patients.[11] A 1991 study in Thailand estimated that annual costs for inpatient and outpatient AIDS treatment ranged from $658 to $1,016 per person.[12] Table 11.5 summarizes cost estimates from the study. Overall, inpatient services accounted for 97 to 98 percent of annual costs per patient, and outpatient services accounted for the remaining

$US (millions)

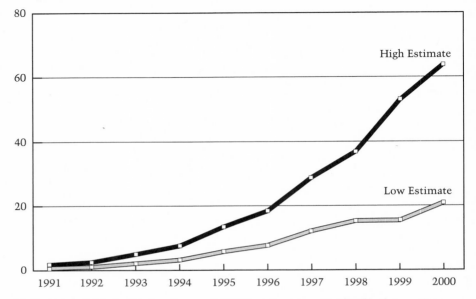

Figure 11.4. Projected annual cost of AIDS patient care in Thailand, inpatient
and outpatient, 1991-2000.
Source: M. Viravaidya, S. Obremskey and C. Myers, "The economic impact of AIDS on
Thailand," Harvard School of Public Health, Department of Population and International
Health, Working Paper no. 4 (March, 1992).

2 to 3 percent. Drugs accounted for approximately 9 percent of annual
costs assuming no AZT was supplied.

The estimate of $1,016 as the cost of AIDS treatment for one year
represents more than 50 percent of average annual household income.
Since few people in Thailand have health insurance, the government
and individuals pay for the bulk of AIDS care. Nationally, total inpatient and outpatient costs for AIDS in 1991 ranged from $710,000 and
$1,752,000, but projections indicated that this could reach $20 million
to nearly $65 million by the year 2000 (see Figure 11.4). Thailand
currently has approximately 75,000 hospital beds. While about one
percent of total bed days were required for AIDS in 1991, by the year
2000, up to 12 percent of hospital bed days will be required for AIDS.

The Caribbean, South America, and Central America

Annual medical costs per AIDS case vary widely in the Caribbean, South American and Central American nations, such as Jamaica, Barbados, Brazil, and Mexico, as well as in Puerto Rico.[13,14,15] In general, the per person costs for AIDS are significantly higher than for African countries. In Mexico, for example, the costs are reported to range from $1,430 to $7,350, or from 72 percent to 369 percent of per capital GNP. A study of the impact of AIDS on health services in Mexico suggested that the social security system, which provided resources for 39 percent of AIDS cases in 1987, will be more heavily affected than the public health system.[16]

In Puerto Rico, a cost analysis provided a rationale for planning and allocating resources.[17] In San Juan, the number of AIDS patients is projected to reach 2,500 in 1992, and by the year 2000, there may be up to 50,000 AIDS cases. The cost of care was projected to be $93 million in 1992, rising to $2 billion by the year 2000. Approximately 86 percent of these costs were for inpatient care. Thus, AIDS threatens to overwhelm the health care system in San Juan. As a result of these projections, increased outpatient facilities have been developed.

━━━━━━━ · · ·

INDUSTRIALIZED COUNTRIES

The cost of AIDS care in the industrialized world is characterized by wide differences in magnitude and a continuing shift toward outpatient care. Unlike developing countries where locations of care delivery tend to determine the scale of care costs, the large variations among and within countries, such as the United States, France, and Switzerland, reflect differences in types of costs reported, methods of reporting costs, definitions of AIDS, stages of disease, and patient groups examined.[18,19] The trend of the past several years to shift from inpatient to outpatient care in some industrialized countries adds to this broad range of costs. For example, whereas for some countries total inpatient care costs on a per day basis have stabilized, the total cost of outpatient services and outpatient drugs has grown enormously.[20] In the state of California it has been estimated that, in 1986, 13.6 percent of AIDS-related medical costs were attributable to out-

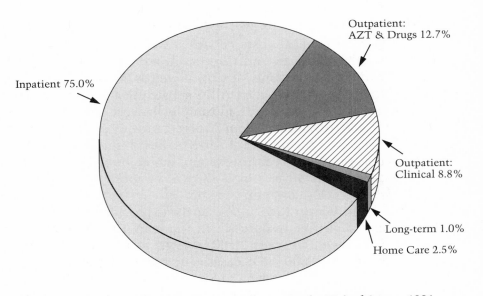

Outpatient:
AZT & Drugs 12.7%

Inpatient 75.0%

Outpatient:
Clinical 8.8%

Long-term 1.0%

Home Care 2.5%

Figure 11.5. Components of AIDS care and costs in the United States, 1991 (percent of costs).
Source: F. Hellinger, "Forecasting the medical care costs of the HIV epidemic," *Inquiry* 28 (Fall 1991): 213-25.

patient care; by 1989, this had nearly doubled to 25 percent.[21] A similar trend has been reported in France where, in early 1988, 80 percent of persons with AIDS were treated on an inpatient basis. However, by mid-1990, this had decreased to about 25 percent.[22] By the end of 1990, an estimated 62 percent of the 2,577 persons reported to have AIDS in that year received outpatient care, and an estimated 1,500 HIV-infected persons without AIDS also utilized outpatient services.[23]

In 1991, the U.S. health care system provided medical care (both inpatient and outpatient), counseling and nursing (including home care), and social, welfare, or long-term support to approximately 275,000 persons infected with HIV and 137,400 persons with AIDS.[24] Most of this care was provided in the formal health care system comprising hospitals, clinics, hospices, and long-term care facilities. Of total costs, nearly 75 percent were for inpatient hospital care. Outpatient hospital services included 12.7 percent of costs for AZT and other drugs and 8.8 percent for clinical services. Home care accounted for 2.5 percent and long-term care and support 1 percent of total costs (see Figure 11.5).

As the epidemic progresses, there has been a general trend toward increasing lifetime costs. In 1986, the average life expectancy for a person with AIDS was 13 months following diagnosis; today, it is an average of 22 months. Thus, an increase in life expectancy for people with AIDS, although partially offset by decreases in annual costs for treating AIDS patients, has increased the lifetime costs of medical treatment for an individual with AIDS in the United States.[25] The average cost of treating a person with AIDS (inpatient and outpatient) was $32,000 per year, and the annual cost of treating a person with HIV but not AIDS was estimated at $5,150.[26]

The cost of HIV and AIDS care in the United States in 1991 was estimated at $5.8 billion, including $4.4 billion for people with AIDS and $1.4 billion for HIV-infected persons without AIDS. This sum represented less than 1 percent of total U.S. health care expenditures in 1991. However, the estimation of this national cost assumed that over 137,000 people with AIDS were alive during any part of the calendar year in 1991. The Centers for Disease Control is currently revising downwards its previous estimates of people with AIDS to a number that could be significantly less than the original estimate.

AIDS in the World estimates that in the United States and Canada, almost 57,000 new cases of AIDS had occurred in 1991. However, the number of person-years of care (the care of one person for the full year) was estimated at 66,000, taking into account the need for care by people who were diagnosed with AIDS in 1991 and earlier. Multiplying the estimated person-years of care by the annual treatment cost of $31,995 (in constant 1990 U.S. dollars) for the United States and Canada, *AIDS in the World* calculated care costs of approximately U.S. $2.1 billion in 1991. No estimate was made of the cost of treatment of people with HIV diseases not meeting the AIDS diagnostic criteria.

Further in this section, the methodology used to estimate the cost of AIDS care in North America and the rest of the world from 1990 through 1995 will be presented.

In France, the government reportedly spent $370 million (FF 2 billion) for hospital-based care of persons with AIDS in 1990.[27] Hospital costs for AIDS were projected to be $555.6 million in 1992, compared with a total 1990 national health budget for France of $102 billion. Hospital-related expenditures accounted for approximately 40 percent of the total national health budget, or about $40.8 billion. Therefore, hospital-based AIDS care represented about 1 percent of all hospital expenditures and less than 1 percent of total national health expenditures. Of all hospital-based expenditures related to AIDS, 74 percent was for short hospital stays, 17 percent for day care, and the remaining 9 percent for longer hospital stays, consultations, and home care.

Certain diseases associated with HIV infections could greatly benefit from prophylactic treatment. For example, regular inhalation of Pentamidine or oral administration of Co-trimoxazole, alone or in association with other therapies, could have a significant impact on the primary prevention of *Pneumocystis carinii* pneumonia (PCP). The cost of such an approach has been studied in France (see Box 11.1). The monthly cost of PCP prevention per person ranged from $40 to $219, depending on the drugs used and the extent of laboratory follow-up. Operational and cost-effectiveness studies are needed to determine the place that prophylactic therapies for opportunistic infections must occupy in industrialized and developing country settings.

In Switzerland, approximately $68.4 million (SFr 95.76 million) of direct personal costs were estimated to have been expended in 1990 to care for almost 1,200 persons with AIDS.[43] Meeting the annual medical, counseling, and support needs for a person with AIDS was estimated to cost approximately $57,000 (SFr 80,000).

THE GLOBAL COST OF AIDS

What is the global cost of AIDS care and prevention, and how does this cost compare to spending for other diseases? Societies are continually forced to make difficult resource allocation decisions within and across programs. Politics, cultural values, religious influences, and economic considerations all influence this process. One measure for comparing the cost of different diseases is the cost per year of life saved.[44,45] This represents the cost of extending a life by one year as the result of a medical intervention. In some industrialized countries, providing care for persons with AIDS costs significantly less than the cost per year of life saved from many procedures, such as renal dialysis, coronary bypass surgery, and screening mammography (see Figure 11.6). The annual cost of inpatient and outpatient care for a person with AIDS costs 26 percent less than a liver transplant and 30 percent less than renal dialysis in the United States. However, AIDS is generally a fatal disease, and persons are not expected to live more than a few years even with treatment. In addition, multiple drug use can significantly increase the cost of AIDS treatment.

Comparing the cost of AIDS care to the costs of other diseases is even more difficult in developing countries because of a lack of data, inconsistencies in methodologies, and differences in treatment protocols. A partial analysis can be done using tuberculosis and leprosy for comparison. Like AIDS in adults, both have long latency periods and require long-term care. However, unlike AIDS, tuberculosis and leprosy can be cured. A twelve-month chemotherapy regimen for treating pulmonary tuberculosis in Tanzania was reported to cost about $123 in 1986.[46] Costs for leprosy vary by type of leprosy and country.

Box 11.1: Pneumocystis Carinii Pneumonia in France

Shahin Gharakhanian, ical Assistant, and Dr. 'y Rozenbaum, Head, partment of Tropical and ectious Diseases, thschild Hospital, Paris

Pneumocystis carinii pneumonia (PCP) is the first clinical manifestation of AIDS in 35 percent of patients in France and occurs in about 60 percent of people with HIV-infection. The estimated number of patients with PCP in France, in the absence of prophylaxis, is expected to be about 3,000 in 1992.[28]

Since 1977, it has been known that chemoprophylaxis against PCP is effective in immunologically incompetent people,[29,30] and in Paris, chemoprophylaxis for prevention of PCP relapse has been the rule since 1985 in some, but not all, centers caring for people with AIDS.[31] Prophylaxis for PCP has been officially endorsed[32] for HIV-infected patients with a CD4 cell count of less than 200 per μl, and a statement of consensus concerning pneumocystosis was published and widely distributed in 1990.[33]

However, PCP is still relatively common among people with AIDS in France (see Table 11.A), and a clear downward trend has not been observed (see Figure 11.A).[34] The median survival of patients with PCP as the sole opportunistic infection is 17.6 months (sem. = 2.5 m).[35]

Three different retrospective, hospital-based studies in the regions of Paris and Nantes, carried out during 1989–1992, attempted to look into this problem.[36,37,38] A total of 130 patients with PCP were identified; 30 to 35 percent were not known to be

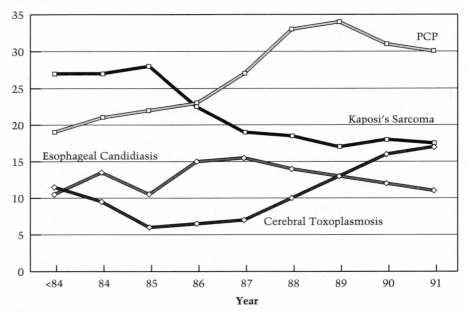

Percent

Figure 11.A. Evolution of the frequency of the main AIDS-related opportunistic diseases (as the only manifestation) in France (12-31-91).
Source: Surveillance du SIDA en France (situation au 31 decembre 1991) (1992).

HIV-positive, and among those with PCP who knew of their HIV-infection, 20 to 37 percent received no medical follow-up. In one of those studies, 21 percent of HIV-positive patients were not offered PCP prevention by their physician.[39] Furthermore, among patients admitted to the intensive care unit for PCP, HIV status was unknown in 75 percent of the cases. Another study[40] attempted to evaluate through interviews the social characteristics of patients currently developing PCP. In that study, patients cited fear of HIV testing and unawareness of the efficacy of prophylaxis as barriers to treatment, in addition to lack of information from physicians and inadequate medical follow-up.

The economic aspects of prophylaxis have been studied in France.[41] Costs are covered by the usual and/or specific hospital and social security funding. Table 11.B summarizes the monthly cost of different prophylactic options as well

Table 11.A: Frequency of PCP among adult AIDS cases by year of diagnosis in France

Year	No. of new AIDS cases	% of cases developing PCP
1983	87	18.4
1984	218	28.0
1985	541	29.6
1986	1,188	32.2
1987	2,109	35.3
1988	2,905	35.6
1989	3,563	33.8
1990[a]	3,796	30.1
1991[a]	3,001	30.5
Total	17,408	32.5

Source: "Surveillance du SIDA en France (situation au 31 décembre 1991)," *BEH* 6 (1992).
a. Provisional data.

Table 11.B: Monthly cost of preventing *Pneumocystis carinii* pneumonia (PCP) and total cost per case prevented (1990 French francs and equivalent $U.S.)

Prophylaxis option	Monthly cost FFr ($U.S.)	Cost/case of PCP prevented over a 26-month period CD4 < 200/μl FFr ($U.S.)[a]
Inhalations[b] at home without help	250 ($42)	18,830 ($3,138)
Inhalations at home with help	635 ($106)	44,900 ($7,483)
Inhalations during a hospital consultation (min.)	295 ($49)	21,880 ($3,647)
Inhalations during a hospital consultation (max.)	495 ($83)	44,780 ($7,463)
Inhalations at the hospital day clinic (min.)	870 ($140)	60,810 ($10,135)
Inhalations at the hospital day clinic (max.)	1,010 ($168)	70,290 ($11,715)
Co-trimoxazole only	98 ($16)	13,840 ($2,307)
Co-trimoxazole + folinic acid supplement	418 ($70)	35,510 ($5,918)
Co-trimoxazole + folinic acid supplement + laboratory tests	1,313 ($219)	59,750 ($9,958)

Source: A. Fiori and A. Triomphe, "L'évaluation économique du coût et du traitement de la pneumocystose," *Médecine des Maladies Infectieuses* 20 août–septembre (1990):414–19.
Note: In 1990 6 FFr = 1 $U.S.
a. Amount in francs rounded to nearest 0.
b. Inhalations = Pentamidine.

---

as the cost of preventing PCP in a patient with less than 200 CD4 cells per μl over a 26-month period.

Despite adequate scientific background, availability of at least two acceptable drugs,[42] as well as adequate medical resources, PCP continues to be a major opportunistic infection in France with considerable morbidity, affecting the long-term survival of HIV-infected patients. Although much has been achieved, the effective control of the AIDS epidemic requires a clear nationwide policy on the primary prevention of opportunistic infections. Financial aspects have not been identified as a major hurdle for the generalization of PCP prophylaxis in France. This information should be directed to the public and the medical profession, the majority of whom still believe that no therapy is available, and thus, no pressing reason to promote voluntary HIV testing, to monitor the condition of persons diagnosed with HIV infection and to treat them before the onset of full-blown AIDS. The primary prevention of one or, better, several infections can contribute to extending the length and improving the quality of life of people with HIV infection.

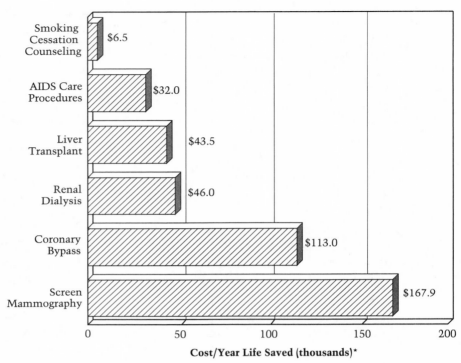

*Costs in 1988 dollars, excluding AIDS care (1990).

Figure 11.6. Cost of medical, surgical or public health intervention or screening procedure required to save one year of life compared with cost of AIDS care, United States.

Sources: K. Schulman, et al., "Cost effectiveness of low-dose Zidovudine therapy for asymptomatic patients with human immunodeficiency virus (HIV) infection," *Annals of Internal Medicine* 114 (9) (1991): 798-802; and A. Scitovsky, M. Cline and D. Abrams, "Effects of the use of AZT on the medical care costs of persons with AIDS in the first 12 months," *Journal of Acquired Immune Deficiency Syndromes* 3 (9) (1990): 904-15.

However, on average, treatment for Paucibacillary leprosy (80 percent of leprosy cases) is reported to cost about $8 for a six-month treatment regimen, including drugs, delivery, and supervision. Treatment of multibacillary leprosy is reported to cost about $35 per year. This means that the average annual cost of $393 for treatment of AIDS in sub-Saharan Africa makes it significantly more expensive than treatment for either tuberculosis or leprosy.

Comparing medical cost estimates among different countries is also problematic. Among the factors that must be addressed are questions of data validity, variations in treatment protocols across countries, response of patient populations to receiving care, accessibility of care, severity of disease, use of public versus private hospitals and clinics, and others. National-level aggregations and averages often mask significant local variations in care and support. Although national-level averages are useful for planning and comparisons, they can obscure the needs and care of particularly vulnerable populations.[47,48]

For example, in San Francisco, many men with AIDS are well-educated, have jobs that may provide insurance coverage, and have good access to health care systems. The gay movement continues to mobilize resources, provide support systems, and politicize the issue of AIDS in support of the needs of those affected.[49,50] Conversely, many injection drug users (IDU) in New York City are from economically disadvantaged minorities. Many are uninsured, have few social support networks, and lack political structure and organization. Therefore, their needs are less likely to be known, and they are less likely to receive necessary types of care. In Europe, meeting the needs of IDUs is compounded by the problem of their mobility. IDUs may move through Germany, Switzerland, Italy, and other European countries.

AIDS in the World made an attempt to estimate the worldwide cost of AIDS care during the period 1990 through 1995. However, because of the paucity of data, this estimate did not include cost estimates for HIV infection nor the cost of care for pediatric AIDS.

The first step was to estimate, for each year, the number of adults with AIDS who were alive. This was done for each of the 10 Geographic Areas of Affinity (GAAs). Next, different annual survival rates were applied depending on whether they included more affluent countries (GAAs 1, 2, 3, and 9) or less affluent countries (other GAAs). These rates are presented in Appendix 2.2. The result of these calculations enabled estimation of person-years of care required in each GAA from 1990 through 1995. The estimation assumes that all persons needing care have access to it.

The next step was to estimate the direct personal costs: for one person, for one year of care. These unit costs, which varied across GAA, were derived using two methods. Where country-specific data

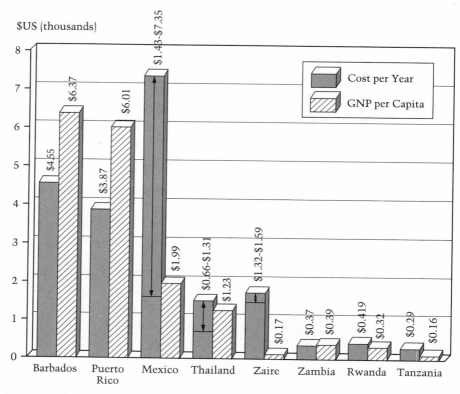

$US (thousands)

Figure 11.7. Cost per year of inpatient care per AIDS case versus per capita GNP, 1986-1991.
Source: See Table 11.4 for country sources.

were available, the unit cost was assumed to represent the value of a person-year of care within that country. Cost studies, followed up by *AIDS in the World* inquiries, provided cost data for a number of affluent, industrialized countries (Table 11.4). In fact, cost information was available for countries which account for a large proportion of the AIDS cases in the industrialized (affluent) world.

In countries where cost data were unavailable, an alternative method had to be applied. Researchers have estimated that, in developing countries, the annual cost of care for a person with AIDS can

Table 11.6: Estimated global cost of AIDS prevention and care by Geographic Area of Affinity, 1990

GAA	Person-years of care	% of global total	Cost per person-year (1990 $U.S.)	Total cost, adults (millions 1990 $U.S.)	% of global total	Costs (millions 1990 $U.S.)	% of global total	Total, care and prevention (millions 1990 $U.S.)	Ratio of care-to-prevention costs
		Care				Prevention			
1	56,000	18.8	31,995	1,792	72.0	746	53	2,538	2.4:1
2	23,000	7.7	22,391	515	20.7	512	36	1,027	1.0:1
3	1,000	0.3	14,015	14	0.6	59	4	73	0.2:1
4	23,500	7.9	1,992	47	1.9	11	1	57	4.5:1
5	178,000	59.8	393	70	2.8	39	3	109	1.8:1
6	6,000	2.0	2,157	13	0.5	11	1	24	1.2:1
7	500	0.2	1,520	1	0.0	13	1	14	0.06:1
8	500	0.2	2,446	1	0.0	6	0	7	0.2:1
9	1,000	0.3	23,160	23	0.9	4	0	27	6.3:1
10	8,000	2.7	1,700	14	0.5	9	1	22	1.6:1
Total	297,500	100		2,490	100	1,410	100	3,898	1.8:1

Source: AIDS in the World survey of national AIDS programs.

be approximated by the per capita GNP or a derivative of GNP (see Figure 11.7).[51,52] Therefore, per capita GNP was used for a large number of countries for which cost studies had not been undertaken. These included many developing countries and also some industrialized, less affluent ones, such as those in Eastern Europe. Although less reliable as a surrogate for care-costs in industrialized, affluent countries, the same methodology was used where cost studies did not exist.

Total annual costs for each Geographic Area of Affinity were calculated by summing up the costs in each Area. Calculations were made using constant 1990 U.S. dollars, assuming fixed individual AIDS care costs during the period 1990 through 1995. Estimates of AIDS care costs in 1990 and projections for 1992 and 1995 were made for each GAA (see Tables 11.6, 11.7, and 11.8). Figure 11.8 shows the

Table 11.7: Estimated global cost of AIDS care by Geographic Area of Affinity (GAA), 1992

GAA	Person-years of care	% of global total	Cost per person-year of care (1990 $U.S.)	Total cost AIDS care, adults (millions, 1990 $U.S.)	% of global total
1	74,000	17.1	31,995	2,368	67.5
2	38,000	8.8	22,391	851	24.3
3	1,600	0.4	14,015	22	0.6
4	33,000	7.6	1,992	65	1.9
5	254,000	58.7	393	100	2.8
6	10,000	2.3	2,157	22	0.6
7	1,500	0.3	1,520	2	0.1
8	1,000	0.2	2,446	2	0.1
9	1,800	0.4	23,160	42	1.2
10	18,000	4.2	1,700	31	0.9
Total	432,900	100.0		3,505	100.0

Source: *AIDS in the World* survey of national AIDS programs.

Table 11.8: Estimated global cost of AIDS care by Geographic Area of Affinity as of 1995

GAA	Person-years of care	% of global total	Cost per person-year of care (1990 $U.S.)	Total cost AIDS care, adults (millions 1990 $U.S.)	% of global total
1	93,000	15.0	31,995	2,976	61.5
2	63,000	10.2	22,391	1,411	29.1
3	2,500	0.4	14,015	35	0.7
4	45,000	7.3	1,992	90	1.9
5	357,000	57.7	393	140	2.9
6	15,000	2.4	2,157	32	0.7
7	1,400	0.2	1,520	2	0.0
8	1,800	0.3	2,446	4	0.1
9	3,800	0.6	23,160	88	1.8
10	36,300	5.9	1,700	62	1.3
Total	618,800	100		4,840	100

Source: *AIDS in the World*, 1992.

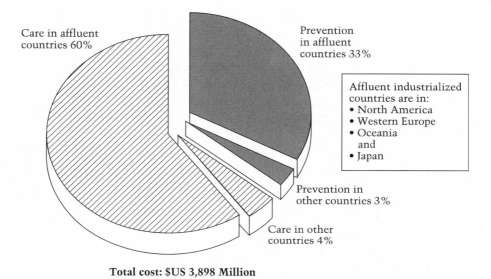

Care in affluent
countries 60%

Prevention
in affluent
countries 33%

Affluent industrialized
countries are in:
• North America
• Western Europe
• Oceania
  and
• Japan

Prevention in
other countries 3%

Care in other
countries 4%

Total cost: $US 3,898 Million

Figure 11.8. Estimated global costs of AIDS prevention and care in the world, 1990. Share by affluent and other countries.

estimated global cost of AIDS prevention and care for 1990 of $3.9 billion. Of this amount, affluent countries account for 93 percent of the total cost; care in affluent countries accounts for 60 percent of total costs.

A factor which, due to the lack of data, could not be included in the estimations was the rate of access to and use of a full year of care by adults with AIDS. For example, in the United States, approximately 29 percent of people with AIDS in 1990/1991 were uninsured, many of whom were among the socially marginalized. About 40 percent of people with AIDS were covered by Medicaid. However, in order to benefit from Medicaid coverage, an individual must meet stringent eligibility criteria. For most people with HIV disease, eligibility for Medicaid is through disability, which requires a clinical diagnosis of AIDS. The U.S. National Commission on AIDS established that Medicaid was generally available only to very poor individuals and only during the later stages of HIV disease. These factors affect the degree to which advantage will be taken by people with AIDS of a full year of care opportunities. In order to adjust for these factors, it would be necessary to apply a utilization factor which in one scenario could be as low as 70 percent in the United States and 80 percent in Western Europe (1990). Application of an access factor would significantly affect the total cost in those affluent countries which represent the majority of worldwide care costs. In such a scenario, North America and Europe would still account for the vast majority (89 percent) of world spending on AIDS care for adults, although these areas accounted for less than 30 percent of the world's people with AIDS.[53]

In 1990, the ratio between costs of medical care and prevention ranged widely among GAAs. Highest care-to-prevention spending ratios were in North East Asia (6.3:1), Latin America (4.5:1), and North America (2.4:1). In three GAAs, the care-to-prevention ratio favored prevention: Eastern Europe (0.06:1) and the South East Mediterranean and Oceania (0.2:1). However, interpreting these ratios is complicated. For example, high care-to-prevention ratios in Latin America may reflect increasing costs for people with AIDS against a background of inadequate prevention efforts, whereas the high ratio in North East Asia reflects both a tiny number of AIDS cases requiring care plus inadequate attention to HIV prevention. The low care-to-prevention ratios in Eastern Europe and the South East Mediterranean are more indicative of a small number of people with AIDS than of a major commitment to prevention.

In 1992, an estimated 432,900 person-years of care will be needed on a worldwide basis. This is projected to cost $3.5 billion (in 1990 U.S. dollars) as shown in Table 11.7. About 26 percent of worldwide person-years of care will be in North America and Western Europe as shown in Figure 11.9. However, these areas will account for almost 92 percent of worldwide costs. North America alone, with 17 percent of person-years of care, will represent over 67 percent of worldwide costs. Conversely, almost 59 percent of person-years of care will be in sub-Saharan Africa; yet they are projected to account for less than 3 percent of worldwide medical costs for treatment, unless major efforts are promptly made to expand AIDS care efforts and mobilize the needed resources. (For a comparison of estimated global costs of AIDS prevention, care, and research, see Figure 8.8.)

Worldwide, in 1995, the projected cost of adult AIDS care will be nearly double the estimated cost in 1990 (Table 11.8). This trend

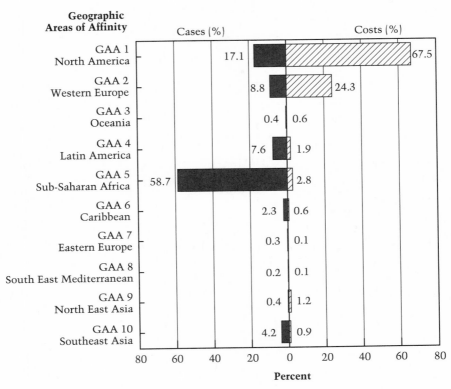

Figure 11.9. Proportional contribution of ten Geographic Areas of Affinity to projected adult AIDS cases needing care in 1992 and projected percent of cost of AIDS care in the world.
Source: AIDS in the World, 1992.

highlights the urgent need for strategic planning for AIDS care and related health and social services. During the period 1990–1995, the global cost of adult AIDS care could reach a total of $22.2 billion, of which less than 10 percent would occur in less affluent countries and over 90 percent in industrialized, affluent countries (Table 11.9 and Figure 11.10).

Further research and closer monitoring are needed to refine cost estimates and projections. These will be critical for decisions on resource allocation at national and international levels. It will be

Table 11.9: Estimated number of person-years of AIDS care and related costs in more affluent and less affluent countries 1990–1995

Year	Person-years of AIDS care			Cost of AIDS care (millions 1990 $U.S.)		
	More affluent countries[a]	Less affluent countries	Annual world total	More affluent countries[a]	Less affluent countries	Annual world total
1990	81,000 (27%)	216,500 (73%)	297,500	2,345 (94%)	144 (6%)	2,489
1991	98,000 (27%)	267,200 (73%)	365,200	2,818 (94%)	180 (6%)	2,997
1992	115,000 (27%)	317,900 (73%)	432,900	3,290 (94%)	215 (6%)	3,505
1993	130,000 (26%)	364,900 (74%)	494,900	3,681 (93%)	269 (7%)	3,950
1994	145,000 (26%)	411,900 (74%)	556,900	4,072 (93%)	323 (7%)	4,395
1995	160,000 (26%)	458,800 (74%)	618,800	4,463 (92%)	377 (8%)	4,840
Total	729,000 (26%)	2,037,200 (74%)	2,766,200	20,669 (93%)	1,508 (7%)	22,176

Source: AIDS in the World, 1992.

a. More affluent countries include all countries in GAA 1 (North America), GAA 2 (Western Europe), and GAA 3 (Oceania), and countries in GAA 9 where most cases are expected to occur through 1995, in particular, Japan.

Note: Estimates for 1991, 1993, and 1994 were interpolated from 1990, 1991, and 1995 calculations.

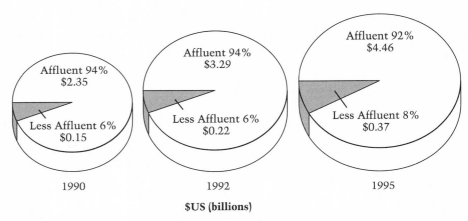

$US (billions)

Figure 11.10. Estimated AIDS care costs for adults and percent distribution of cost in affluent industrialized countries and in other countries in 1990, 1992, and 1995.

important to incorporate in these analyses the cost of pediatric care and the treatment of HIV-related diseases which do not fully meet the AIDS diagnostic criteria.

As the number of AIDS cases continues to rise relentlessly around the world, more and more countries will begin to feel the weight of this rapidly expanding epidemic on health care systems. In the case of some industrialized countries, many people with AIDS already lack the ability to pay for care, because they do not have health insurance or have exhausted their resources. In developing countries, uninsured and impoverished people with AIDS have already begun to overburden often aging or inadequate medical systems and infrastructures. Despite shifting strategies for AIDS care, many health care systems in the world today are already staggered by the impact of AIDS. The response of governments and societies over the coming years will determine whether these systems meet the needs imposed by AIDS or collapse under their weight.

CHAPTER TWELVE

. . . .

Funding the Global AIDS Strategy

chapter was
▪ared by the Editors
IDS in the World, in
▪boration with Joel
▪y, M.P.H., of the
▪artment of National
▪th and Welfare
▪ada).

In 1987, the World Health Organization created the global AIDS strat-egy, which was universally adopted as the blueprint for international and national efforts against AIDS. This chapter of *AIDS in the World, 1992*, focuses on the financial support provided for implementation of the global AIDS strategy, including resources for international ac-tivities and for HIV/AIDS prevention and care activities in the devel-oping world.

Prior to 1986, none of the wealthy (industrialized) nations funded AIDS prevention and care programs in the developing world. Part of the responsibility for this delay lies with the United Nations system, which was slow to identify the AIDS pandemic as an important global problem. However, the delay also reflected confusion within official development assistance (ODA) agencies concerning the extent and seriousness of the AIDS pandemic, uncertainties about how to proceed in funding for AIDS prevention and care activities, and concern that AIDS would divert funding from existing health priorities and proj-ects.

In 1986, about $200,000 was contributed by ODA and interna-tional agencies to developing countries for AIDS work. During the next five years, from 1987 through 1991, approximately $864 million was contributed in support of the global AIDS strategy, increasing from approximately $53 million in 1987 to more than $255 million in 1990. However, in 1991, available data show a decline, for the first

Table 12.1: Multilateral and bilateral donors' support to the global AIDS strategy, 1986–1991, as reported in June 1992 (millions $U.S.)

Country[a]	Multilateral WHO-GPA	Multi/Bi through WHO/GPA	Bilateral	Total	Cumulative %
United States	87.060	5.271	145.000	237.331	35.3
Sweden	52.738	9.575	35.226	97.539	49.8
Canada	23.312	1.573	45.615	70.500	60.2
United Kingdom	37.424	10.372	11.544	59.340	69.0
Norway	16.391	12.603	12.454	41.448	75.1
France	4.349	0.245	34.329	38.923	80.9
Denmark	14.479	2.517	19.900	36.896	86.4
Germany	4.100	2.806	21.345	28.251	90.7
Netherlands	17.858	1.045	3.829	22.732	94.0
Switzerland	10.255	—	3.595	13.850	96.0
Japan	7.500	0.600	—	8.100	97.3
Finland	3.513	—	0.569	4.082	97.9
Australia	1.661	0.059	1.923	3.643	98.5
USSR	3.550	—	—	3.550	99.0
Italy	1.749	—	1.796	3.545	99.5
Belgium	0.987	0.057	—	1.044	99.7
Spain	—	—	0.800	0.800	99.7
New Zealand	0.336	—	—	0.336	99.9
Austria	0.158	—	—	0.158	99.9
Kuwait	0.050	—	—	0.050	100.0
Subtotal	287.470	46.723	337.925	672.118	

time, in total ODA contributions for AIDS prevention and care in the developing world.

.   .   .

WHO PROVIDES THE OFFICIAL DEVELOPMENT ASSISTANCE FOR AIDS?

The $864 million figure estimated to have been mobilized worldwide in support of developing countries' AIDS programs includes $847.6 million in contributions reported for the period 1986 to 1991 as of June 1992, and $16.5 million to adjust for delayed reporting by several ODAs on bilateral financing. (Details are provided in Table 12.3.) The

Table 12.1 (cont.): Multilateral and bilateral donors' support to the global AIDS strategy, 1986–1991, as reported in June 1992 (millions $U.S.)

Other agencies	To WHO/GPA	To country programs through WHO/GPA	To country programs	Total
IBRD[b]	3.027	—	—	3.027
Sasakawa Foundation	1.626	—	—	1.626
IBM	1.500	—	—	1.500
World AIDS Foundation	0.846	—	—	0.846
Swiss Red Cross	0.033	0.100	—	0.133
UNDP	4.133	15.996	21.523	41.652
World Bank	—	—	55.805	55.805
EEC	—	0.040	48.000	48.040
UNICEF	—	0.064	7.017	7.081
UNFPA	—	0.415	—	0.415
Miscellaneous and interest	15.423	—	—	15.423
Subtotal	26.561	16.615	132.345	175.521
Total	314.031	63.338	470.270	847.639

Sources: WHO/GPA Financial Information on 1991 Income and Obligations (April 30, 1991); WHO/GPA summary data, Donor Contributions for Specified Countries from 1987 to June 30, 1991 (updated July 31, 1991); correspondence from OECD to *AIDS in the World* (October 18, 1991); Support Program on AIDS for Developing Countries, Ministry of Economic Cooperation, Federal Republic of Germany (1991); correspondence from Sasakawa Memorial Health Foundation to Global AIDS Commission (January 17, 1992); Commission of European Communities, *AIDS Control Programme Report* (1987–1991); correspondence from UNDP to the Global AIDS Commission (October 3, 1991); data from WHO/GPA Management Committee, Ad Hoc Working Group (1992).

a. Countries are ranked by total contributions.

b. The amount from the International Bank for Reconstruction and Development is listed separately because it was entirely in the form of multilateral aid to WHO/GPA.

Note: EEC = European Economic Community; IBM = International Business Machines; IBRD = International Bank for Reconstruction and Development (part of the World Bank); UNDP = United Nations Development Program; UNFPA = United Nations Population Fund.

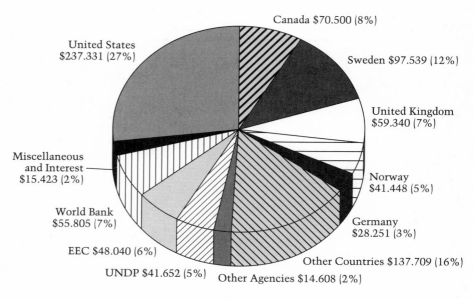

Total $847.639 (millions $US)

Figure 12.1. Principal donors 1986-1991, global AIDS strategy.
Source: AIDS in the World, 1992.

Box 12.1: Who Are the Official Development Assistance Agencies?

Source: The World Bank, *World Development Report 1991: The Challenge of Development* (New York, 1991).

Eighteen countries are members of the Organization for Economic Cooperation and Development (OECD[a]); most have their own official development assistance (ODA) agency through which public development assistance funds are generally channeled. The list of major ODA agencies includes the United States Agency for International Development (USAID); the Swedish International Development Agency (SIDA); the Canadian International Development Agency (CIDA); the Danish International Development Agency (DANIDA); and the United

Kingdom's Overseas Development Authority (ODA).

In 1990, a total of $US 54.1 billion in official development assistance was provided by the OECD countries, with the United States making the largest single contribution ($US 11.4 billion), followed by Japan and France. As early as 1970, the United Nations proposed that each country contribute 0.7 percent of its gross national product to development assistance. In 1990, 5 countries (Norway, Sweden, Netherlands, Denmark, and France) exceeded this target, and nine countries fell below the halfway mark of 0.35 percent (in descending order: Australia, Italy, Japan, Switzerland, the United Kingdom, Austria, New

analysis in this section is based on the $847.6 million in reported contributions only.

Support for the global AIDS strategy from 1986 to 1991 was reported to total $847.6 million (see Table 12.1 and Figure 12.1). ODA funding represented 79 percent of all support for the global AIDS strategy during this period. A total of 20 countries provided ODA for AIDS, including most countries in the Organization for Economic Cooperation and Development (OECD), plus the former Soviet Union and Kuwait. (A brief profile of the ODA agencies is found in Box 12.1.) The largest single contributor was the United States (35.3 percent); 8 countries in North America and Western Europe together provided 91 percent of all ODA funding for AIDS.

In addition to the World Health Organization (WHO), 4 United Nations agencies have contributed to support of the global AIDS strategy: the United Nations Development Program (UNDP); the United Nations Children's Fund (UNICEF); the United Nations Population Fund (UNFPA); and the World Bank (Table 12.1). Together, these agencies contributed $104.9 million, or 12 percent of the total resources during this period. Additional contributions have been made

---

Zealand, the United States, and Ireland).

Two final notes: first, domestic political pressure generally results in spending substantial portions of ODA in the donor country itself, or for purchase of donor country products or hiring of donor country citizens. Second, overall, only about 5 percent of ODA resources are targeted for health.

OPEC (the Organization of Petroleum Exporting Countries)[b] provides a second major source of ODA. In 1989, Saudi Arabia's ODA represented 2.7 percent of gross national product; for other OPEC countries, with the exception of Libya (0.52 percent) and Kuwait (0.41 percent), the ODA contributions were negligible (0.08 percent or less of GNP).

---

a. List of OECD countries

Australia	Italy
Austria	Japan
Belgium	New Zealand
Canada	Netherlands
Denmark	Norway
Finland	Sweden
France	Switzerland
Germany	United Kingdom
Ireland	United States

b. List of OPEC countries

Algeria	Nigeria
Iran	Qatar
Iraq	Saudi Arabia
Kuwait	United Arab Emirates
Libya	Venezuela

Box 12.2: Funds Channeled by NGOs to Developing Country Projects

Sources: Correspondence from the Ford Foundation to *AIDS in the World* (December 5, 1991), the Norwegian Red Cross (November 15, 1991), CARITAS Internationalis (November 22, 1991), HIVOS (Humanistic Institute for Cooperation with Developing Countries, Holland) (November 25, 1991), Action AIDS (November 22, 1991), and CARE, December 12, 1991.

Some funding is provided by nongovernmental organizations (NGOs) in support of national AIDS prevention and control projects in developing nations. The financial information provided below (all in millions of U.S. dollars) includes only money channeled by these groups to the projects, but it does not include money for projects on which these NGOs act as executing or implementing agencies. (This listing of NGOs is not meant to be complete. Rather, it is illustrative of the broad range of NGOs involved in providing support as part of the global AIDS strategy.)

Ford Foundation

1988	$1.088
1989	$1.345
1990	$1.390
1991[a]	$1.578
	$5.401

CARITAS Internationalis

1988	$0.147
1989	$0.490
1990	$0.491
1991	$0.257
	$1.385

Action AIDS

1987–1990	$0.103

The Public Welfare Foundation (Washington, D.C.)

1988	$0.040
1989	$0.184
1990	$0.316
1991[b]	$0.048
	$0.588

Norwegian Red Cross

1985	$0.002
1986	$0.248
1987	$0.332
1988	$0.881
1989	$0.651
1990	$1.531
	$3.645

HIVOS (Humanistic Institute for Cooperation with Developing Countries, Holland)

1990	$0.130
1991	$0.335
	$0.465

CARE[c]

	$0.050

American Foundation for AIDS Research (AmFAR)

1988–1991	$0.800

Atkinson Foundation (San Francisco)

1988–1991 cumulative	$0.030

---

a. As of November 27, 1991.
b. 1st quarter only.
c. CARE does not generally use its unrestricted monies to fund projects. Therefore, only a limited amount has been used as seed monies for AIDS-related projects. However, CARE does function as the executing or implementing agency for a number of AIDS-related projects funded by government donor agencies.

by the United Nations Educational, Scientific and Cultural Organization (UNESCO), the International Labor Organization (ILO), and the United Nations Population Division. However, these contributions have been relatively small and generally involved staff, travel, and internal project funding.

In July 1987, the Commission of European Communities created a special AIDS program to support developing country activities, which provided 6 percent of total resources during the period 1986 to 1991. Contributions were also made by private companies, foundations, and nongovernmental organizations (NGOs). With the several exceptions noted in Table 12.1 (all of which provided funding to WHO), the full scope and diversity of these contributions are not known at this time and have, therefore, not been included in this analysis. Further information on the financial contributions of selected NGOs and corporations is provided in Boxes 12.2 and 12.3.

A brief explanation of terms is required to understand the analysis of support for the global AIDS strategy. The major routes for providing funds from ODA agencies are these:

1. The *multilateral* approach involves funds given by ODA agencies to the United Nations or any of its specialized agencies; of these, the most important during this period is WHO. Multilateral funds can either be unspecified (to be used as the UN agency decides) or specified (for a specific project or purpose).

Box 12.3: Support by Corporations to the Global AIDS Strategy

urce: AIDS Funding: A ide to Giving by undations and Charitable ganizations. Report on rnational AIDS intmaking (published by iders Concerned about)S, 1991) (supported by Ford Foundation, Levi auss Foundation, and the . Fels Fund).

Listed below are examples of donations of funds and products (in kind) from corporations in support of the global AIDS strategy (for the year 1990 unless otherwise indicated).

Burroughs Wellcome: $400,000 per year in products to developing countries

Levi Strauss: $83,000 (1989–1991)
Thai Military Bank: $1 million to Thai National AIDS Program
Bangkok Bank: $1.1 million to Thai National AIDS Program
Avon: $50,000 to Thai National AIDS Program
American International Insurance: $150,000 to Thai National AIDS Program

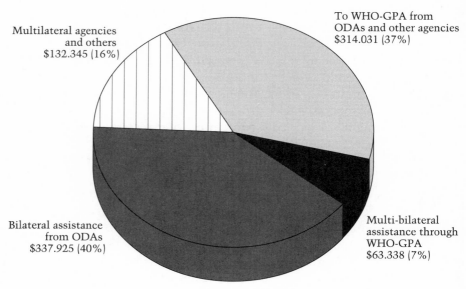

Multilateral agencies
and others
$132.345 (16%)

To WHO-GPA from
ODAs and other agencies
$314.031 (37%)

Bilateral assistance
from ODAs
$337.925 (40%)

Multi-bilateral
assistance through
WHO-GPA
$63.338 (7%)

Total $847.639 (millions $US)

Figure 12.2. Global AIDS strategy, governments and official multilateral agencies, 1987-1991.
Source: AIDS in the World, 1992.

2. The *bilateral* approach involves a transfer of funds directly from the ODA agency to a developing country (e.g., Canada to Thailand; France to Senegal).

3. The *multilateral-bilateral* (*multi-bi* for short) approach allows ODA agencies to channel funds through WHO to a specific country. In 1987, WHO created this third option to help increase support from ODA agencies for countries in desperate need of resources for AIDS work. For example, through a multi-bi arrangement, Sweden could support a national AIDS program in a country in which its ODA agency (the Swedish International Development Agency) did not have an office by channeling the funds through WHO.

As seen in Figure 12.2, of the $847.6 million provided in support of the Global AIDS Strategy from 1986 to 1991, the largest portion ($337.9 million, or 40 percent) was bilateral assistance; next most important involved multilateral assistance through WHO ($314 mil-

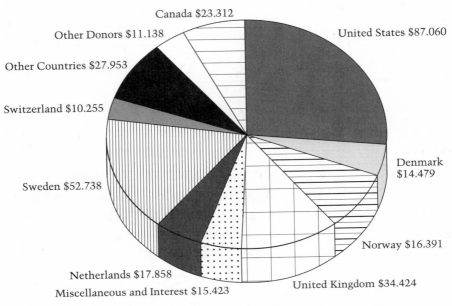

Canada $23.312

Other Donors $11.138

Other Countries $27.953

Switzerland $10.255

Sweden $52.738

United States $87.060

Denmark $14.479

Norway $16.391

Netherlands $17.858

Miscellaneous and Interest $15.423

United Kingdom $34.424

Total $314.031 (millions $US)*

Figure 12.3. Major donors to WHO-GPA, 1987-1991.
Source: AIDS in the World, 1992.
*Difference between this figure and total of individual contributions is due to rounding-off

lion, 37 percent); followed by support by multilateral agencies other than WHO ($132.3 million, 16 percent); multilateral-bilateral support of $63.3 million accounted for the remaining seven percent. Therefore, approximately one-half of all support for the global AIDS strategy was provided *to* or *through* WHO.

· · ·

SUPPORT TO THE WORLD HEALTH ORGANIZATION

From 1987 to 1991, a total of $314 million was provided to the WHO Global Programme on AIDS (WHO/GPA) for global activities. Of this total, $287.5 million (91 percent) was provided by ODA agencies (donor countries), and the remaining $26.6 million (9 percent) was made available by other donors, including miscellaneous income and accrued interest (see Figure 12.3 and Table 12.2).

Funding the Global AIDS Strategy 519

Table 12.2: Multilateral contributions to WHO/GPA global activities, 1987–1991 (inclusive) ($U.S.)

Source of income	Contributions					Cumulative total
	1987	*1988*	*1989*	*1990*	*1991*	
Country						
Australia	—	380,400	375,300	687,932	217,140	1,660,772
Austria	47,720	—	32,099	33,991	44,860	158,670
Belgium	—	—	191,635	516,304	279,392	987,331
Canada	3,732,323	4,076,885	3,795,456	7,774,130	3,933,566	23,312,360
Denmark	2,179,124	3,131,675	2,959,258	3,322,692	2,886,331	14,479,080
Finland	66,200	987,256	703,284	878,073	878,294	3,513,107
France	169,491	328,579	1,557,103	1,092,028	1,201,351	4,348,552
Germany	76,823	792,723	317,373	327,708	2,585,355	4,099,982
Italy	—	—	1,272,867	—	476,190	1,749,057
Japan	—	1,450,000	1,750,000	2,100,000	2,220,000	7,500,000
Kuwait	—	—	50,000	—	—	50,000
Netherlands	3,752,384	3,309,186	3,050,566	3,615,641	4,130,609	17,858,386
New Zealand	—	335,971	—	—	—	335,971
Norway	1,828,867	2,380,839	2,229,389	4,268,900	5,682,509	16,390,504
Sweden	5,058,376	14,268,602	8,596,868	16,821,178	7,993,666	52,738,690
Switzerland	—	3,875,969	—	4,309,777	2,068,966	10,254,712
United Kingdom	5,193,893	8,215,707	7,274,536	8,469,575	8,266,680	37,423,391

Five countries (United States, Sweden, United Kingdom, Canada, and the Netherlands) contributed 76 percent of all external support to WHO/GPA; 90 percent of support to WHO was received from only 8 countries (above 5 plus Norway, Denmark, and Switzerland) (see Table 12.2).

After increasing dramatically to $30.3 million in 1987, funding for WHO/GPA more than doubled in 1988 ($63.47 million), then plateaued for 1989 ($65.5 million) before increasing substantially in 1990 ($82.39 million).

Table 12.2 (cont.): Multilateral contributions to WHO/GPA global activities, 1987–1991 (inclusive) ($U.S.)

| Source of income | Contributions | | | | | Cumulative total |
	1987	1988	1989	1990	1991	
United States	6,640,500	11,056,000	25,652,580	20,710,888	23,000,000	87,059,968
USSR	798,849	821,557	765,111	823,181	341,128	3,549,826
Subtotal	29,544,550	55,411,349	60,576,425	75,751,998	66,186,037	287,470,359
Other agencies						
UNDP	150,000	2,909,750	282,500	508,500	282,500	4,133,250
Swiss Red Cross	—	—	—	—	32,895	32,895
IBRD	—	—	1,000,000	1,000,000	1,000,000	3,000,000
IBM	—	1,500,000	—	—	—	1,500,000
Sasakawa Foundation	—	875,500	—	—	750,000	1,625,500
World AIDS Foundation	—	—	—	592,530	253,374	845,904
Miscellaneous	168,496	33,724	15,387	7,707	96,075	321,389
Interest and other income	391,090	2,740,606	3,633,167	4,530,712	3,806,198	15,101,773
Subtotal	709,586	8,059,580	4,931,054	6,639,449	6,221,042	26,560,711
Total	30,254,136	63,470,929	65,507,479	82,391,447	72,407,079	314,031,070

Sources: See Table 12.1.

However, in 1991, for the first time, contributions received by WHO/GPA declined, by approximately $9.9 million (12.1%) to $72.41 million. In addition to this decrease in funding, funds were provided to WHO/GPA in the later part of the year, resulting in a slowdown of activities due to uncertainty concerning the level of available funding. In fact, the level of income in 1991 was insufficient to carry out the full proposed budget and the GPA was obliged to implement a contingency budget and program, set at 72 percent of the original 1991 proposed budget.

Table 12.3: Bilateral assistance for AIDS prevention programs, 1986–1991, reported as of June 1992, and adjusted for delayed reporting (millions $U.S.)[a]

Donor country[b]	1986	1987	1988	1989	1990[c]	1991[c]	Total	Percent	Cumulative %
United States	0.00	11.40	25.70	24.30	30.80	52.80	145.00	38	38.0
Canada	0.01	1.70	4.00	3.50	36.40	N/A	45.61	12	50.0
Sweden	0.00	0.00	0.10	8.50	11.40	15.20	35.20	9	59.0
France	0.00	2.20	1.70	8.30	9.40	12.80	34.40	9	68.0
Germany[d]	0.00	0.00	7.00	7.00	7.30	N/A	21.30	6	74.0
Denmark	0.00	0.00	0.00	6.70	0.90	12.30	19.90	5	79.0
Norway	0.10	0.00	0.00	0.20	12.20	N/A	12.50	3	82.0
United Kingdom	0.00	0.00	0.00	4.20	3.40	3.90	11.50	3	85.0
Netherlands	0.00	0.00	0.50	0.50	1.70	1.10	3.80	1	86.0
Switzerland	0.00	3.40	0.20	0.00	0.10	N/A	3.70	1	87.0
Australia	0.00	0.00	0.00	0.20	1.80	N/A	2.00	1	88.0
Italy	0.00	0.00	0.40	1.40	N/A	N/A	1.80	0	88.5
Spain	0.00	0.00	0.00	0.20	0.30	0.30	0.80	0	88.7
Finland	0.00	0.20	0.00	0.30	N/A	N/A	0.50	0	88.8
Subtotal	0.11	18.90	39.60	65.30	115.70	98.40	338.01	88	88.0
EEC[d]	0.00	0.00	0.00	12.00	18.00	18.00	48.00	12	100.0
Total (reported)	0.11	18.90	39.60	77.30	133.70	116.40	386.01	100	100.0
Adjusted total[c]	0.11	18.90	39.60	77.30	136.37	130.37	402.65		

Sources: Correspondence from OECD to *AIDS in the World* (October 18, 1991); Support Program on AIDS for Developing Countries, Ministry of Economic Cooperation, Federal Republic of Germany; (1991); USAID HIV/AIDS Prevention Program, FY 1990, Funding Summary (August 5, 1991); correspondence from Canadian International Development Agency, Cumulative List, AIDS Control Projects (September 1991); Commission of the European Communities—AIDS Control Program Report: 1987–1991; data from WHO/GPA Management Committee, Ad Hoc Working Group (June 1992).
Note: N/A = data not available.
a. Some countries provided figures by year of commitment; others noted year of disbursement. This table lists the higher figure provided.
b. Countries are ranked by total contributions.
c. Figures presented for 1990 and 1991 are estimated to represent 98% and 88%, respectively, of bilateral resources made available in each of these years because of delayed reporting. The totals for 1990 and 1991 have therefore been adjusted by a factor of 1.02 and 1.12, respectively.
d. Years of commitment were not specified. Funds were apportioned against each year covered by respective reports.

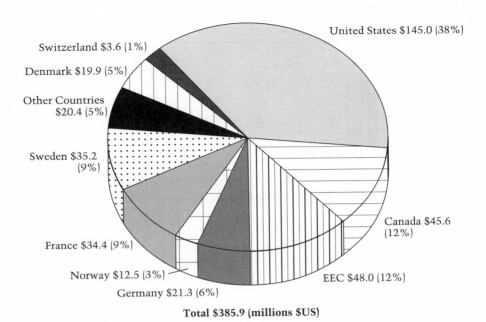

United States $145.0 (38%)

Switzerland $3.6 (1%)

Denmark $19.9 (5%)

Other Countries $20.4 (5%)

Sweden $35.2 (9%)

France $34.4 (9%)

Norway $12.5 (3%)

Germany $21.3 (6%)

Canada $45.6 (12%)

EEC $48.0 (12%)

Total $385.9 (millions $US)

Figure 12.4. Bilateral assistance as reported by principal donors, 1986-1990.
Source: AIDS in the World, 1992.

In addition to direct support for WHO/GPA, a total of $63.3 million was provided to WHO/GPA as multilateral-bilateral funds, for support to specified national AIDS programs (Table 12.1). Of this amount, approximately $47 million was provided by 12 ODA agencies (3 largest contributors: Norway, United Kingdom, and Sweden). The remaining multi-bi resources were contributed by other multilateral agencies (principally UNDP).

■■■■■ . . .

DIRECT ODA SUPPORT (BILATERAL) FOR NATIONAL AIDS PROGRAMS

From 1986 to 1991, 14 countries contributed $338 million as bilateral support to national AIDS programs; in addition, the EEC provided $48 million in direct support for AIDS work in developing countries (Table 12.3). Major donors choosing the bilateral route for support to national

Table 12.4: Funding of the global AIDS strategy by official development assistance agencies (ODAs) and international organizations, 1986–1991 (millions $U.S.)

Donor source	1986	1987	1988	1989	1990[a]	1991[a]	Total	%
WHO/Multilateral[b]	0.00	30.25	63.47	65.51	82.39	72.41	314.03	36
Bilateral[c]	0.11	18.90	39.60	77.30	136.37	130.37	402.65	47
Multi/bilateral[d]	0.00	2.40	16.20	13.10	14.90	16.70	63.30	7
World Bank[e]	0.10	1.90	13.20	30.00	10.60	N/A	55.80	6
UNDP and UNICEF[f]	0.00	0.00	0.00	0.00	11.20	17.30	28.50	3
Total[g]	0.21	53.45	132.47	185.91	255.47	236.78	864.28	100

Sources: See Table 12.1.

a. Bilateral contributions for 1990 and 1991 have been adjusted to compensate for delayed reporting.

b. Includes all contributions to the WHO Global Programme on AIDS.

c. Bilateral support to country programs by ODAs and EEC.

d. Contributions through WHO/GPA by ODA and other international agencies, including UNDP and UNICEF.

e. This contribution is in the form of a low interest loan, not a grant, to recipient countries. A loan to India that was negotiated in 1991 (to be formalized in 1992) is not shown.

f. In the absence of data, the annual breakdown of funds was estimated by *AIDS in the World*.

g. Direct contributions by NGOs, foundations, and the private sector to country programs are not included. Because of rounding of numbers, totals may not exactly match those in earlier tables in this chapter.

AIDS programs included (in descending order): United States, Canada, Sweden, France, Germany, and Denmark; these 6 countries plus the EEC accounted for 91 percent of all bilateral support reported as of June 1992 for the period 1986–1991 (Figure 12.4).

After adjustment for delayed reporting in 1990–1991, bilateral funding for AIDS increased almost sevenfold from 1987 to 1990. While in 1987–1988 the ratio of multilateral-to-bilateral support remained constant (approximately 60:40), in 1990–1991 the situation was reversed, with bilateral ODA contributions exceeding contributions to WHO/GPA (40:60).

■■■■■ . . .

INDUSTRIALIZED COUNTRY SUPPORT FOR DEVELOPING COUNTRY AIDS PROGRAMS

In 1990, total ODA from the OECD countries for all development activities was $54.1 billion. In 1990, the estimated total support by

Table 12.5: Per capita contributions to the global AIDS strategy by donor countries, 1986–1991

Country	Population (millions)	Contribution (millions $U.S.)	Per capita contribution ($U.S.)
Sweden	8.5	97.539	11.48
Norway	4.2	41.448	9.86
Denmark	5.1	36.896	7.23
Canada	26.2	70.500	2.69
Switzerland	6.6	13.850	2.10
Netherlands	14.8	22.732	1.54
United Kingdom	57.2	59.340	1.04
United States	248.8	237.331	0.95
Finland	5.0	4.082	0.82
France	56.2	38.923	0.69
Germany	62.2	28.251	0.45
Australia	16.8	3.643	0.21
New Zealand	3.3	0.336	0.10
Belgium	10.0	1.044	0.10
Japan	123.1	8.100	0.07
Italy	57.5	3.545	0.06
Kuwait	2.0	0.050	0.03
Austria	7.6	0.158	0.02
USSR	275.0	3.550	0.01

Sources: Population: World Bank, *World Development Report 1991*; contributions: see Table 12.1.

Table 12.6: Official development assistance (ODA) from OECD and OPEC members and development assistance for AIDS programs

Country	ODA as % of GNP, 1989	Total net flow (millions $U.S.)	AIDS assistance provided, 1986–1991[a]
OECD			
Norway	1.04	917	Yes
Sweden	0.97	1,799	Yes
Denmark	0.94	937	Yes
Netherlands	0.94	2,094	Yes
France	0.78	7,450	Yes
Finland	0.63	706	Yes
Belgium	0.46	703	Yes
Canada	0.44	2,320	Yes
Italy	0.42	3,613	Yes
Germany	0.41	4,949	Yes
Australia	0.38	1,020	Yes
Japan	0.32	8,949	Yes
United Kingdom	0.31	2,587	Yes
Switzerland	0.30	558	Yes
Austria	0.23	283	Yes
New Zealand	0.22	87	Yes
Ireland	0.17	49	No

these OECD countries to the global AIDS strategy (contributions to WHO and other UN agencies plus direct assistance to developing countries) totaled approximately $175 million. Thus, contributions to the global effort against AIDS represented 0.32 percent of all ODA provided in 1990.

Table 12.5 expresses the total contribution of each industrialized nation to the global AIDS strategy on a per capita basis through 1991. When contributions through the EEC are not included, only 7 nations

Table 12.6 (cont.): Official development assistance (ODA) from OECD and OPEC members and development assistance for AIDS programs

Country	ODA as % of GNP, 1989	Total net flow (millions $U.S.)	AIDS assistance provided, 1986–1991[a]
United States	0.15	7,676	Yes
OPEC			
Saudi Arabia	2.70	2,098	No
Libya	0.52	129	No
Kuwait	0.41	108	Yes
Qatar	0.08	4	No
Venezuela	0.04	49	No
Nigeria	0.03	14	No
Algeria	0.02	13	No
Iran	0.02	39	No
Iraq	−0.05	−28	No
United Arab Emirates	−0.07	−17	No

Sources: World Bank, *World Development Report 1991*; WHO/GPA Financial Information on 1991 Income and Obligations (April 30, 1992); WHO/GPA summary data: Donor Contributions for Specified Countries from 1987 to June 30, 1991 (updated July 31, 1991); correspondence from OECD to *AIDS in the World* (October 18, 1991); Support Program on AIDS for Developing Countries, Ministry of Economic Cooperation, Federal Republic of Germany (1991); USAID HIV/AIDS Prevention Program, FY 1990, Funding Summary (August 5, 1991); correspondence from Canadian International Development Agency, Cumulative List—AIDS Control Projects (September 1991).

a. Cumulative multilateral, bilateral, and multilateral assistance to national AIDS programs as noted in Table 12.2.

contributed more than $1 per capita directly to the global AIDS effort; the three most generous nations were Sweden, Norway, and Denmark. Only 8 OECD and OPEC members provide more than 0.5 percent of their GNP for all kinds of official development assistance (see Table 12.6). While all OECD countries, except Ireland, direct some of this assistance to support AIDS programs in the developing world, only one OPEC member (Kuwait, with a one-time contribution of $50,000 in 1989) has so far done so.

RESPONSE TO THE UNITED NATIONS SYSTEM

In the early stages of the global mobilization, donors were channeling a larger portion of their resources through WHO. Since 1990, there continues to be a shift toward bilateral funding of the global AIDS strategy.

Excluding the World Bank (a lender and not .a grant agency), UNDP provided the most support for AIDS prevention and control during the period 1987–91 (total, $41.7 million) (see Table 12.1). UNICEF's expenditure of $7.1 million in 1990 and 1991 understates the organization's actual contributions, as AIDS efforts may be integrated within ongoing UNICEF programs. Similarly, the contribution of the UNFPA of $400,000 only reflects designated AIDS efforts. Nevertheless, including AIDS and AIDS-related programs in UNESCO, ILO, the UN Population Division, and others, the total UN expenditure on AIDS (excluding WHO and the World Bank) during the period 1986–91 is estimated at $50 million.

By 1990, the World Bank had committed $55.8 million for AIDS prevention and control projects in 13 countries (10 in Africa, 2 in the Americas, 1 in Asia), of which the largest was a $19 million project in Zaire (see Table 12.7). In 1991, with a major new planned loan to India, the World Bank may become the second largest single financial contributor to AIDS prevention and control after the United States.

WHICH COUNTRIES RECEIVE SUPPORT?

Bilateral support from ODA agencies is generally targeted to a limited number of countries considered to be of special interest to the donor country, usually for a combination of historic, economic, and political reasons. Thus, as of January 1, 1992 for example, while five major ODA agencies made bilateral or multi-bi contributions to Thailand (Canada, France, Germany, Japan, United States), only the United States makes bilateral contributions to the Philippines, and none contribute to Burma. Similarly, 7 ODA agencies provide bilateral support to Kenya (Canada, Denmark, Finland, Norway, Sweden, United Kingdom, United States), while Togo receives support only from Germany and the United States.

Table 12.7: World Bank support for AIDS prevention and control, 1986–1990 (millions $U.S.)[a]

Recipient country	1986	1987	1988	1989	1990	Total
Niger	0.150					
Zimbabwe		1.900				
Burundi			1.900			
Guinea			1.000			
Uganda			1.000			
Brazil			9.300			
Guinea-Bissau				0.055		
Nigeria				1.000		
Zaire				19.000		
Indonesia				9.900		
Lesotho					0.900	
Morocco					8.000	
Haiti					1.700	
Total	0.150	1.900	13.200	29.955	10.600	55.805

Source: Correspondence from World Bank, Population, Health and Nutrition Division, Population and Human Resources Department, to *AIDS in the World* (October 17, 1991).
    a. No figure reported for 1991. Figures are expressed in the year of commitment. Projects are multiyear projects, and not all funds were necessarily disbursed in the year of commitment. The World Bank has also provided support to other health or social sector development projects that, although they may not have included a specific AIDS component, do provide support to some AIDS- and STD-related activities.

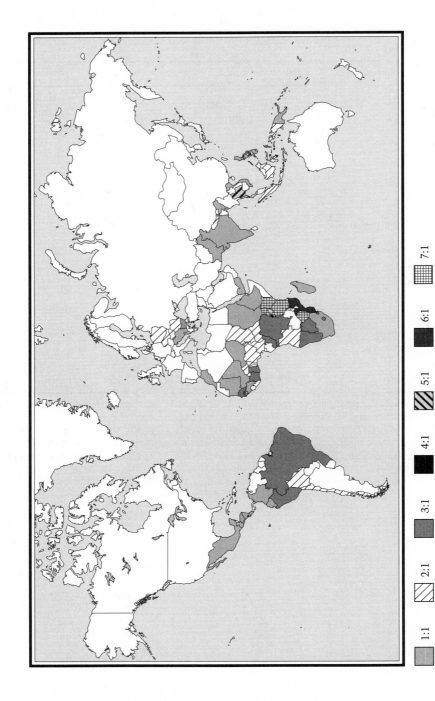

Figure 12.5. Global AIDS strategy donor country: recipient country ratio.

| 1:1 | 2:1 | 3:1 | 4:1 | 5:1 | 6:1 | 7:1 |

There are 4 countries that receive support from 7 donors, 2 that receive funds from 6 donors, 1 country that has 5 donors, two with four donors, 13 with 3 donors, 24 with 2 donors, and 37 countries receiving bilateral assistance from only one donor (see Figure 12.5). Appendix 12.1 shows the developing countries receiving bilateral assistance from each donor nation.

HOW MUCH DO DEVELOPING COUNTRIES CONTRIBUTE?

A recent study carried out by WHO/GPA (November 1991) examined the mix of external support and domestic contributions to the national AIDS programs in developing countries. In 7 of the 9 countries examined, the "governments were not at all or very insignificantly sharing the resource burden for AIDS control."* Notable exceptions were Ethiopia and Thailand, where the national governments were funding almost half of their programs.

The profiles of 6 selected countries (Table 12.8) suggest that developing country governments have not yet shifted substantial resources to their national AIDS programs.

FUNDING GAPS—ALREADY APPARENT

In 1991, for the first time since the global mobilization against AIDS began, international resources made available by wealthy countries to developing ones in support of their AIDS prevention and control effort, have declined, even after adjustment for delayed financial reporting in 1990–1991 (see Figure 12.6). Resources made available to WHO/GPA for 1991 have not been sufficient to fully finance its contingency budget (72 percent of the initially proposed budget). Meanwhile, bilateral funding has not kept up with the pace dictated by expanding needs in the developing world. Unless a major effort is made, the gap in AIDS prevention and care capacity between wealthy and developing countries—already large—will continue to grow.

In addition, pressures on ODA budgets will increase, including

---

*Quote from Interim Financial Report, WHO/Global Programme on AIDS, November 1991.

Table 12.8: Profiles of expenditure activity in selected countries, 1989

Item	Cameroon	Egypt	Mexico	Nigeria	Trinidad and Tobago	Zambia
Defense	6.7%	14.4%	2.2%	2.8%	N/A	0.0%
Education	12.0%	11.9%	12.3%	2.8%	N/A	8.6%
Health	3.4%	2.5%	1.7%	0.8%	N/A	7.4%
Total government expenditures as % of GNP	20.9%	40.2%	21.2%	28.1%	36.9%	20.0%
GNP/capita ($U.S.)	$1,000	$640	$2,010	$250	$3,230	$390
Total government expenditures (millions $U.S.)	$2,424.4	$13,056	$36,050	$7,994	$1,549	$608.4
Total government health expenditure (millions $U.S.)	$762.4	$65.3	$613	$63.9	$24.7	$45.0
Government expenditure per capita on health ($U.S.)	$65.72	$1.28	$7.24	$0.61	$19.00	$5.79
National AIDS budget (millions $U.S.)	$3.1	$1.3	$2.487	$1.5	$0.292	$5.5
% of government health expenditures (1988) on AIDS (1991)	0.4%	1.9%	0.4%	2.3%	1.2%	12.0%

Sources: World Bank, World Development Report 1991, tables I and II; *AIDS in the World* survey, 1991–92.

Note: N/A = data not available.

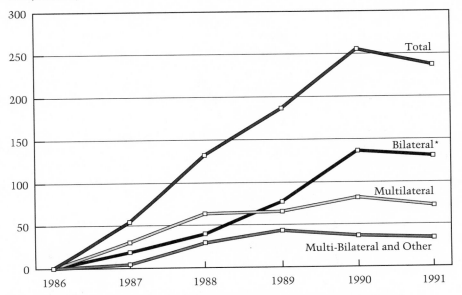

Figure 12.6. Funding of the Global AIDS Strategy, 1986-1991, decline in international financing.
*Adjustment of 1990 and 1991 reported bilateral contributions have been made to account for delayed reporting by ODAs.
Source: AIDS in the World, 1992.

competition for ODA funds by Central and Eastern European nations (see Box 12.4).

■ ■ ■ ■ ■ ■   .   .   .

COMMENTS AND EMERGING CONCERNS

No agency has assumed responsibility for collecting data on international and national contributions to AIDS prevention and care in the developing world. Therefore, the basic questions of how much? from whom? and to whom? can only be addressed by collecting data from many diverse sources.

A review of these figures suggests several major conceptual and data gaps in existing approaches for funding of AIDS programs in developing countries:

- What are the medium- and longer-term needs of national AIDS programs?
- What is the anticipated cost of AIDS prevention and care in developing countries?
- What are the responsibilities of national, bilateral, multilateral, and nongovernmental systems and organizations for support of AIDS prevention and care in the developing world?
- How can the burden of support for developing countries be most equitably shared?

In summary, in the absence of a clear strategy based on measurable targets and outcomes, the international system for supporting AIDS prevention and control at the national level may be degenerating into a series of short-term, uncoordinated, and reactive responses, increasingly subjected to domestic and foreign policy pressures rather than guided by the need for prevention and control of the global epidemic.

Box 12.4: Eastern and Central Europe: Support for National AIDS Prevention and Control Programs

source: Correspondence in WHO Regional Office Europe to *AIDS in the World* (November 15, 1991).

The changes over the last 24 months in Central and Eastern Europe may have significant impact on patterns of development assistance. This region presents a very attractive investment opportunity for foreign aid, as well as new opportunities for the development of political and economic influence by the major industrialized nations.

Given this situation, there is the possibility that ODA agencies will see their budgets limited, as governments direct funding to programs that support trade and investment opportunities with Eastern and Central Europe, as opposed to providing assistance funding for programs in the developing world.

With the reality of slow economic growth in the industrialized countries and the resultant constraints on foreign aid budgets, the nations of Eastern and Central Europe will have a competitive advantage, in terms of investment opportunities, over the countries of the developing world.

Currently, short- and medium-term national AIDS plans are being developed for the countries of this region. The two-year budgetary project for this group of seven countries (Albania, Bulgaria, Czechoslovakia, Hungary, Poland, Romania, and Yugoslavia) has been projected at $1,595 million by the WHO Regional Office for Europe. Of this amount, approximately $1 million has been pledged.

Donor	Amount
Netherlands	$474,000
USSR	400,000
United Kingdom (U.K.)	60,000
	$934,000
Nongovernmental Organization (U.K.-based)	$ 75,000
Total (millions $U.S.)	$ 1.009

Approximate budget 1990 and 1991	Amount
Albania	$250,000
Bulgaria	143,000
Czechoslovakia	168,000
Hungary	220,000
Poland	168,000
Romania	500,000
Yugoslavia	146,000
Total (millions $U.S.)	$ 1.595

CHAPTER THIRTEEN

AIDS and Human Rights

The heated, intense dialogue between public health and human rights has been one of the most important and unanticipated outcomes of the first decade of the AIDS pandemic. Discrimination has been identified as both counterproductive for public health program effectiveness and as a major underlying cause of ill health worldwide. It is reasonable to speak of a "revolution" in thinking about health through its inextricable connection with human rights. Yet, the temptation to return to so-called traditional public health approaches is also strong and will intensify as the number of people with AIDS and the economic impact of the pandemic increase during the 1990s. As a result, some people speak of the need to end the special treatment accorded to HIV prevention (translation: special treatment = strong emphasis on human rights as a key component of public health strategies). Rather, as the challenges of AIDS and other major public health problems of the future involve behavior—individual and collective—the value of incorporating human rights norms within public health practice will increase. Can the insights and new approaches pioneered in the context of AIDS be sustained, as well as extended to other health problems?

—The Editors

This chapter was written by Katarina Tomasevski, a fellow at the Danish Center for Human Rights, Copenhagen, Denmark, with the collaboration of Sofia Gruskin, Dean's Fellow, Center for the Study of Human Rights, Columbia University, New York; Zita Lazzarini, a public health attorney in Boston working on international health and human rights issues; and Aart Hendriks, a legal researcher attached to the Faculty of Law, University of Utrecht, the Netherlands.

AIDS is the first worldwide epidemic to occur in the modern era of human rights. For the first time, public health practitioners are being held to a dual standard in the design and implementation of public health programs, in this case to prevent HIV transmission. Programs must be effective in public health terms, but in addition they must respect and respond to human rights norms.

The first decade of AIDS was strongly marked by the dialogue, and often by a conflict, between so-called traditional public health approaches and pressures to respect human rights norms. Now, at the beginning of the second decade, there is a noticeable decline in international attention to the human rights aspects of HIV/AIDS prevention and care. After a period in which the rights of people with AIDS and those infected with HIV had come to be acknowledged, there is again increasing pressure for restrictive legislation. Discrimination and a lack of protection of human rights and dignity are rising, fueled by economic, social, and political instability, resurgent complacency, prejudice, denial, and an unwillingness or inability to address discrimination in all its forms.

The relationship between HIV/AIDS prevention and care and human rights can be considered in two ways. First, there are possible pressures and problems related to human rights that are created by the choice or manner of implementation of public health measures. This is the more traditional arena in which public health and human rights issues have been negotiated. Second, during the past decade it became clear that societal discrimination in all its forms creates increased vulnerability to HIV infection. Therefore, efforts to protect human rights and to promote human dignity are extremely important for protecting public health in the HIV/AIDS pandemic.

Protection against epidemics is one of the main tasks of the public authorities emanating from the human right to health.* In addition, public health has been accepted as a legitimate ground for limiting human rights in international human rights law.[1] Incorporating

---

*The International Covenant on Economic, Social and Cultural Rights includes "the prevention, treatment and control of epidemic . . . diseases" among the steps that States Parties should undertake toward the full realization of the right to health. *Human Rights: A Compilation of International Instruments* (New York: United Nations, 1988) 12.

human rights into public health responses to epidemics has not been easy. Public health developed through centuries by relying on coercion, compulsion, and restriction[2] and, therefore, does not readily adjust to the requirements of human rights.[3]

The ways in which many national authorities have responded to the AIDS epidemic have created a wide range of human rights problems by imposing coercive or restrictive AIDS control measures. Virtually every measure of disease control has human rights implications: public health surveillance may seek and record the personal identity of infected persons, and people identified as *carriers* may be subjected to isolation and quarantine. Even how a disease is classified may lead to compulsory medical examination or hospitalization, depending on local or national disease control legislation. Because many public health measures are coercive, compulsory, or restrictive, they must be authorized by law. Public health laws thus specify what individuals must do (vaccination, for example)[4] and what they must not do (by defining offenses against public health, including the transmission of infectious diseases).*

Whether it is AIDS or any other epidemic, the bulk of public health measures deal with the identification of the affected groups and individuals and with safeguards against further spread of disease. This approach is reflected in the terminology used in AIDS prevention and control: such terms as *strategy, surveillance, agent,* and *combat* clearly convey the message of fighting an enemy. Not surprisingly, language became one of the many contentious issues during the first decade of dialogue between public health and human rights.†

---

*Cf. Criminal law and criminological questions raised by the propagation of infectious diseases, including AIDS. Report submitted by the Portuguese delegation, *16th Conference of European Ministers of Justice, Lisbon, 21–22 June 1988,* Council of Europe, MJU-16 (88) 1 (1988).

†In 1983, Peter Seitzman stated, speaking in the name of people with AIDS: "We are victims and not the guilty" [*New York Native,* 3–16 January 1983, 23], but the term *victim* was soon rejected by those to whom it referred, and the United States PWA Coalition declared at the second AIDS Forum in Denver in 1983: "We condemn attempts to label us as 'victims,' which implies defeat, and we are only occasionally 'patients,' which implies passivity, helplessness and dependence upon the care of others. We are 'people with AIDS.'" [*Surviving and Thriving with AIDS,* ed. M. Callen (New York: PWA Coalition, 1987)].

As in all other areas of human rights, movements to reinforce their universality emerge in response to violations. Before AIDS, public health laws and measures were rarely, if ever, reviewed by human rights criteria, either in individual countries or by the international human rights bodies. When the AIDS pandemic triggered a whole gamut of coercive and restrictive public health measures, many proved to be incompatible with human rights,[5] and this provided an incentive for in-depth examinations of public health from the viewpoint of human rights.[6]

The second area of dialogue between human rights and public health responses to the HIV/AIDS pandemic arose when it became clear that a discriminatory social environment was counterproductive for HIV information/education and prevention programs. Threats and coercion toward HIV-infected people had the effect of driving people with risk behaviors away from the health and social services created to help prevent HIV transmission. Thus, from a practical viewpoint, discrimination was viewed as a danger to public health.

However, as understanding of the pandemic evolved, the relationship between societal discrimination or marginalization and the risk of becoming HIV infected became more evident. Being excluded from

---

Box 13.1: The Difficulty of Ranking Countries by Human Rights Criteria

The Editors

This first issue of *AIDS in the World* has refrained from ranking countries by human rights criteria. Most human rights organizations (notably Amnesty International) refuse to rank countries because availability of information correlates negatively with the gravity of problems: where formal complaints of human rights violations are numerous (in the Netherlands or Canada, for example), this is actually evidence of their openness and of the extent to which those countries have incorporated the principles of human rights protection into their social framework.

However, the paucity of complaints of HIV/AIDS-related violations also suggests that human rights norms relevant to HIV/AIDS have not yet been clearly articulated and may be unknown both to the violators and the victimized.

The second edition of *AIDS in the World* will address this issue. It will combine data on the binding international human rights norms by country with data on AIDS prevention and control measures that should conform to these norms. This will provide a framework to describe and help monitor HIV/AIDS-related human rights violations in the world.

the mainstream of society, or being discriminated against on grounds of race/ethnicity, national origin, religion, gender, or sexual preference, led to an increase in the risk of HIV infection. Thus, during the first decade of work against AIDS, the positive contribution that improving protection of human rights could have for public health became evident. This was a further challenge to the public health tradition that emphasizes individual duties and obligations rather than rights and freedoms.

THE PATTERN OF HUMAN RIGHTS PROBLEMS

This section focuses on the first part of the public health-human rights equation: burdens on human rights created by public health programs. Unfortunately, no worldwide review of AIDS-related human rights problems has yet been made to indicate what acts constitute human rights violations (Box 13.1).*

Although the United Nations appointed a Special Rapporteur in 1989 to study AIDS-related discrimination,[7] his reports have described human rights problems as these emerge in responding to AIDS, but not the pattern of human rights violations.[8] That same year the European Parliament called for the establishment of a unit to monitor AIDS-related discrimination in its resolution on the fight against AIDS, but no monitoring scheme has yet been established.[9] This does not amount to saying that intergovernmental bodies have done nothing. The numerous international policy documents on the human rights aspects of AIDS are a good indicator of the nature and scope of the threat that responses to AIDS have created for human rights.[10] In many countries where coercive and discriminatory AIDS control measures have been carried out by the public health authorities, they have

*Few comparative surveys of AIDS control measures from the viewpoint of the applicable international human rights standards have been carried out: R. Cohen and L. S. Wiseberg, *Double Jeopardy—Threat to Life and Human Rights. Discrimination against Persons with AIDS* (Cambridge, Mass.: Human Rights Internet, Harvard Law School, 1990); *The 3rd Epidemic. Repercussions of the Fear of AIDS* (London: PANOS Institute, 1990); M. Breum and A. Hendriks, eds., *AIDS and Human Rights. An International Perspective* (Copenhagen: Danish Center for Human Rights, 1988).

provoked much criticism and opposition. Discriminatory practices by insurance companies, private employers, or medical practitioners, victimizing HIV-infected people and people with AIDS, have been tolerated in many countries, leading to demands that public authorities fulfill their obligations under international law and provide protection against discrimination.

In summary, information on both public and private practices that may violate human rights norms remains fragmentary.[11,12]

In addition, fear of AIDS has prompted the public to support coercive and restrictive measures that may not have been tolerated in other areas. Thus, public opinion surveys often show relatively strong support for discrimination against HIV-infected people,[13] while the widespread view that AIDS is a self-inflicted disease further reinforces discriminatory attitudes.[14] Paradoxically, fear of public exposure is an additional reason for the paucity of information. The people who are victimized are often too frightened of stigmatization to seek redress. Silence, as is well known in human rights work generally, enables violations to continue unchallenged. Nevertheless, existing information suggests that virtually all human rights and fundamental freedoms have been affected: from access to education, employment, and health care; to freedom of expression, assembly, and association; to freedom of movement; and to the protection of the basic human rights of prisoners, children, or refugees.

The general global pattern of human rights violations has been repeated in the context of AIDS: violations have been at their worst for people least able to assert and protect their rights, such as prisoners, commercial sex workers, asylum seekers, or drug-dependent persons. They have become targets of compulsory or coercive AIDS control measures, and this has created an additional need to link AIDS with broad human rights work.

Finally, fresh problems have also arisen in the context of the HIV/AIDS pandemic: fear of contagion has been used to discriminate against people who are or might be HIV-positive and those associated with them, thereby creating new grounds for discrimination—the status of potential infectiousness[15]—and the consequent need for human rights safeguards.[16] The lack of an explicit international prohibition of discrimination on the grounds of health status has led to national interpretations whose nature and scope varied widely.[17]

Moreover, the high costs of medical and social assistance to people with AIDS[18] have tended to reinforce discriminatory practices, particularly in employment[19] and related health insurance.[20] Nevertheless, opposition to coercive, compulsory, restrictive, and, in particular, discriminatory HIV/AIDS control measures has been widespread, even worldwide. Many of these measures have been successfully challenged, often by invoking human rights (Box 13.2).

Human Rights Aspects of National Responses to AIDS: National Laws, Policies, and Practices

In the first decade, 1981–1990, 104 countries adopted some AIDS-related legislation (see Figures 13.1 and 13.2). Thus, "where technology is still unable to provide a solution to the spread of disease, people look to the law."[21]

As illustrated in Table 13.1, the period 1985–87 represented the peak of the global epidemic of AIDS legislation: the cumulative number of countries with laws on AIDS more than quadrupled, from 18 at the beginning of 1985, to 78 by the end of 1987. In the United States

Box 13.2: The AIDS Litigation Project: Lens on Public Policy

y Gostin, J.D., Execu-
Director, American
ety of Law and Medi-
, and Lane Porter, J.D.,
H., Chair, International
th Committee, Section
ternational Law,
rican Bar Association

Courts and human rights commissions work like a lens to magnify public policy and social tensions. Examination of cases brought before these bodies reveals conflicts in values likely to emerge as major issues in the future, requiring resolution by legislatures and health officials. In an attempt to gain insight into the contemporary history of the HIV epidemic, the AIDS Litigation Project undertook a review of legal cases brought before courts and human rights commissions in the United States at the federal, state, and local levels.[a]

The AIDS Litigation Project review found numerous, often highly publicized cases of criminal law being used to prosecute persons for allegedly exposing others to HIV, through having sex without disclosing their serological status, or biting, spitting on, or splattering their blood on others. However, the largest proportion of cases concerned alleged discrimination in employment settings, schools, and, increasingly, in the health care system. Employment discrimination was clustered among health care workers, people who work with children—such as teachers, foster parents, and day care workers—and food handlers, but it persists across a broad spectrum of occupations. Court decisions did not tolerate exclusion of HIV-infected children from ordinary schools; however, they did require the school, parents, and child to comply

Number of Countries

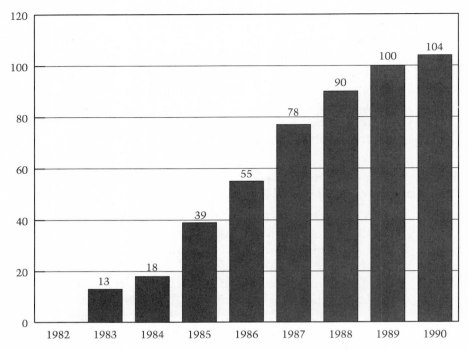

Figure 13.1. Cumulative number of countries adopting AIDS legislation.

with specified safeguards against possible transmission. Courts and the Americans with Disabilities Act (ADA), which comes into effect in 1992, have reaffirmed that all stages of HIV disease are a disability for the purposes of discrimination law.

Health care discrimination cases mainly involved claims that health providers or facilities refused to treat patients, referred them, or treated them badly because they were infected with HIV. These refusals occurred both in relation to invasive procedures, such as surgery, and noninvasive therapy, such as psychiatry and chiropractics. In some cases, AIDS care professionals were refused premises in which to offer their services to persons

with HIV/AIDS. A growing number of claims also involved testing of and limitations on the right to practice among HIV-infected health care workers. In these cases, decisions were most likely to uphold reasonable restrictions on the practice of invasive procedures and to strike down testing and restrictions for noninvasive procedures.

Finally, a rising number of court cases on the validity of insurance policies highlighted the potentially unresolvable conflict between insurers' desire to discriminate against people with higher risk and the rights of a person with HIV to adequate insurance protection.

According to the survey,

Number of Countries

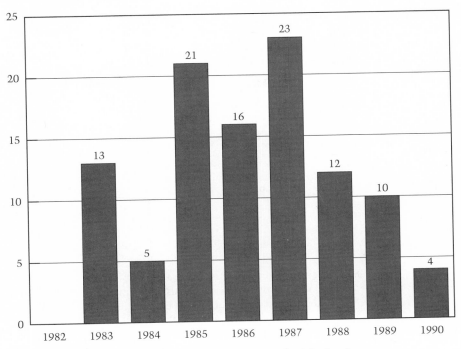

Figure 13.2. Number of countries adopting AIDS legislation by year.

discrimination against persons with HIV in the areas of employment, education, housing, and public accommodation is declining, due in large part to increased public knowledge and changing attitudes toward people infected with HIV, as well as rigorous enforcement of laws to protect people with disabilities. However, complaints about discrimination in health care, nursing, and social services have predominated in recent years. The patterns of discrimination can be expected to shift further as the epidemic affects increasing numbers of injection drug users, who have been traditionally underserved by health care systems because of their socioeconomic status and the lack of expertise and willingness among many health care professionals to treat drug abuse. The findings of the AIDS Litigation Project support the hypothesis that the combined impact of education, law enforcement, and increased tolerance can reduce discrimination against persons with HIV and, thereby, help advance public health.

a. The AIDS Litigation Project, supported by the National AIDS Program Office, U.S. Public Health Service, collected and analyzed data through June 1989 (Project I), with additional data collected through June 1991 (Project II).

Table 13.1: Countries adopting first AIDS legislation, 1983–1990

Year	Country	Number of countries
1983	Austria, Canada, Denmark, France, Germany/West, Greece, Israel, Italy, New Zealand, Norway, Sweden, Turkey, United States	13
1984	Australia, Chile, Luxembourg, Uruguay, Venezuela	5
1985	Bahamas, Barbados, Belgium, Bermuda, Brazil, Congo, Costa Rica, Ecuador, Finland, French Polynesia, Hungary, Malaysia, Panama, Paraguay, Peru, Romania, Singapore, Spain, Thailand, United Arab Emirates, United Kingdom	21
1986	China, Cuba, Egypt, Grenada, Guatemala, Iceland, Kuwait, Malta, Mexico, Monaco, Mozambique, Philippines, Poland, Portugal, Switzerland, Yugoslavia	16
1987	Belize, Brunei Darussalam, Bulgaria, Burundi, Cyprus, Dominican Republic, El Salvador, Iraq, Jordan, Kenya, Republic of Korea, Liberia, Libya, Liechtenstein, Mauritius, Netherlands, Niger, Papua New Guinea, South Africa, Sudan, Syria, Togo, USSR	23
1988	Bulgaria, Chad, Colombia, Comores, Czechoslovakia, Equatorial Guinea, Guinea, Hong Kong, Japan, Mali, Sri Lanka, Suriname	12
1989	Algeria, Bolivia, Guinea-Bissau, India, Mongolia, Nicaragua, Rwanda, Tunisia, Vietnam, Yemen	10
1990	Argentina, Bahrain, Madagascar, Senegal	4
		104

Sources: K. Tomasevski, Survey of national AIDS legislation, *Regional Consultation on Ethical and Legal Aspects, Seoul, 23–25 July 1990* (World Health Organization, Regional Office for Western Pacific); K. Tomasevski, AIDS and human rights: An overview of repressive and liberal legislation, *Liberation Development,* special issue (September 1990); K. Tomasevski, "AIDS and human rights. Part 1: National responses to AIDS," in *Collected Courses of the Academy of European Law. Second Session, Florence, 1991,* ed. A. Cassesse and A. Clapham; W. J. Curran, L. Gostin, and Z. Lazzarini, *International Survey of Legislation Relating to the AIDS Epidemic* (conducted in behalf of WHO Global Programme on AIDS) (forthcoming).

alone, more than 180 laws relating to HIV/AIDS were enacted in the period 1985–87,[22] while more than 840 bills appeared before state legislatures, including 450 in a single year (1987).[23] Since this peak, there has been a marked slowing in the adoption of AIDS legislation.

The first national AIDS legislation was passed in 1983, less than 2 years after AIDS had become known and 2 years before a test for HIV became widely available. This first legislation, requiring the reporting of suspected and confirmed cases of AIDS, was enacted in Sweden on March 8, 1983, and was followed by similar laws in several European countries.[24] Most often this early legislation established safeguards to promote blood safety (through donor referral) and introduced compulsory notification for cases of AIDS.[25] Yet, until 1985, no country adopted a comprehensive law on AIDS, in part because a test for HIV infection had not yet been developed.

Analysis of subsequent laws reveals that the availability of a test to detect antibodies to HIV[26] was the driving force behind the legislation. Most of these laws dealt directly with testing, and many authorized public health authorities to carry out compulsory tests. The legal authorization to isolate people, detain them or force them into hospitals often appeared alongside provisions for compulsory testing. Although only Cuba[27] has officially adopted mandatory and automatic hospitalization of all HIV-infected people, many other countries have passed laws empowering public health authorities to resort to restrictive measures (see Table 13.2 and Figure 13.3). These include placing HIV-infected people under surveillance, isolation or segregation, mandatory hospitalization, or imposing specific restrictions on their behavior.[28] Information on the actual application of such restrictions is not available for many countries.

Specific factors that influenced the adoption of AIDS legislation in individual countries cannot be easily identified. As illustrated by the Chronology of AIDS Legislation at the end of this chapter, Western industrialized countries were the first and the most active in this regard. Latin American and Asian countries soon followed, and in Africa AIDS legislation emerged later. The common assumption that countries adopted AIDS legislation because of a high prevalence of HIV and/or large numbers of AIDS cases is not confirmed. Countries without a single reported case of AIDS or of HIV infection adopted AIDS-related laws (e.g., Vietnam and Mongolia). As will be discussed

Table 13.2: Countries imposing restrictions based on HIV/AIDS status as of 1991

Placement under surveillance	Hospitalization/isolation	
Angola	China	Monaco
Burma	Chile	Panama
China	Cuba	Poland
Czechoslovakia	Dominica	Romania
Hungary	Finland	South Africa
Japan	Korea	Sweden
Jordan	Kuwait	United Kingdom
Korea, Republic	Malaysia	Vietnam
Mexico	Malta	
Norway		
Peru		
USSR		

Sources: Same as Table 13.1.

later, excessive AIDS control measures have been adopted in certain countries not as a response to HIV/AIDS inside their own borders but ostensibly to prevent its importation.

. . .

DISEASE CLASSIFICATION

Disease classification is one of many public health measures that are considered *technical,* yet it has direct consequences for human rights. Classification of a disease as contagious, communicable, transmissible, infectious, or sexually transmitted is only the beginning of a process entailing the application of previously existing laws that may mandate compulsory medical examination or hospitalization, restrictions on travel or immigration, or isolation. For example, the (failed) California Proposition 64 in 1985 sought to increase the powers of the public health authorities by classifying AIDS as an "infectious, contagious and communicable disease."[29] Classification can also lead to stigma, as evidenced by the frequent so-called analogies between AIDS and leprosy.[30]

The relation of disease classification to human rights has only recently been addressed. In 1990, for example, the European Parlia-

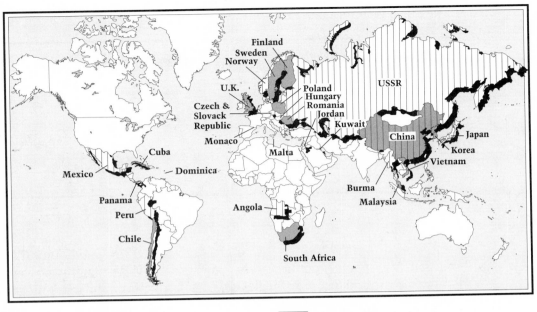

▦ Placement under surveillance	▦ Hospitalization/isolation

Figure 13.3. Countries imposing restrictions based on HIV/AIDS status, as of 1991.

ment emphasized that "it is impossible to accept discrimination based on a disease which is transmissible but not contagious."[31] Also in 1990, the New York State Public Health Council refused to classify HIV infection as sexually transmissible "because such a declaration would trigger certain statutory requirements permitting isolation and quarantine, reporting, testing and contact tracing."[32] Even though the scientific literature has pleaded for consistency and precision in disease classification,[33] there is still no uniformity regarding AIDS and HIV infection. Some countries classify HIV/AIDS as a communicable disease, others as an infectious disease, still others as a viral disease. Many countries have classified AIDS as a sexually transmitted disease (STD). (See Table 13.3.)

The World Health Organization (WHO) seems to have passively endorsed this approach, arguing that most HIV infections are acquired

Table 13.3: Countries classifying HIV/AIDS as a sexually transmitted disease as of 1991

Algeria	Iceland	Senegal
Bhutan	Madagascar	Sri Lanka
Brazil	Malawi	Swaziland
Bulgaria	Mexico	Sweden
Chile	Nepal	Syria
Dominican Republic	Nicaragua	Thailand
El Salvador	Panama	Trinidad and Tobago
Guatemala	Papua New Guinea	Uruguay
Guinea	Poland	Vietnam
Hungary	Romania	

Sources: See Table 13.1.

and transmitted sexually.* From the human rights viewpoint, this classification gives public health authorities wide-ranging powers under already existing STD legislation.[34] The coercive and compulsory measures envisaged in STD laws are broad, and the stigma associated with sexually transmitted diseases means that these laws are rarely challenged.

The main feature of legislation on STDs is the effort to prevent the spread of infection by denying rights to infected individuals.[35] Yet for all their powers, the traditional measures for controlling sexually transmitted diseases have been generally ineffective in halting their spread, while often harming the people affected by them.[36] Nevertheless, they have been faithfully and generally unthinkingly applied to AIDS: compulsory examination, contact tracing, restrictive measures against carriers to prevent further transmission, compulsory treatment and/or hospitalization, and extensive case finding through pre-

---

*The WHO has justified the linking of AIDS and STD control as follows: "The predominant mode of transmission of both human immunodeficiency virus (HIV) and other STD is sexual, although other routes of transmission for both include blood, blood products, donated organs or tissue, and through an infected mother to her fetus or newborn infant. . . . Many of the measures for preventing sexual transmission of HIV and STD are the same, as are the target audiences for these interventions." Consensus statement from the Consultation on Global Strategies for Co-ordination of AIDS and STD Control Programmes, Geneva, 11–13 July 1990, WHO/GPA/INF/90.2 (1990) 1.

marital and prenatal screening. Every prohibition and sanction relating to transmission of HIV infection and/or exposure of others to risk of HIV infection has been adopted from preexisting STD laws.[37] Moreover, immigration regulations once enacted for STDs have been applied to AIDS in order to exclude persons who are HIV infected, thus reviving "certificates of freedom from venereal disease."[38]

▬▬▬▬▬   · · ·

HIV TESTING

Most countries adopting legislation have given public health authorities powers to carry out epidemiologic surveillance. The exercise of such powers is often discretionary and seldom includes procedures to prevent human rights violations. Most countries have been unwilling to analyze the compatibility of public health measures with human rights.[39]

Public health surveillance* involves an assessment of the existing distribution and scope of infection and its likely spread in the population and is an important first step in responding to a disease. As people infected with HIV can remain asymptomatic for a very long time and because HIV infection can only be detected with a specific test, testing became the central issue in public health surveillance. However, for this specific purpose it is sufficient to know *how many* people are infected; it is not necessary to learn the identity of these infected people. Thus, as WHO declared in 1987, if testing was to be used to identify specific infected individuals, voluntariness—free and informed consent—was an indispensable precondition, and it had to be accompanied by counseling and protection of confidentiality.[40] These safeguards needed a powerful advocate, because the history of public health shows that compulsory and coercive measures have consistently been applied in a discriminatory manner.[41] This was particularly apparent when an epidemic concentrated in specific pop-

---

*According to the WHO, "public health surveillance is the collection of information of sufficient accuracy and completeness regarding the distribution and spread of infection to be pertinent to the design, implementation, or monitoring of prevention and control programmes and activities." *Unlinked anonymous screening for the public health surveillance of HIV infections. Proposed international guidelines*, Geneva, June 1989.

Table 13.4: Mass HIV screening in countries with low HIV prevalence as of 1991

Target population	Country
General population	Cuba: 75% of population screened Bulgaria: 45% of population screened USSR: 30% of population screened
Specific categories	Burma, China, India, Indonesia, Jordan, Korea (DPR), Kuwait, Nepal, Oman, Pakistan, Papua New Guinea, Sri Lanka, Syria, Tunisia, Vietnam

Sources: See Table 13.1.

ulations, where the identification of carriers was part of the stigmatization of these populations as "sources of infection."[42] Whenever an epidemic was transmitted sexually, this stigmatization was associated with the attribution of blame and by scapegoating.[43]

In addition, *surveillance* is a term often associated with intrusions into individual privacy; in some cases, people have been required to undergo HIV testing and have even been subjected to testing without being asked.[44] Information on people identified as HIV infected has been and still is made available to the police or immigration authorities, to employers or insurance companies, and even to the media. Thus, the question of involuntary testing emerged early and forcefully in the AIDS pandemic,[45] and testing remains at the center of controversies relating to AIDS prevention and control.

■   .   .   .

TARGETS OF MASS TESTING

The worldwide pattern of HIV testing policies and practices gives a good indication of the orientation of HIV/AIDS prevention and control. Few countries have attempted to screen their entire population, but this apparently reflects prohibitive cost and complex logistics rather than human rights considerations. As seen in Table 13.4, at least 3 countries, Bulgaria, Cuba, and the former USSR, initiated mass screening for a large part of their population. Today, Cuba remains the only country to pursue this approach.

In some countries, large numbers of HIV tests have been performed without evidence that consent had been obtained or confidentiality preserved. Low-prevalence countries where large-scale testing has been carried out are listed. These are principally Asian and Middle Eastern countries, and the power to carry out testing has been accompanied by provisions for placing restrictions on people found to be HIV infected.

In virtually all countries, the selectiveness of HIV testing has raised important human rights problems. The choice of groups or categories to be tested has not always reflected the epidemiological pattern of HIV/AIDS nor the dominant mode of HIV transmission. Compulsory and mass HIV testing has targeted a variety of groups, including: returning nationals, resident aliens, aliens entering the country, military personnel, police officers, drug users, commercial sex workers, prisoners, people with hemophilia, pregnant women, children of HIV-infected mothers, and patients in hospitals. Some countries mandated compulsory HIV testing of unspecified high-risk groups (often involving homosexuals, commercial sex workers, and drug users),* although seroprevalence studies among such high-risk groups might have shown that they were presently neither high-risk nor groups.[46] Captive populations (prisoners, refugees in closed camps, women attending antenatal clinics, STD patients, military recruits) have been subjected to compulsory HIV testing in many countries and in large numbers. Such groups are within the reach of public health authorities, and because safeguards against compulsory and/or coercive measures are ineffective and nonexistent, they are often unable to refuse HIV testing.

Tables 13.5–13.8 list the most frequent targets of mass HIV testing by category and by country. Prisoners have been targeted in the largest number of countries (30), followed by STD patients (23), pregnant women (23), and returning nationals (20).

Much effort has been devoted to preventing the so-called importation of HIV/AIDS. Some countries have imposed AIDS-free certificates or an HIV test as a condition for entry. Despite the widespread

---

*Sudan has defined high-risk groups to include the following categories: "STD patients, prostitutes, truck drivers, military recruits, displaced populations, refugees, street children, and prisoners." National Medium-term Plan for the Prevention and Control of AIDS, Ministry of Health, Khartoum, October 1989.

Table 13.5: Countries screening specified "high-risk groups" as of 1991

"High-risk" groups	Countries
Commercial sex workers	Belize, DPR Korea, Indonesia
Prisoners	Bhutan, Bulgaria, Burma, Cape Verde, Costa Rica, Dominican Republic, Hungary, Indonesia, Italy, Jordan, Kenya, Kuwait, Mali, Mexico, Nepal, Niger, Nigeria, Oman, Pakistan, Papua New Guinea, Sierra Leone, Sri Lanka, Sudan, Syria, Thailand, Tunisia, United States, Uruguay, Vietnam, Yugoslavia
Drug-dependent people	Bulgaria, Burma, Czechoslovakia, Hungary, Indonesia, Italy, Kuwait, Nepal, Oman, Pakistan, Sri Lanka, Syria, Thailand, Tunisia, USSR, Vietnam
Homosexuals	Bulgaria, Burma, Dominican Republic, El Salvador, Guatemala, Indonesia, Kuwait, Oman, Papua New Guinea, Philippines, Sierra Leone, Suriname, Syria, Tunisia, USSR

Sources: See Table 13.1.

belief that such requirements are oriented toward international travelers, most actually target migrant workers, applicants for long-term residence, and even returning nationals.

The AIDS pandemic was a test case for upholding the International Health Regulations, which were first adopted in 1969 by the World Health Assembly as a binding international instrument to prevent unnecessary restrictions on international traffic. Widespread noncompliance with the spirit and wording of the Regulations, however, drew public attention to their existence. They stand out as the sole international legal instrument providing safeguards against excessive restrictions on international movement imposed under the pretext of fighting AIDS.

In 1985, WHO implicitly confirmed that breaches of International Health Regulations were taking place when it stated that "no country bound by the Regulations may refuse entry into its territory to a person who fails to provide a medical certificate stating that he or she

Table 13.6: Countries screening users of health services as of 1991

Pregnant women	Belize, Bhutan, Burma, Cape Verde, Dominican Republic, DPR Korea, Guinea Bissau, India, Lesotho, Mali, Mexico, Nepal, Niger, Nigeria, Pakistan, Papua New Guinea, Sierra Leone, Sri Lanka, Sudan, Syria, Uruguay, Zaire, Zambia
Patients with sexually transmitted diseases	Belize, Bhutan, Botswana, Burkina Faso, Burma, Côte d'Ivoire, Dominican Republic, Hungary, Indonesia, Kuwait, Nepal, Niger, Nigeria, Oman, Papua New Guinea, Philippines, Sierra Leone, Sri Lanka, Sudan, Suriname, Trinidad and Tobago, Vietnam, Zambia
All hospitalized patients	Botswana, Burkina Faso, Burma, Côte d'Ivoire, Mali, Nigeria, Sri Lanka, Vietnam
Patients with tuberculosis	Belize, Bhutan, Botswana, Burkina Faso, Chad, Côte d'Ivoire, Dominican Republic, Guinea Bissau, Lesotho, Sierra Leone, Suriname, Uruguay, Zaire
Patients with hepatitis B	Jordan, Pakistan
Mental patients	Pakistan, Philippines
Recipients of blood transfusions	DPR Korea, India, Jordan, Oman, Pakistan, Syria, Tunisia, Vietnam
People with hemophilia	Kuwait, Mexico, Pakistan, Panama, Sri Lanka, Syria, Tunisia, USSR

is not carrying the AIDS virus."[47] Later that year it added, "It must be vigorously stressed that to require such certificates, let alone to insist on blood tests on arrival, would be totally contrary to the International Health Regulations."[48] Nevertheless, the Regulations have continued to be breached, and the WHO has not taken clear action to identify instances of noncompliance and to promote compliance with the sole binding international instrument the Organization has produced.

More than 50 countries have imposed such restrictions,[49] in defiance of explicit provisions of International Health Regulations, which has prompted widespread criticism.[50] The first prohibition of entry for

Table 13.7: Countries screening migrants and travelers as of 1991

Returning nationals	Bhutan, Bulgaria, Burma, China, Cuba, Czechoslovakia, Hungary, Iraq, Jordan, Korea (DPR), Korea (Republic of), Mongolia, Pakistan, Philippines, Poland, Syria, Tunisia, USSR, Vietnam, Yugoslavia
Immigrants	Argentina, Australia, Burma, China, Costa Rica, Cuba, Hungary, Iraq, Republic of Korea, Mongolia, Philippines, South Africa, Syria, Thailand, United States, USSR
Applicants for long-term residence	Belize, Bulgaria, China, Costa Rica, Czechoslovakia, Germany (Bavaria), Jordan, Republic of Korea, Kuwait, Pakistan, Philippines, Poland, Syria, Thailand, Turks and Caicos Islands, United Arab Emirates, United States, USSR
Foreign residents	Bulgaria, Costa Rica, Dominican Republic, Germany (Bavaria), Iraq, Kuwait, Mongolia, Pakistan, Philippines, South Africa, Syria, Tunisia, USSR
Migrant workers	Bhutan, Czechoslovakia, Dominica, Dominican Republic, Jordan, Kuwait, Libya, Philippines, South Africa, Spain, Sri Lanka, St. Vincent and Grenadines, Suriname, Syria, Turks and Caicos Islands, United Arab Emirates, Vietnam
Foreign students	China, Czechoslovakia, Hungary, India, Kuwait, Poland, Syria, Tunisia, USSR
Applicants for asylum	Philippines, Spain, United States
Refugees	Belize, Hong Kong, Pakistan, Philippines, Sudan, Vietnam

Sources: See Table 13.1.

Table 13.8: Countries screening occupational categories as of 1991

Seafarers	Burma, China, Republic of Korea, Pakistan, Philippines, Sierra Leone, Sri Lanka, Tunisia, Vietnam
Military	Bhutan, Cape Verde, France, Kenya, Kuwait, Pakistan, Sudan, Thailand, United States, Yemen
Police	Bhutan, Burma, Cape Verde, Italy, Kuwait, Nigeria, Oman
Civil servants	Germany (Bavaria), Kuwait, United States
Scholarship holders	Belgium, Greece, Guinea Bissau, Finland, Sri Lanka
Students	Bhutan, Dominican Republic, Jordan, Kenya, Pakistan, Zambia
Airline personnel	Czechoslovakia, Kuwait
Tourist personnel	Cape Verde, DPR Korea, Sri Lanka, Tunisia
Truck drivers	Bhutan, Sierra Leone, Sudan
Entertainers	Cyprus, DPR Korea, Indonesia, Philippines, Vietnam
Health personnel	Botswana, Burma, Cape Verde, Jordan, Kenya, Pakistan, Papua New Guinea, Philippines, Sri Lanka, Syria, Zaire

Source: See Table 13.1.

HIV-infected people, introduced by Saudi Arabia early in 1986, was widely reported in the press. An official protest to the WHO was made by the United Kingdom, invoking the Regulations.* Although no public records are available on the WHO's response, it appears that this controversy was not resolved, nor has an effort been made to uphold the application of the Regulations and prevent states from breaching them. AIDS-free certificates have been introduced as well, contrary to Article 81 of the Regulations, which prohibits the require-

---

*In March 1986, Saudi Arabia introduced the requirement for all foreign visitors to present "certificates showing that visitors are free of AIDS," and the Government of the United Kingdom lodged a complaint to WHO, stating that this requirement was a breach of the International Health Regulations. "Saudi Arabian visa regulation—UK protest," *AIDS Newsletter*, Bureau of Hygiene & Tropical Diseases, London, vol. 1, No. 3 (7 March 1986):1.

ment of any health document, other than those envisaged by the Regulations themselves, in international traffic.

━━━━━ .   .   .

NOTIFICATION

Notification to health authorities of cases of communicable diseases is another traditional public health measure[51] that, while appearing to be technical, has significant implications for human rights. Public health laws may require physicians to report a *case* (anonymously) or *the patient* (by including his or her personal identity). Where identity is to be revealed, human rights problems regularly emerge, but they are rarely anticipated when disease notification is legislated.[52] Only within the Council of Europe[53] have the human rights implications of such public health laws and practices, especially those involving confidential data, been the object of international protection; meanwhile, the United Nations is still elaborating a set of recommended standards.[54] This issue became the object of intense professional and public debate in the context of the AIDS pandemic.[55]

Many countries have sought to ascertain who is HIV infected by making personal identity part of the obligatory notification of cases of AIDS and results of HIV tests. Thus, two different public health approaches—epidemiological surveillance and case finding—have been merged; this has had detrimental consequences for both approaches and also for the protection of human rights. When noti-

---

Box 13.3: The Legacy of Hans-Paul Verhoef

Richard Rector, Health Educator, Copenhagen, Denmark

On April 2, 1989, a Dutch man named Hans-Paul Verhoef was detained by U.S. officials for posing a *serious threat* to the public health in the United States. Verhoef, an educator and AIDS activist, was trying to enter the United States to attend an international meeting. When customs officials discovered AZT in his luggage, Verhoef confirmed that he had AIDS. His detention captured headlines and focused wide public attention on American travel policy towards people with AIDS for the first time.

Before Verhoef's detention, most people were not aware of American regulations restricting entry of people with AIDS and HIV into the country. International Conferences on AIDS were scheduled to be held in Montreal, Canada, in 1989 and in San Francisco in 1990, and planning and preparations proceeded although both countries had restrictive regulations or

fication is by name, protection of confidentiality is essential to prevent stigmatization and discrimination. Only a few countries have made notification anonymous, and only a few have added special safeguards for confidentiality where the required notification of AIDS and HIV infection included personal identities.[56] Yet, the disclosure of personal identity of HIV-infected people has brought about their loss of employment, housing, insurance, residence, and work permits; both social ostracism and suicide rates have increased.[57] Notification to public authorities of the names of people who are HIV infected without necessarily showing any symptoms, but who are able to infect others, creates an extremely complex and inherently controversial issue.

▬▬▬▬ .   .   .

COUNTERPRODUCTIVENESS OF COMPULSORY TESTING

Evidence from a number of countries demonstrates that the lack of safeguards for confidentiality in HIV testing, and for avoiding discrimination against persons who are found to be infected, results in decreased participation in testing programs. For example, a study of patients consenting to or declining HIV testing at a clinic for sexually transmitted diseases in New Mexico (USA), carried out in 1986–88, revealed that people declining to be tested were 5 to 8 times more likely to be HIV infected.[58] Researchers subsequently established that the main reasons for refusal were concerns about confidentiality and

---

practices regarding the disease to be discussed.

Hans-Paul Verhoef died fifteen months after his confrontation with the U.S. government, but his legacy lives on. Although the restrictive U.S. policies have not changed, complacency about this issue was shattered. The VIII International Conference on AIDS—originally scheduled to be held in Boston in 1992—was held instead in Amsterdam as a protest over the regulations that led to Verhoef's detention. Other

conferences on AIDS have been canceled or boycotted because of restrictive AIDS policies, and the attitudes of governments are now a key factor in deciding the future locations of such important meetings. Hans-Paul Verhoef proved that individuals are not powerless to speak out against restrictive, short-sighted, and ill-founded policies on AIDS. This is a tribute to Verhoef, whose legacy continues in the actions and deeds of all those struggling for solidarity, unity, and equity in the fight against AIDS.

fear of stigmatization if knowledge of HIV infection became known. In a survey carried out in March 1989 in San Francisco, "the vast majority of men said they would consent to required testing if anti-discrimination laws were in place."[59]

In 1987, publicity about proposed legislation on HIV/AIDS in Japan, which included provisions for disclosing personal identity, led to a decline in attendance at STD clinics. Attitudes toward HIV testing in Japan were further examined in 1988 to determine whether notification of personal identity to the authorities would deter people from HIV testing. More than 30 percent of respondents indicated their preference for HIV testing without such notification.[60]

In 1987, in the German state of Bavaria participation in AIDS education programs declined following the announcement of forth-coming restrictive measures.[61] Negative effects of the legal enactment classifying AIDS as an STD have also been documented in Sweden: ". . . a 30 percent drop occurred in attendance at the units that perform HIV screening in conjunction with the enactment."[62]

A good example of the ineffectiveness of compulsory HIV testing was the introduction and the subsequent rescindment of compulsory premarital testing for HIV. Beginning in 1987, applicants for marriage in the state of Louisiana (USA) were required to undergo HIV testing. The requirement was repealed two years later after a review confirmed that compulsory premarital screening was wasteful and ineffective. In the state of Illinois (USA), mandatory premarital testing took effect on January 1, 1988.[63] During 1988, the number of applicants for marriage licenses in Illinois declined by 22 percent. Out of 155,000 applicants who were tested for HIV, only 26 were HIV-positive; the cost was $208,000 for every HIV-positive result obtained.[64] The Illinois requirement for premarital HIV testing was revoked in 1989.[65]

The beginning of democratization in Eastern Europe brought about not only a change in responding to AIDS, but also more complete information on the policies and practices of the previous regimes. In March 1989, the WHO Regional Office for Europe commented: "Through mandatory screening of risk groups, Bulgaria, Czechoslovakia, Poland and Hungary seem to know almost all infected persons in their countries, but still this type of information might be misleading, as was recently confirmed by the incident of HIV-infection in Elista, USSR."[66] At around the same time, the president of the USSR Academy of Medical Sciences publicly declared that the screening of 18 million people in 1988 had not been cost-effective. The compulsory screening of 4 million pregnant women had identified 6 HIV-positive women, and voluntary anonymous testing of 19,000 people had identified 4. Thus, the voluntary testing program was more than 1,000 times more efficient than was compulsory screening.[67] As an example of recent change in AIDS policies reflecting broader societal evolution, in March 1991, compulsory HIV testing was abolished in Bulgaria.

THE PRIMACY OF NONDISCRIMINATION

In public health and in human rights work, nondiscrimination has been indentified as the key to integrating human rights concerns and AIDS prevention and control efforts. In October 1989, the Council of Europe stated: "[an explicit policy] should state unequivocally that HIV-infected individuals have the right to enjoy the same civil and social rights as the non-infected, while bearing ethical, civil and legal responsibilities to contain transmission."[68] This not only reinforced the prohibition of discrimination under international human rights law, but it also provided an incentive to broaden the prohibition, particularly by urging that it be extended to cover the grounds for discrimination that were used in the context of AIDS: sexual orientation,[69] and state of health, especially disability.[70]

As always in human rights, legislation to protect individual rights and freedoms has been a reaction to violations. The first antidiscrimination legislation appeared in the United States, starting with the Los Angeles AIDS Discrimination Ordinance in June 1985;[71] by 1988, many states had adopted antidiscrimination laws.[72]

Yet, as with human rights legislation in any other area, the mere adoption of an antidiscrimination provision does not necessarily signify a commitment to human rights protection. Nor should it be presumed that nondiscrimination is applied and enforced. It is too well known in human rights work that words are not necessarily matched by deeds. It is, however, important to stress that prohibitions of AIDS-related discrimination were a symbolic but indicative signpost of an advance in human rights protection.

The Comores adopted its first AIDS law in November 1988. This legislation gives the National AIDS Control Committee a particular mandate to ensure that citizens' rights are protected and that the national AIDS program conforms to the WHO Global AIDS Strategy. The AIDS legislation of Argentina (Law on AIDS No. 23 of 16 August 1990) states that no AIDS-related regulations may be adopted if they would infringe on personal dignity or result in discriminatory or marginalizing effects for those affected or likely to be affected. It requires respect of individual dignity, medical confidentiality, and privacy and prohibits marginalization, degradation, and humiliation of persons affected by HIV/AIDS. Similarly, the USSR Law on Prevention of AIDS of April 23, 1990, states in Article 8(4):

> Dismissal from work, refusal of work, refusal of admission to medical and educational establishments, refusal to admit children to pre-school establishments, the restriction of other rights, and limitation of the legitimate interests of such individuals solely on the grounds that they are carriers of the virus or are suffering from AIDS, as well as restrictions of the right to accommodation and other rights

---

Box 13.4: HIV/AIDS-Related Violence

Sofia Gruskin, J.D., Dean's Fellow, Center for the Study of Human Rights, Columbia University, New York

The AIDS pandemic has sparked a particular type of hate crime: attacks on people because of an illness. Even though most people realize that HIV cannot be spread by casual contact, hatred, and blame aroused by the disease have spurred attacks ranging from the verbal to the physical and even lethal. Often, the people attacked are either suspected of being ill or are somehow linked to the disease: gay men, lesbians, straight men and women, people who are HIV infected, people with AIDS. These attacks usually occur on the street, although there have been documented assaults by landlords, family members, and neighbors.

AIDS-specific violence is just that: it generally involves a verbal reference to the disease. For some people, the fear of AIDS has provided a powerful, if misguided, rationalization for attacks on traditionally stigmatized groups, particularly gay men and female sex workers. In the United States, for example, such violence is often accompanied by the language of homophobia and racism.

The National Gay and Lesbian Task Force in the United States reports that violent attacks against gay men and lesbians increased by 31 percent from 1990 to 1991, and verbal harassment by 61 percent involving 2,405 incidents ranging from verbal abuse to murder. Twelve percent of all the reported attacks either involved reference to AIDS or were directed

and legitimate interests of relatives and close associates of an infected person, shall be prohibited.

The Japanese AIDS Prevention Law of December 23, 1988, stipulates in Article 2(3) that the authorities "shall give consideration to protecting the human rights of AIDS patients"; it continues in Article 3 by saying that "the public shall ensure that the human rights of AIDS patients" shall not be endangered. In Kuwait, the Committee to Combat AIDS has been asked to "propose the arrangements and procedures to ensure safeguarding the rights and personal liberties of victims in the framework of social values and conventions."[73]

Even when not included in national AIDS legislation, the need to respect human rights has been frequently mentioned in national debates on AIDS laws and policies. Contrary to the frequent remark that human rights are Western, several examples from Asia demonstrate that universality of human rights has involved worldwide calls for their observance.

For example, in September 1989, the Ministry of Public Health of Thailand proposed a draft law on AIDS that included provisions for

---

against people with obvious signs of the disease. "Anti-gay violence has reached epidemic proportions," said Kevin Berrill, author of the report. "People are getting the message that gay equals AIDS, that it's OK to hate those people and that it's OK to do something about it."

Traditional human rights institutions monitor compliance for a host of human rights violations. But they often fail to monitor attacks against individuals based on their real or perceived HIV status. Even nongovernmental and community-based organizations that have examined HIV/AIDS as a health issue and as a basis for discrimination have failed to examine HIV status as a motivation for victimization. The only organization to address the issue directly is the Gay and Lesbian Anti-Violence Project in New York City. Until other organizations around the world begin to monitor human rights violations occurring on the basis of HIV/AIDS, such hate crimes will continue unreported and unabated.

A new program is being formed to address, respond to, and study HIV/AIDS-related violations of human rights and dignity. The program is being organized by several institutions, including the Danish Center for Human Rights, the International Federation of Red Cross and Red Crescent Societies, the McGill Center for Medicine, Law and Ethics, and the Global AIDS Policy Coalition.
—The Editors

Box 13.5: Chronology of International Policies on the Human Rights Aspects of AIDS Prevention and Control

October 1, 1981 Resolution 756 (1981) on discrimination against homosexuals adopted by the Parliamentary Assembly of the Council of Europe

June 23, 1983 Recommendation No R (83) 8 of the Committee of Ministers to Member States on Preventing the Possible Transmission of Acquired Immune Deficiency Syndrome (AIDS) from Affected Blood Donors to Patients Receiving Blood (Council of Europe)

November 23, 1983 Resolution 812 (1983) on the Acquired Immune Deficiency Syndrome (AIDS) of the Parliamentary Assembly of the Council of Europe

September 13, 1985 Recommendation No R (85) 12 of the Committee of Ministers to Member States on the Screening of Blood Donors for the Presence of AIDS Markers [Council of Europe]

May 29, 1986 Resolution of the representatives of the Governments of Member States meeting within the Council on AIDS [EEC, OJ C 184]

March 3, 1987 WHO Consultation on International Travel and HIV Infection (Doc. WHO/SPA/GLO/87.1)

May 15, 1987 Global Strategy for the Prevention and Control of AIDS (Res. WHA40.26)

May 15, 1987 Conclusions of the Council and of the Governments of the

Member States meeting within the Council concerning AIDS [EEC, OJ C 178]

May 21, 1987 WHO Meeting on Criteria That Must be Considered in Planning and Implementing HIV Screening Programs (Doc. WHO/SPA/GLO/87.2)

June 6, 1987 HIV Infection and Health Workers (Doc. SPA/INF/87.6)

July 27, 1987 Conclusions of the Council and of the representatives of the Governments of the Member States meeting with the Council concerning AIDS [EEC, OJ C 197]

July 30, 1987 UNFPA Guidelines on AIDS (Doc. UNFPA/CM/87/38)

September 17, 1987 *Note verbale* from the WHO Director-General on the prevention of HIV transmission through skin-piercing procedures (Doc. C.L.30.1987)

October 27, 1987 Prevention and control of AIDS (UNGA res. 42/8)

November 18, 1987 Consensus Statement of WHO Consultation on Prevention and Control of AIDS in Prisons (Doc. WHO/SPA/INF/87.14)

November 26, 1987 Recommendation No R (87) 25 of the Committee of Ministers to Member States on a Common European Health Policy to Fight the Acquired Immunodeficiency Syndrome (AIDS) [Council of Europe]

December 1, 1987 Social Aspects of AIDS Prevention and Control Programs (Doc. WHO/SPA/GLO/87.2)

1988 WHO Statement on Screening of International Travellers for Infection with Human Immunodeficiency Virus (Doc. WHO/GPA/INF/88.3) .

January 1988 WHO Meeting on HIV Infection and Drug Injecting Intervention Strategies (Doc. WHO/GPA/SBR/89.1)

January 28, 1988 London Declaration on AIDS Prevention of the World Summit of Ministers of Health

February 15, 1988 UNHCR health policy on AIDS (Doc. UNHCR/IOM/21/88)

May 13, 1988 Avoidance of discrimination in relation to HIV-infected people and people with AIDS (Res. WHA41.24)

May 17, 1988 WHO Global Blood Safety Initiative Meeting (Doc. WHO/GPA/DIR/88.9)

May 31, 1988 Conclusions of the Council of the European Communities concerning AIDS

June 29, 1988 Consensus Statement of WHO/ILO Consultation on AIDS and the Workplace (Doc. WHO/GPA/INF/88.7)

June 30, 1988 Recommendation 1080 (1988) on a Co-ordinated European Health Policy to Prevent the Spread of AIDS in Prisons [Council of Europe, Parliamentary Assembly]

September 1, 1988 Discrimination against persons with the HIV virus or suffering from AIDS [Decision 1988/111 of the Sub-Commission for Prevention of Discrimination and Protection of Minorities]

October 27, 1988 Prevention and control of acquired immunodeficiency syndrome (AIDS) [UNGA res. 43/15]

November 23, 1988 Resolution of the Council and of the Ministers of Education meeting within the Council concerning health education in schools [EEC, OJ C 3]

December 15, 1988 Conclusions of the Council and the Ministers for Health of the Member States meeting with the Council concerning AIDS [EEC, OJ C 28]

December 15, 1988 Conclusions of the Council and the Ministers for Health of the Member States meeting with the Council concerning AIDS and the place of work [EEC, OJ C 28]

January 1989 Heterosexual Transmission of HIV and Certain Common Social Situations (Doc. WHO/GPA/INF/89.5)

January 1989 Consensus Statement of WHO Consultation on Partner Notification for Preventing HIV Transmission (Doc. WHO/GPA/INF/89)

March 2, 1989 Consensus Statement of WHO Consultation on Criteria for International Testing of Candidate HIV Vaccines (Doc. GPA/INF/89.8)

March 2, 1989 Nondiscrimination in the field of health [United Nations Commission on Human Rights, res. 1989/11]

March 30, 1989 Resolution of the European Parliament on the fight against AIDS [OJ C 158]

March 31, 1989 Attention to applicable international law [WHO

Global Commission on AIDS (Doc. GPA/GCA(1)/89.1)]

May 16, 1989 Conclusions of the Council and the Ministers for Health of the Member States meeting with the Council regarding the prevention of AIDS in intravenous drug users [EEC, OJ C 185]

May 26, 1989 Resolution of the European Parliament on the fight against AIDS [Doc. A2–35/89]

July 6, 1989 Consensus Statement of WHO Consultation on HIV Epidemiology and Prostitution (Doc. WHO/GPA/INF/89.11)

July 28, 1989 Final Document of the International Consultation on AIDS and Human Rights [U.N.Doc. HR/AIDS/1989/3]

August 31, 1989 Discrimination against HIV-infected people or people with AIDS [Sub-Commission on the Prevention of Discrimination and Protection of Minorities, res. 1989/18]

September 29, 1989 Recommendation 1116 (1989) on AIDS and human rights [Council of Europe, Parliamentary Assembly]

October 24, 1989 Recommendation No R (89) 14 of the Committee of Ministers to Member States on the ethical issues of HIV infection in the health care and social settings [Council of Europe]

November 30, 1989 Paris Declaration on women, children, and AIDS

December 22, 1989 Prevention and control of acquired immunodeficiency syndrome (AIDS) [UNGA res. 44/233]

December 22, 1989 Resolution of the Council and the Ministers for Health of the Member States meeting within the Council on the fight against AIDS [EEC, OJ C 10]

February 1, 1990 Avoidance of discrimination against women in national strategies for the prevention and control of AIDS [CEDAW, General Recommendation No. 15]

March 7, 1990 Discrimination against HIV-infected people or people with AIDS [United Nations Commission on Human Rights, decision 1990/65]

May 11, 1990 *Note verbale* of the WHO Director-General referring to avoidance of discrimination in national AIDS programs worldwide (Doc. C.L.7.1990)

August 31, 1990 Infection with human immunodeficiency virus (HIV) and acquired immunodeficiency syndrome (AIDS) in prison [Resolution 18 of the Eighth United Nations Congress on the Prevention of Crime and the Treatment of Offenders]

June 4, 1991 Europe against AIDS Plan for Action adopted by the EEC Commission

compulsory screening of high-risk groups and registration and detention of HIV-positive people (which were contrary to the prohibition
of discrimination against people with AIDS contained in the same
draft).[74] Public hearings on this proposed law were held in November
1989, and the *Bangkok Post* reported that all those who took part in
the hearings stressed that the rights of people with HIV/AIDS must
be protected;[75] the draft was said to violate human rights and that it
"resembles one of Hitler's laws."[76] Recent reports of the evolving
response to AIDS in Thailand noted the establishment of an ethical
committee mandated to define "the legal rights of the infected people."[77]

In India in December 1989, the Bombay High Court rejected a
petition by two mothers to release their HIV-infected sons, detained
in Goa under public health law.* The Court noted that "isolation
results in social ostracism and encroaches on the individual's liberty,"
but added that isolation was necessary because of fear of AIDS
amongst the public: "An error on the safer side may be more agreeable
since the dimension of AIDS created a fear psychosis."[78] Less than
two years later, the Indian courts overruled the detention of a large
number of commercial sex workers, forcibly tested for antibodies to
HIV, thus signifying a change in the interpretation of Indian law.

INTERNATIONAL RESPONSES: AIDS AND HUMAN RIGHTS

At the global level, AIDS was seen during the first years of the pandemic as a disease of the rich, confined to the Western industrialized
countries. Indeed, one of the first internal memoranda concerning
AIDS written at the WHO in 1983 stated that there was no need for
the Organization to become involved because AIDS "is being very
well taken care of by some of the richest countries in the world where
there is the manpower and knowhow and where most of the patients
are to be found."[79] In Europe, a common policy of responding to AIDS
was developed in 1983. By 1985, the evidence that AIDS was a global

---

*The Goa Public Health (Amendment) Act of 5 June 1989 gave health officers
powers to "remove or cause to be removed" to hospital or "other place" any
person suffering from an infectious disease or any person who appears to the
health officer to be suffering from an infectious disease.

problem started becoming available. By the end of the 1980s, the first, erroneous image of the pandemic was corrected: it was shown that AIDS was generally and increasingly a disease of poverty rather than wealth, "a misery seeking missile" as described by the PANOS Institute.[80] According to WHO, "the developing countries are increasingly bearing the brunt of the pandemic: by the year 2000 they will have over 90 percent of the world's HIV infections and AIDS cases."[81]

The global response to AIDS included an emphasis on human rights from the very beginning. In May 1987, at the time when the global strategy for the prevention and control of AIDS was being elaborated, the director of the Global Programme on AIDS spoke about the need to counter "the epidemic of social, economic, political and cultural reaction and response to AIDS and HIV infection."[82] In his address to the General Assembly on October 20, 1987, the Secretary-General of the United Nations said the fight against AIDS "is also a fight against fear, against prejudice and against irrational action born of ignorance,"[83] and he added later "that the world should make war *against AIDS*, and *not* against *people* with AIDS."[84]

The need to respect human rights in responding to HIV/AIDS was first affirmed by the Council of Europe, then by the World Health Assembly, then by the United Nations Commission on Human Rights and its Sub-Commission on the Prevention of Discrimination and Protection of Minorities. These policy statements and positions were followed by a vast number of organizations, intergovernmental and nongovernmental, international and national, which adopted explicit policies or guidelines on the human rights aspects of AIDS.

In its statement on the social aspects of AIDS prevention and control, WHO's Global Programme on AIDS said that "AIDS prevention and control strategies can be implemented effectively and efficiently . . . in a manner that respects and protects human rights" and added that "there is no public health rationale to justify isolation, quarantine, or any discriminatory measures based solely on the fact that a person is suspected or known to be HIV infected . . . [and] failure to prevent discrimination may endanger public health."[85] By incorporating human rights into its global AIDS strategy, the World Health Organization set a genuine precedent in the history of responding to disease.

The fact that international health as well as human rights bodies affirmed the application of human rights merits emphasis. The Global Commission on AIDS, established by the WHO, stated that no "blanket exemption from observance of human rights obligations" may be accepted in combating AIDS,[86] and the 1989 International Consultation on AIDS and Human Rights concluded that exemptions from observance of human rights could not be justified simply by claiming that they were required for public health reasons.[87] The United Nations Commission on Human Rights reaffirmed that the prohibition of discrimination on the grounds of health applies universally, restating that all people are "equal before the law and entitled to equal protection of the law from all discrimination and from all incitement to discrimination relating to their state of health."[88]

When the global AIDS strategy was first formulated in 1987, WHO stressed that transmission of HIV was preventable and that every individual had the responsibility to prevent contracting or transmitting HIV infection.[89] This was reinforced a year later in the World Health Assembly resolution on the avoidance of discrimination in relation to HIV-infected people and people with AIDS, by emphasizing "the responsibility of individuals not to put themselves or others at risk of infection with HIV."[90] Detailed provisions on individual responsibilities, as a corollary to the human rights guarantees, have been elaborated by the Council of Europe. Its recommendation in November 1987, on the common European health policy on AIDS, stated that health education should emphasize that "the individual is responsible for the outcome of his behavior towards himself, others and the society" and that sex education "should encourage individuals to assume responsibility for their health by becoming aware of risks and benefits inherent in various lifestyles."[91]

Restrictive or repressive measures have not been endorsed by WHO and have been explicitly rejected by the Council of Europe, because of the "impossibility of imposing behavior modification."[92] The Council of Europe's recommendation on AIDS in prison, for example, stated in 1988 that "unless future scientific findings should indicate otherwise, HIV-infected prisoners [should] not [be] isolated or segregated, provided they do not act irresponsibly."[93] The 1989 International Consultation on AIDS and Human Rights developed a link between informed and responsible behavior and protection against discrimination, based on the notion of empowerment. It emphasized in 1989 the need "for protection of the human rights of those specially at risk for exposure to HIV so that they will be empowered to protect themselves. By so doing, they are enabled to fulfill their responsibility to protect others."[94]

ACTION BY THE INTERNATIONAL HUMAN RIGHTS SYSTEM

The concordance between the targets of so-called conventional and AIDS-related human rights violations has exposed the *lacunae* in the international human rights system. The reasons for insufficient human rights protection in general were the same as those for AIDS-related violations of human rights. The protection of basic rights of some marginalized categories, such as drug users or commercial sex workers, was insufficient, and the protection of prisoners' rights, although representing a large proportion of human rights litigation, nationally and internationally, still too often left prisoners without effective protection. In countries where national human rights protection was fairly effective in conventional areas, it was not always extended to AIDS-related issues immediately and fully. As Justice Michael Kirby of the Supreme Court of Australia wrote in 1989:

> Democratically elected governments, under the pressure to be seen to be doing something effective in the face of a major epidemic, may be tempted to legislate against particular groups. Migrants, prisoners, drug users and prostitutes, in particular, lack an effective voice to dissuade lawmakers from provision of laws discriminating against them.[95]

The functioning of human rights protection at the global level is influenced by two main factors: the increasingly widespread knowledge that governments may be condemned internationally for the way they treat their population; and the limitations of the intergovernmental human rights system.

The two most pressing international issues in AIDS-related human rights issues have been the following:

1. Thus far there has been no international litigation in AIDS-related human rights problems, even in cases that may have set precedents that could have applied globally as authoritatively determined min-

imum standards that all governments should be required to observe. One reason for this is the relative lack of involvement in AIDS-related issues by the main international human rights organizations, coupled with the relative lack of knowledge about human rights standards and procedures on the part of the main AIDS organizations.

2. AIDS-related human rights activism, sharing the orientation of mainstream human rights, has focused on the visible and purposeful governmental acts that jeopardize individual privacy, liberty, and protection against discrimination. Human rights obligations stemming from the right to health care, to social assistance, or from the necessity to improve the enjoyment of human rights through international co-operation have been neglected.

More broadly, during the past forty years, the United Nations' human rights work evolved from defining human rights violations, to condemning governments violating human rights, to developing procedures to prevent violations. The first steps, in the 1940s to the 1960s, established the main substantive global human rights standards. It is worth recalling that the United Nations Commission on Human Rights started in 1947 by explicitly rejecting consideration of complaints for human rights violations.[96] Yet, by the 1970s it became possible to institute international complaints procedures, and individuals became able to pursue internationally demands to investigate and condemn human rights violations by their own government. Critics of the international human rights system regularly emphasize that not all governments violating human rights are condemned, but seldom stress the importance of this profound change: the government is no longer the judge in its own case, and it can be held accountable internationally for what it does to its own people. Thus, the dominant mode of human rights work has been denunciatory: governments are singled out for condemnation.

Yet, condemning governments for human rights violations is neither the end nor the necessary means of human rights work. However (in)effectively it is done in an intergovernmental system, it always comes too late. Hence, procedures were developed to prevent the occurrence of those human rights violations that are universally accepted as violations—torture, summary and arbitrary executions, and disappearances. Yet, ideas about what constitutes violations of economic, social, and cultural rights remain vague. Similarly, assistance to facilitate "recovery from adverse consequences of a repressive regime"[97] constitutes a minuscule component of the United Nations human rights activities.

The international human rights bodies have included AIDS-related questions in their dialogue with government over the implementation of human rights treaties. However, these questions have simply elicited descriptions of policies and practice; self-audit by governments rarely includes information on actions (or omissions) that could constitute violations of human rights.

The United Nations Committee on Economic, Social and Cultural Rights has also added questions relating to AIDS in its consideration of States' reports on the implementation of the right to health. For example, in discussing the report of Denmark, the Committee elicited the following description: "The official emphasis was on prevention through information. As to patients already infected by the virus, he described the efforts undertaken by his Government which, while attempting to avoid the spread of the disease, respected the rights of those affected by relying on voluntary treatment, consent at all stages and anonymity."[98]

The Government of the Netherlands included AIDS in its report under the Covenant and emphasized individual responsibility as the key to AIDS prevention: "The legislation under preparation focuses to a large extent on reducing, where possible, the role of the State, with a view to maximizing individuals' responsibility for themselves and for their own health care. In this way it is hoped to increase the self-reliance of individuals within society."[99]

A striking feature of the existing examination of AIDS-related human rights problems by the human rights bodies is their focus on good examples. This is an inevitable outcome of the reliance on governments as the sole source of information. For obvious reasons, governments seldom report on their own violations of human rights. Information on violations comes from their victims and regularly from nongovernmental organizations. These sources have not yet taken up the challenge of AIDS-related violations.

In conclusion, the dialogue between public health and human rights—pioneered in many ways through work on HIV/AIDS—will continue to be critical both for HIV/AIDS prevention and care and for improved understanding of public health in the modern world. During the coming decade, both major elements of the dialogue will be pursued: the need to prevent and respond to violations of human rights occurring in public health work; and the broader, more positive approach of promoting public health through protection and promotion of human rights and dignity. The quality and scope of this dialogue will be critical for the future of global public health.

PART THREE

. . . .

Global Vulnerability

CHAPTER FOURTEEN

· ·

Assessing Vulnerability to HIV Infection and AIDS

Faced with the HIV/AIDS pandemic, people often react by distancing themselves from the problem. Many people believe that today, and even tomorrow, their risk of becoming HIV infected or having a loved one become HIV infected may be essentially zero. Is it?

To confront a dynamic, volatile epidemic, a more thorough appreciation of vulnerability and a more useful approach to assess current and future vulnerability to HIV are needed. *AIDS in the World* had developed a framework for critically assessing vulnerability to HIV infection and AIDS that is essential both for understanding the history of the HIV pandemic and for predicting its future course.

Vulnerability to HIV Infection

At a biological level, all people are vulnerable to HIV infection: if exposed to the virus through sexual intercourse or through blood, any person can apparently become HIV infected. If any innate, biological basis of total resistance to HIV infection exists, it has yet to be discovered.

In addition to biological vulnerability, there is a fundamental epidemiological reality: HIV requires specific, identifiable actions (behaviors) for transmission to occur. To become infected with HIV, or to transmit it to another person, visible actions must occur involving two or more participants. Precisely because these are visible, specific, and concrete, the transmission of HIV can also be prevented through specific behaviors.

Table 14.1: Definitions of individual vulnerability to HIV/AIDS

In absolute terms: unprotected

In relative terms: exposed to a higher-than-average risk

In epidemiological terms: exposed to higher risk of HIV infection

In medical terms: unable to avail the optimal level and quality of medical care

In operational terms: requiring a higher degree of protection and care

In human rights terms: exposed to the risk of discrimination or unfair treatment challenging basic principles of equity and human dignity

In social terms: deprived of some or all social rights or services

In economic terms: because of financial constraints, unable to offset the risk of infection or to access the optimal level and quality of care

In political terms: unable to achieve full representation or lacking political power

Beyond these two human common denominators—biological susceptibility to infection and the limited, behavior-based modes of HIV transmission—lie the forces, factors, and influences that will diminish, sustain, or accelerate the progress of the HIV epidemic throughout the world.

Individual behavior is the ultimate determinant of vulnerability to HIV infection; therefore, a focus on the individual is necessary, although clearly not sufficient. Individual behavior is both mutable and societally connected, varying over a person's lifetime (e.g., sexual behavior at adolescence, middle, and old age), changing in response to personal history and experience, and strongly influenced throughout by key individuals (family, lovers, friends), communities, and larger societal and cultural entities, such as religions and nation states. Therefore, when assessing vulnerability, it is important to take into account the community, national, and even international factors that could influence personal vulnerability over the course of a life (see Table 14.1).

Vulnerability versus Empowerment

A thorough examination of the individual behaviors that expose people to HIV infection, including the community and larger societal dimensions of these behaviors, leads to a central conclusion: personal empowerment is the antithesis of vulnerability.

Worldwide experience during the past decade has demonstrated that successful HIV prevention—empowerment for HIV prevention—requires three elements: information/education; health and social services; and a supportive social environment (see Chapter 9 on prevention). Personal vulnerability to HIV infection increases with a lack of accurate, relevant, and comprehensible information about HIV. Personal vulnerability increases when the individual is not concerned or sufficiently motivated regarding the danger of HIV infection. Personal vulnerability also increases when the individual lacks skills, the access to needed services, supplies, or equipment, and the power or confidence to sustain or implement behavior changes.

Given the nature of HIV/AIDS, the ultimate task of prevention is individual empowerment: societies cannot administer HIV prevention (except through ensuring a safe blood supply) to a passive population, as water can be made safer, or air cleaner. HIV prevention requires individuals empowered to learn and to respond.

Framework of Analysis

An analysis of factors limiting empowerment for HIV prevention, and thereby increasing vulnerability to HIV, requires first a careful inventory and assessment of the behaviors through which HIV can spread. Once these behaviors are recognized, the key questions become: How can the preconditions for reducing personal vulnerability to HIV infection be met? How can communities and countries best promote individuals' empowerment for HIV prevention?

In practice, this process will be mediated through two sets of factors: access to information/education and to health and social services that depend on the quality and nature of the community or national AIDS programs; and the broad societal influences that increase, sustain, or reduce personal empowerment (see Figure 14.1).

Once having considered individual vulnerability to HIV transmission and AIDS, community and national vulnerability will be assessed as an interacting function of AIDS programs and broader societal features. From these elements, an index will be constructed to help assess any community's or nation's vulnerability—past, present, and future.

As the HIV pandemic will be determined by human behavior

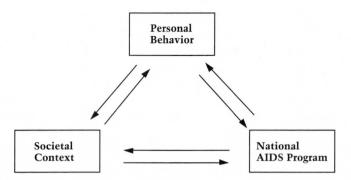

Figure 14.1. Vulnerability to HIV infection.

(individual and collective), so the world map of vulnerability is drawn, and the future of the pandemic will be determined by the specific response of communities, nations, and the global community to HIV/AIDS and by the broader, preexisting societal characteristics that increase, stabilize, or suppress personal empowerment.

PART I: INDIVIDUAL VULNERABILITY

Assumptions Underlying the Index of Individual Vulnerability

Several assumptions underlie the concept of individual vulnerability in HIV prevention and HIV/AIDS care.

Assumption 1: Every person who is not infected with HIV has a potential degree of vulnerability to the infection and its consequences, which may not be significant at present but which may increase as the environment within which the individual evolves challenges personal values or deprives him or her of the means to attain and sustain the lowest possible level of vulnerability.

Assumption 2: Individuals who are or will become infected with HIV are vulnerable to unwarranted morbidity, disability, or mortality if optimal health services and social support are denied to them.

Assumption 3: Preconditions of a cognitive, behavioral, and social nature will affect the degree to which each person will be vulnerable to being infected with HIV, to transmitting the infection to others, or to suffering from inadequate health care or social support.

In the following sections, a description of individual vulnerability is followed by examples of cognitive, behavioral, and social preconditions for decreasing vulnerability.

By applying the scale below, a realistic self-appraisal of individual vulnerability can be made. No scoring system is proposed here. For each individual, the intent of this assessment is to address six questions. It must be recognized that some people may have low self-awareness and empowerment and therefore may not have the ability to perform such a self-appraisal.

- How vulnerable am I to HIV infection and AIDS?
- What are the preconditions for reducing my vulnerability, and which of these have not been met?
- To what extent can I reduce this vulnerability?
- What can I do to generate changes in the social and health services to reduce my vulnerability?
- What can I do to generate the societal changes in my environment that are necessary to reduce my vulnerability?
- How can my individual or collective actions facilitate these changes?

Sexual Transmission of HIV

Individual vulnerability

Minimum vulnerability exists when the person:

- is/will be sexually inactive or abstinent, or will practice nonpenetrative sex

Vulnerability increases as the person:

- has/will have penetrative sex with one sexual partner who is not infected and does/will not have any other concurrent sexual partner (mutual monogamy)
- adheres to safer sex practices

- does not adhere to safer sex practices

Preconditions to decreasing vulnerability

Cognitive

- awareness of modes and risk of sexual transmission of HIV and prevention methods for HIV and other sexually transmitted diseases (STDs)
- awareness of past and present vulnerability of sexual partner(s) to HIV infection

Behavioral

Self-determined sexual behavior:
- sustained sexual abstinence
- practice of safer sex
- monogamy
- reduction in the number of sexual partners

Role perception:
- self-esteem
- responsibility toward present and future sexual partner(s), dependants, and offspring(s)

Skills acquisition:
- appropriate use of condom
- practice of nonpenetrative sex
- skills of negotiation about sexual practice

Social

Social status:
- power to negotiate with regular partner
- power to negotiate with occasional partners

Access to:
- information
- condoms
- safer sexual partners
- voluntary, confidential testing and counseling
- alternate source of income (sex workers)
- diagnosis and treatment of STDs

HIV transmission through injection drug use

Individual vulnerability

Minimum vulnerability exists when the person:

- does not use any substance (including alcohol or any other substance, through any route) that would diminish self-control or the ability to resist peer pressure to engage in risk behavior.

Vulnerability increases as the person:

- uses any ingesting or inhaling substance to the extent of diminishing self-control, decision making, or power to negotiate
- uses injection drugs without ever sharing injecting equipment
- uses injection drugs and shares injection equipment

Preconditions to decreasing vulnerability

Cognitive

- awareness of risks attributable to use of substances, including injection drug use
- awareness of approaches to demand and harm reduction and treatment options

Behavioral

Role perception:
- restoration of self-esteem
- determination to resist peer pressure to substance use

Skills acquisition:
- dose reduction
- shift to less harmful substance
- use of sterile injection equipment
- cleansing of injection equipment
- skills of negotiation about drug injection and/or sharing of nonsterile equipment

Social

Access to:
- information

- sterile injection equipment
- less harmful substance
- treatment
- voluntary, confidential testing and counseling

HIV transmission through blood and blood products

Individual vulnerability

Minimum vulnerability exists when the person:

- does not receive blood, blood products, or organ transplants and is not subjected to invasive surgical procedures.

Vulnerability increases as the person:

- receives blood, blood products, or organ transplants after appropriate screening for HIV or is subjected to invasive surgical procedure with adherence to infection control practices
- is subjected to medical injection or invasive surgical procedure without adherence to infection control practices
- receives blood, blood products, or organ transplants that have not been appropriately screened for HIV

Preconditions to decreasing vulnerability

Cognitive

- awareness of risk attributable to blood transfusion, blood products, and organ transplants and nonadherence to infection control procedures in the health care setting
- reduction of personal need for blood transfusion through improved lifestyle, prevention and treatment of parasitic infections, and pregnancy monitoring

Behavioral

Skills:
- sterilization practices by those who self-administer medical drugs

Social

Access to:
- information

- health and nutrition status in which needs for transfusion or injections are reduced
- services that offer safe blood, blood products, and organ transplants and where infection control procedures are enforced

HIV transmission from mother to fetus/infant

Individual vulnerability

Mimimum vulnerability of a fetus/newborn to acquiring HIV infection exists when:

- the mother is not infected with HIV before, during, or after pregnancy.

Vulnerability increases as:

- the biological mother is infected with HIV prior to conception but remains asymptomatic during pregnancy
- the biological mother acquires HIV infection during pregnancy or develops symptoms of AIDS during pregnancy
- the mother becomes HIV infected immediately prior to or during breastfeeding period

Preconditions to decreasing vulnerability

Cognitive

- partners' awareness of pre/perinatal transmission risk
- partners' awareness of contraception methods

Behavioral

Role perception:
- partners' responsibility toward offspring

Skills:
- partners' appropriate use of contraceptives to prevent pregnancy, if so desired

Self-determined sexual behavior:
- reinforcement of safer sexual practices during pregnancy and period of breastfeeding

Social

Access by partners to:
- information
- supportive maternal and child health services
- voluntary, confidential testing and counseling
- contraceptives
- safe alternatives to breast milk when so desired
- pregnancy termination
- means of defense of the person's right of reproduction
- a supportive environment for HIV-infected children

Inadequate care and social support

Individual vulnerability

Minimum vulnerability to inadequate health care or social support exists when the person:

- has complete access to prevention services and treatment of opportunistic infections, malignancies, and AIDS, and retains the full range of social and economic rights including confidentiality, privacy, equity in employment, housing, insurance, and free movement.

Vulnerability increases as the person:

- retains the full range of individual and social rights, but, given competing priorities in the allocation of funds to the health and social sectors, health care and social support are restricted by what the state defines as affordable
- has to forfeit certain social rights in order to access the desired level of care
- is deprived of any of the individual or social rights or has no access to affordable medical, psychological, or social welfare care and support

Preconditions to decreasing vulnerability

Cognitive

- awareness of the needs of people with HIV and AIDS and the present and future gaps in meeting these needs

- knowledge by people with HIV of clinical manifestations of HIV infection and AIDS
- knowledge by people with HIV of ways to reduce the frequency and severity of opportunistic infections
- knowledge of available services
- awareness of ways to induce national policy and program change

Behavioral

Skills:
- capacity of people with HIV and AIDS to access preventive measures
- capacity of people with HIV and AIDS to benefit from health and social support and to establish and defend their individual rights

Role perception:
- personal commitment to consider HIV and AIDS as an unprecedented pandemic and to respond to it on the local level
- personal commitment to address HIV and AIDS as a global issue
- commitment to promote health as a universal right

Social

- commitment to exercise pressure on the social system so that sufficient attention and resources are dedicated to health

Access to:
- supportive health and social services
- existing health insurance schemes
- information on coping with HIV infection and AIDS, on a personal and community level

These examples help to identify unmet needs for reducing individual vulnerability and promoting individual empowerment. However, the response to these needs requires an effective national AIDS program and is dependent upon broad, underlying societal features. Therefore, the analysis must shift to the collective level to describe the context within which HIV prevention, HIV/AIDS care, and individual empowerment are (or are not) occurring.

Table 14.2: Indexes of national AIDS program capacity to reduce vulnerability to HIV/AIDS

Index 1. Voicing commitment

Commitment is reflected by:
  Acknowledging AIDS at the highest executive level
  Creating programs
  Creating a multidisciplinary, multisectoral national AIDS advisory
    committee that reports to and interacts with the forum where policies are
    formulated and decisions are made
  Including HIV/AIDS prevention and control in the development plan,
    national budget, or organization's mandate

Index 2. Translating commitment into action

Ensuring consistency between policies and strategies endorsed in international
arenas and domestic policies and activities for:
  Providing information and education
  Providing health and social services
  Creating and reinforcing a supportive social environment, with special
    attention to human rights
  Upholding international solidarity through the exchange of information,
    knowledge, skills, and resources and participating in international
    governmental and nongovernmental networks

Index 3. Coalition building

Partnership between governmental and nongovernmental sectors in policy de-
velopment and program implementation, as reflected in:
  A jointly stated policy and a mutually agreed on agenda delineating the re-
    spective roles and responsibilities of the governmental and nongovernmental
    partners
  A delegation of authority and resources by the governmental to nongovern-
    mental programs and, in return, a commitment by the nongovernmental
    sector to adhere to mutually agreed on policies
  The participation of people affected by the pandemic in program develop-
    ment and implementation

Index 4. Planning and coordinating

Establishment of a comprehensive plan:
  Stating objectives, targets, strategies, and evaluation criteria
  Focusing on the modes of HIV transmission relevant to the populations at
    risk and preparing a detailed plan of action
  Specifying population groups that would benefit from the program and those
    that will not be reached
  Establishing functional links and ties with primary health care and social
    services
  Providing a mechanism for domestic and international coordination

Table 14.2 (cont.): Indexes of national AIDS program capacity to reduce vulnerability to HIV/AIDS

Index 5. Managing

Strengthening program management through:
    Training and deployment of needed human resources
    Efficiently using existing structures and services
    Undertaking innovative and dynamic action

Index 6. Responding to prevention needs

Responding to individual and collective needs by:
    Providing information, supplies, equipment, prevention, and social services
    Prioritizing interventions according to risks and resources

Index 7. Responding to care needs

Responding to individual and collective needs for care by:
    Expanding coverage and increasing the quality of medical services
    Prioritizing interventions according to needs and resources

Index 8. Securing financial resources

Securing needed financial resources and accounting for their use by:
    Mobilizing resources nationally and internationally
    Developing and operating a reliable accounting system

Index 9. Sustaining the effort

Ensuring the sustainability and self-reliance of effective programs by:
    Setting a course of action that reflects the needs and aspirations of the
        community served
    Concentrating on long-term activities that require minimal external support

Index 10. Evaluating progress

Improving program efficiency by periodically:
    Monitoring and evaluating program's process and progress
    Applying evaluation findings in reorienting program direction

Index 11. Evaluating impact

Improving policies and enhancing programs' cost effectiveness by:
    Conducting periodic evaluations of the program's impact on behavioral and
        epidemiological trends
    Applying evaluation findings to policy and program development

PART II: COLLECTIVE VULNERABILITY

National AIDS Programs

A primary function of national AIDS programs is to provide information and education about HIV/AIDS. Global experience has shown that the details of program design and implementation are vital and a most critical element is audience participation in all phases. Furthermore, the combination of broad informational efforts that introduce basic issues and create a positive climate for discussion and the more intensive, targeted activities is essential. In general, information/education programs must be comprehensive, sustained and coherent.

In order to support and sustain the implementation of intentions derived from the information/education process AIDS programs must also ensure that needed health and social services are accessible. The details of needed health and social services are community specific. Integration of these health and social services into the existing (or strengthened) health and social system is the goal.

The role of national AIDS programs in promoting and ensuring a supportive social environment occurs at several levels. A positive and receptive climate for information/education and use of health and social services is required. HIV/AIDS must also be *normalized* as a health problem so that the stigma attached to people who are infected and ill is reduced. A broader understanding must be developed about the need to prevent discrimination against HIV-infected people, people with AIDS, and people with at risk behaviors.

At both the functional and structural level, the capacity of a national AIDS program to reduce individual and collective vulnerability to HIV/AIDS can be assessed using the indexes in Table 14.2, which can be locally adapted where needed. By using these indexes and applying a scoring system, a national AIDS program, a governmental, nongovernmental, or private program can be ranked.

Societal Status

Although most measures of individual empowerment are interconnected, *AIDS in the World* has selected 8 indicators to reflect societal status and realities. Combining these measures with the assessment of the national AIDS program produces an index of national vulnerability to HIV/AIDS. Table 14.3 lists and defines the indexes selected by *AIDS in the World* for this analysis. Additional definitions and values can be found in the United Nations Development Program's (UNDP) *Human Development Report,* 1991 (New York: Oxford University Press).

Application of a Societal Vulnerability Scoring System

- For each of the indexes, numerical values were defined and then grouped as "Low," "Medium," and "High" (see Table 14.4). A score of 1 was given for "Low"; 2 for "Medium"; and 3 for "High."
- Since not all countries had data available for all 8 indicators, only those countries with 6 or more complete indexes were ranked. The remaining countries were designated as having "Insufficient Data."
- HDI (Index 8) was given a weight of 3; all others were given a weight of 1.
- The addition of weighted values for each index and each country totaled from a minimum of 11 to a maximum of 30 allows for ranking of societal vulnerability to HIV/AIDS:

Score	Societal Vulnerability Scale
11–18	High vulnerability
19–26	Medium vulnerability
27–30	Low vulnerability

Table 14.5 provides the indexes for 37 selected countries surveyed by *AIDS in the World.* These countries which are drawn from the ten Geographic Areas of Affinity include 15 industrialized and 22 developing countries.

Table 14.6 shows the results when the above scoring scheme is applied to divide countries into three categories of societal vulnerability to HIV/AIDS: high, medium, and low vulnerability.

Bringing It Together: National Vulnerability

National vulnerability can be assessed through a two-dimensional matrix, which is comprised of national AIDS program scores and the index of societal vulnerability (Figure 14.2). Countries with the highest vulnerability have both a low-quality national AIDS program and

Table 14.3: Index of societal vulnerability to HIV/AIDS

Information/education will be influenced by:

- Educational attainment, which reflects such basic variables as the % of adults who are literate and mean years of schooling. This index is incorporated in the Human Development Index (HDI), listed as Index 8 below.

- *Index 1:* Access to information. Measured by the number of:

Radios per capita	For developing countries: radios per capita, 1986–1988
Televisions per 1,000	For industrialized countries: the number of televisions per 1,000 persons, 1986–1988

Health and social services are reflected by:

- *Index 2:* Health expenses measured by:

% GNP	For developing countries: as % of Gross National Product (GNP), public expenditures on hospitals, health centers, clinics, health insurance schemes, and family planning programs, 1986
% GDP	For industrialized countries: as % of Gross Domestic Product (GDP), total expenditures on hospitals, health centers, clinics, health insurance schemes, and family planning programs, 1987

- *Index 3:* Access to health services — % of a country's population with access to health services, 1985–1987

- *Index 4:* Under-5 mortality — The probability of dying between birth and age 5, calculated by the annual number of children under age 5 who die per 1,000 live births

A supportive and empowering environment is reflected by:

- Gross Domestic Product (GDP) per capita: per capita, total for final use of output of goods and services produced by an economy by both residents and nonresidents, regardless of the allocation to domestic and foreign claims. This index is incorporated in the Human Development Index (HDI), listed as Index 8 below.

Table 14.3 (cont.): Index of societal vulnerability to HIV/AIDS

- *Index 5:*
  Total female score

This is a combined indicator that measures the overall condition of women in individual countries, reflecting the gender gap. Of the maximum score of 100, 75 points are based on women's status and 25 points reflect the gender gap.

- *Index 6*
  Human Freedom Index

A composite indicator of freedom comprised of 40 separate indicators that include some of the following: freedom from arbitrary rule, illegal arrest, unwarranted attack on person or property; right to life, liberty, security, ethnic and gender equality, rule of law, freedom of assembly, movement, thought, religion, speech; right to work, free choice of jobs, adequate standard of living; right to participate in community life and organize opposition parties or trade union groups.

Scoring: 0–10 = Low freedom ranking
11–30 = Medium freedom ranking
31–40 = High freedom ranking

- *Index 7:*
  Ratio of military expenditures to health and education spending

Ratio of military expenditure to combined education and health expenditure, 1986

- *Index 8:*
  Human Development Index

In order to quantify a country's development beyond the GNP and to more fully capture how economic growth translates into human well-being, the Human Development Index (HDI) measures development by combining annual income per capita, life expectancy, adult literacy, and mean years of schooling.

Sources: 1991 United Nations Human Development Report; World Bank Database (1991); Population Crisis Committee, "Country Rankings of the Status of Women: Poor, Powerless, and Pregnant" (1988).

Table 14.4: Values and weights applied to societal vulnerability indexes

Indexes	High vulnerability	Medium vulnerability	Low vulnerability	Weight
1 Access to information				
Developing: radios per capita	<10	10–19	≥20	1
Industrialized: televisions per 1,000	<200	200–299	≥300	1
2 Health expenditures				
Developing: % GNP	<1%	1.0–1.9%	≥2%	1
Industrialized: % GDP	<1%	1.0–4.9%	≥5%	1
3 Access to health care	<50%	50–99%	100%	1
4 Under-5 mortality	≥100%	50–99%	<50%	1
5 Total female score	0–49.9	50–69.9	≥70	1
6 Human Freedom Index (HFI)	<10	10–29	≥30	1
7 Ratio of military expenditure to health and education spending	≥50%	25–49%	<25%	1
8 Human Development Index (HDI)	<.500	.500–.899	≥.900	3
Total				12

Table 14.5: Societal vulnerability index in 37 countries surveyed by *AIDS in the World*, 1992

Country	Access to information: Radio or TV[a]	Health expenditures as % GNP/ GDP[b]	% with access to health care	Under-5 mortality	Total female score	Human Freedom Index	Ratio military expenditure to health/education	Human Development Index	Vulnerability rating
Argentina	3	2	2	3	2	2	2	2	Medium
Australia	3	3	3	3	3	3	3	3	Low
Cameroon	2	1	1	1	1	1	2	1	High
Canada	3	3	3	3	3	3	3	3	Low
China	2	2	N/A	3	2	1	1	2	Medium
Colombia	2	1	2	2	2	2	2	2	Medium
Congo	2	3	2	1	N/A	N/A	1	1	High
Côte d'Ivoire	2	2	1	1	N/A	N/A	3	1	High
Czechoslovakia	2	2	3	3	3	1	N/A	1	High
Egypt	3	2	N/A	2	1	2	1	1	High
Ethiopia	2	2	1	1	N/A	1	1	1	High
France	N/A	3	3	3	3	3	2	3	Low
Germany	3	3	3	3	3	3	3	3	Low
Haiti	1	1	2	1	1	1	1	1	High
India	1	1	N/A	1	1	2	1	1	High
Italy	N/A	3	3	3	3	2	3	3	Low
Japan	3	3	3	3	2	3	3	3	Low
Mexico	3	2	N/A	2	2	2	3	2	Medium
Morocco	3	1	2	1	1	1	1	1	High
Netherlands	3	3	3	3	3	3	3	3	Low
Nigeria	2	1	1	1	1	2	1	1	High
Norway	3	3	3	3	3	3	3	3	Low
Pakistan	1	1	2	1	1	1	1	1	High
Poland	2	2	3	3	3	2	2	2	Medium
Rwanda	1	1	1	1	1	N/A	1	1	High
Saint Lucia	3	N/A	N/A	N/A	N/A	N/A	N/A	2	Insufficient data
Senegal	2	2	1	1	1	2	2	1	High
Sweden	3	3	3	3	3	3	3	3	Low
Switzerland	3	3	3	3	3	3	3	3	Low
Tanzania	1	2	2	1	1	2	1	1	High
Thailand	2	2	2	3	2	2	1	2	Medium
Trinidad and Tobago	3	3	2	3	2	2	3	2	Medium
Uganda	2	1	2	1	N/A	N/A	1	1	High
United Kingdom	3	3	3	3	3	3	2	3	Low
United States	3	3	3	3	3	3	2	3	Low
USSR	3	2	3	3	3	1	N/A	3	Low
Zambia	1	2	2	1	1	1	1	1	High

Note: N/A = data not available.

a. For developing countries, access to information is measured by radios; for industrialized countries, the units of measurement are televisions (TV).

b. GNP is the unit used for developing countries, GDP the unit for industrialized countries.

Table 14.6: Societal vulnerability index for countries and areas

High (n = 57)

Algeria	Egypt[a]	Madagascar	Rwanda[a]
Angola	Ethiopia[a]	Malawi	Senegal[a]
Bangladesh	Gabon	Mali	Somalia
Benin	Ghana	Mauritania	South Africa
Bolivia	Guatemala	Morocco[a]	Sudan
Burkina Faso	Guinea	Mozambique	Syria
Burma	Haiti[a]	Nepal	Tanzania[a]
Burundi	Honduras	Niger	Togo
Cameroon[a]	India[a]	Nigeria[a]	Turkey
Central African	Indonesia	Pakistan[a]	Uganda[a]
Republic	Iraq	Papua New	Yemen
Chad	Kenya	Guinea	Zaire
Congo[a]	Lesotho	Paraguay	Zambia[a]
Côte d'Ivoire[a]	Liberia	Peru	Zimbabwe
Czechoslovakia[a]	Libya	Philippines	

Medium (n = 39)

Argentina[a]	Dominican Republic	Kuwait	Saudi Arabia
Austria	Ecuador	Malaysia	Singapore
Botswana	El Salvador	Mauritius	Sri Lanka
Brazil	Greece	Mexico[a]	Thailand[a]
Bulgaria	Iran	Nicaragua	Trinidad and Tobago[a]
Chile	Israel	Oman	Tunisia
China[a]	Jamaica	Panama	United Arab Emirates
Colombia[a]	Jordan	Poland[a]	Venezuela
Costa Rica	Korea, DPR	Portugal	Yugoslavia
Cuba	Korea, Republic of	Romania	

Low (n = 21)

Australia[a]	Germany[a]	Netherlands[a]	Switzerland[a]
Belgium	Hungary	New Zealand	United Kingdom[a]
Canada[a]	Ireland	Norway[a]	Uruguay
Denmark	Italy[a]	Spain	United States[a]
Finland	Japan[a]	Sweden[a]	USSR[a]
France[a]			

Table 14.6 (cont.): Societal vulnerability index for countries and areas

Missing data (n = 76)

Afghanistan	Cyprus	Luxembourg	St. Lucia[a]
Albania	Djibouti	Macao	St. Vincent
American Samoa	Dominica	Maldives	Samoa
Andorra	Equatorial Guinea	Malta	San Marino
Anguilla	Federated States of	Mariana Islands	São Tomé and
Antigua and	Micronesia	Marshall Islands	Príncipe
Barbuda	Fiji	Martinique	Seychelles
Bahamas	French Guiana	Monoco	Sierra Leone
Bahrain	French Polynesia	Mongolia	Solomon Islands
Barbados	Gambia	Montserrat	Suriname
Belize	Grenada	Namibia	Swaziland
Bermuda	Guadeloupe	Nauru	Tokelau
Bhutan	Guam	Netherlands	Tonga
British Virgin	Guinea-Bissau	Antilles	Turks and Caicos
Islands	Guyana	New Caledonia	Islands
Brunei	Hong Kong	Niue	Tuvalu
Cambodia	Iceland	Palau	Vanuatu
Cape Verde	Kiribati	Qatar	Vatican City
Cayman Islands	Lao PDR	Reunion	Vietnam
Comoros	Lebanon	St. Kitts and	Wallis and Fortuna
Cook Islands	Liechtenstein	Nevis	

a. Country surveyed by *AIDS in the World, 1992*.

a high index of societal vulnerability; countries with the lowest vulnerability possess both effective national AIDS programs and a low index of societal vulnerability. Though no entity can reach zero vulnerability (V_0), the V_0 point should be considered the goal. The closer the country is placed to V_0, the lower the national vulnerability to HIV/AIDS.

Figure 14.3 illustrates the interaction between the index of societal vulnerability and national AIDS programs. For example: India, with a high index of societal vulnerability, will find itself along the continuum India-C to India-A, depending on the quality of its national AIDS program. Ultimately, however, even with an excellent national AIDS program, the country cannot approach substantially closer to V_0 without societal changes to lower its index of societal vulnerability. In a second example, because Sweden has a low index of societal

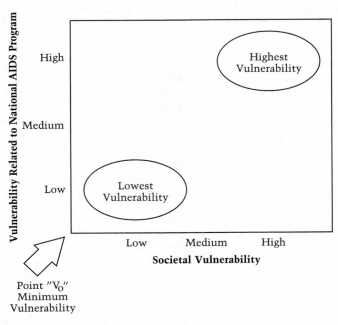

Figure 14.2. National vulnerability to HIV/AIDS.

vulnerability, the quality of its program will determine where, along the continuum Sweden-C to Sweden-A, its national vulnerability to HIV/AIDS will be located.

Incorporating Individual Vulnerability into the Model

Once the societal environment and national AIDS program strength are determined, the ultimate capacity to reduce vulnerability rests with the individual. Even though people are exposed to a similar quality national AIDS program and live within a similar societal environment, individual needs for information, education, health and social services, and support from the social environment will vary. Figure 14.4 illustrates this interaction between person, program, and society. Within a country, the vulnerability of a person depends on:

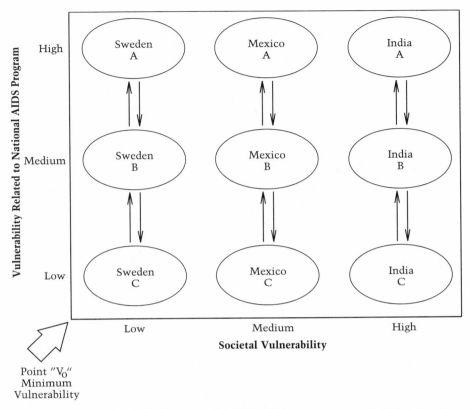

Figure 14.3. Interaction between national AIDS program strength and societal support in reducing vulnerability.

1. the strength of the national program in relation to the particular behaviors or conditions that place this person at risk of HIV infection or inadequate care (shown on axis A); and
2. the degree of societal support (or lack thereof) in relation to this person's particular behaviors or the conditions in this country (shown in axis B). Individual efforts to move toward the point of minimum vulnerability to HIV/AIDS (Point V_0) will be constrained by program and societal limitations. Lowering one's vulnerability involves behavior change while acting to improve programs and societal conditions.

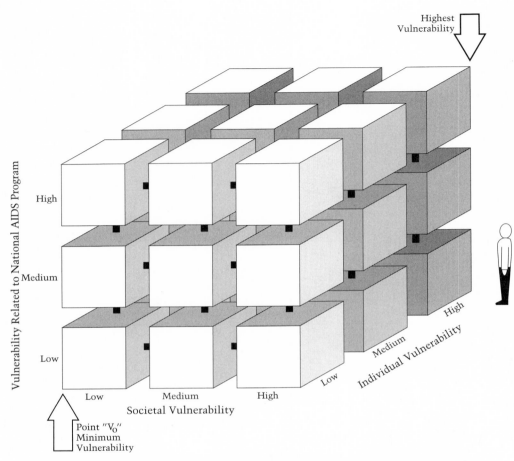

Figure 14.4. Interaction between individual, national AIDS program, and societal vulnerability.

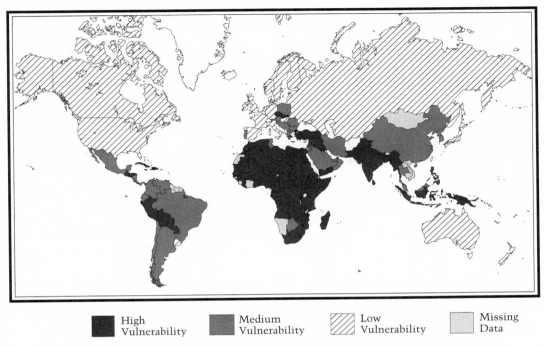

| High Vulnerability | Medium Vulnerability | Low Vulnerability | Missing Data |

Figure 14.5. Map of the world indicating high, medium, and low societal vulnerability to HIV/AIDS, by country.

World Vulnerability to Further Spread of HIV

Beginning next year, *AIDS in the World* will provide a world index of countries classified according to the capacity of their program and societal commitment to reduce individual and collective vulnerability to HIV/AIDS. However, country societal vulnerability can already be mapped out applying the criteria already given.

As a first indicator of danger zones for HIV spread, Figure 14.5 is a map of the world indicating 57 countries having a high societal vulnerability to HIV/AIDS. The largest number of these countries (34) are in sub-Saharan Africa, 9 are in the South East Mediterranean, 6 are in Southeast Asia, 5 are in Latin America, and 1 each is in Oceania, the Caribbean, and Eastern Europe.

Regardless of the current status of their HIV experience, each of these 57 countries must be considered at high risk for introduction and spread of HIV infection. Therefore, countries that have thus far escaped the brunt of the HIV/AIDS pandemic, including Indonesia, Egypt, Pakistan, Nigeria, Bangladesh, Afghanistan, and Somalia, must act now—for the warning signs are clear.

Thirty-nine countries are at a substantial yet somewhat lower level of societal vulnerability. If this group of countries is considered the next-most vulnerable to HIV/AIDS, the likely evolution of HIV/AIDS geography will clearly move toward Latin America (11 countries), the South East Mediterranean (8), the Caribbean (4), Asia (4 in Southeast Asia; 3, including China, in North East Asia), sub-Saharan Africa (2), Eastern Europe (4), and Western Europe (3).

Countries that do not have an overall high vulnerability should be evaluated in relation to societal features that are connected to their risk behaviors or conditions, and relative to the program elements directed to them.

AIDS in the World strongly encourages communities and national groups to assess their community and national situation, either by using the criteria proposed in this chapter or by modifying and developing improved criteria and indicators.

In future years, *AIDS in the World* will refine national programs and societal vulnerability indexes in order to maintain an updated world map of vulnerability to the HIV/AIDS pandemic. *AIDS in the World* will also propose an index of vulnerability applicable to communities and groups that may be far more vulnerable than their own national (aggregate) vulnerability index may suggest.

PART FOUR

. . . .

Critical Issues

CHAPTER FIFTEEN

The Shape of the Pandemic

![marker] . . .

TRENDS IN THE UNITED STATES AND EUROPE

Laurence Slutsker, Jean-Baptiste Brunet, John M. Karon, and James W. Curran

.urence Slutsker, M.D.,
hn M. Karon, Ph.D.,
d James W. Curran,
.D., are at the Division
HIV/AIDS, National
enter for Infectious
seases, Centers for
sease Control, Public
ealth Service, U.S.
epartment of Health and
uman Services.
ean-Baptiste Brunet is at
e European Center for
e Epidemiological
onitoring of AIDS,
ôpital National de
aint-Maurice, France.

In 1981, the first cases of acquired immunodeficiency syndrome (AIDS) were reported from Los Angeles in 5 homosexual men.[1] In the ensuing 10 years, more than 200,000 AIDS cases have been reported in the United States,[2] and 65,000 in Europe.[3] In the United States, approximately 1 million persons are infected with the human immunodeficiency virus (HIV),[4] and the number infected in Europe is estimated at 500,000. Worldwide, the number of HIV-infected persons was estimated by the World Health Organization (WHO) to be 8 to 10 million in 1991.[5]

Although the number of persons with AIDS in industrialized countries is large, it is apparent that the majority of cases have yet to develop. After 10 years of the epidemic in the industrialized world, the number of persons currently alive with AIDS represents a small proportion of those with HIV infection. For example, of the estimated 1 million HIV-infected persons in the United States, approximately 90,000 are currently living with AIDS. Three factors may contribute to an increased prevalence of AIDS in industrialized countries in the coming decade: the large number of HIV-infected individuals who have not yet developed AIDS, the prolonged survival of AIDS patients receiving both antiretroviral therapy and prophylaxis and treatment for opportunistic diseases, and the continued incidence of HIV infection and transmission.

AIDS cases in the United States continue to occur predominantly in men who have sex with men (MSWM). In Europe, however, since 1990, equal proportions of AIDS cases have been reported associated with MSWM and injection drug users (IDUs). Emerging patterns suggest that HIV infection and AIDS are becoming increasingly important in different population subgroups and in different geographic areas. This section reviews the trends in HIV/AIDS incidence and prevalence in the United States and Europe and highlights how the epidemiology of AIDS is evolving in these areas as the epidemic moves into its second decade.

Blood and Blood Products

In the United States, through December 1991, 6,512 (6,060 adults; 452 infants/children) AIDS cases (3.2 percent) were reported in persons exposed to HIV through receipt of blood or blood products, of whom 29 percent had a history of hemophilia or other coagulation disorders and 71 percent had a history of transfusion cases.[6] In Europe, 6.2 percent of cases have been reported associated with this mode of exposure.[7]

Trends have changed in regard to cases associated with transfusion of blood and blood products. In the United States, the proportion of AIDS cases with a history of hemophilia or other coagulation disorder has remained relatively stable over time at 2 to 3 percent. Of the first 100,000 reported cases of AIDS in the United States (June 1981–August 1989), the proportion associated with transfusion was 2.5 percent for adults and 11 percent for children; in the second 100,000 reported cases (September 1989–December 1991), these proportions decreased to 1.9 and 5.6 percent, respectively.[8]

In Europe, the proportion of transfusion-associated cases has declined from 5.7 percent of AIDS cases diagnosed in 1983 to 1.7 percent of those diagnosed in 1991. If the 559 transfusion-related AIDS cases from Romania are included among the 1,493 transfusion-related cases diagnosed in Europe in the last 3 years, then the percentage of transfusion-associated cases in the region has been stable at 3 percent over these 3 years. Rates of infection in European people with hemophilia vary from less than 10 percent in eastern countries and Belgium to more than 40 percent in France and Germany and 80 percent in Spain.[9]

HIV-antibody screening of all blood donations and heat treatment of factor concentrates have dramatically reduced HIV transmission through blood components and clotting factors. Nearly all newly reported cases associated with infected blood or blood products reflect transmission from products received prior to the availability of screening for HIV antibody in 1985.[10]

Thus, the incidence of transfusion-associated AIDS in industrialized countries has stabilized or begun to decline and will most likely continue to decline through the next decade. In industrialized countries with large numbers of AIDS cases, this exposure category contributes a relatively small number of cases to the total. This suggests that the impact on overall trends in AIDS incidence of the decline in transfusion-associated cases will be minimal in these countries.

Homosexual/Bisexual Men

In the United States, 58 percent of all AIDS cases have been reported among men who report sexual contact with other men (MSWM) who are not known injection drug users (IDUs). Of all cases reported in the United States in 1991, 53 percent were MSWM who were not IDUs. In Europe, 42 percent of all AIDS cases have been reported in MSWM; this percentage varies from less than 20 percent in Italy and Spain to more than 75 percent in the Federation of Czech and Slovak Republics, Denmark, Finland, the Netherlands, and the United Kingdom. In Western Europe, AIDS incidence in MSWM increased rapidly until 1987 and moderately thereafter.

In New York City, San Francisco, and Los Angeles, AIDS incidence among MSWM increased much less rapidly after 1986.[11] For example, in New York City, incidence was roughly constant from mid-1986 to mid-1990; in 1989, the annual AIDS incidence decreased by 4 percent. Over the same time periods, the annual AIDS incidence in San Francisco increased by only 6 percent and 8 percent, respectively; the corresponding changes in Los Angeles were 11 percent and 2 percent, respectively. In contrast, from 1984 to 1986, the annual increase in the AIDS incidence in these 3 cities among MSWM ranged from 43 to 113 percent.

A similar change in the rate of increase in incidence is noted in other urban areas in the United States with a population of at least 1 million. In these areas, annual increases in incidence in AIDS in MSWM declined from 15 to 20 percent in 1988 and 1989 to 5 percent during the first three quarters of 1990. The incidence trend in 36 of these cities is a composite of several types of trends. Increases in incidence slowed markedly in some areas. In Washington, D.C., for example, incidence in 1988–1990 was at most 10 percent greater than in the previous year; similarly, in Newark, New Jersey, and in Boston, Massachusetts, incidence in 1989 was at most 5 percent greater than in 1988 and did not increase in 1990. In contrast, marked increases in AIDS incidence among MSWM continue in other large urban areas (e.g., Detroit, Michigan, and San Diego, California), where the incidence in both 1989 and 1990 was at least 14 percent greater than in the previous year. In smaller urban and rural areas, incidence trends among MSWM continued to increase.

Trends in AIDS incidence among MSWM vary by racial/ethnic group. In both New York and Los Angeles, incidence has plateaued among non-Hispanic whites, non-Hispanic blacks, and Hispanics, with the plateau occurring a year earlier (1988) among non-Hispanic whites. Outside New York, San Francisco, and Los Angeles, incidence among non-Hispanic white MSWM may be leveling. However, there is no evidence yet that a similar plateau is occurring among non-white MSWM; the annual AIDS incidence in non-Hispanic black MSWM outside New York City, San Francisco, and Los Angeles continues to increase (26 percent in 1989 and an additional 12 percent in 1990). Similar increases occurred in Hispanic MSWM (21 percent and 14 percent, respectively).

The overall leveling in annual AIDS incidence in MSWM may be due to several factors, including a previous decline in the incidence of HIV infection and a slowing in the progression to AIDS in HIV-infected persons due to antiretroviral therapy and prophylaxis against *Pneumocystis carinii* pneumonia. In support of significant behavior changes, evidence from San Francisco and elsewhere in the early 1980s indicates a decline in the number of nonsteady sexual partners and a decrease in specific sexual practices, including receptive anal intercourse.[12] Similarly, rates of rectal and pharyngeal gonorrhea have declined among men aged 15–44 years in New York, San Francisco, and many other cities.[13]

Increasing use of antiretroviral therapy with zidovudine and prophylaxis for *Pneumocystis carinii* pneumonia often delay the onset of AIDS.[14] In the United States, many HIV-infected persons, including MSWM, received zidovudine before they had developed AIDS under a limited distribution program in 1987; many of these men lived in large urban areas in New York, New Jersey, or California. Zidovudine treatment of these men could have resulted in delayed development of AIDS in some individuals in this group, contributing to the observed plateau in reported AIDS incidence. To the extent that this is a contributing factor, the leveling may be somewhat misleading, as morbidity and mortality attributable to AIDS in this group may only be delayed rather than decreased.

Although AIDS incidence trends among MSWM summarized here are encouraging, these should be interpreted with caution. Recent evidence suggests that some MSWM, particularly adolescents and minorities, do not maintain safe sex practices.[15] This observation is supported by a recent rise in rates of gonorrhea among sexually active homosexual/bisexual men in King County, Washington.[16] In addition, HIV seroconversion continues to be detected in cohorts of homosexual men in major metropolitan areas and in small communities.[17]

In Europe, recent data on gonorrhea among MSWM from London, Leeds, and Amsterdam suggest that sexual practices associated with a high risk of acquiring HIV infection have recently increased.[18] In London, the incidence of HIV infection among MSWM undergoing repeated antibody testing from 1988 to 1990 was 4.6 seroconversions per 100 person-years.[19] In France, 9 percent of MSWM who tested HIV negative in 1989 were found to be HIV positive in the first quarter of 1991 upon presentation for treatment of an acute sexually transmitted disease (STD) at an STD clinic.[20] These data, and the high HIV seroprevalence rates in cohorts of MSWM, indicate that HIV transmission in homosexual and bisexual men will continue. Prevention efforts must be maintained and targeted at those who remain at greatest risk, including minority MSWM.

Injection Drug Users (IDUs)

After MSWM, IDUs comprise the largest exposure category among persons with AIDS in the industrialized world. In the United States, through December 1991, 58,888 AIDS cases had been reported among

IDUs, representing 29 percent of all adult cases.[21] Of these, 13,135 (22 percent) were also homosexual or bisexual men. Fifty percent of women with AIDS and 27 percent of men with AIDS were IDUs. In Europe, 22,810 cases have been reported among IDUs, including 1,156 homosexual or bisexual IDU males.[22] IDUs represented 39 percent of all adult AIDS cases diagnosed in Europe in 1991; 36 percent of AIDS cases among men and 56 percent of those among women were associated with this risk group.

Though cases of AIDS among IDUs have been reported from every state in the United States, rates vary widely by geographic area. In 1988, rates of IDU-associated AIDS (includes AIDS in IDUs, sex partners of IDUs, and children born to mothers who were IDUs or sex partners of IDUs) in excess of 10 cases per 100,000 population were reported from Puerto Rico, New Jersey, New York, and the District of Columbia.[23]

In the United States, the growth in incidence of AIDS in female and heterosexual male IDUs began to decline in mid-1987. When examined by geographic region, this pattern is a composite of a plateau in incidence in New York City and New Jersey, with a continued linear increase in incidence in this exposure category elsewhere in the United States.[24] In men with a history of both IDU and sexual contact with other men, the growth in AIDS incidence has been declining since late 1986 and appears to have leveled in early 1989.

In contrast to the incidence trend seen in IDUs in the Northeast, the proportion of AIDS cases attributable to IDUs or sexual partners of IDUs is increasing in the southeastern United States (Alabama, Florida, Georgia, Mississippi, North Carolina, and South Carolina). From 1984 to 1986, this region accounted for 9.2 percent of U.S. AIDS cases associated with being an IDU and 15.5 percent of AIDS cases associated with being a sexual partner of an IDU; from 1987 to 1989, these proportions increased to 13.8 percent and 27.9 percent, respectively.[25] Seventy-five percent of IDUs and sexual partners of IDUs with AIDS in this region are African-American, compared with 22 percent of the population. More than half of these cases and 75 percent of the population in the southeastern United States reside in rural or in smaller (population less than 1 million) metropolitan areas.

In Europe, 69 percent of AIDS cases among IDUs have been diagnosed in Italy and Spain, where IDUs comprise more than 60 percent of all AIDS cases. In contrast, IDUs account for less than 10 percent of reported cases in northern countries like Denmark, Sweden, the Netherlands, and the United Kingdom. AIDS incidence in Spain and Italy increased rapidly between 1984 and 1988 and has leveled off since 1989. In the northern countries, there has been moderate growth in the incidence of AIDS among IDUs since the beginning of the epidemic.

HIV seroprevalence studies of IDUs entering drug treatment programs in the United States from 1988 to 1990 at different geographic locations show a wide variation in rates by geographic area, with highest rates in the Northeast (14–39 percent) and lowest rates along the West Coast (0–5 percent).[26] Significant increases in rates over the 3-year period were noted in Boston (Northeast) and Chicago (North central), while rates elsewhere varied with no overall increase or decrease noted. In New York City, HIV seroprevalence among cohorts of IDUs have shown a leveling, with HIV antibody detected in 59 percent and 52 percent of subjects in 1987 and 1988, respectively.[27] Difference in infection rates among IDUs by geographic area remains incompletely explained, but may be related to differences in access to drug treatment, differences in needle sharing practices, or other factors.[28]

HIV seroprevalence among IDUs in many geographic areas in the United States appears to have leveled. However, the prevalence of high-risk behaviors (i.e., sharing needles, not cleaning needles, having sexual contact with partners who are IDUs) remains high, and in IDU populations in Los Angeles, New York City, and Chicago, it did not decline appreciably over a 3-year observation period.[29] However, in some IDU populations (Trenton, New Jersey), the prevalence of risk behavior did decline. Finally, the majority of IDUs in the United States are not yet in treatment, due in part to a chronic shortage in treatment capacity.

Large variations in HIV seroprevalence among IDUs are also found in European countries, but rates vary widely at national levels, depending on characteristics of tested subjects and location of studies.[30] For example, in Scotland, prevalence rates up to 60 percent were found among IDUs in Edinburgh, whereas in England and Wales, these rates were always lower than 5 percent.[31] In Italy, HIV seroprevalence among IDUs in different communities varies from 10 percent to over

60 percent.[32] Although seroprevalence rates appear stable in most countries in Western Europe, studies conducted in Amsterdam and Rome document new infections in cohorts of IDUs. Incidence rates in these cities were 5 per 100 person-years in 1988–89, although this rate was 2 to 3 times lower than that seen in previous years.[33] Of particular concern are countries in Europe where HIV infection among IDU populations may have only recently been introduced. For example, HIV serosurveys among IDUs in Poland, which has reported only 78 AIDS cases, have shown an increase from no HIV-positive IDUs among 1,632 tested between 1985 and 1987 to 1 percent infected among 1,424 tested in 1988 and 9 percent among 4,738 tested in 1990.[34]

Current HIV prevention efforts targeted toward IDUs are far from sufficient and need to be expanded; these efforts should target sexual transmission among IDUs, as well as needle transmission, and increase the availability of treatment. The explosive HIV epidemics in IDUs observed in some cities in the United States and other countries (e.g., Italy, Scotland) indicate the serious potential for rapid spread of HIV into low prevalence areas and underline the need for successful prevention efforts in IDUs.

Heterosexual Contact

Of additional concern in the industrialized world is the increasing incidence of AIDS cases associated with heterosexual transmission. Through December 1991, 11,936 cases of AIDS in the United States were reported to be associated with heterosexual contact, representing 6 percent of all cases.[35] In the United States, in each of the last 5 years, the percentage increase in annual AIDS incidence in this group has been higher than that of any other exposure category.[36] Diagnosed cases in this group increased 41 percent from 1989 to 1990,[37] while corresponding increases were no more than 8 percent in adults in each of the other exposure categories. Projections suggest that AIDS incidence related to heterosexual contact will more than double from 1990 to 1995.[38]

In Europe, half of the 5,655 AIDS cases reported associated with heterosexual transmission through December 1991 have been diagnosed in the last 2 years. These cases represented 7 percent of all adult cases diagnosed in 1987 and nearly 11 percent of those diagnosed in 1991. In Belgium, of a total of 1,046 AIDS cases, 42 percent were reported to have been associated with heterosexual transmission; the majority of these have occurred in African immigrants or Belgians who had lived in African countries. Overall, 46 percent of heterosexual cases have had sexual contact with partners originating from or having lived in countries where sexual transmission among heterosexuals is frequent. However, this percentage has decreased from 90 percent among heterosexual cases diagnosed in 1985 to 39 percent in 1991.

Heterosexual transmission is of particular importance among women in industrialized countries. Among women reported with AIDS in the United States, heterosexual contact is the second most frequently reported exposure category and accounts for 34 percent of all reported cases. Most heterosexual contact cases in women are related to sexual contact with an HIV-infected IDU; however, the proportion of women reported exposed through heterosexual contact where the risk of the infected partner was not specified increased from 3 percent in 1983–84 to 16 percent in 1989–90.[39]

Seroprevalence studies among young women suggest that transmission of HIV is continuing. In the United States, a national survey of childbearing women indicated the overall seroprevalence was 1.5 per 1,000 childbearing women, with rates as high as 5–6 per 1,000 childbearing women in some northeastern states.[40] In Europe, unlinked anonymous HIV serosurveys of delivering pregnant women showed a prevalence rate of 0.27 percent in Paris, 0.20–0.33 percent in industrialized regions of Italy, and 0.14 percent in London.[41]

Among disadvantaged adolescents (aged 16–21 years) applying for work in the Job Corps in the United States, the rate of infection was only slightly lower among women than men (3.2 vs. 3.7 per 1,000); among those aged 16 and 17, seroprevalence was higher among women (2.3 per 1,000) than men (1.5 per 1,000).[42] It is unlikely that injection drug use among young women would explain this low male-to-female ratio, because 2 to 3 times more male than female high-school students report injecting drugs and sharing needles.[43] Rather, the narrow gap between HIV infection prevalence in young men and women is consistent with the epidemiology of traditional STDs, suggesting that heterosexual transmission may have contributed to the relatively high rates of HIV infection among females in this group.

Heterosexual transmission of HIV may be linked both to drug use and STDs. Genital ulcerative diseases, such as chancroid, syphilis, and perhaps other STDs, have been noted to facilitate acquisition and transmission of HIV.[44] In the United States, the incidence of primary and secondary syphilis increased 61 percent from 1985 to 1989, with the greatest increase (176 percent) in African-American women.[45] Spread of syphilis, as well as gonorrhea and chancroid, has been linked in some situations to use of illegal drugs, especially crack cocaine, through drug-related high-risk sexual behaviors, such as having sex with multiple partners for money or drugs.[46] Thus, approaches to limit heterosexual transmission of HIV, syphilis, and other STDs in the United States may require additional resources for programs for STD-infected sex workers, drug users, and their sexual contacts.

Infants and Children

Through December 1991, 3,471 children under 13 years of age were reported with AIDS in the United States. Most (85 percent) of the children with AIDS were reported as having been infected perinatally; 8 percent had received contaminated blood components, and 5 percent were infected during treatment for hemophilia or other coagulation disorders.[47] Whereas the proportion of children infected through receipt of contaminated blood products has declined recently, cases associated with perinatal transmission have shown an increase. The first 100,000 persons reported with AIDS in the United States included 1,683 children, of whom 81 percent were born to mothers with or at risk for HIV infection; among the 1,702 children in the second 100,000 reported cases, 87 percent were reported to have been exposed in this manner.[48] Of the mothers, 49 percent were reported to be IDUs, and 37 percent were sexual partners of infected men, most of whom (55 percent) were IDUs.

Among the 2,918 pediatric AIDS cases reported in Europe through December 1991, 54 percent were diagnosed in Romania; most were reported infected through transfusion of unscreened blood and through reuse of inadequately sterilized needles and syringes.[49]

Seroprevalence data have provided estimates of the number of infected infants delivered in the United States. Based on a national survey among delivering women, an estimated 6,079 HIV-infected women delivered an infant in 1989.[50] Assuming a perinatal transmission rate of 25 percent, an estimated 1,500 HIV-infected infants were delivered during 1989. This number is larger than the cumulative total of perinatally acquired AIDS cases reported in the United States from

1981 through 1988, indicating that substantial increases in the numbers of perinatally acquired AIDS cases can be expected in the coming years. Prevention strategies must be focused not only on women who are IDUs or sex partners of IDUs, but also on all sexually active men and women, including adolescents.

Conclusions

As prophylaxis and treatment for opportunistic diseases improve, and as ever larger numbers of patients receive antiretroviral therapy with zidovudine and other drugs still under development, it can be expected that the number of persons living with severe HIV-related immunosuppression and/or AIDS will increase. In the United States, the Centers for Disease Control estimated that by January 1, 1992, approximately 90,000 persons would be living with AIDS, and an additional 55,000–65,000 persons would be diagnosed with AIDS during 1992. Moreover, it is estimated that at the beginning of 1992 in the United States, there were 100,000–140,000 HIV-infected individuals with severe immunosuppression (CD4+ lymphocyte count <200/µl) and no AIDS-defining illness.[51] A substantial increase in resources will be needed to provide both acute medical therapy and long-term care for these individuals.

The continued evolution of the epidemic in the industrialized world will bring new and difficult challenges. One such challenge in the United States is the increasing magnitude of tuberculosis (TB) as a public health problem. The number of cases of TB reported annually in the United States declined steadily from 1953 to 1984, but then increased by 3 percent in 1986, 5 percent in 1989, and 9 percent in 1990.[52] The contribution of HIV-related TB morbidity to total TB morbidity is not precisely known, but HIV infection appears to have had a substantial impact in some areas. For example, 5 percent of AIDS patients in New York City and 10 percent of AIDS patients in Florida had a history of TB; conversely, rates of HIV seropositivity among non-Asian adult TB patients in Seattle and San Francisco were 23 percent and 29 percent, respectively.[53] Closely related to the resurgence of TB in the United States is the emerging problem of multidrug resistant tuberculosis (MDR-TB). The recent occurrence of outbreaks of MDR-TB in HIV-infected patients underscores both the difficulty of diagnosing TB infection in these patients and problems inherent in delayed recognition of drug resistance, as well as the unusually high susceptibility of HIV-infected persons to severe clinical TB when they become infected with *Mycobacterium tuberculosis*.[54] In addition, these outbreaks highlight the importance of implementing infection-control precautions to prevent transmission of TB to patients and health care workers.

In Europe, there is increasing concern regarding the recently reported increase in STDs among MSWM in western countries where AIDS incidence was stabilizing. In eastern countries, another emerging problem is the recent documented spread of HIV among IDUs. The profound economic, political, social, and cultural changes in Eastern Europe may have substantial and unpredictable effects on sexual behavior and drug use. In addition, the outbreak in Romania of nosocomial HIV infection among children highlights the risk of transmission in hospital settings when shortages of injecting and sterilizing equipment occur.

Because of the large number of persons already infected with HIV and evidence that transmission is ongoing, morbidity and mortality due to HIV infection and AIDS will pose an increasingly formidable challenge. The AIDS epidemic is far from winding down in industrialized societies. On the contrary, dealing with the inexorably growing burden of HIV-related morbidity in developed societies will require even greater compassion and commitment of resources for prevention and treatment as the epidemic moves into the 1990s.

■■■ . . .

IS BREAST FEEDING AT RISK? THE CHALLENGE OF AIDS

Jody Heymann

Dr. Jody Heymann is currently a MacArthur Foundation Fellow at the Center for Population and Development Studies at Harvard University, Boston, Massachusetts.

Since the first case reports of possible HIV transmission through breast milk, concerns have been raised about the continued safety of breast feeding, particularly in the developing world. The stakes are high. Breast feeding has saved millions of children's lives worldwide. If breast feeding were to decline precipitously, child mortality could double or triple in many parts of the world. If the risk of HIV transmission through breast feeding is substantial, many more hundreds of thousands of infants could be additionally infected with HIV.

In 1987, the World Health Organization (WHO) stated that HIV-infected women should continue to breast-feed where "safe enough" feeding alternatives were unavailable. Although these recommendations were clear and supportive of the continuation of breast feeding in developing countries, their ramifications for the industrialized countries were less clear. Several major health institutions in industrialized countries, including the U.S. Centers for Disease Control (CDC) and the United Kingdom's Department of Health, have recommended against breast feeding for HIV-infected women. The United Kingdom went even further, advising women who may be at high risk of HIV infection, but who had not been diagnosed as infected, against breast feeding.

Information that is becoming available may profoundly influence our understanding of the circumstances under which bottle and breast feeding should be recommended to HIV-infected mothers. This section reviews current knowledge about the risks of HIV transmission via breast feeding and the benefits of breast feeding; it then proposes recommendations for future practice and research.

HIV Transmission via Breast Milk

Initial concern about postnatal transmission (transmission from HIV-infected mother to infant after childbirth) was raised when HIV was found in colostrum and breast milk.[55] However, finding the virus in breast milk did not mean that breast feeding would become a significant transmission route. Several reasons were proposed for this, including the inability of HIV to survive in the inhospitable environment of the digestive tract and the presence of anti-HIV antibodies in breast milk.[56]

Experience with other viruses in breast milk is varied. For example, both cytomegalovirus and HTLV-1 are commonly transmitted via breast milk. While rubella and hepatitis B virus have been detected in breast milk, breast feeding does not appear to be a common mode of transmission for either.[57]

Debate over the extent of HIV transmission via breast feeding grew heated as transmission was documented in case reports on 4 continents.[58] Although these reports provided evidence that HIV can and has been transmitted via breast milk, the extent and precise circumstances of transmission remained unknown.

Some studies have focused on infants whose mothers became HIV infected after giving birth as a means of differentiating postnatal transmission from prenatal and connatal (during the process of childbirth) transmission. In Zambia, one study of mothers infected with HIV after childbirth showed that 3 of their 19 breast-fed infants (16 percent) became HIV infected.[59] In another study, in Rwanda, in which maternal infection was believed to have occurred postnatally, 36 to 53 percent of breast-fed infants became HIV infected.[60] In a third study, 3 of 11 breast-fed infants born to postnatally infected mothers developed HIV infection.[61] All of these studies suggest a high HIV transmission rate via breast feeding for infants of mothers who are postnatally infected, but it is not clear how far these studies can be generalized to apply to infants of mothers already infected with HIV prior to or even during pregnancy. Women who have either been infected recently or have advanced HIV disease may be much more infectious through breast milk than are women with an intermediate stage of infection because of the peak levels of virus in the blood that occur soon after infection and late in the course of illness.

Other studies have tried to assess the risk of postnatal HIV transmission by comparing breast- and bottle-fed infants born to women with varying stages of HIV infection. Among children born to HIV-infected mothers in France, 5 out of 6 breast-fed infants became infected, compared with only 25 out of 99 bottle-fed infants. While the difference was statistically significant, the confidence interval on the actual transmission rate was large because so few breast-fed infants were studied. A recent study, following the progress of 560 infants born to HIV-infected mothers, found breast-fed infants to have nearly double the HIV infection rate of bottle-fed infants (42.9 percent as compared with 22.4 percent).[62]

Different rates found in different studies may be influenced by unidentified cofactors, recent HIV infection, advanced AIDS or a low CD4 count in the mother.[63] Although studies have drawn a variety of conclusions regarding the rate of postnatal transmission, there is profound concern that the transmission rate from mothers infected around the time of childbirth, or after childbirth may be as high as 20 percent to 35 percent. Whether women with long-standing HIV infection will prove to be as infectious is not yet known.

Benefits of Breast Feeding

If there were no risk in bottle feeding and no additional benefits to breast feeding, recommendations against breast feeding by HIV-infected women could be made comfortably. Yet bottle feeding has been associated with markedly increased mortality among infants and children, particularly in developing countries.

Studies in Bangladesh found increased mortality for bottle-fed children up to the age of 3.[64] The negative synergism of poor sanitation and bottle feeding on infant health leading to diarrhea and malnutrition has been well documented.[65] The studies often suggest a 1.5- to 5-fold increase in relative risk of mortality among bottle-fed children.[66]

Although death from diarrheal diseases is much less common in industrialized countries, it does occur. In the United States between 1979 and 1987, 1,588 infants between the ages of 1 month and 4 years died from infectious diarrhea.[67] An increased fatality rate from diarrhea has been documented among bottle-fed children in the United States, Canada, and the United Kingdom, as well as in developing countries.[68]

In addition to reducing infant and child mortality, breast feeding has been associated with reduced morbidity from other infectious diseases, including pneumonia, otitis media, bacteremia, and meningitis.[69] Whether breast feeding is the critical factor in all cases remains unclear due to the lack of controlled studies. For example, some authors believe that different rates of smoking among bottle- and breast-feeding mothers may explain the apparent association of bottle feeding with an increase in respiratory infections.[70]

The relationship between bottle feeding, infectious diseases, and malnutrition explains only in part the reason breast feeding is associated with greater child survival. In many parts of the world, breast feeding is also a major factor leading to reduced fertility rates.[71] In some populations, the decrease in fertility is directly attributable to the hormonal changes that occur when a woman breast feeds. In other populations, the drop in fertility rates reflects the cultural practice of sexual abstinence during breast feeding.[72]

In sub-Saharan Africa, breast feeding reduces fertility by 4 births per woman; the reduction due to contraception is less than 1 birth per woman. If breast feeding in sub-Saharan Africa were decreased by as little as 25 percent, then contraceptive use would have to increase by nearly 150 percent in order to keep fertility rates constant. However, the international variation is great. In Asia and the Pacific, it would take a 23 percent increase in contraceptive use to offset a 25 percent decrease in breast feeding; in Latin America, only a 5 percent increase would be required.[73]

Therefore, before changing current recommendations about breast feeding based on HIV-related concerns, it is important to consider the significant benefits of child spacing on the health of both women and children. If breast feeding were decreased without a concomitant increase in contraceptive use, more mothers and children would die. The association between child mortality and child spacing has been well documented. Although this association is confounded by the fact that breast feeding is associated with increased child spacing and decreased child mortality, child spacing has been found to affect the health of both mothers and children.[74]

Special Considerations

It is not yet known whether HIV-infected mothers confer the same health protection to their infants by breast feeding as do HIV-negative mothers. Immunologically, breast milk from immunocompromised mothers and mothers with advanced HIV disease may not be as beneficial as is milk from immunocompetent mothers. From a nutritional standpoint, women with AIDS will be much more at risk of malnutrition or wasting than the general population. Studies have shown that mortality is high among infants of malnourished women, partly due to decreased breast milk production as well as lower initial birth weight.[75]

Impact on Women

For too long, the debate over breast feeding has focussed primarily on infants. The mother's health, well being, and survival must also be considered. Yet in this area, perilously little is known. Past studies have questioned whether pregnancy accelerates the progression of HIV disease. Studies should examine the impact of breast feeding on the mother's immune status, nutritional condition, and HIV-disease progression. Nutrition is particularly important for symptomatic HIV-infected women, given that they are more likely to start breast feeding malnourished and that a malnourished mother's nutritional status can suffer while she is producing milk for the newborn.[76]

Recommendations

Why not simply say that HIV-infected women should breast feed where bottle feeding is not safe enough? The trouble comes from defining safe enough. This section proposes recommendations under two sets of assumptions. In the first scenario, HIV transmission via breast milk is estimated to be low (5 percent) for all infants, except those born to mothers who become infected while breast feeding; for these women, a transmission rate of 25 percent is consistent with available data. In the second scenario, all HIV-infected women (regardless of when they were infected) are assumed to have a 25 percent likelihood of HIV transmission via breast milk.

In both scenarios, bottle-fed infants are considered to have a threefold increase in risk (relative risk RR=3) of child mortality compared with breast-fed infants. This is consistent with available research, but as discussed earlier, the exact relative risk is unknown and may vary by setting. The thresholds for making different recommendations that are presented in the following figures were derived using decision analysis. These algorithms consider the two basic scenarios described here; in each, the entry point depends on whether voluntary HIV testing and counseling are available and/or chosen. The methodology is similar to that described previously,[77] but the results have been updated to include the best available data as of January 1992.

This approach considers the safety of bottle feeding in different localities according to the area's baseline child mortality rate (CMR). Others have suggested that as CMR increases, the relative risk of bottle feeding also increases. This postulate can be reasonably grounded in evidence that poverty and poor sanitation increase both CMR and relative risk. Even where the relative risk of bottle feeding is constant, the overall attributable risk of bottle feeding will increase as CMR increases.

The goal of these two scenarios (see Figures 15.1 and 15.2) is to illustrate how rational recommendations can be formulated to take account of conditions at a local level.* Given the great variation in

---

* Recommendations are a function of the relative risk of bottle feeding, and these charts are meant only to give sample recommendations for scenarios consistent with available information.

Flow Charts I and II assume that the postnatal HIV transmission rate is 25 percent for perinatally and postnatally infected women and 5 percent for women with pre-existing HIV infections.

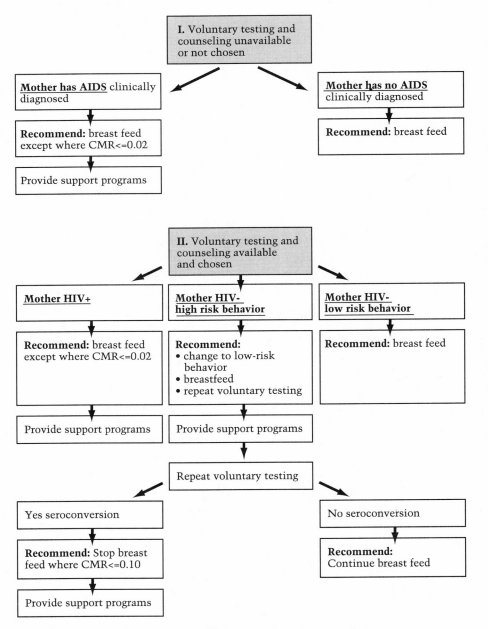

Figure 15.1. Elements to consider in formulating recommendations on breastfeeding in relation to HIV infection: scenario one.

Flow Charts I and II assume that the postnatal HIV transmission rate is 25 percent for all HIV-infected women.

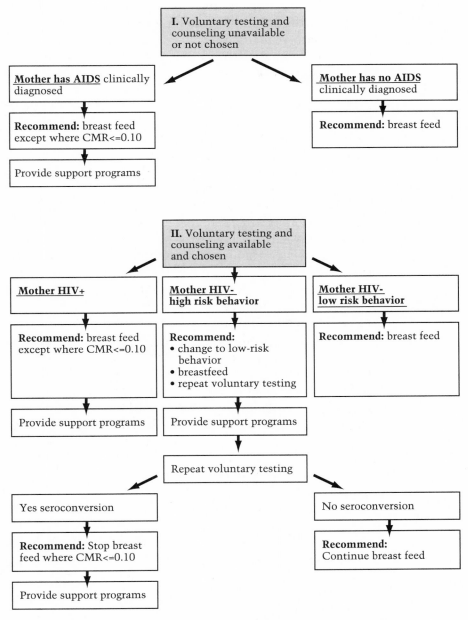

Figure 15.2. Elements to consider in formulating recommendations on breastfeeding in relation to HIV infection: scenario two.

the risk of bottle feeding within individual countries and between different regions and subpopulations, local rather than national recommendations may be preferable. Specific strategies can then be developed for the smallest areas for which data on CMR and HIV infection rates are available.

The following critical notes must be made about these and any set of recommendations:

- These recommendations, like others currently in effect worldwide, are based on the infant's welfare. Recommendations also need to reflect the health and welfare of the mother. It is not yet possible to do this with confidence, for information is lacking on the effect of feeding practices on the health of the HIV-infected mother. Such information needs to be gathered and incorporated immediately.
- In the absence of voluntary HIV testing, even if the rate of postnatal transmission is found to be 25 percent, breast feeding must be recommended to all women without clinical AIDS. This recommendation draws on the fact that the risk to infants of bottle feeding by uninfected women outweighs the potential benefits to children of HIV-infected women.[78] If postnatal transmission is found to be high, then prenatal and pregnancy voluntary testing programs should be strongly encouraged. In addition to enabling better counseling in regard to infant feeding, voluntary testing could improve counseling about contraception and safer sexual practices for adults and initiation of preventive treatment for HIV-infected women.
- Wherever the risks of bottle feeding are found to be less than those of breast feeding, bottle feeding should be recommended if mothers are known to be HIV-infected. To minimize the negative consequences of bottle feeding, women should also be educated about methods for decreasing child mortality from diarrhea and other infectious diseases and about contraceptive options. Given the well-documented efficacy of programs in reducing mortality from diarrheal disease,[79] educational programs would clearly benefit all children.
- Even under circumstances where bottle feeding is found to be less risky than breast feeding, bottle feeding should be recommended only to families who can afford it and have access to it. As obvious as this statement may seem, bottle feeding is too often introduced to families who lack adequate access or resources to continue the

practice. Commercial formula has been shown to take up a dramatic amount of a poor family's income,[80] without any clear evidence that it is better for the child than cheaper powdered milk.

- If and when it does become available, neonatal HIV testing will improve the ability to make sound and safe recommendations about feeding practices. If accurate neonatal HIV testing were available, maternal breast feeding could be recommended for infants found to be already infected with HIV. A retrospective study suggested that HIV-infected infants who were breast fed progressed more slowly to AIDS than did bottle-fed infants, although their rates of developing AIDS were equivalent by age 5.[81]

- Wet nursing could be confidently recommended for infant and wet nurse pairs who were both known to be HIV negative. Wet nursing is a much safer alternative to breast feeding than is bottle feeding. Given the potential risk of HIV transmission from infant to nursing woman in the presence of mouth sores and breast lesions,[82] recommendations cannot be made as confidently for infants whose infection status is unknown (as is currently always the case because of technical limitations in testing). Where a potential wet nurse has not been tested voluntarily, recommendations should depend on the probability of the wet nurse's being HIV infected and the relative risk of bottle feeding in the particular setting.

- In these recommendations, women with AIDS and those with asymptomatic HIV infection are treated alike because there are insufficient data to make separate recommendations. In the future, different recommendations may be possible that take into account varying risks for mother and child. As discussed earlier, the consequences for a mother with AIDS who is already nutritionally and immunologically compromised may prove to be significant. Postnatal transmission may prove to be as high from women with AIDS as from those mothers who are postnatally infected, yet low among asymptomatic HIV-infected women who have been infected for a long time. Alternatively, immunologic differences between early infection and late disease may prove significant and lead to different transmission rates.

Conclusions

In the vast majority of developing country settings, the benefits of breast feeding continue to outweigh the risks, even for infants of women known to be HIV infected. Although women who become HIV infected after childbirth while breast feeding may be an exception to this rule, it is rare that a woman will be discovered to have been newly infected while she is still breast feeding. The apparently higher risk of postnatal mother-to-infant transmission by women infected with HIV after delivery provides added reason for education about safer sexual and behavioral practices both during and after pregnancy which would benefit both children and parents.

In the majority of industrialized country settings—with lower child mortality rates, better sanitation, higher average income, greater access to breast milk substitutes and health care services, and consequently lower relative risk of bottle feeding—women who are known to be HIV infected should be advised that bottle feeding may present a lower risk to their infants than does breast feeding. The risks and benefits of breast feeding should also be discussed with women who are at high risk of becoming infected postnatally. Programs to prevent postnatal infection of women are as important as they are in developing country settings, for the welfare of both the mother and the child.

Although great progress has been made in understanding both the risks and the benefits of breast feeding by the HIV-infected mother, much more knowledge is needed. Although temporary recommendations must be made, recommendations that involve hundreds of thousands of lives should be based, as much as possible, on a tightly woven fabric of knowledge rather than on a net of ignorance. (See Table 15.1.)

Research on a number of central issues must be a high priority:

1. *What is the rate of HIV transmission to infants via breast feeding by HIV-infected women?* Studies in this area are sensitive but even with the cost of services necessary to conduct such a study ethically included,* the cost of such research would clearly be justified by

---

*Until a reliable neonatal test for HIV infection is available, studies will depend on comparing cohorts who are breast fed and bottle fed. To conduct such studies ethically, given the risks that accompany bottle feeding, the bottle-feeding, mother-infant control pairs in randomized trials should be given an adequate amount of formula, access to safe water, and special support services to prevent infectious or nutritional complications, as well as to treat any that occur. Such services would not alter the validity of the results as the purpose of the study would be to determine HIV transmission rates, not risk of bottle feeding.

Table 15.1: Effect of maternal infection status and feeding choices on maternal and child outcomes: Many unanswered questions

Maternal and child outcomes	HIV– mother		HIV+ mother	
	Breast feeding[a]	No breast feeding	Breast feeding[a]	No breast feeding
Risk of postnatal transmission of HIV to previously HIV– child	N/A	N/A	Increase	Decrease
Rapidity of onset of HIV disease for child born HIV+	N/A	N/A	Decrease	Increase
Risk of developing AIDS for child born HIV+	N/A	N/A	Same	Same
Morbidity and mortality from infectious diseases for HIV– child	Decrease	Increase	?	?
Nutritional status of HIV– child	Increase	Decrease	?	?
Risk of mortality for HIV– child associated with close birth spacing of siblings	Decrease	Increase	?	?
Maternal fertility	Decrease	Increase	?	?
Maternal risk of morbidity or mortality associated with large number of pregnancies	Decrease	Increase	?	?
Progression of HIV in infected mother	N/A	N/A	?	?
Nutritional status of mother	Depends on prior maternal health, nutrition, and food resources		?	?

Source: AIDS in the World, 1992.
Note: N/A = not applicable; ? = currently unknown.
a. Breast feeding by the biological mother.

the hundreds of thousands of children who are exposed to the risk of postnatal HIV transmission every year.

2. *What cofactors strongly influence that rate?* Among other factors, the amount of time since the onset of maternal HIV infection and maternal immune status should be studied. Future recommendations regarding breast feeding may vary according to stage of maternal infection and other maternal characteristics.

3. *What are the effects of different feeding options on the HIV-infected woman?* Thus far, the debate has looked only at the infant. The mother must be treated as an equally important human being, with examination of the impact of different feeding options on her health and well being.

4. *What are the effects of different feeding options on other members of the family?* In regions where the cost of bottle feeding may consume a large portion of the family income, bottle feeding can mean less money for other family members for food, schooling, health, and other expenditures. The economic impact on families in different circumstances should be considered, with concern for the health of the entire family. Where bottle feeding is necessary, it is also important to compare the costs and benefits of formula against much cheaper powdered milk.

5. *What can be done to make breast feeding and bottle feeding safer for the HIV-infected woman?* First, the nutritional, contraceptive, and other health and personal effects of different feeding methods on the mother must be understood. If conflicts between the health needs of mother and child arise, then programs need to be developed to minimize them so that the recommended feeding practice is healthy for both mother and child.

6. *Are the risks and benefits of breast feeding constant, decreasing, or increasing over time? Is colostrum more likely to transmit HIV than later milk, or vice versa?* If either the risks or benefits of breast feeding are not found to be constant over time, the optimal recommendations could involve either early breast feeding of short duration or disposal of early milk followed by late onset of breast feeding. Limiting the duration of breast feeding could be considered if the protective benefits of breast feeding decrease more rapidly than does the risk of HIV transmission via breast feeding.

7. *An effective and inexpensive means of determining an infant's HIV infection status at birth is essential.* Clearly, such a test would

make it possible to determine the rate of postnatal HIV transmission under a variety of conditions. Furthermore, if we knew which infants were HIV infected at birth, wet nursing could be recommended for HIV-negative infants and breast feeding by the mother for HIV-infected infants.

Tragically, even if adult HIV transmission stopped today, millions of unborn children would still be exposed to HIV in the years to come. At present, the mother-infant pair is one of the most vulnerable to HIV infection and to our own ignorance. With millions of women and children vulnerable over the coming decade, the time, energy, and funds must be invested both in research and services to make safer alternatives available to women and children worldwide.

■■■■■   .   .   .

PERINATAL HIV TRANSMISSION

Marc Lallemant, Normand Lapointe, Pierre M'Pelé, and Sophie Lallemant-Le Coeur

c Lallemant, M.D.,
artment of Cancer
ogy, Harvard School
ublic Health, Boston,
sachusetts, and
TOM, Paris, France;
nand Lapointe, M.D.,
de service de la
que d'immunologie,
tre Maternel et
ntile sur le SIDA,
ital Sainte-Justine,
treal, Canada; Pierre
elé, M.D., Director,
onal AIDS
gramme, Ministry of
th, Brazzaville,
go; and Sophie
emant-Le Coeur, M.D.,
artment of Cancer
ogy, Harvard School
ublic Health, and
ERM, Paris, France.

The question of whether infected mothers will give birth to infected infants has attracted enormous emotional attention in the HIV/AIDS pandemic. In addition to the moral stigmas that are sometimes associated with HIV infection, women have also had to bear another—that they, and they alone, may be held *responsible* for their children's infection.

If the emotion surrounding the issue makes it a test case of society's approach to the HIV/AIDS pandemic, the scientific challenge is no less acute. Babies do not come into this world complete with their own ready-made immune systems. They inherit some antibodies from their mothers; others they develop themselves. It takes more than a year for a child's immune system to mature, and this process is by no means uniform. Some maternal antibodies disappear more quickly than others; some of the child's own antibodies take longer to develop than do others.

Herein lies a central difficulty confronting researchers seeking to uncover how HIV passes from mother to child: how can they tell if it has passed at all? Although a reliable indicator of HIV infection in an adult, the presence of HIV antibodies provides no reliable indication about an infant's HIV status. And because newborns lack fully developed immune systems, they naturally remain at high risk of contracting—and dying from—some of the opportunistic infections normally associated with HIV, particularly during the first 15 months of life.

Matters become even more complex when the focus shifts to understanding how prevention might work. The obvious point of departure here is to establish when the infection passes from mother to child. Research indicates not just a variety of possibilities, but, indeed, a variety of actual ways and times in which the critical transmission can take place: at various times during pregnancy, during childbirth (in labor and in delivery—both natural and cesarean section); and later, through breast feeding. Prevention itself encompasses both lessening the risk of transmission and delaying the onset of HIV-related disease in the child.

Today, 10 years after the first reports of children with HIV/AIDS and despite a tremendous increase in our knowledge of HIV and AIDS, a virtually uncontrollable pandemic continues to progress. Many questions remain to be fully answered: What, precisely, is the risk of perinatal HIV transmission? What are the factors influencing this transmission? Does pregnancy affect the course of HIV infection, and conversely, does HIV influence the evolution and outcome of pregnancy? What strategies could prevent or control the perinatal transmission of HIV?

History

As early as 1982, children with AIDS were reported in North America and Europe, only a few months after AIDS had been described as a new disease in adults by the U.S. Centers for Disease Control (CDC).[83] Even though the description differed from that of genetic immune deficiencies, these reports were initially received with skepticism by the medical community, in part because these cases had been identified almost simultaneously in different geographical areas under widely differing circumstances. In San Francisco, an infant had received several blood transfusions; in New York and Newark, the majority of the cases were children born to mothers who used injection drugs; in Montreal and Miami, most of the children were of Caribbean origin.[84] Even though the virus responsible for the disease had not yet been identified, the pediatricians involved were certain that the children had been infected either by their mothers during pregnancy or through blood transfusions.[85]

The first descriptions of AIDS in Africa also met with skepticism as the cases did not belong to any known risk group. In addition, the cases could be explained by endemic infectious, parasitic, or deficiency diseases, occurring in countries where the origin of a disease is usually difficult to establish.[86] (It was later discovered that some infants born to parents originating from Zaire, Rwanda, Burundi, and Haiti had been infected by HIV as early as 1981.)

Mother-to-child HIV transmission was soon recognized as the main cause of HIV infection in children, although a few of these cases resulted from transfusions of blood or blood-related products. Subsequently, the use of contaminated medical equipment was identified as having been responsible for local HIV epidemics in Romania and the former Soviet Union.

General prevention guidelines were introduced soon after the first pediatric cases were described.[87] These guidelines included primary prevention—advice on safer sex, injection drug behavior, and tighter control of blood donations. Considered responsible for most cases of pediatric HIV infections, women were often seen as *vectors* for infections, not only to their children but also to their male sexual partners. Programs aimed at women with multiple sexual partners, commercial sex workers, and female injection drug users nearly always stigmatized their behavior, even though in most cases, these women had been infected by their habitual sexual partner. Finally, despite the absence of clear data, seropositive women were told that pregnancy would accelerate their progression toward AIDS and were encouraged to accept abortion or even sterilization.

The Present Situation

According to the most recent data, the average HIV prevalence in women in sub-Saharan Africa is approximately 25 per thousand (or 2.5 percent), which is 35 times the prevalence rate in western European countries and 18 times the rate in the United States.[88] *AIDS in the World*'s best estimates indicate that in 1992, 4.7 million women worldwide will have been infected. Eighty-three percent of these women, totaling more than 3.9 million, will be in sub-Saharan Africa. AIDS cases in women number more than half a million, and AIDS has become the leading cause of death among women aged 20 to 40 in major sub-Saharan African, western European, and American cities.

A great deal of knowledge about vertical (mother-to-child) HIV transmission must be acquired to reduce pediatric HIV infections. It is known that only a given number of HIV-infected women will transmit the virus to their children, although little knowledge exists about the risks, the influencing factors involved, and the precise mechanisms of this transmission.

In fact, the primary difficulty is diagnosing HIV infection itself in infants born to HIV-infected mothers. Anti-HIV antibodies are transferred by a mother to her fetus and may still be detected for months after birth, even though the infant is not actually infected.

Box 15.1: HIV Infection in Infants Still a Difficult Diagnosis

Three factors complicate diagnosis of HIV infection in newborns and infants with seropositive mothers:

- First, the seropositive mother will pass certain types of anti-HIV antibodies to the fetus. Some of these will persist well into the child's second year of life, making serological diagnosis difficult before the age of 15 to 18 months even if the infant is uninfected;
- Second, a relatively high proportion of HIV-infected infants present few or no symptoms during their first year of life; and
- Third, during the first 15 months of life, children face a high incidence of diseases (pneumonia, enteritis, malnutrition) that are difficult to differentiate clinically from HIV infection. This is especially true in tropical countries where many HIV-infected children may die before reaching health care facilities where

diagnosis could have been established.[a]

Diagnosis of mother-to-child HIV transmission in newborns, infants, and young children rests, therefore, on a combination of the following epidemiological, clinical, and biological elements, which are seldom all available in developing countries:

1. *Indirect evidence* includes maternal seropositivity; symptoms in the child that are compatible with pediatric HIV infection; and immune system perturbations, such as reduction of the CD4 count and CD4/CD8 ratio and increase of immunoglobulins or a rise in beta-2 microglobulin. These are indicators of HIV infection in children, but they are often moderately altered during the first months of life.[b]

2. *Antibody evidence.* The immune system produces three types of antibody to HIV: immunoglobulins A (IgA), G (IgG), and M (IgM). All three have different characteristics.

IgG is the only one that crosses the

Conversely, infants may die from HIV-related disease before being diagnosed (Box 15.1).

Risks of HIV Mother-to-Child Transmission

A number of studies have attempted to evaluate the risks of mother-to-child transmission.[89] But it is not easy to draw general conclusions from them, both because HIV is difficult to diagnose in infants and because the studies were designed in different ways. A general difficulty is that exposed children must be immediately enrolled in a prospective study no later than on the first day of life.

At present, six U.S. studies have been published, showing mother-to-infant transmission rates ranging from 7 to 42 percent; a study in

---

placenta, so testing must wait until the child is around 18 months old, by which time the mother's antibodies will have disappeared and the child's own antibodies can be detected. IgM antibodies are the first to appear in response to HIV; as they do not cross the placenta, they do indicate that the infant is infected. However, they appear for only a few weeks after initial infection and are almost always missed by visual diagnostic procedures;[c] IgA antibodies, which follow IgM, do not cross the placenta either and remain permanent. They can also be detected in a relatively specific and sensitive way in HIV-infected infants—but, with current technology, not before around the sixth month of life.[d]

One new technique relies not on testing the blood serum itself, but on culturing the cells that produce the antibodies. Though sensitive and specific, in vitro anti-HIV antibody production (IVAP and Elispot) is useful only after the sixth month of life.[e]

3. *Direct evidence.* This is obtained

by finding the virus itself in any one of three ways. The first, viral culture, is costly, time consuming (up to two months), and requires laboratories with highly advanced technology. This method also lacks sensitivity during the first few weeks of life.[f] The second, known as P24 antigenemia, detects a specific fragment of the virus. The test can be performed simply with commercially available kits, and although it provides direct proof of viral presence, it is, unfortunately, not a sensitive test in the newborn (although a positive result is generally indicative of a poor prognosis).[g]

Finally, there is a polymerase chain reaction (PCR), which can take a small snippet of viral DNA that has been incorporated in the host's genome and multiply it until it becomes easily identifiable. This test is still mainly used in research. Several studies have shown that results from PCR testing correlate well both with results from viral culturing and with clinical indicators of infection.[h]

A slightly modified technique using

Montreal, Canada, showed a rate of 34 percent; another in Haiti found a rate of 24 percent. (See Table 15.2.)

Four European studies found mother-to-infant transmission rates of 33 percent in Italy, 27 percent in France, and 7 percent in Spain. The collaborative European survey, carried out in 8 countries, reported a transmission rate of 24 percent in 100 children 2 years ago; more recently, this ongoing study reported a rate of 12.9 percent in a total of 372 children. The latest analysis of the French study uncovered a similar trend, with a transmission rate now estimated at below 20 percent.

Studies in African countries have generally found higher rates of transmission, from 25 percent in the Central African Republic to more

---

blood collected on blotting paper (DBS-PCR) seems to enhance PCR sensitivity.[i] Because it requires very small quantities of blood that can be easily collected, this technique could be especially valuable in developing countries.

a. M. Lallemant, S. Lallemant-Le Coeur, D. Cheynier, et al., "Mother-child transmission of HIV and infant survival in Brazzaville, Congo," *AIDS* 3 (1989):643–46.

b. S. Blanche, C. Rouzioux, M. L. Guihard Moscato, et al., "A prospective study of infants born to women seropositive for human immunodeficiency virus type 1," *New England Journal of Medicine* 320 (1989):1643–48; M. C. Garcia Rodriguez, F. Omenaca, A. Ferreira, et al., "Immunological followup in children born to HIV-1 infected mothers," *Acta Paediatrica Scandinavica* 80 (1991):1183–91.

c. C. Gaetano, G. Scano, M. Carconari, et al., "Delayed and defective anti-HIV IgM response in infants," *Lancet* 1 (1987):631; M. Fauvel, J. Lecompte, J. Samson, et al., "Investigation of radioimmunoprecipitation assay for the detection of IgM specific HIV antibody," *Canadian Journal of Infectious Diseases* (in press).

d. B. J. Weiblen, E. R. Coper, S. H. Landesman, et al., "Early diagnosis of HIV infection in infants by detection of IgA HIV antibodies," *Lancet* 335 (1990):988–90.

e. A. Amadori, A. De Rossi, C. Giaquinto, et al., "In vitro production of HIV-specific antibody in children at risk of AIDS," *Lancet* 1 (1988):852–54; A. De Rossi, A. Amadori, L. Chiedo-Bianci, et al., "Polymerase chain reaction and in-vitro antibody production for early diagnosis of paediatric HIV infection," *Lancet* 2 (1988):278.

f. A. Alimenti, K. Luzuriaga, B. Stechenberg, and J. L. Sullivan, "Quantitation of human immunodeficiency virus in vertically infected infants and children," *Journal of Pediatrics* 119 (1991):225–29.

g. M. Ellaurie and A. Rubinstein, "Correlation of serum antigen and antibody concentration with clinical features in HIV infection," *Archives of Diseases in Children* 66 (1991):200–03.

h. M. F. Rogers, C. Y. Ou, M. Rayfield, et al., "Use of the polymerase chain reaction for early detection of the proviral sequences of human immunodeficiency virus in infants born to seropositive mothers," *New England Journal of Medicine* 320 (1989):1649–54; P. S. Weintrub, P. P. Ulrich, J. R. Edwards, et al., "Use of polymerase chain for the early detection of HIV infection in the infants of HIV-seropositive women," *AIDS* 5 (1991):881–84; F. Laure, V. Courgnaud, C. Rouzioux, et al., "Detection of HIV-1 DNA in infants and children by means of the polymerase chain reaction," *Lancet* 2 (1988):538–41.

i. S. Cassol, T. Salas, M. Arella, et al., "Use of dried blood spots in the detection of HIV-1 by the polymerase chain reaction (PCR)," *Journal of Clinical Microbiology*, April 1991:667–71; S. Cassol, N. Lapointe, T. Salas, et al., "Diagnosis of vertical HIV-1 transmission using the polymerase chain reaction and dried blood spot specimens," *Journal of Acquired Immune Deficiency Syndromes* 5 (2)(1992):13–19.

Table 15.2: Examples of cohort studies on mother-to-child transmission, 1986–1992

Country	Period of study	Number in study	Rate of trans- mission (%)	Reference
Zaire (Kinshasa)	1986–1990	92	39%	Ryder et al.
Congo (Brazzaville)	1987 to present	118	42%	Lallemant et al.
Rwanda (Kigali)	1989 to present	218	30%	Lepage et al.
Zambia (Lusaka)		205 (109 followed up to 24 months)	39%	Hira et al.
Kenya (Nairobi)		361 (79 followed up to 15 months)	39%	Datta et al.
Central African Republic (Bangui)	1988–89	139	23%	Bouquety et al.
United States (New Haven)		62	26%	Andinam et al.
United States (Miami)		82	30%	Hutto et al.
United States (New York)		33	21%	Mayers et al.
Haiti (Cité Soleil)		230	24%	Halsey et al.
France	1987 to present	117	27%	Blanche et al.
Europe	1987 to present	372	13%	European coll. study
Spain (Madrid)	1989	87	7%	Garcia Rodriguez et al.

Sources: Spain: M. C. Garcia Rodriguez, F. Omenaca, A. Ferreira, et al., "Immunological followup in children born to HIV-1 infected mothers," *Acta Paediatrica Scandinavica* 80 (1991):1183-91; all other references: see Chapter 15, note 89.

Note: These examples show the wide diversity in the rates of transmission found in cohort studies, possibly in part as a result of study design (time of inclusion, followup, and definitions of HIV infection) or differences in populations.

than 40 percent in Congo. These results must be compared with caution: the inclusion criteria varied from one study to another; the number of people who dropped out of the studies was sometimes high; and HIV diagnosis in newborns was not always based on the same clinical or biological criteria.

Little is known about perinatal transmission of HIV-2, the other retrovirus responsible for AIDS, found mainly in West Africa. Mother-to-child transmission of this virus seems to occur less frequently than in the case of HIV-1. Of 25 infants born to HIV-2-infected mothers in France, none were infected,[90] in the Ivory Coast, of 34 infants born to infected mothers, only 1 was infected.[91]

The Elusive Moment for Perinatal Transmission

It is essential to know the timing of mother-to-child HIV transmission during pregnancy and/or during the first months of life in order to implement effective preventive measures.[92] Experience with other viruses indicates a range of possibilities: rubella virus, for example, may be transmitted across the placenta, but only in the early stages of pregnancy; hepatitis B virus is transmitted mainly during birth; HTLV-1 (another human retrovirus) is transmitted through breast feeding in the first few months of life.

We now know that fetuses can be infected with HIV as early as 8 weeks after conception.[93] By then, they already have the receptors that enable HIV to penetrate their T cells. However, HIV transmission also seems to occur at a later stage in pregnancy, as indicated by both the absence of clinical signs of infection in the newborn[94] and the low numbers of viruses in the blood, which, therefore, creates difficulties in detection by polymerase chain reaction (PCR) or viral culture.[95]

Some children not infected during pregnancy probably become infected during birth. This is further suggested by results in studies of twin pregnancies.[96] The rate of discordant twins (one infected, the other not) was reported to be slightly lower when the twins are identical. It was further suggested that the first twin to be born is significantly more likely to be infected than is the second, whether the birth is natural or by cesarean section. This suggests that fetuses are infected either at a late stage of pregnancy or during birth itself.

Why should this be? One explanation could be that the first child is subjected to a longer—and thus more stressful—labor than is the second. Furthermore, recent analysis of the collaborative European study has shown that children who were delivered by cesarean section were less likely to become infected than were children who were delivered naturally.[97]

Although HIV has been identified in breast milk, it is difficult to ascertain the risk of HIV transmission by breast feeding in a child who was exposed to the virus during pregnancy and parturition. The first suggestion of this mode of transmission was in 1985 in a child whose only source of exposure to HIV was the breast milk of his mother who had contracted the virus after a blood transfusion following delivery.[98] Since then, other cases have been reported.[99]

There have been several cases of apparent postnatal HIV transmission in children whose mothers seroconverted after delivery.[100] In a study in Kigali, Rwanda, half of the women documented as seronegative at the time of delivery but seroconverted after delivery apparently transmitted HIV to their newborns. If cases where mothers who seroconverted within 3 months after delivery were set aside because they might have transmitted the virus to their fetuses during pregnancy, the postnatal mother-to-infant transmission rate would be estimated to be 36 percent.[101]

However, these two situations (infection of the mother through blood transfusion or heterosexual intercourse following delivery) are very specific, and the results cannot be applied to the rest of breast-feeding seropositive mothers. In fact, these children were breast-fed by women who were in the process of seroconverting, and therefore, had particularly high levels of viral activity. At this time, their children had no passively transmitted immunity (through breast milk or blood) that could have prevented transmission by HIV.[102] Breast-feeding seronegative women, therefore, need to be offered advice on avoiding infection, especially in high-incidence areas.

Even though we now know that mother-to-child transmission can occur during pregnancy, delivery, or after birth, the precise mechanisms of such transmission remain to be established. Further, children infected at an early stage may have the bleakest prognosis and may die during their first year. If true, this could explain the phenomenon, seen in industrialized countries and in Africa, of some HIV-infected infants developing AIDS and dying very rapidly, whereas others live much longer with a no less persistent, but less aggressive, disease.[103]

Other Factors Associated with Perinatal Transmission

The quantification of individual risks of mother-to-child HIV transmission during pregnancy may have significant impact on treatment and may help guide appropriate counseling, and assist expectant mothers to decide on the course of pregnancy. The different factors that appear to influence transmission are the characteristics of the mother's infection (her clinical or immune status during pregnancy, and her immune response to the virus), the placental barrier, the virus itself, and the child's clinical status during exposure to HIV.

Some prospective studies have monitored women during successive pregnancies. These studies have identified women with *high-transmission* and women with *low-transmission* status. For example, in a study from Kinshasa, Zaire, women who have already transmitted HIV to their children have a 50 percent risk of transmitting HIV during the next pregnancy, compared to a 10 percent risk in women who had not transmitted HIV during the first pregnancy.[104]

A number of mechanisms may help explain this phenomenon. The first is the stage of HIV infection in the mother. Several studies show an increased risk of mother-to-child HIV transmission when the mother's infection is already advanced or when it occurs during pregnancy or postpartum.[105] The second is the mother's immune status, which closely reflects the clinical stage of the disease. A study in Kinshasa, Zaire, supported by others, found close correlation between the CD4 count and perinatal transmission risks: the lower the CD4 count (and accordingly, the weaker the immune system), the higher the risk of transmission.[106] If CD4 counts were carried out widely on women in Africa, they would provide a more reliable way of evaluating the mother-to-child transmission risks and facilitate comparison with studies in industrialized countries. Studies from different groups show that the highest transmission risks are associated with the highest viral activity.[107]

In 1989, several teams reported that the presence of neutralizing antibodies in pregnant women was correlated with the absence of mother-to-child HIV transmission.[108] The protective nature of these antibodies has been the subject of great controversy, as this suggested not only that transmission could be predicted but also that preventive measures could be developed. For example, if these antibodies could be isolated, their administration in pregnant women or in children at birth could help prevent transmission in a manner similar to experience with the hepatitis B virus. Unfortunately, most studies have failed to confirm these results.[109]

Studies are presently being carried out on the relationship between perinatal transmission of HIV and the presence of antibodies directed against other areas of viral proteins. These studies are also investigating the link between HIV transmission and the antibody-dependent cytotoxicity (ADCC) as well as cytotoxic T-cell lymphocytes (CTL). Above all, these studies underline the need for a better understanding of the moment and the mechanisms of HIV transmission (cell-free or cell-associated viruses, for example).

The integrity of the placental barrier is a key part of the hypothesis that mother-to-child HIV transmission occurs when free viruses cross the placenta. Sexually transmitted diseases (STDs), malaria, or other viral infections, may provoke chorio-amniotitis—lesions in the amniotic sac—that may, in turn, make the placenta more permeable to HIV. This concept is supported by a study from Kinshasa, Zaire, in which transmission rates were twice as high in HIV-infected women with chorio-amniotitis compared to other seropositive women (39 percent as opposed to 15 percent).[110] Infections of the placenta may be more frequent in Africa than in Europe or North America and may provide an explanation for the particularly high transmission rates found in Africa. Of greater pertinence, perhaps, is that due to a greater frequency of pregnancy and less access to contraception seropositive women in Africa are more likely than women elsewhere to have babies at a more advanced stage of infection.

Viral strains differ greatly, suggesting that some strains may be more easily transmitted. A recent study showed that transmitted strains could undergo selection. Rare viral strains in the mothers were the strains most commonly found in their infected children.[111] The speed at which cultured HIV strains replicate may also be associated with a greater or lesser degree of transmission. In fact, HIV-1 and HIV-2 are closely related retroviruses that behave very differently.

Finally, it is reasonable to ask whether the general condition of the fetus or the newborn makes it more or less vulnerable to HIV. At the moment, there is very little evidence either way. Only one study showed an association between prematurity and increased risk of prenatal transmission, but prematurity may be a consequence of HIV infection, not a cause.

Limited Effects of Pregnancy on the Natural Course of HIV Infection in Women

In 1987, a retrospective study on the evolution of pregnancy in HIV-seropositive women who gave birth to children infected with HIV found that disease progression over a period of 2 1/2 years was significantly higher than expected. But this is not as strange as it might seem, because they were most often identified retrospectively, through their infected children. Furthermore, women who have delivered an HIV-infected infant represent a special group and are not typical of all HIV-infected pregnant women. The same bias could also explain similar results from retrospective studies.

Prospective studies, following women over time, have yielded conflicting results. For example, one study noted that in the case of HIV-infected women, the normal lowering of the immune response during pregnancy was not followed by the usual rise after delivery. On the other hand, prospective studies in New York and France found that women who carried their pregnancy to term, women who aborted, and women who were not pregnant progressed to AIDS at the same rate.[112]

A Complication-Free Pregnancy, Provided It Is Closely Monitored

Studies from industrialized countries are contradictory, partly due to added risk factors that may affect the course of pregnancy and its outcome, for example injection drug use. Equally, results obtained from African studies, in which drug injection was not a factor, may be applicable in the developing world but not in countries where pregnant women are less likely to suffer from infections, parasites, or malnutrition.

A study in Kenya showed a high correlation between HIV serostatus in women and occurrence of miscarriage and stillbirth. Syphilis was the only other STD in this study associated with a failure to carry to term.[113] A study in Malawi showed that among women who had several previous pregnancies, miscarriages were linked to HIV infection, independent of past history of STDs.[114] A similar result was reported in Kigali, Rwanda.[115] One problem with these studies, however, is that they were carried out on a case-control basis: the search for HIV infection began only after the problem in pregnancy, so that a causal relationship between HIV and poor pregnancy outcome could not be established. Prospective studies could confirm these results. However, these studies are particularly difficult to carry out, as women must be included in the study at a very early stage of pregnancy. To date, it appears that the influence of HIV infection on the course of pregnancy is small.

Education, Information, and Counseling

In the absence of any clinical method, prevention of mother-to-child transmission has to depend on education. This must cover behavior in teenagers before they become sexually active, the use of condoms in discordant couples, voluntary testing and counseling before or during pregnancy, and systematic screening during pregnancy and delivery.

In the field of voluntary antenatal HIV testing and counseling, it has become increasingly clear that couples facing the reality of HIV infection may react contrary to what guidelines advocate. Although approximately 30 percent of children born to seropositive mothers are likely to be infected, this fact does not necessarily lead women to consider contraception or abortion. The issue of contraception and abortion often arises when fetal genetic anomaly is suspected. But HIV further complicates the dilemma because one or both of the parents may die prematurely.[116] In the United States, women using injection drugs were studied during rehabilitation programs. It appeared that knowledge of serostatus seldom influenced decisions about whether to continue pregnancies. Some women chose to continue their pregnancy, even though they had sought abortion during a previous pregnancy and now knew that they were HIV seropositive.[117] Similar observations were made in Africa, in a completely different cultural environment.[118]

Attitudes toward antenatal screening and counseling have evolved considerably. At first, women/mothers were seen only as transmitting a deadly virus to their innocent child. Studies in high-risk groups and similar social and behavioral research have helped to show that the mother and father are as much victims of the disease as the child itself. Decisions about contraception are very complex; childbirth is not an isolated event but rather occurs within a specific emotional, social, and cultural framework. New issues raised by HIV infection will have to be answered, and decisions will have to be made concerning the future of the child, the mother, the couple, and the family within this particular framework.

Declaration of seropositivity may jeopardize not only a woman's health, but also her place in society. Her role, that of her spouse, and those of the grandparents and the other children may be deeply altered. The real issues in counseling are the right to information and time to understand and plan for the future.[119] Counseling involves certain fundamental ethical principles, including the need to respect the individual's right to autonomy. Unfortunately, prenatal screening and counseling do not always take place under sufficiently good conditions. Health personnel, faced with a deep feeling of powerlessness themselves, may be tempted not to address the critical issues.

If testing is involuntary, counseling hardly stands a chance of success. Women may understandably question the confidentiality of the procedure or feel that the final responsibility for the decision is not their own. Often, they do not feel sure of benefiting from medical care during and after pregnancy. They may fear that their child will be taken away from them (in some countries, half the children born to mothers who use injection drugs are given up for adoption). These

---

Box 15.2: Drugs to Combat AIDS in Adults and Children

Early treatment by AZT or ddI lowers the risk of progression toward symptomatic HIV infection.[a] Preliminary studies are being conducted on ddI and ddC in single-agent therapy or in association with other drugs.

Prophylaxis against opportunistic infections is a new element in AIDS care. The incidence of pneumocystis pneumonia may be significantly reduced by oral drug therapy.[b] Mortality due to pneumocystis pneumonia is so high during the first year of life that prophylaxis is clearly beneficial.[c] Similarly, monthly administration of immunoglobulins effectively reduces the risk of bacterial infection in children without symptoms of HIV-related disease.[d] There is a growing trend toward tuberculosis prophylaxis, which is known to be effective.[e]

Published data on treating children infected with HIV at birth are still limited. Weight gain, decreased lymph node and liver size, and increased CD4 cell counts have been generally reported together with limited bone marrow toxicity. Remarkably, several studies have shown that AZT significantly improved intellectual and motor-skill development in children

are among the reasons that some women, suspecting or knowing that they are infected by HIV, only seek medical examination at the very last minute, when they know that it is too late for a safe and legal abortion.

Preventing Mother-to-Child HIV Transmission

Whether or not the transmission of HIV can be completely prevented in pregnancy, one thing is clear: it is not easily transmitted. Therefore, it seems logical that one could attempt to lessen the risk by intervening during pregnancy, at birth, or during the first few months of the child's life. And, indeed, it should soon be possible for pregnant women to consider several possibilities, including participation in therapeutic trials. Several trials involving drug dosage, mode of administration, toxicity, tolerance, and efficacy are currently entering their initial phase (Box 15.2).

The goals are to prevent mother-to-child transmission of HIV and to treat perinatally infected children as early as possible. However, it takes years for experimental drugs to be tested before they are approved and used in therapy, and until recently, a drug was seldom given to children before it had been successfully tested in adults. For example, Zidovudine had been approved for the experimental treat-

with AIDS or AIDS-related complex. (See Box 15.3.)

a. R. E. McKinney, P. A. Pizzo, G. B. Scott, et al., "Safety and tolerance of intermittent intravenous and oral zidovudine therapy in human immunodeficiency virus infected pediatric patients: A phase 1 study," *Journal of Pediatrics* 116 (1990):641–47; K. M. Butler, R. M. Husson, F. M. Balis, et al., "Dideoxyinosine in children with symptomatic human immunodeficiency virus infection," *New England Journal of Medicine* 324 (1991):137–44.
b. Centers for Disease Control, "Guidelines for prophylaxis against *Pneumocystis carinii* pneumonia for persons infected with human immunodeficiency virus," *Morbidity and Mortality Weekly Report* 38 Suppl. (5) (1989):1–9.
c. P. A. Pizzo, K. Butler, F. Balis, et al., "Dideoxycytidine alone and in an alternating schedule with zidovudine in children with symptomatic human immunodeficiency virus

infection," *Journal of Pediatrics* 117 (5) (1990):799–808; Centers for Disease Control, "Guidelines for prophylaxis against *Pneumocystis carinii* pneumonia for children infected with human immunodeficiency virus," *Morbidity and Mortality Weekly Report* 40(RR-2) (1991):1–13.
d. National Institute of Child Health and Human Development, Intravenous Immunoglobulin Study Group, "Intravenous immune globulin for the prevention of bacterial infections in children with symptomatic human immunodeficiency virus infection," *New England Journal of Medicine* 325 (2) (1991):73–80.
e. P. A. Selwyn, D. Hartel, V. A. Lewis, et al., "A prospective study of the risk of tuberculosis among intravenous drug users with human immunodeficiency virus infection," *New England Journal of Medicine* 320 (1989):545–50; Centers for Disease Control, "The use of preventive therapy for tuberculosis infection in the United States," *Morbidity and Mortality Weekly Report* 39 (1990):9–12.

ment of adult AIDS care two years prior to approval for use in children (Box 15.3). In contrast, ddI was approved in only a few months.

Treatment of asymptomatic children, especially newborns, raises other issues. As discussed earlier, there are difficulties associated with diagnosis in the newborn. Special consideration must therefore be given to the dilemma of the advantages of treating infected children early, set against the dangers of toxic chemotherapy to HIV-free children, should they be treated. This gives particular importance to early diagnosis and identification of the exact moment of mother-to-child HIV transmission.

Therapeutic trials that compare drugs such as AZT known to be effective with placebos raise extremely complex ethical problems. Additionally, the efficacy of these drugs together with their toxicity

---

Box 15.3: Bantsimba's Story

Bantsimba, a 5-year-old girl of African origin, was diagnosed in Montreal as being infected with HIV. Her general condition was satisfactory, and she met all criteria to benefit from zidovudine. Her pleasant disposition and cooperation allowed detailed continuous assessment of her psychological and motor-skill development (McCarthy scale). During the first evaluation, her overall score was 65 and her verbal, quantitative, and motor-skill score was 32, or more than two standard-deviations below average. Her perceptual score was even lower. She could distinguish neither colors nor shapes, and her drawings were immature. She could not correctly name the parts of her body. The child's mother had a secondary education, took very good care of her daughter, and had no major health or financial problems, despite the fact that she was raising her child alone. She monitored her daughter's progress closely and gave the child her medication regularly.

Within a few months after starting zidovudine treatment, Bantsimba's condition improved noticeably. She entered kindergarten, was well accepted by her classmates, and did not fall behind. On reevaluation, her performance had greatly improved. Her overall score was now 83, her verbal score was 40, and her quantitative score was 39, which was only one standard deviation below the average. Her perceptual score had improved by 20 points. The child's drawings had greatly matured, and she was now able to distinguish shapes and colors.

One is reminded of this child's fragility when, after three months of follow-up, she returned to the hospital with acute pneumonia. Her condition deteriorated so quickly that her life was threatened, but she overcame this challenge. She becomes even better integrated in her surroundings with each passing day.

and side effects during treatment of asymptomatic infants and newborns might be virtually impossible to evaluate without a control group. This is especially true if preventive steps using toxic drugs (e.g., zidovudine) were to be taken during pregnancy.

However, a number of preliminary studies aimed at assessing the appropriate dosage and approximate toxicity of several drugs are under way or completed. One trial looked at the toxicity and the pharmacological dynamics of genetically engineered CD4-immunoglobulin G used in HIV-positive women during their third trimester of pregnancy (GENETEC, ACTG 146). Another is evaluating zidovudine use in women in labor and in the newborn (ACTG 082), including trials on the effectiveness of zidovudine in preventing transmission when given to both the mother from the seventh month of pregnancy and the infant until 6 weeks (ACTG 076). Finally, there is a study evaluating the passive immunization of pregnant women by administering immunoglobulins.[120]

In certain countries, the United States, for example, women have only recently become eligible to participate in experimental therapeutic protocols. Recognizing the importance and specificity of AIDS in women has also been a lengthy process. Despite the hopes generated by these therapeutic approaches, the central issues in preventing transmission are closely tied to a woman's role and status in society: her ability to protect herself from infection, her access to treatment, and her control over her own fertility. The rights and prerogatives of HIV-infected women, their children, or their partners receive scant respect throughout the world. Has the time come when entire societies are capable of mobilizing over a cause on which their survival depends?

■ ■ ■ . . .

DOES MALE CIRCUMCISION PREVENT HIV INFECTION?

Rachel Royce

It is very difficult to be certain about the circumcision-HIV relationship, and the translation from epidemiological studies to programs for HIV prevention is not a simple process. How much research or of what quality and extent are required before intervention studies are warranted? Despite provocative data suggesting an increased risk of

HIV or STD acquisition among uncircumcised men, there has been a distinct lack of enthusiasm for even small pilot studies of male circumcision as a prevention strategy.

—The Editors

Dr. Rachel Royce is a research fellow in the Department of Biostatistics at the Harvard School of Public Health, Boston, Massachusetts.

Since the late 1800s, it has been repeatedly reported that men with sexually transmitted diseases (STDs) are more likely to be uncircumcised than are men without STDs. Modern investigators have reported that uncircumcised men were more likely than circumcised men to be infected with gonorrhea or syphilis, less likely to have genital warts, and equally likely to have herpes virus infections.[121]

Recently, several investigators reported that uncircumcised men may be more susceptible to HIV infection than are circumcised men. At least one researcher believes the evidence may be compelling enough to warrant considering circumcision for HIV prevention among men at high risk.[122] Yet given the costs, potential risks, and sociocultural issues involved, it is extremely important to review and interpret the evidence regarding circumcision and HIV infection and to consider some of the problems faced by investigators of this issue.

Table 15.3 summarizes the published articles and abstracts on circumcision and HIV infection obtained through (1) Medline search of the medical literature from 1981 through 1991; (2) review of the bibliographies of all articles obtained; and (3) review of abstracts from the III through the VII International Conference on AIDS. Of the 12 published papers, 9 used a cross-sectional design, 2 were ecological studies, and 1 was prospective.

Ecological Studies

Two ecological studies have used ethnographic data on circumcision practices in Africa and correlated these practices with HIV seroprevalence data.[123] Both studies provide evidence for an association between increased HIV prevalence and lack of circumcision. A serious flaw of these studies, however, is that the seroprevalence data is measured in each capitol city or in other specific locations, but the prevalence of circumcision is determined for the country as a whole. The results of these studies are provocative but problematic because the correlation was determined on a population level, and it is unknown if the correlation exists for individuals in the population.

Table 15.3: The association of male circumcision and HIV infection in published studies

Country	Year	Population	Methods	Association (p-value, 95% CI)	Reference
Cross-sectional design					
Rwanda	1988	Kigali hospital-based partner study, woman index (n = 150 couples)	Comparing concordant HIV positive couples to concordant HIV negative couples. Overall Relative Prevalence	1.1 (p = .64)	Carael et al.
Kenya	1988	Nairobi STD clinic, male attenders with GUD (n = 115)	Overall Relative Prevalence (RP)	1.7 (p = .01)	Greenblatt et al.
			Adjusted for GUD, number of sexual partners, ethnic identity, and several other potential confounders.	NA (p > .05)	
Kenya	1988	Nairobi STD clinic, male attenders with prostitute contact (n = 340)	Overall Relative Prevalence	2.4 (1.3–4.3)	Simonsen et al.
			Adjusted for travel, prostitute contact: No history of GUD. Odds Ratio	5.2 (1.6–18.8)	
			History of GUD Odds Ratio	8.2 (2.2–30.0)	
Zambia	1990	Lusaka STD clinic, male attenders (n = 610)	Matched on age and lifetime number of sexual partners. Overall Relative Prevalence	1.4 (p = .04)(.9–2.2)	Hira et al.
Rwanda	1991	Kigali prenatal/pediatric clinic women attenders (n = 1,458)	Indirect measurement of circumcision in male partner		Allen et al.
			Overall Relative Prevalence	1.1 (p = .45)	
			Among Muslim women Relative Prevalence	2.7 (p = .002)	

Table 15.3 (cont.): The association of male circumcision and HIV infection in published studies

Country	Year	Population	Methods	Association (p-value, 95% CI)	Reference
Prospective design					
Kenya	1989	Nairobi STD clinic, HIV seronegative male attenders with prostitute contact (n = 293)	Overall Relative Cumulative Incidence Adjusted for presenting GUD, prostitute contact more than once. Odds Ratio	8.1 (p < .001) 8.2 (3.0–23.0)	Cameron et al.
Ecologic design					
Africa	1989	U.S. Census Bureau and ethnographic data from 37 countries.	Linear regression correlation coefficient	.90 (< .001)	Bongaarts et al.
Africa	1990	U.S. Census Bureau and ethnographic data from 41 countries	Graphing methods. 5 countries ratio of HIV seroprevalence according to circum-cision prevalence.	NA (< .01)	Moses et al.
Published abstracts					
United States	1987	Miami partner study. Origin of index cases unstated (n = 92 couples)	Comparing concor-dant couples with all discordant couples. Odds Ratio	9.6 (< .04)	Fischl et al.
Kenya	1990	Nairobi partner study of HIV positive STD attenders and partners (n = 90 couples)	Comparing concordant couples with all discordant couples. Relative Prevalence	1.6 (p = .08)	Moss et al.
United States	1989	New York City STD clinic attenders (n = 1,726)	Adjusted for race, number of partners, presenting STD, and other factors. Odds Ratio	NA (p > .05)	Surick et al.

Table 15.3 (cont.): The association of male circumcision and HIV infection in published studies

Country	Year	Population	Methods	Association (p-value, 95% CI)	Reference
Kenya	1990	Nairobi family planning clinic women attenders (n = 726)	Indirect measurement of circumcision in male partner. Adjusted for woman's age at first intercourse, her lifetime number of partners, her history of STDs and transfusions. Odds Ratio	3.7[a] (1.5–9.0)	Hunter et al.
Uganda	1991	Mulago partner study, STD clinic attenders (n = 132 couples)	Comparing concordant couples with discordant couples with man HIV seronegative. Odds Ratio	5.4 (1.1–27.0[b])	Hellman et al.

Note: CI = confidence interval; GUD = genital ulcer disease; NA = data not available.

a. Measuring the association of male circumcision with female HIV infection status also evaluates transmission to women according to male circumcision status. Assumes only one primary male partner.

b. Upper bound of the 957. CI is corrected. Originally, it is listed as 2.7, which is smaller than the Odds Ratio point estimate.

Sources: M. Carael, P. H. Van de Perre, P. H. Lepage, et al., "Human immunodeficiency virus transmission among heterosexual couples in Central Africa," *AIDS* 2 (1988):201–05; R. M. Greenblatt, S. A. Lukehart, F. A. Plummer, et al., "Genital ulceration as a risk factor for human immunodeficiency virus infection," *AIDS* 2 (1988):47–50; J. N. Simonsen, D. W. Cameron, M. N. Gakinya, et al., "Human immunodeficiency virus infection in men with sexually transmitted diseases," *New England Journal of Medicine* 319 (1988):274–78; S. K. Hira, H. Kamanga, R. Macuacua, et al., "Genital ulcers and male circumcision as risk factors for acquiring HIV-1 in Zambia" (letter), *Journal of Infectious Diseases* 3 (1990):584–85; S. Allen, C. Lindan, A. Srufilira, et al., "Human immunodeficiency virus infection in urban Rwanda: Demographic and behavioral correlates in a representative sample of childbearing women," *Journal of the American Medical Association* 266 (1991): 1657–63; W. D. Cameron, N. J. Simonsen, L. J. D'Costa, et al., "Female to male transmission of human immunodeficiency virus type 1: Risk factors for seroconversion in men," *Lancet* 2 (1989):403–07; J. Bongaarts, P. Reining, P. Way, and F. Conant, "The relationship between male circumcision and HIV infection in African populations," *AIDS* 3 (1989): 373–77; S. Moses, J. E. Gradley, N. J. D. Nagelkerke, et al., "Geographical patterns of male circumcision practices in Africa: Association with HIV seroprevalence," *International Journal of Epidemiology* 19 (1990):693–97; M. A. Fischl, T. Fayne, S. Flanagan, et al., Seroprevalence and risks of HIV infections in spouses of persons infected with HIV, presented at the IV International Conference on AIDS, Stockholm, Sweden, June 1988; G. B. Moss, L. J. D'Costa, F. A. Plummer, et al., HIV transmission in stable sexual partnerships in Kenya, presented at the VI International Conference on AIDS, Montreal, Canada, June 1989; I. Surick, M. McLaughlin, and M. Chiasson, HIV infection and circumcision status, ibid; D. Hunter, N. Maggwa, J. Mati, et al, Risk factors for HIV transmission in women attending family planning clinics in Nairobi, presented at the VI International Conference on AIDS, San Francisco, June 1990. N. S. Hellmann, S. D. Desmond-Hellmann, P. Nsubuga, et al., Risk factors for HIV infection among Ugandan couples, presented at the VII International Conference on AIDS, Florence, Italy, June 1991.

Cross-Sectional Studies

Five of 9 cross-sectional studies found a significant negative association between circumcision and HIV infection. For example, in an analysis of men with an STD who came to the Nairobi STD clinic following recent contact with female sex workers, circumcised men were less likely to have an HIV infection than were uncircumcised men.[124] Among men with a history of genital ulcer disease (GUD), there was no association of HIV infection with circumcision status, whereas among men with no history of GUD, there was a strong association. The interaction among GUD, circumcision, and HIV infection is shown in more detail in Table 15.4.

Similarly, at an STD clinic in Lusaka, Zambia, the correlation between HIV seroprevalence and circumcision was examined in 590 uncircumcised clinic attenders and 20 circumcised attenders.[125] Compared with the circumcised group, uncircumcised men were 1.4 times more likely to be HIV infected. However, in a study from Kigali, Rwanda, no association was found between circumcision and HIV serostatus among 150 couples with and without HIV infection.[126]

One prospective cohort study has been published on circumcision and HIV transmission in Nairobi, Kenya.[127] The 293 HIV-seronegative men described in a cross-sectional study[128] were followed to identify new HIV infections among those men diagnosed with an STD and who had recent contact with sex workers. There were 24 HIV seroconversions during follow up, of which 75 percent occurred among uncircumcised men. Overall, uncircumcised compared with circumcised men had an eightfold increased risk of becoming HIV infected. As in the cross-sectional study of this same population, there was statistical interaction between GUD and circumcision status (see Table 15.4).

Methodologic Issues

The majority of the studies support an association between circumcision status and HIV infection. However, the studies must be interpreted cautiously because they may contain unavoidable confounding, which tends to produce an association even if one did not actually exist or to make a weak association stronger. The large potential for confounding results from the sexual transmission of HIV. Among the

Table 15.4: Relationship between circumcision, genital ulcer disease (GUD),[a] and HIV infection in an STD clinic in Nairobi, Kenya

	Cross-sectional study (n = 338)			Prospective study (n = 293)		
	HIV prevalence		Relative prelavence	HIV cumulative incidence		Relative risk
	%	n		%	n	
No GUD						
Circumcised	2.5	5	1.0	0.8	1	1.0
Uncircumcised	16.1	9	6.5	8.7	2	10.4
GUD						
Circumcised	30.0	15	12.1	5.3	5	6.4
Uncircumcised	25.8	8	10.4	28.6	16	34.3
Total	—	37	—	—	24	—

Source: Cross-sectional data from J. N. Simonsen et al., "Human immunodeficiency virus infection in men with sexually transmitted diseases," *New England Journal of Medicine* 319 (1988):274–78; prospective data from W. D. Cameron et al., "Female to male transmission of human immunodeficiency virus type 1: Risk factors for seroconversion in men,"*Lancet* 2 (1989):403–07.

a. GUD in the cross-sectional study is history of genital ulcer disease and in the prospective study is presentation at baseline with genital ulcer disease.

sexual practices that may act as confounders (associated both with circumcision status and with HIV transmission) are (1) number of partners; (2) frequency of contact with partners; (3) partner selection, which determines mixing patterns between high- and low-risk partners; and (4) specific high-risk sexual practices.

Circumcision is usually socially and culturally determined, not the result of individual choice. Because sexual behavior is also greatly influenced by social and cultural factors, circumcision may be associated with sexual practices and sexual preferences, including mixing patterns. For example, in Kenya, where the Kikuyu men are circumcised and the Luos men are not, it is possible that tribal membership (and thus circumcision status) could affect prostitute selection and use, especially in Nairobi, which is home to the Kikuyu but not the Luos, who come from the northwestern part of the country. If the

Luos tended to select a class of prostitutes with a higher prevalence of HIV infection, this could result in a spurious association between circumcision and HIV infection.

Genital ulcer disease is another potential confounder because it is also associated with both HIV acquisition and noncircumcision. History or presence of GUD may be a marker for unmeasured high-risk sexual behavior and/or a marker of an increased probability of exposure to HIV-infected partners.

Besides acting as a marker for increased risk of exposure to HIV in men attending the STD clinic, GUD may also lie along the causal pathway between circumcision and HIV infection if (1) an intact foreskin increases the probability of GUD and (2) the presence of GUD increases the probability of infection given exposure to HIV. Therefore, a clearer understanding of the biological role of GUD in HIV infection may be required before the relationship among GUD, HIV, and circumcision can be adequately understood.

Summary

Despite the provocative results of several studies, it would be premature to launch major campaigns for male circumcision for the purpose of preventing HIV transmission. If the association between lack of circumcision and HIV infection is not an artifact resulting from confounding, it is critical to define the biological basis of the association. It is possible that after sexual contact with HIV, the presence of the foreskin increases the duration of survival of the virus and thus the probability of infection, or that the foreskin and the friction of sexual contact create microlesions on the glans of the penis. It is also possible that the foreskin does not directly increase the susceptibility to HIV, but increases the risk of contracting GUD or increases the duration of GUD. If GUD, in turn, increases the risk of acquiring HIV infection, then circumcision could still be an effective preventive measure. Even if it may be very difficult to change circumcision practices, knowledge about the specific effects of the foreskin may lead to recommendations for care of the genitals after sexual activity that could potentially reduce the risk of HIV infection and infection with other STDs.

In areas where the epidemic of infection is making new inroads—Asia and the Indian subcontinent—circumcision is uncommon. If the HIV and circumcision association is valid, the potential impact of intervention on the course of the pandemic could be quite large.

MAINTENANCE OF HIV RISK REDUCTION AMONG GAY-IDENTIFIED MEN

Ron Stall, Maria Ekstrand, Mitchell E. Cohen, Gary Dowsett, Gottfried van Griensven, Graham Hart, and Jeffrey Kelly

Stall and Maria
rand, Center for AIDS
ention Studies,
ersity of California,
Francisco; Mitchell E.
en, Harvard School of
ic Health, Boston,
sachusetts; Gary
sett, National Centre
IIV Social Research,
quarie University
Sydney, Australia;
fried van Griensven,
artment of Public
th, Amsterdam,
erlands; Graham
, University College
Middlesex School of
icine, London, United
dom; and Jeffrey
, Medical College of
onsin, Milwaukee.

Homosexual men in the United States were the first focus of attention when the HIV/AIDS epidemic began, and their communities were the first to develop prevention education programs. As safer sex became a by-word and men changed their sexual behavior, and dramatic declines in seroconversion were reported in the gay community. Now, however, alarming data are emerging: maintenance of safer sex practices may not be permanent.

Cohort studies in the gay community have provided the most comprehensive longitudinal data available during the HIV/AIDS epidemic and essential insights into the progression of HIV and AIDS. They have also documented the unprecedented changes in sexual behavior among gay-identified men over the past decade and the reasons for those changes.[129] However, most studies have only examined declines in the prevalence of risk within entire samples from one year to the next, not the proportion of individuals who have remained consistently safe over long periods of time, that is, those who have maintained safer sex practices.

The HIV epidemic has several characteristics that highlight the importance of maintaining risk reduction. First, the long period of time between initial infection with HIV and the expression of serious AIDS symptoms means that HIV-infected individuals must consistently restrict their sexual expression to only those acts that are safe if they are to avoid possible transmission of HIV to their sexual partners. Second, each unsafe sexual act that occurs in subpopulations with a high concentration of HIV infection—among them, urban gay males for whom there exists greater probability of transmission per unprotected sexual act—conveys much more risk for HIV transmission than does a comparable act in populations with low HIV seroprevalence. Therefore, both initiation of risk reduction efforts and long-term maintenance of behavioral risk reduction must become nearly universal. An understanding of the experience of gay men's long-term behavioral risk reduction is of compelling importance to global HIV prevention efforts.

Maintenance (and nonmaintenance) of sexual risk reduction over time has been analyzed in several studies. The first, using longitudinal data from the San Francisco Men's Health Study, found that whereas 10 percent of the cohort exhibited a pattern of consistently risky sex, 16 percent had a pattern of reinitiation of unprotected insertive anal intercourse and 12 percent reinitiated unprotected receptive anal intercourse after a period of exclusively safe sex.[130] In another study, using data from the AIDS Behavioral Research Project, a San Francisco cohort followed annually since 1984, the pattern of inconsistent safe and unsafe sex was 8 times more common than a pattern of consistent high-risk sex, indicating that long-term maintenance of safer sex is at least as important an issue as initiation of behavioral risk reduction.[131] At the time, HIV prevention efforts for gay men were concerned almost exclusively with the initiation of safer sex techniques, so this finding was of considerable importance. Using data from a third San Francisco cohort defined in 1984 (The Communication Technologies longitudinal survey), approximately half of the men who had previously made a commitment to themselves never to have unprotected anal intercourse were found to have done so during the previous year.[132]

Other longitudinal studies have also been used to detect how the prevalence of reinitiating risky sexual behavior varies over time. After a six-month measurement period, 4 percent of the North American seronegative men in a cohort study did not maintain safe sex.[133] A set of independent British and Australian studies—both long-term follow-up studies with 2 waves of data collection each—yielded very similar results. Using year-long measurement periods, British investigations found at 2 waves of data collection that 40 percent of their sample practiced safer sex, 16 percent moved from unsafe to safer behaviors, 37 percent remained risky and 7 percent changed from safer to unsafe behaviors.[134] In Sydney, Australia, 43 percent of a study sample practiced safer sex only at two waves of data collection, 25 percent moved to safer sex practices at the second wave, 6 percent moved from safer to risky sex at the second wave, and 26 percent had unprotected anal intercourse at both waves.[135] The Australian study did note, however, significantly lower levels of unprotected anal intercourse between casual partners than between regular partners, especially those with the same HIV serostatus. In a Dutch cohort study based on annual measures of risk from 1984 to 1991,[136] 6 percent of their sample was consistently safe, 46 percent changed to safer behaviors, 19 percent moved from safer to risky behaviors, and 29 percent was risky at every interview period.

Variability in the reported rates of maintenance and nonmaintenance of safer sexual techniques is to be expected, given the studies' differences in sampling methods, measurement of sexual risk, time periods of observation, number of observations over time, and different health promotion strategies (see Chapter 9, "Prevention"). There were also variations in the effects of death and attrition and possible underlying differences in the prevalence of risk-taking behaviors across different populations of gay men. Nevertheless, despite these important methodological differences, it is clear that the proportion of gay men reinitiating riskier sexual behaviors after a period of practicing safer sexual behaviors has increased, and that this behavioral pattern is a likely source of increased HIV transmission.

Research based on self-reported behavior can be criticized on 2 points. The first is methodological (concerning the reliability of measuring self-reported behavior), and the other is the fact that behavioral risk does not necessarily result in HIV infection. Therefore, longitudinal studies of HIV seroconversion among gay men are also relevant to the issue of maintenance of behavioral risk reduction over time.

The largest of these studies reports data from the Multicenter AIDS Cohort Study (MACS) conducted among gay-identified men in 4 large U.S. cities.[137] This study did detect overall annual declines in seroconversion among the more than 3,000 men who were HIV negative at the start of the study. However, this trend was set during the first 3 years of the 5-year period of observation, and no further declines in seroconversion were detected after year 3 of the study. The MACS reported especially disturbing trends from Chicago, where the incidence of new infections *increased* during the last year of the observation to over 1 percent per year. Despite the declines in HIV seroconversion observed during this time period, and despite the extensive health education interventions given this group of gay men, 11.3 percent of the men who were initially HIV negative seroconverted over the 5-year period.

In England, Amsterdam, and San Francisco, researchers found somewhat higher annual rates of HIV seroconversion among gay men than those reported in the MACS study. Among four cohorts of gay men who initially tested negative in British HIV-testing centers, rates of new HIV infection ranged from 2.3 per 100 person-years to 4.6 per 100 person-years.[138] In a cohort of gay men in Amsterdam in 1990, HIV seroconversions increased to 2.8 percent a year, after a decline from 8.9 percent in 1985 to 1 percent in 1989.[139] This group also found a significant increase in the prevalence of receptive anal intercourse among the men who recently seroconverted. In comparison, among the men who remained HIV seronegative, rates of receptive anal intercourse had declined. Finally, the AIDS Office of the City and County of San Francisco, reporting on findings from a series of independent data sets, concluded that new infections among younger gay men, ethnic minority gay men, and "older gay and bisexual men who have relapsed into unsafe sexual behaviors" constituted a "second wave" of new HIV infections.[140] The rate of new infection among gay and bisexual men was estimated to be 2 percent a year, increasing San Francisco's population of approximately 25,000 HIV-seropositive gay male residents by some 650 men each year.

Thus both self-reported sexual behavior and HIV seroconversion data support the argument that maintenance of sexual behavior change is an important issue. Whatever the rates of non-maintenance of safe sex among gay men may be, understanding the conditions under which gay men do not maintain safer sex techniques has a more direct prevention application. Several correlates of seroconversion have been identified: young age, a lower level of education, lower socioeconomic status, and ethnic minority status.[141] Behavioral factors related to maintaining safer sex have also been identified: having a greater number of sexual partners, and having had unprotected sex with someone diagnosed with AIDS before 1984.[142] Several studies (although not all) have also found that drug use and alcohol use are related to not maintaining safer sex.[143]

In addition to demographic correlates, several studies have identified psychosocial factors related to having unprotected anal sex, including low self-efficacy, depression, and the need for love.[144] Certain cognitive factors have also been identified, particularly negative attitudes about condoms and identifying anal sex as a favorite act.[145]

Although identifying these correlates within ongoing studies is interesting, it should be emphasized that these analyses have been conducted in studies not specifically designed to study nonmaintenance of safer sex over time. The effort and expense of forming new cohorts of gay men specifically to study maintenance issues appear to be justified, especially as the earlier cohorts age. Given that most analyses to date have proceeded relatively atheoretically, researchers should also consider designing exploratory, inductive, and retrospective research to identify conditions that favor long-term safer sex.

The documented return to unsafe sexual practices is not easily explained. Studies based on cognitive risk-taking theories (health belief models, for example) have not been very predictive of behavior change. After a decade of changing social norms, new approaches and recommendations must be developed to target men who have not adopted or not maintained safer sexual behaviors both as individuals and as partners. These new approaches are likely to emphasize the role of partners, peers, and community in an effort to create an environment encouraging safer sex.

As the gay community has the longest continually documented epidemiological and behavioral history with HIV/AIDS, the trends it reflects can serve as an early warning system for other communities. The second wave of HIV infection emerging today among gay and bisexual men should alert other communities that have made substantial change (sex workers, for example, or individual groups of drug users). For those concerned with HIV/AIDS control, the message from the gay community is that prevention calls for sustained and innovative approaches and long-term resource commitments.

· · ·

GENDER, KNOWLEDGE, AND RESPONSIBILITY

Elizabeth Reid

zabeth Reid is the
rector of the HIV and
evelopment Programme
the United Nations
evelopment Programme
NDP).

One of the most striking features of the response to the HIV epidemic to date is how few of the policies and programs are related to women's real-life situations. The daily lives of women and the complex network of relationships and structures that shape them are well known and well documented. Nevertheless, current theories, research agendas, policies, and programs have neither been grounded in nor informed by these experiences. This failure to take into account existing knowledge or sources of knowledge, to seek to understand and explore relevant facts and strategies, is a failure of *epistemic responsibility.*

Epistemic responsibility is marked by an openness to the acquisition of knowledge and a certain kind of orientation to the world and to one's knowledge-seeking self within it.* Certain kinds of knowledge are contingent on experience, which itself is mediated by an individual's gender, ethnicity, class, academic discipline, and geographic location. The value of what is known depends on the alternatives or perspectives considered. If assumptions have not been questioned and alternative sources of knowledge sought, then such knowledge can be faulted. Not only can claims to knowledge be verified, but also claimants can be faulted for not having looked enough or for the way they come to knowledge.

The concept of epistemic responsibility has already been used in the context of the HIV epidemic. It has been accepted that those in charge of blood and blood-product services in a number of countries can be held accountable for not exercising their responsibility to know or to take existing knowledge and techniques into account, which, for example, could have significantly lessened the contamination of the blood supply before HIV test kits were available. Individuals and the systems within which they operate can and should be held responsible for their lack of interest, commitment, or sense of urgency.

Responsible knowledge of human experience in general, and of women's experiences in particular, is essential to effective HIV-related research, policy, and program development. Because the cost of ineffectiveness in these areas is an increasing toll of human despair, destitution, illness, and death, epistemic responsibility is also a moral imperative.

This article focuses on the urgent need to ensure that women's knowledge and their varying life situations are systematically taken into consideration in the formulation of responses to the epidemic. Clearly, HIV-related research, policies, and programs must be grounded in human experiences, that is, experiences of men and boys as well as women and girls. However, to a great extent, the life

---

*The author is indebted to Professor Lorraine Code (1988) for an elaboration of the concept of epistemic responsibility and its relevance as a means of measuring the adequacy of theories.

situations of men and boys have been more accessible to those responsible for developing HIV programs. The reason for this differential access begs exploration and provides the justification for the specific focus on women's experiences.

Thus far in the HIV pandemic, nearly 5 million women are infected, ill, or dead. The majority of these women are 10 to 30 years old, with the highest prevalence among those aged 15 to 25 years. In developing countries, the proportion of women to men is almost equal or rapidly becoming so.[146] Elsewhere, the proportion is also approaching 1 to 1, although more slowly.

Most women are at risk of infection by sexual transmission. Yet strategies advocating prevention of HIV via sexual transmission have offered women relatively little or no protection from infection.[147] Prevention strategies in general, and information, education, and communication (IEC) messages in particular, have focused on the reduction of the number of sexual partners, fidelity within relationships, safer sexual practices (particularly the use of condoms), and more recently, the treatment of sexually transmitted diseases (STDs). However, these measures, grounded in men's physique, life styles, and experiences rather than in women's, should be directed at men as they provide inadequate means by which women can protect themselves from HIV infection.

Advocating the reduction of sexual partners as a prevention strategy is irrelevant to the lives of women who have no sexual partner other than their husband or regular partner. Where women do have multiple sexual partners, this may be a choice forced on them by economic necessity. As long as the socioeconomic system gives women few opportunities for economic independence, women will not be able to adopt this strategy.

The second strategy, faithfulness within relationships, is not enforceable by women. Some people estimate that between 50 and 80 percent of all infected women in Africa have had no sexual partners other than their husbands. Whereas women may choose their own behavior with regard to fidelity, their male partner's behavior usually lies beyond their control. Condom use could be an important prevention strategy for women who cannot negotiate the nature of their relationships. However, condoms are used by men; women can only ask for their use. Thus, the same structural determinant of women's lives as described earlier means that they may have no power to control the use of condoms or to negotiate abstinence.

Advocating the treatment of STDs as a prevention strategy can be similarly faulted. Rarely are these services provided in culturally acceptable circumstances; they need to be paid for in cash and are usually neither easily accessible nor provided by women. The probability of infection by the virus during unprotected intercourse with an infected partner may be significantly increased when there are lesions, inflammation, secretions, or scarification of the genital area. In men's lives, such conditions are usually caused by the presence of sexually transmitted infections, and again, this has determined the research and intervention agendas. But even in men, it is possible that such factors as lack of circumcision may cause conditions that increase the likelihood of infection or increase infectiousness. Better understanding is needed.

For women, the situation is more complex. Lesions, inflammations, or scarifications may be caused not only by sexually transferred pathogens, but also by sexual practices, cultural practices (in particular, infibulation and severe forms of circumcision), genito-urinary tract infections, and other common conditions (e.g., fistulas) arising from women's reproductive role. An estimated 84 million women and girls have been infibulated or circumcised worldwide, causing conditions of the genital area that could place them at high risk of infection if intercourse takes place with an infected man. More than 1 million women will suffer disabling illness and conditions from reproductive-related causes this year.[148] These disabilities are higher among poor women everywhere, and 99 percent occur in developing countries.

Many of these conditions, including most sexually transmitted infections in women, are treatable.* Some will require changes in cultural practices, such as child brides, pregnancies in young girls or reproductively immature young women, assaultive sexuality (including rape and incest), and other sexual practices causing lesions or inflammation.

The social, sexual, and economic subordination of women places them at risk of HIV infection in different ways from men. Strategies must differ when addressing those at risk of infection through behav-

---

*For many sexually transmitted infections in women, the problem is one of diagnosis rather than treatment.

ior or circumstances that they can control and those at risk of infection through behavior or circumstances that they cannot control. The current prevention strategies have failed, particularly for young women who become infected immediately on commencing sexual activity. For those young women, the circumstances in which they become sexually active allow them little opportunity for choice or control. The unsafe behaviors are often determined or controlled by other people.

For prevention or behavior change strategies to protect women, they must fit their lives at two levels. On one hand, they must be based on the actual contexts of women's sexuality; at the individual level, they must be strategies women can exercise and control.

Few possible strategies fulfill these conditions. The diaphragm plus spermicide may protect both women and men from HIV infection and other STDs, and when necessary, can be used privately and secretly by women.[149] However, little or no research has been done in this area. Indeed, not enough is known about how the virus enters a woman's genital tract, whether infection occurs at the level of the vagina, the cervix, or the uterus, or about how infected women infect men.

The female condom (see Chapter 16) effectively protects both women and men, although it cannot be used without the man's knowledge. However, it has not yet been aggressively advocated, and means to make it more affordable and accessible have not been explored.

All genital conditions that may facilitate HIV transmission should become a focus of attention. Treatable conditions should be treated. Although many women have genital conditions that could be treated, an insignificant number of these women attend STD services. In fact, very few women receive internal exams in their lifetime, despite repeated pregnancies.[150]

The protective strategy most widely adopted by women is talking to their sexual partners and attempting to help them see the importance of protecting themselves from infection and the consequences for their families of not doing so.[151] This is a strategy that may best be undertaken by women collectively. Individually, women may feel and be powerless, but together, women can change community norms for both women's and men's behaviors.[152]

If these strategies are not available or effective, possibly the only other strategy is leaving the marriage. This is happening with increasing frequency in seriously affected areas. However, it is an effective protective strategy only if the woman is then able to support herself and her children (if able to take them with her) by means other than sex work.

If no strategies adequately fulfill the two conditions identified here, this must be clearly acknowledged, and the focus of behavior change strategies sought elsewhere: in men's sexuality and life situations or in communities. Changing men's behavior and changing community standards to support the required behavior changes are the most effective ways to protect women and their children from infection.

Prevention strategies advocated to date have not emerged from or responded adequately to women's experiences; they were not even based on a complete knowledge of human experience—of men's as well as women's. Yet all of the facts about women's and men's lives on which this analysis is based are well documented.

Both the experience and the knowledge of an individual are shaped by gender. It is, therefore, necessary to find appropriate ways of learning women's experiences and the structures that shape them and to develop research priorities, policies, and programs that retain contiguity with these experiences. What men and women know differs because their experiences are different.*

Areas where gender difference may preclude the possibilities of common knowledge include pregnancy and childbirth, sexuality, parenting, strictly gender-specific tasks, and in certain circumstances, some psychological and emotional states. This is not to argue that such knowledge is necessarily or intrinsically gender-based, but that where experiences are not available to one gender, knowledge arising from these experiences is not readily accessible. Men could be knowledgeable about growing manioc, tending the sick, nurturing children, and expressing grief through crying. Where they are not, this is a matter of choice, not of necessity.

---

*This is not to argue that all women or all men know these aspects of their lives in the same way. It is a point about the lack of such experience and direct knowledge across gender.

The need to draw on women's knowledge and to remain in touch with the reality of women's lives will become more critical as the epidemic intensifies. As the limits of the capacity of institutionally based services to cope become clear, community- and family-based services are being advocated.[153] The terms *community-based* and *family-based* obscure the reality that these services are provided by women: caring for the sick, feeding and caring for the elderly and the young, healing the traumatized, and easing grief. Women do the work of holding together families, communities, and their societies. Furthermore, to the extent that caring for the sick and the dependent means women's exclusion from the labor market, their economic and emotional dependence and their inability to protect themselves from HIV infection will be reinforced.

Policies that build on and reinforce the assumption or the stereotypes of women as care givers presume the availability of women to undertake these tasks. However, as demand will increase for women's labor as nurturers, networkers, copers, and carers, the economic and demographic changes induced by high young adult mortality rates will simultaneously increase the need for women's participation in productive labor.

These considerations must be taken into account as strategies are sought to satisfy the increasing demand for care and support services and the expressed desire of the infected and the survivors to remain within their communities. Care must be recognized as a collective responsibility of all involved: governments and communities, men and women, families and communities. Each has a role to play in the provision of support services to carers or in direct care provision. These strategies may vary from place to place, but the responsibility for them must be collectively exercised.

Unfortunately, a limited perspective has dominated the HIV research and program agendas, irrespective of discipline: epidemiology, clinical research and trials, intervention design, biological research, behavioral research, and economics.[154] There are three contributing factors. First, the early research populations were infected men; second, male researchers have predominated in all disciplines; and third, because of the severe inequalities of wealth between the industrialized and developing worlds, all early research populations were drawn from industrialized countries. It should be remembered that there were more infected women than gay men or men with hemophilia in the world at every stage of the epidemic. Women have been missing from clinical trials; they have been tested without consent and denied access to the results; they have not been informed that their husbands are infected; their clinical conditions have not been included in case definitions or research priorities; stereotypes of prostitutes or wives have closed off possibilities of communication and understanding.

Most HIV research touches experiences that are gender specific—sexuality, reproduction, labor, domestic responsibilities, and oppression. A serious constraint to progress is that women are more aware than men that experience and knowledge are gender-based,* that social, political, moral, research, policy, program, and other agendas are drawn up on the basis of men's experiences. As a result, the relevance of women's perspectives may not be realized by those developing responses to the epidemic, and gender specificity may not be seen as critical to the outcome.

This can lead to a failure to search further in the face of dissonant facts, to set aside stereotypes, and to search for knowledge. For example, the prevalence of HIV infection is highest in young women aged 15 to 25 but peaks in men about 10 years later. This consistent difference between women and men was known as early as 1986.

However, only rarely in the literature have the possible causes of this difference been explored. Some argue that this difference is due to the fact that sexual partnerships are usually formed between older men and younger women.[155] This is likely a contributing factor but not the complete explanation.

Why do young women between 15 and 25 have significantly higher rates of HIV infection than young men in the same age group? Both groups are sexually active, although young men more so than young women.[156] Both groups have sexually transmitted infections, though once again, young men more than young women. Young women often have different sexually transmitted infections than

---

*Professor Anne Jacobson, University of Houston, Texas, noted that men may have to be reminded to worry about their daughters. It seems more difficult for men to believe that there is any perspective on the world different from theirs. I am indebted to Professor Jacobson for assisting in clarifying the conceptual issues in this section.

young men. Both older men and young men form sexual partnerships with the women who are sexually active in this young age group. Nevertheless, these facts do not adequately explain why the rate of infection is so high at the onset of sexual activity. The question can be rephrased: Why are more young women infected than older pre-menopausal women?[157] In one South African study, 50 percent of all infected women were aged 15 to 19 years, had limited sexual experience, and had significantly higher rates of infection than did young men of the same age and women of all age groups; similar patterns were found in a study of the Rakai district in rural Uganda.[158]

In this case, the principle of epistemic responsibility would require urgent and high-priority exploration of possible determining causes of this high infection rate in young women. As frequency of sexual intercourse with infected men is insufficient to explain the data, it is highly probable that the condition of the genital tract in young women significantly increases the likelihood of transmission whenever unprotected sexual contact occurs. The efficacy of HIV transmission to young women may be increased by:

- sexually transmitted infections found in young women and/or other infections of their genital area
- cervical ectopy in young, sexually active women
- hormonal changes at the onset of menstruation and during the menstrual cycle
- changes in the anatomy of the genital tract as young women reach puberty
- immaturity of the genital tract in postpubertal young women

The biology of the female genital tract remains poorly understood. We know more about the cellular structure of lungs, for example, or about the increased protection from HIV infection offered by an intact genital mucosa in monkeys.[159] In young women, the explanation for their shocking rates of HIV infection may be a combination of some or all of these or other factors. The research agenda is in urgent need of realignment.

Because so many facets of the HIV epidemic are gender specific, gender-specific experience and knowledge must be made accessible so it can shape and reshape theory and practice. Women's gender-specific experiences and knowledge can be accessible by ensuring that women, as well as men, shape and determine the agendas, through first-person narratives or through the devolution of responsibility for interventions to women and their communities.

First-person narratives provide access that can be subtle and various. Some stories from the epidemic are now being told, a few by women.[160] They can bring to light different perspectives and points of view and make them accessible across gender. These narratives present and interpret the relationship between the individual and society and the dynamics of power between women and men. They provide glimpses into men's lives as well as women's and relate individual experience to social and economic structures.

First-person narratives increase understanding. However, listening to and interpreting such narratives, whether as stories, on film, or in consultations, is an acquired capacity. The interpreter must be sensitive to the narrator's purpose in telling her story. Interpretation demands a profound respect for the narrator, for what she says, and for the lives from which the stories are drawn.

Narratives can identify new research areas and program needs. For example, stories told by women of the discrimination and rejection they encountered when a newborn child was diagnosed with HIV have led to the proposal that couples be counseled, informed, and tested together.[161] Patterns and structural factors will emerge as more women's voices are heard.

Narratives, however, do not capture systems of relationships that affect individuals but whose locus lies beyond the individual and her realm of vision. The relationships between poverty and infection status may form a critical part of the narrative, but the relationships between structural adjustment programs, poverty, and the tragedy of being infected may not. Narratives need to be complemented by system-level analyses. A full understanding of the nature and impact of the epidemic requires both kinds of analysis.

The second way in which women's gender-specific knowledge can be made accessible is through devolving responsibility for program development and delivery to women. Solutions must be found for men's refusal to protect themselves and for women's powerlessness to prevent themselves from becoming infected.[162] Women's knowledge and experiences are essential to the development of effective solutions.

A critical strategy of this epidemic will be to ensure that women's perceptions, experiences, and capacities are able to be expressed, valued, understood, and acted on. In so doing, the discontinuity between HIV-related experiences and HIV-related research and programs will be mitigated. Once it is recognized that knowledge of human experiences in general, and women's experiences in particular, is essential to developing effective responses to the epidemic, and once people are more at ease and more skilled at acquiring or expressing that knowledge, we can face the coming decades with increased hope. Programs grounded in human experiences can best address the 3 central areas of the epidemic: changing attitudes and behavior; caring for the affected; and maintaining the social and economic infrastructure of seriously affected communities and countries.

■■■■■■■   .   .   .

CHILDREN AND AIDS

Mike Bailey

e Bailey is an HIV and
elopment consultant
l has worked for Save
Children Fund, United
gdom, as a policy
iser.

HIV infection is predicted to become a major cause of death among children by the end of the century, yet the pandemic is still perceived as largely an adult issue. When the initial impact of HIV becomes apparent in a particular country, the effects on children are not immediately obvious. Sick adults are noticed first, and infected adults are identified through testing and screening programs. In contrast, infants infected with HIV die early, usually without being diagnosed. When parents have AIDS, the effect on their children is cumulative and not easy to see at first. These children receive less nutrition, have to leave school, assume adult responsibilities, face the trauma of the death of their parent(s), or carry the stigma of being labeled *AIDS orphans*. Those children who lose their parents and grow up outside a family environment are more likely to become sexually active early, to get sexually transmitted infections and to become infected with HIV. Thus, despite the increasingly apparent impact of HIV, the effect on children remains, as with so many other health problems, overlooked.

The statistics on children and HIV are alarming: according to *AIDS in the World* projections, by 1995, more than 2.2 million children worldwide will have been infected with HIV; over 1.4 million of the infected children will have died. In a study of 10 countries in Central and East Africa, the United Nations Children's Fund (UNICEF) projected that by 1999, AIDS will have orphaned nearly 11 percent of the population of those countries and will account for an increase of as much as 43 percent in deaths of children under 5.[163] The epidemic has had a profound impact on children, especially in the developing nations: in the orphanages of Port-au-Prince, Haiti, more than half the children under 18 months of age are infected with HIV; in São Paulo, Brazil, 9 percent of children tested in state institutions were infected; in the Rakai district of Uganda, 12.5 percent of the children under 18 are orphans—two-thirds of them because of HIV.[164]

Even though they account for more than half the world's population, children are kept powerless by adults, professionals, and societies. They have little or no influence on how family, community, and society respond to the pandemic, yet they are uniquely vulnerable to its impact on their health and nutrition, their well being and material support, their emotional development, education, and sexuality; in short, on the quality and duration of their lives. (See Table 15.5.)

The Impact of the Pandemic on Children

Children in Society—Health Care, Education, and Sexuality: HIV is a direct threat to children. The extent of the risk they face and of their vulnerability will vary with the country or region of birth, the family's socioeconomic status, and how that status changes in the years between a child's birth and entry to adulthood. Generally, a child's vulnerability to HIV infection increases as the family's socioeconomic status decreases. Children not infected perinatally face the possibility of subsequent infection through breast milk if their mothers have HIV (see the article on breast feeding in this chapter). All children are at risk of HIV through contaminated blood transfusions, unsterile skin piercing instruments, and/or sexual activities—whether coercive or consensual. Few children, if any, have the control over their lives to avoid these risks.

The impact of the epidemic on children is amplified by the fact that it adds to competing priorities within the family and within the health sector, as well as between the health and other social service sectors. In parts of the developing world, health services face an

Table 15.5: AIDS and children: Impact and response

	The child in a world faced with the HIV pandemic	The child with HIV-infected parent(s)	The child with HIV infection and AIDS
Impact			
Health and nutrition Well-being Material support	Competing priorities within health sector Competing priorities between health/ social sector and other sectors Impact of pandemic on availability of service and support	Loss of family income Priority allocation of available resources to support infected parents/siblings Poverty	Disease Stunted growth Disability Death
Emotional, affecting development	Fear Loss of childhood	Fear Loss of childhood Living through parents' disease and death	Child facing own illness and death
Education	Strained educa-tional resources Absenteeism/illness of educators	Reduced ability of parents to provide sustained support/ guidance	Discontinued access to education Possible effect of HIV trauma on skill/ knowledge acquisition
Sexuality	Misperception of risk/protection Misconception of sex	Street kids: survival and sexual abuse/injection drug use	Hopelessness, fear, and feeling of rejection
Response			
Family, community, and societal support		Family response Community response Institutional response	Primary health care/ referral Insertion in community Societal/material support
Policies/ programs	Prevention Social support International cooperation Health care Solidarity	Support to HIV-affected families Nondiscriminatory	Support of HIV infected children Nondiscriminatory isolation
Tomorrow's world	Term impact of HIV on human relations/ economy Reallocation of priorities		

increasing burden of terminally ill patients, serious economic strain, and staff illness and death. This compounds the difficulty of providing maternal and child care in general, let alone for mothers and children infected with HIV. For example, in some areas of Africa with already very limited facilities for tertiary health care, young adult men with AIDS are displacing women, children, and the elderly from the few available hospital beds.

Pressure is also building on educational services. Schools are competing for dwindling public funds, while HIV is slowly eroding their private financial base. The full impact of this trend has yet to be felt. As increasing numbers of families have their structure undermined by the impact of HIV, more and more children will leave school—either because their parent or guardian can no longer afford the fees or because they must stay at home to work. Girls are the most likely to leave school first. What money is spent is likely to go to educate male children. Once a family begins to rely on a child's labor, it is highly unlikely he or she will ever return to school. (Ironically, orphans are more likely than other poor children to have their school fees paid. Several organizations have responded to the increase in the number of orphans by setting up funds to ensure that they stay in school. Unfortunately, this does not speak to some of the core problems of orphanhood. It also singles out orphans for preferential treatment, which can cause resentment and add to their stigmatization.)

In addition to the strain on educational and health care services, simply living with HIV can have serious psychological effects on children. These effects are most severe for children orphaned because of AIDS, but wherever the virus is widespread, children are likely to face the trauma of watching someone close to them sicken and die. In effect, children are at risk of losing their childhood.

The implications of HIV also put increased stress on the always delicate subject of children's sexuality. Mounting pressure to provide children with information that will help them avoid HIV infection confronts traditional attitudes toward children's sexuality. In many societies, people don't speak about sex, and children, particularly girls, become sexually active (whether by choice or by force) without having any understanding of their bodies or their sexuality. Resistance to early and universal sex education for children is widespread, although this is beginning to change in some areas. Parents generally do not like to think of their children as being sexually aware, fearing that if they are aware, they will become active. This denial keeps children ignorant about the risks. Sadly, those children most vulnerable to HIV infection—victims of sexual abuse, street children, those sold into sex work, the children of sex workers,* and young girls whose cultures and societies deny them the right to say no to males—are also most likely to be deprived of the information, education, and support that could help them avoid infection with HIV.

Children in HIV-Infected Families—Becoming an Orphan: HIV infection in a family has multiple ramifications. A family's socioeconomic standing influences both the likelihood that one or more members will be infected with HIV and how adversely the family will be affected. Effects on the poorest families are the most immediate and the most extreme, but whatever the degree of impact, children are the largest group of affected dependents. If, for example, the husband is initially infected with HIV, it is likely that his wife will become infected as well, in which case she has a 1-in-3 chance with each pregnancy of bearing an infected child. Whether her child is infected or not, that child will face future health problems if she is too ill to breast-feed or provide care and nurture. Resources used to cope with the effects of HIV in the family drain its savings and reduce the productivity of individual members. An infected infant will need treatment and care, putting an additional burden on the family budget and on the time and energy of siblings and the parents. The schooling of siblings may have to be curtailed.

When productive family members die, survivors are placed at a greater disadvantage. If the father dies first, traditions of patrilineal inheritance may deny his wife and children their right to stay where they have been living. Such displacement, or simply extreme poverty, may force female family members, including younger girls, into commercial sex work. When both parents die, the children may be taken in by their extended family or cared for by older siblings. For others, the options are institutionalization or life in the streets, where they

---

*Redd Barna of Norwegian Save the Children estimates that there are nearly 5 million children of sex workers in India alone and tens of millions worldwide.

will be extremely vulnerable to HIV infection. Being orphaned by AIDS may also impose on a child the additional stigma of suspected infection. The savage irony of HIV is that its effects intensify the socioeconomic conditions in which it is most easily transmitted.

Children who lose one or both parents to AIDS experience psychological trauma that can be devastating. The experience is not directly analogous to, say, the death of a parent in war or by accident. Instead, children are likely to spend 6 months to several years living with a parent who slowly deteriorates and who has chronic infections and constant diarrhea. In addition, pressures from outside the family, such as discrimination and isolation, can add to the trauma and reinforce their growing disaffection. Parenting socializes children, so the younger the orphan, the more likely he or she is to pass into adulthood with a poor outlook and an inadequate social orientation, in addition to material disadvantage. Rural children who are not taken in by families in their village may drift to urban areas, where they are unlikely to find any support services. It is difficult not to conclude that HIV will increasingly generate an urban underclass of unsocialized young adults; as they try to function in an environment already disrupted by the consequences of HIV, they will be neither socially stable nor productive in the labor force.

Although the phenomenon of children whose parents have died of AIDS is also affecting western cities like New York City, the problem is currently most acute in Africa. The World Health Organization (WHO) predicts that there will be 10 million unaccompanied (orphaned, abandoned, runaway) children in sub-Saharan Africa due to HIV by the end of the century—3 times the current estimate from all other causes.

Particularly in rural areas, orphans have usually been adopted by members of their immediate or extended family, but as the number of orphans increases, this tradition is coming under increasing strain. HIV tends to cluster in families and to target the relatively young adults who might otherwise take responsibility for orphans. Grandparents, who once thought their children would care for them in old age, are finding themselves raising a second generation of children that they may be ill-equipped, both physically and financially, to handle.

Children living in the streets face different problems. There are an estimated 100 million street children today.[165] Population growth, urbanization, and HIV continue to swell that number. They may be able to fend for themselves, but they have few options for survival. The implications for the spread of HIV among them are alarming. For boys, theft and extortion may be supplemented by sex work. For girls, the choice of prostitution is often made for them if they are subjected to sexual abuse and rape. Street children who inject drugs also face the additional risk of HIV transmission from shared needles. The children living in the golden triangle area, where injectable drugs are more readily available than any other intoxicant, are at special risk. In Manipur, India, for example, the prevalence of HIV infection went from 0 percent to approximately 50 percent in just 1 year in a population of 15,000 injection drug users, the majority of whom were adolescent males.[166]

The Child with HIV—The Costs of Sickness and Care: The course of HIV infection in infants is different from that in adults. Infected children progress to disease and death much more rapidly than do adults. Whether HIV is acquired perinatally, from breast milk, or through some other means, 50 percent of infected infants are likely to die before age 2, and an additional 30 percent will likely die before they are 5. Because their symptoms often mimic other childhood diseases of the poor, their infection is usually unrecognized.

A typical HIV-infected infant suffers chronic diarrhea, fever, and respiratory infection. Many are unable to absorb nutrients and lose or fail to gain weight. Growth is stunted. If, as is common in the developing world, the infant's serostatus is unknown, the mother may think he or she has a disease the local clinic can treat. When the infant fails to respond to standard interventions, she may lose confidence in the clinic. Either prior to or after seeking health clinic care, the child is likely to receive care from traditional healers, often at high financial cost. Diagnosis of HIV infection is important because the child can be allowed home with treatment, if necessary, for TB or oral thrush. Though requiring time, energy, and resources, home care is better for the child's quality of life than is being in the unfamiliar surroundings of a hospital. It is also better for the child's siblings to have their parents at home and not away with the sick child. Overall, home care is better for the family budget and also allows optimal use of restricted hospital resources.

Responding to the Impact of AIDS on Children

It is difficult to design effective responses to these problems. In general, but especially when dealing with children, the most successful programs and policies involve and have the support of families and communities. Children's needs have to be addressed on several levels—physical, psychological, medical, educational—all of which are embedded in the matrix of a given society. No matter how great the need, there is no easy way to change social and cultural traditions.

Ideally, long-term infection control planning should be directed toward children, although most efforts will first have to address the attitudes and behavior of adults. While HIV prevention policies cannot really be effective without childhood education, this idea meets with strong resistance in many societies. Families and communities are faced with the stark choice, however, of either rethinking what they teach children about their sexuality or seeing the negative effects of HIV in generations to come.

For children, as in all areas of HIV prevention, the triad of information/education, health and social services, and a supportive societal environment is critical. HIV prevention requires that children learn about their bodies before puberty begins. Girls, especially, need to understand the relationship between sex and power, to see what forces drive adult behavior, to strengthen self-esteem, and to be assured of their right to make sexual decisions. This means helping girls achieve more control over their lives, reducing the double standard that favors boys, and extending general education to all children. Primary schools are the key, both because these are formative years and because many children, especially girls, will receive no further education. Special strategies are needed for children who never attend school and are, thus, even more at risk. They can be approached through youth groups, in the streets, or in the fields or factories where they work— anywhere where contact is possible and trust can be established. But approach is just the first step. The experience of working with street children in Latin America makes it clear that a full range of services has to be provided before any real advantage is gained.

Both practical help and a willingness to examine and change

social customs will be needed to back up education programs. Support services (e.g., distribution of condoms in sizes to fit boys, opening sexually transmitted infection clinics) are most effective with children if they are free of charge, readily available, and delivered in a nonjudgmental way. The impact of HIV will be particularly severe wherever culture and religion continue to put strict limits on access to health care for women. Girls will also be less at risk if the growing trend toward early marriage to older men can be reversed. HIV has increased the premium men put on youth and virginity, and in some societies under pressure from HIV, younger girls are being sought out because they are perceived as uninfected.

Changing cultural traditions will be difficult, especially in rural areas. Yet HIV is creating strong pressures, and policymakers *can* help shape the response. Uganda's education ministry, for example, has pioneered a countrywide syllabus on sex education and self-esteem development for both the primary and secondary schools. UNICEF considers this program a model for other countries in East and Central Africa. Other regions will need to find effective approaches to sex education that suit their cultures. In Asia, for example, sex is often not discussed, and it will take political and social will to implement prevention programs. Without that will, HIV will continue to spread unchecked.

Addressing Physical Needs: Uninfected children orphaned by HIV need to be fed, clothed, housed, and educated, preferably within families and within their own villages or neighborhoods. Placing the child with a family member is ideal, but if this is impossible, adoption or fostering are preferred. Institutions have a role only as a last resort. Institutionalization usually means the child must be relocated, eventually leaving the orphan in a strange place with few social skills.

Programs that focus on orphans need to perform a delicate balancing act, for the children need most to be treated as normal in abnormal circumstances. It is difficult enough to integrate orphans into families and communities where there is no tradition of fostering or adoption outside the natural family. The problem is compounded by making them conspicuous (and perhaps resented) because they are the only children in the foster family with shoes or whose school fees are paid, thanks to relief programs.

Policy is also urgently needed to help and protect the rights of children at high risk who are on the streets and/or working in commercial sex. They face not only infection by sexual transmission and sharing needles but also incarceration because of policies that criminalize their activities and drive them farther from sources of help. In many countries, children are incarcerated with adults if they are arrested. This commonly means rape and violence for boys and girls alike. Anti-slavery International estimates that there are 100,000 street children imprisoned every year, often with adults.

Addressing Psychological Needs: Teams from Save the Children (U.K.) working with AIDS orphans in the Rakai district of Uganda and with war orphans in Liberia, found that both groups had the same range of psychological problems and needed counseling and rehabilitation in order to function in society again.

Both individuals and families need nondiscriminatory community support that does not create an added burden of ostracism or isolation. To date, counseling survivors has not been a priority—groups, such as The AIDS Support Organization (TASO) in Uganda, that provide counseling have been overburdened by the immediate and obvious needs of people living with HIV. But there is a growing realization that providing psychological help to the much larger number of survivors around each person with AIDS, including orphans, is in society's long-range interest.

Addressing the Health Care Needs of Parents and Children with HIV: It is important that HIV infection in infants and children be properly diagnosed, because the medical care given to HIV-infected children and the advice given their parents differ from that for other childhood illnesses. In many cases, home treatment rather than hospitalization is appropriate for an HIV-infected child. This reduces the burden on the family and avoids filling scarce hospital beds.

Although the annual per capita health care budget in most developing countries is extremely small ($3 in Uganda, for example), there are strong social as well as humanitarian arguments for spending time and money on parents and children with AIDS. Medical interventions that relieve pain, treat symptoms, and improve the patients' quality of life are socially healing. By ameliorating the symptoms, families can feel they have some control over the disease. Medical policy that prolongs the life of parents with HIV is important for their children's future welfare. It has been suggested that for perhaps $50 a year, the life of an adult with AIDS in Africa can be extended by 1 to 2 years. This can give the parents more time to provide for their children's future; the children will be older when their parents die and will have the benefit of 1 to 2 more years of parenting.

Developing the primary health care (PHC) structure is important for both health education and counseling programs. The PHC strategy of reaching out into the community with trained, community-based health workers is well suited for reaching families with HIV prevention information and for providing care and support.

Looking to the Future

With more and more children becoming infected or ill with AIDS, what stands between the grim reality of today and an even bleaker tomorrow? Policies and programs to empower children and to change some of the most fundamental social inequities must be created; short-term approaches and narrowly targeted programs are not only wasteful and inefficient, but also miss the opportunity to begin to control the spread of HIV. No matter how good a sex education syllabus is, it is ineffective if parents, religious and community leaders, and the health care system clinics do not support its message.

The long-term impact of HIV on human relations and the world economy call for a reallocation of priorities. The only effective way to prevent transmission is to change the conditions of disadvantage that make people more vulnerable to infection. Programs emphasizing care and support within the community can begin to make these changes, for the process of caring strengthens communities and creates an environment of hope that makes sustained attitude and behavior change possible.

DEMENTIA AND OTHER NEUROLOGICAL MANIFESTATIONS OF HIV/AIDS

Justin C. McArthur

Justin C. McArthur, M.B.B.S., M.P.H., is Associate Professor of Neurology and Epidemiology at Johns Hopkins University, Baltimore, Maryland.

The profile of dementia worldwide is changing because of AIDS. HIV dementia is probably now and most certainly will become the most common cause of dementia in people between the ages of 20 and 50 in the United States and Europe, and probably also in developing countries.*

It appears that HIV enters the brain shortly after infection, but it does not begin to cause the mental disorders associated with HIV dementia and other neurological manifestations until much later, with the development of immune deficiency and AIDS. HIV dementia differs from, for example, the more familiar Alzheimer's disease. It strikes people in their most productive years and causes a relatively brief, but often intense illness. The precise implications of this new disease are still unclear, but they are suggested by these questions: How will a large increase in young people with both AIDS-related opportunistic infections and dementia affect the health care system? How will the incidence and impact of dementia differ between the developed and developing nations?

The Profile of HIV Dementia

The pathogenesis of HIV dementia remains uncertain. Researchers are looking at the virus itself, including tropism and replication properties, as well as neurotoxins or cytokines released by infected macrophages, as possible causes of the neurological disorders associated with HIV. It is clear that marked immunological suppression seems

---

*There is little information about the incidence and prevalence of HIV dementia in developing countries. There is evidence that it occurs in Africa and Southeast Asia, but precise figures are unavailable. Most of the relevant investigations have been carried out in western countries on samples of well-educated, homosexual or bisexual men. Generalizing from these results is uncertain at best. The World Health Organization's ongoing study on the neuropsychiatric aspects of HIV infection in cities on 5 continents should provide needed data on dementia in the developing world.

to be necessary for dementia to develop, though only about 30 percent of severely immunosuppressed people develop the HIV dementia syndrome.

Unpublished data from the Multicenter AIDS Cohort Study, an ongoing epidemiological study of the natural history of HIV infection in homosexual and bisexual men in the United States, show that the risk of developing HIV dementia at the onset of AIDS is 4 percent. Contingent on survival, the risk of dementia increases to about 8 percent within 6 months after onset of AIDS, 11 percent within 12 months, and 19 percent within 2 years. In general, the implication of this study is that the chance of someone infected with HIV exhibiting dementia increases approximately 10 percent for each year of survival after a diagnosis of AIDS.

Currently, the period of survival after AIDS diagnosis is between 2 and 3 years in the United States. Thus, today, the majority of individuals with AIDS will not develop HIV dementia. However, survival of people with AIDS is increasing, and the frequency of HIV dementia can, therefore, be expected to rise as individuals with AIDS live longer.

For individuals with HIV dementia, not only is the quantity of life affected in terms of reduced survival times compared to non-dementia AIDS illnesses (median survival with dementia is only about 6 months), but quality of life is obviously strongly affected as well. The course of HIV dementia is variable, and currently there is no way to predict the pace of its progression. It may progress rapidly to severe deterioration and death, or there may be prolonged periods of stability. Intercurrent illnesses and infections may precipitate delirium and mental clouding. The onset of HIV dementia is insidious and may include forgetfulness, mental slowing, loss of concentration, social withdrawal, and loss of coordination. In the late stages of the disease, however, there is significant, global deterioration of cognitive and motor functions and severe psychomotor retardation. These symptoms are likely to be present at the same time as systemic AIDS-related opportunistic infections, further complicating treatment.

The impact of antiretroviral therapy on the frequency and the course of HIV dementia is under active study. Some studies have suggested that the incidence of HIV dementia has declined with use of AZT.[167] Information from various trials of AZT in HIV dementia has shown that there can be measurable improvement in neurocognitive performance, lasting at least several months. In this setting, the usefulness of ddI and ddC remains unproven, and the limited brain penetrance of those compounds may limit their effect. Information is needed on the optimal AZT regimen for treating HIV dementia, along with better data on whether early antiretroviral treatment may prevent development of dementia.

Dementia and Public Policy

The strongest and most common public concern about HIV dementia is whether it poses any threat to public safety, and questions have been raised about the value of routine or even mandatory HIV screening. Numerous studies have examined the neurocognitive performance of individuals infected with HIV. Different tests have been employed, with different criteria for so-called abnormality and varied sample sizes. Most have focused on well-educated homosexual men in the United States and have only tested performance cross-sectionally.

The largest studies, with appropriate controls, have found that during the asymptomatic phase of HIV infection, there is no significantly increased rate of neurocognitive impairment. Smaller studies, using more liberal criteria, have suggested that mild neurocognitive abnormalities can be detected in asymptomatic carriers, but the clinical relevance of these observations remains obscure. More important, 2 studies examining longitudinal neurocognitive performance in homosexual men and male and female injection drug users have shown no decline during 2 years of follow-up.[168] These findings—namely, that HIV dementia should not be expected to occur frequently in otherwise asymptomatic individuals—have important implications for the many millions of people who are asymptomatic and infected with HIV. Therefore, the most recent studies support the 1990 conclusion by the World Health Organization (WHO) expert meeting that "there is no justification for HIV-1 serological screening of asymptomatic people as a strategy to detect [cognitive] impairment in the workplace or in any other context."[169] The question of HIV testing will no doubt remain controversial and may be raised again as improved treatment and prolonged life span increase the possibility that signs of clinical dementia may appear before any other AIDS-defining disease.

The Impact on Health Care and Diagnostic Facilities

Current evidence indicates clearly that the impact of HIV-associated mental disorders on health services will be dramatic. It is still unclear whether care will require specialized inpatient AIDS units or will best be provided within general psychiatric or medical facilities. What is certain is that the burden on treatment and diagnostic and care services will increase significantly.

Assuming approximately 400,000 cumulative AIDS cases in the United States by the end of 1993, and a 30 percent prevalence of dementia, about 120,000 individuals can be expected to have developed HIV dementia by that date. To put this in perspective, Alzheimer's disease, which contributes about half the total number of all dementia cases in the industrialized world, develops in about 150,000 Americans annually. In the United States, HIV may add approximately 30,000 additional cases of dementia each year.

In addition to the increase in sheer numbers of patients needing neurological and psychiatric care, there will be added pressure on diagnostic services. In patients with AIDS, a broad range of mental dysfunction, which might mimic AIDS dementia, can be caused by other diseases of the central nervous system (CNS). Depending on the population, between 20 and 30 percent of all individuals with advanced HIV disease will develop an opportunistic infection (or cancer) of the central nervous system. Cytomegalovirus encephalitis, toxoplasmosis, cryptococcal meningitis, and primary CNS lymphoma are the most common of these conditions in the United States. In other parts of the world, tuberculosis meningitis will almost certainly become an important complication of HIV disease.

A number of groups have projected that we will see increasing numbers of these CNS infections as individuals with AIDS live longer.[170] The evaluation of patients with opportunistic CNS infections is complex and time-consuming because expensive and/or invasive tests, such as CT scans, MRIs, or spinal taps, may be required to pinpoint a diagnosis. Diagnosis is vital because treatment varies for the different infections that involve the CNS. For some diseases, such as toxoplasmosis, there are also effective (but as yet unproved) prophylactic agents like pyrimethanine and dapsone. For others, however, such as progressive multifocal leukoencephalopathy (PML), an opportunistic viral infection of the brain, there are none. It has been estimated that AIDS-related CNS lymphomas will become more common than non-AIDS-related astrocytomas (a form of brain tumor) within the next few years,[171] and there are similar projections that AIDS-associated PML will become more frequent than myasthenia gravis.[172]

The implications of these projections for the added burden on sophisticated diagnostic techniques in the industrialized world are sobering. In 1992, some 8,700 cases of AIDS-related brain mass lesions (including toxoplasmosis, primary CNN lymphoma, and PML) are anticipated in the United States. Of these, 60 percent will be toxoplasmosis, 80 percent of which will respond to treatment. Thus, there will be approximately 4,000 other diagnoses and toxoplasma nonresponders whose diagnosis cannot be pinpointed without brain biopsy. Assuming 50 percent of those undiagnosed mass lesions have a brain biopsy performed, about 2,000 such biopsies related to AIDS will be performed in the United States this year, at a cost of approximately $1,000 each. *(The estimated total cost of $2 million is greater than the entire annual AIDS budget of many developing countries.—Eds.)*

Similarly daunting projections can be made for an increase in HIV-related case loads at neuroradiological facilities. Both CT and MRI are widely used to evaluate altered mental state, headache, dementia, and the brain abnormalities characteristic of HIV dementia. No precise figures are available, but it would be reasonable to estimate that, in the United States, the so-called average person with AIDS may undergo between 1 and 3 neuroradiological investigations during the course of his or her HIV disease, with each investigation costing between $500 and $1,000.

Add to these diagnostic costs the expense of short-term but very intensive care for patients with advanced dementia, along with the specialized management problems that may arise with other HIV neurological problems, and the real dimensions of the problem begin to emerge. The demands of HIV dementia and related organic mental disorders will have to be met by both health services and volunteer and community support systems, which may not yet be prepared to assume their new and complex patient care and family support burdens.

Directions of Research

It is essential to improve understanding of pathogenic mechanisms. It seems likely that HIV dementia may result from the release into the brain of several different substances that affect brain function, either by damaging neurons or other specialized cells or by interfering with chemical neurotransmitters. Cytokines may prove to be a crucial link in this process. Second, research is needed to improve the therapy of HIV dementia and to develop new therapeutic strategies.

Finally, learning how to simplify the management of dementia and other neurological disorders associated with HIV infection will be critical, as health care resources decrease despite a growing number of people with HIV/AIDS. As survival for people with AIDS lengthens, we must face the prospect of an epidemic of dementia in young adults, rivaling, in impact, Alzheimer's disease in the older population.

CHAPTER SIXTEEN

Shaping the Response

▬▬▬ . . .

INCREASING ACCESS TO INJECTION EQUIPMENT: SYRINGE EXCHANGE AND OTHER EXAMPLES OF HARM REDUCTION STRATEGIES

Don C. Des Jarlais and Patricia Case

C. Des Jarlais is
tor of Research of
hemical
ndency Institute of
Israel Hospital, New
City, and a member
U.S. Commission
DS; Patricia Case is
tor of the Center for
n Promotion,
tment of Health and
l Behavior, Harvard
ol of Public Health,
n, Massachusetts;
rch assistance
ded by Nakul Jerath,
rd School of Public
h, and Jen Wang,
ational AIDS Center;
ngoing assistance
Jocelyn Woods,
of the International
ng Group on AIDS
he *Injection Drug*
Newsletter, now
defunded, where
of this information
rst reported.

Increasing access to syringes has been the primary global strategy to reduce transmission of HIV among injection drug users (IDUs). Harm reduction strategies are measures designed to minimize the social and health consequences of active injection drug use, such as HIV infection. Examples of harm reduction strategies include drug treatment on demand, low-threshold methadone maintenance programs, provision of housing for IDUs, outreach and education programs, lifting of restrictions on syringes, training pharmacists to provide education when selling syringes, and syringe exchange programs. This section focuses on syringe access strategies as examples of harm reduction.

All syringe access programs are adopted in the interests of public health, but they are shaped by political and social circumstances. The Irish prevention program, for example, has few problems dispensing syringes, but condom distribution is an issue. In Australia, active injection drug users run some of the syringe exchange programs. In the United States, there are large exchange programs, both legal and illegal, but federal funding could not be used to evaluate them until

1992. The Polish syringe exchange program often cannot obtain syringes because of a general supply shortage. And in Zurich, a highly successful program was shut down because the drug market that developed around it interfered with its primary goal—prevention.

Increasing Access to Syringes

Syringe access programs have evolved in tandem with HIV epidemics that are emerging in the IDU populations in more than 30 countries around the world. There are long-established epidemics among IDUs in the United States and in Western Europe, and epidemics are developing in Brazil, Argentina, Burma, China, India, and Eastern Europe.

Unrestricted sales of syringes is the norm in most of the world, yet paradoxically, unrestricted sales alone did not prevent the initial incidence of HIV infection. For example, Thailand had unrestricted sale of syringes for as little as two baht (US $.08), yet HIV incidence rates among injection drug users rose dramatically until IDUs were educated about HIV on a wide scale. Only then did they modify risk behaviors.[1]

Even where there is unrestricted access to syringes, informal policy decisions can restrict sales. In Edinburgh, for example, syringes are legal, but in 1982, the pharmacists' professional association advised pharmacists to limit sales to IDUs as a drug control measure.[2] Users also reported that equipment was removed from them by the police and destroyed.[3] Between 1982 and 1986, when pharmacies again began selling syringes to Edinburgh's IDUs, Edinburgh experienced one of the most rapidly spreading HIV epidemics of any city in the world, with HIV prevalence among IDUs reaching 50 percent within 2 years of introduction of the virus into the city.[4] As this spread occurred in the complicated context of little AIDS awareness, practical restrictions, and legal sanctions, no one factor can be singled out as the cause. In 1986, practical restrictions were lifted. Currently in Edinburgh, there is outreach and education, limited syringe exchange, and unrestricted over-the-counter sales; seroprevalence rates have also stabilized.[5]

Case Studies of Strategies

In response to the increasing incidence of HIV among IDUs, a variety of programs have been implemented to increase access to sterile sy-

Table 16.1: Relative costs of various strategies

	Lifting sales restrictions	Vending machines	Pharmacy program	Syringe exchange
Costs				
Implementation	Low	High	Low	Medium
Maintenance	None	Low	Low	Medium
Staffing	None	Low	None	High
To user	Low	Low	Low	None
Educational opportunities	None	Low	Medium	High
Access to other services	None	None	Low	High
Number of possible locations	High	Low	Medium	Low

ringes. The following case studies illustrate each strategy but are not meant to be comparative. These strategies can be implemented structurally, through policy decisions, or programmatically. Policy modifications, such as lifting restrictions on sales, have low start-up costs and require little staff time to implement legislation and persuade retail outlets to sell syringes to injection drug users. Once implemented, maintaining such a policy as lifted sales restrictions costs little. Relative costs of various strategies are summarized in Table 16.1.

Lifting Restrictions on Sales

Restrictions on sales and possession of syringes have been lifted in France (1987), Australia (1986), Scotland (1988), and New Zealand (1988). Studies of IDUs conducted in France between 1985 and 1987 showed HIV seroprevalence levels of about 40 percent to over 50 percent in different populations, and behavioral studies showed that syringe sharing was common in these groups.[6] Concerned about the emerging epidemic, the French government repealed the prescription laws in May 1987 and allowed unrestricted sales of injection equipment.

The impact of this policy was documented in several studies conducted in France. Interviewing arrestees in Paris, one study found that the use of sterile injection equipment had increased substantially after the repeal of the prescription law.[7]

One problem encountered with the lifting of restrictions in Australia in 1986 was the increase in discarded syringes in public places, as there were no facilities for safe disposal and no incentive, as in strict one-for-one syringe exchange, to return used syringes. However, when the problem was recognized, creative and innovative programs were rapidly developed to reduce biowaste, place disposal units in public places, and give IDUs small, individual disposal containers.[8] One such program, in Sydney, increased the return rate of syringes from 25 to 64 percent.[9]

Pharmacy-Based Interventions

Pharmacy-based interventions combine unrestricted sales with prevention education. Pharmacists and other salespeople not only sell kits that include syringes and other prevention materials but also are trained to deliver HIV prevention messages. These types of interventions have been implemented in Spain,[10] Australia,[11] France,[12] New Zealand,[13] and elsewhere.

By 1991, 80 percent of the AIDS cases in Spain were related to injection drug use. The destruction of the French heroin laboratories in the late seventies led to an increase in heroin manufacture in Spain, with a consequent increase in injected heroin use within the country.[14] In November 1989, in response to the injection-borne HIV epidemic, the Basque Health Service and College of Pharmacists developed an intervention for injection drug users that enhanced existing legal access to syringes and provided both education and additional prevention materials. The Basques developed an anti-AIDS kit and trained pharmacists in AIDS intervention.

The kit included a syringe, condom, plastic container for syringe disposal, and a leaflet on how to sterilize a syringe and clean the skin for injection. Responding to comments from IDUs, two alcohol swabs and distilled water were added. The kit sells for less than the price of an individual condom (50 pesetas, U.S. $.48). One year after its intro-duction, 88 percent of IDUs who used drugs more than once a day were familiar with the kit, and 57 percent of pharmacists sold it. By February 1991, 500,000 kits had been sold.[15]

The advantages of pharmacy-based programs are the prevention message delivered with the sale of injection equipment and the uni-versal access to syringes through commercial outlets. Among the disadvantages are pharmacists' reluctance to have injection drug users in their store, the difficulty of delivering a confidential HIV prevention message when other customers are nearby, and IDUs' lack of access to syringes during hours when the pharmacy is closed.

Vending Machines

The use of vending machines represents a programmatic (as opposed to policymaking) approach to providing access to syringes. Even before the AIDS epidemic, syringes were supplied from a vending machine in Amsterdam for a short time in the early 1970s.[16] Recently, vending machines have been designed to dispense syringes in exchange for money,[17] for a used syringe,[18] or for tokens distributed by social work-ers.[19] Vending machines are in use in Norway, Denmark, and Ger-many[20] and the Netherlands.[21] They are being considered in Aus-tralia.[22]

In Germany, for example, vending machines solved a distribution problem. Syringes are available legally in pharmacies and from med-ical supply houses; yet some outlets are reluctant to sell to injection drug users, and syringes are only sold in multiunit quantities. Fur-thermore, syringes are available from supply houses only during busi-ness hours. The Deutsche AIDS-Hilfe organization responded to this problem by converting two cigarette machines to provide 24 access to an assortment of low-cost syringes. The machines were installed without official permission, but after 2 years of operation, local au-thorities themselves installed new machines. In Germany, vending machines are used in combination with a program that exchanges syringes on a 1-to-1 basis and is perceived to minimize the number of syringes discarded on the street.[23]

Vending machines have the advantage of constant access, partic-ularly late at night, low cost of implementation and maintenance, and user confidentiality. Their disadvantage is that they cannot provide

HIV education, reinforce prevention messages, or integrate injection drug users into a low-threshold care system.

Syringe Exchange

Programs that exchange new, sterile syringes for used syringes are controversial in some countries. Exchange is conducted by outreach workers in a variety of settings—in vehicles and health care clinics, on the streets, or in home visits. Usually, syringes and other materials are provided free of charge, and each exchange involves an encounter with a program staff member. Exchange programs have taken various forms: some distribute needles, others sell syringes as well as exchange them, and still others conduct a strict exchange of one used for each new syringe.

Syringe exchange has several advantages. It removes economic barriers to obtaining sterile equipment for low-income IDUs. It allows exchange personnel to deliver prevention messages, reduces biowaste, and incorporates high-risk IDUs into a helping system. Its disadvantages are the high cost of materials, staff time, and implementation, and the fact that it provides less coverage of the injection drug-using community than do other access programs.

With the lifting of restrictions on sales of syringes in 1986, the Australian National HIV/AIDS strategy included programs to minimize harm among existing users. Currently, programs for IDUs receive a larger share of total education and prevention funding (37.4 percent) than do programs for any other target group. Much of the funding is targeted to government service delivery (82.7 percent, Aus.\$6.6 million, U.S.\$5.2 million).[24]

The Australian state of New South Wales (NSW) opened its first syringe exchange program in 1986 and currently operates 32 primary and 90 secondary needle and syringe outlets that sell, distribute, and exchange needles and syringes and provide condoms, education, and appropriate referrals. Several different kinds of syringe access programs run simultaneously in New South Wales—pharmacy programs, government-sponsored syringe exchange programs, and services operated by nongovernmental agencies.[25]

Different types of services may be used by various subpopulations; for example, recreational or occasional users may prefer the normality of the pharmacy, and such groups as gay IDUs may prefer programs run by nongovernmental organizations (NGOs) that are targeted to their particular group. Peer groups of active IDUs have also received funding in 6 states; in NSW, the New South Wales Users AIDS Association (NUAA), a peer group, received Aus.$288,700 (U.S.$226,000) in 1990–91. These groups conduct peer education, outreach, and advocacy and sometimes run syringe exchange programs. The coverage of the community at risk in NSW is extensive. With full government support, and using a range of strategies and outlets, about 48,000 syringes a week are distributed through syringe exchange programs.[26] With an estimated 10,000–14,000 regular injection drug users in NSW, about 4 syringes per every IDU are distributed each week. There has been a strong commitment of government resources to preventing an IDU epidemic in Australia. Between 1982 and 1990, only 1.7 percent of AIDS cases were heterosexual IDUs, with an additional 1.6 percent attributed to the combined category of homosexual contact and injection drug use. Most survey data suggest that HIV seroprevalence among heterosexual IDUs is below 3 percent, and seroprevalence levels have remained essentially unchanged since 1986.[27]

In contrast, the San Francisco program is an interesting example of how even illegal programs to increase access can have a powerful impact. Prevention Point was started in 1988 by a small group of people whose original intent was to commit civil disobedience for 1 or 2 nights in order to test in the courts the law regarding syringes. Although arrests were made, charges were never pressed. Technically illegal, the program is tolerated by authorities and widely supported by the community. Prevention Point, now in its fourth year of operation, exchanges 12,000 syringes a week, using an exchange protocol that calls for strict 1-to-1 exchange of syringes, but with no limit on the number of exchanges that can be made. Alcohol wipes, bleach, and condoms are also distributed, along with referrals to appropriate services and on-site access to outreach workers from various programs. The program operates at 5 different sites, for a total of 6 hours a week, using all volunteer labor. With an estimated 16,000 IDUs in San Francisco, there are about 75 sterile syringes per 100 IDUs available per week, which is good coverage of the community in light of the constraints on operation. HIV seroprevalence among injection drug users in San Francisco is estimated to be between 14 and 15 percent and has remained stable since 1988.[28]

The current cost of operating the exchange is supported by funds donated by private donors and through benefits organized by organizations, such as ACT-UP. Currently, there is still considerable debate over whether to allow the San Francisco needle exchange program to operate legally, which would require a suspension of state law. The State of California AIDS Leadership Committee, the San Francisco Mayor's Task Force, the mayor of San Francisco, and the San Francisco Health Commission have all recommended and support a comprehensive syringe exchange program. The city's voters have also passed an initiative calling for the deregulation and decriminalization of syringes. Despite strong popular and political support for the program in San Francisco, it is still unclear whether it will be allowed to operate legally.

Who initiates syringe access strategies? Legislative bodies have lifted sales restrictions and repealed paraphernalia laws, thus legalizing syringe access. The medical profession has trained pharmacists to educate IDUs as well as to sell them equipment. Syringe exchange programs have been initiated by governmental and nongovernmental agencies. In some areas, syringe exchange has been organized by IDUs themselves. User self-organization (by current and former IDUs) was seminal in the development of the Australian and Netherlands programs, and it has played an integral role in the development and continuation of the San Francisco syringe exchange program in the United States.[29]

In the United States, most of the operating exchange programs began as acts of civil disobedience. Some are still illegal or unsanctioned, although 2 (Tacoma and Seattle, Washington) developed from unsanctioned into publicly funded programs. Although organized civil disobedience has played a role, it is important to note that syringes have been distributed informally by individual health care personnel since the beginning of the epidemic, often at some personal risk.

Models: What Works Where

Models of increased access that are multifaceted, that target different sectors of the IDU population, and that use a number of strategies are probably the most useful in reducing risk. A number of factors influence the choice of strategies, among them, political climate, supply of injection equipment, and ability to cover the population.

Political Climate: Syringe exchange has often been the strategy of choice in situations where political and legal sanctions work against legalization of unrestricted sales. If there is a perceived need to maintain social or political control over syringe distribution, or over the injection drug user, syringe exchange is implemented or permitted by authorities, but access through sales remains illegal. Syringe exchange is sometimes offered as a strategy to encourage IDUs into drug treatment programs rather than as one part of a multifaceted program supporting HIV prevention among IDUs.

Adequate Supply: Prevention programs based on syringe exchange, pharmacy interventions, and vending machines presuppose the adequate availability of injection equipment. This assumption is sometimes not valid as there may be shortages of syringes due to supply. For example, the Ministries of Health in the Czech Republic report that an estimated 200 million disposable syringes are needed for medical use alone, and the current production is only 80 to 100 million.[30] In this environment, syringe exchange, or an emphasis on single use of syringes, is a very limited solution. An alternative prevention strategy would be unrestricted access combined with intensive education on appropriate disinfection.

Coverage: How efficient syringe exchange can be in decreasing HIV risk behavior depends on how much of the IDU community can be covered. If the program is not large enough to increase the proportion of sterile syringes in the IDU community as a whole, it may have no broad impact on risk behavior or transmission of injection-related disease, although individual participants may benefit.

    Using estimates of IDUs that are necessarily imprecise, Table 16.2 presents some calculations of community coverage, expressed as the number of sterile syringes per 100 injection drug users per week. This is not a comprehensive list of syringe exchange programs; rather, it presents program data for comparison purposes.

    Syringe exchanges, even on a small scale, can have a profound impact on the lives of IDUs who attend regularly. In communities like Lund, Sweden, and Glasgow, Scotland, where the number of exchanged syringes or needles is 20 or 30 per 100 IDUs a week, seroprevalence has stabilized. In these communities, syringe exchange

Table 16.2: Selected examples of syringe exchange programs

Country	Year started	No. of sites	Estimated no. of IDUs in area	Average no. of syringes/needles exchanged per week	No. of syringes/ needles per 100 IDUs per week
Australia					
New South Wales	1986	122	10,000–14,000	48,000	400
Canada					
Montreal	1989	1 + mobile	30,000	3,622	12
Czech Republic					
Prague	1990	1	3,000–5,000	7.5	<1
Nepal					
Kathmandu	1991	8	15,000	225	1.5
Netherlands					
Amsterdam	1984	Many	3,000	13,460	449
Poland					
Warsaw	1989	3	10,000	100	1
Sweden					
Lund	1986	1	1,000	200	20
United Kingdom					
Glasgow	1987	4	9,400	2,635	28
United States					
Boston[a]	1986	Mobile	15,000	600	4
Boulder	1989	Mobile	800	100	12
New Haven	1990	1	2,000	1,000	50
San Francisco[a]	1988	5	16,000	12,000	75
Santa Cruz[a]	1989	2	3,500	260	7
Seattle	1989	3	20,500	8,500	41
Tacoma	1988	3 + mobile	3,000	6,250	208

Sources: A. Wodak, St. Vincent's Hospital, Alcohol and Drug Service, Sydney, Australia, personal communication, 1992; C. Hankins, Montreal Department of Public Health, Canada, personal communication, March 1992; J. Kriz, Chief Public Health Officer, Hlavani Hgienik Cseke Republiky, Prague, Czech Republic, personal communication, 1992; A. Peak, S. Rana, M. Aryal, et al., Risk taking behavior and HIV-1 prevalence among intravenous drug users in Nepal (1992); D. C. Des Jarlais and S. R. Friedman, "AIDS and legal access to sterile drug injection equipment," *Annals of the American Academy of Political and Social Science* (in press, 1992); D. Wiewiora MONAR, Warsaw, Poland, personal communication, December 1991; B. Ljungberg, B. Christensson, K. Tunving, et al., "HIV prevention among injecting drug users: Three years of experience from a syringe exchange program in Sweden," *Journal of the Acquired Immune Deficiency Syndromes* 4 (9)(1991):890–95; L. D. Gruer, J. Cameron, and L. Elliot, A network of evening needle exchanges in health centres in Glasgow, presented at the VII International Conference on AIDS, Florence, Italy, June 1991; J. Parker, National AIDS Brigade, Boston, Mass., personal communication, January 1992; G. Rebchook, Boulder County Health Department, Colo., personal communication, March 1992; E. O'Keefe, New Haven Health Department, Conn., personal communication, 1992; R. Prem, Prevention Point Research Group, San Francisco, Calif., personal communication, March 1992; Ken Vail, Santa Cruz Needle Exchange Program, Calif., personal communication, 1992; N. Harris, Seattle Department of Public Health, Wash., personal communication, March 1992; D. Purchase, Tacoma, Wash., personal communication, 1992.

Note: IDUs = injection drug users.
  a. Illegal exchanges.

is a targeted intervention, directed at low-income, high-risk individuals and offered in conjunction with other communitywide programs providing information, bleach, and increased access to other services.

Coverage is also related to hours of operation and convenient access to sites. Strategies that rely on retail outlets or vending machines may provide extended hours of access to sterile syringes. The importance of nighttime access was noted in a study of 2,417 IDUs in Australia, where 39 percent reported that nighttime hours were the most important time to make syringes available, precisely the time when many exchange programs and retail pharmacies are closed.[31]

Communitywide strategies to increase access to syringes sometimes function in a gray area where the boundary between legal and illegal access is blurred. The primary access strategies discussed here are legal and quasi-legal programs, but there are other strategies as well. One is the phenomenon of the *satellite exchange*. IDUs in programs that exchange unlimited numbers of syringes on a 1-for-1 basis will often exchange many more than are necessary for personal use. In some cities this is encouraged to facilitate user self-responsibility and to increase access at times when the exchange program is closed. For example, a client of the San Francisco syringe exchange routinely exchanges more than 300 syringes at a time, which he/she distributes in Oakland, a nearby city hard hit by HIV and lacking a regular syringe exchange program.[32] Furthering understanding of such syringe supply strategies within the IDU community could improve delivery of sterile syringes, create higher levels of trust, and ease the way for peer-supported prevention messages.

Evaluation

The impact of increased access to syringes has been difficult to assess, especially where strategy has been communitywide or the result of a policy change. Looking at a number of variables can begin to provide a picture of whether a particular strategy has had an impact.

Injection-Related Sequelae: Decreases in injection-related diseases, such as hepatitis B, and incidence of abscesses caused by nonsterile syringes and failure to clean the skin can indicate that high-risk behaviors have been reduced.

Substantial decreases in injection-related hepatitis B cases have been reported in populations exposed to various syringe access strategies, among them, IDUs in Tacoma,[33] Amsterdam,[34] and San Francisco,[35] and among clients of a needle exchange program in Central London.[36] The latter also showed a decrease in the incidence of abscesses.[37]

Multiperson Use of Injection Equipment: Syringe sharing (multiperson use of injection equipment) is considered the primary mode of HIV transmission for injection drug users, and an overall decrease in sharing syringes has been reported in countries that have instituted any kind of increased access to syringes.

Substantial decreases in syringe sharing have been noted by researchers in Amsterdam, where the proportion of IDUs using the syringe exchange program rose from 13 percent to 66.7 percent.[38] In Germany, there was a reported 60 percent reduction in syringe sharing.[39] Similar reductions have been reported among clients of syringe exchanges in San Francisco[40] and Central London.[41]

Increasing coverage of the community with sterile syringes has dramatic effects for nonexchange clients also. Between 1989 and 1990, 6 million syringes were distributed by syringe exchange programs in the United Kingdom. Syringe sharing in a cohort of exchange clients dropped from 36 to 16 percent, but it fell even more dramatically, from 62 to 22 percent, for nonexchange clients. Increased access to syringes appears to have lead to risk reduction for the entire community.[42]

Age and New Injectors: Despite the increased availability of syringes, a study in Amsterdam showed no evidence that people who had not previously injected drugs began to do so. In fact, the mean age of injectors there has risen, and there has been no increase in the overall numbers of injectors. In San Francisco, the age of IDUs in 9 cross sections rose from 34 years in 1986 to 40 years in 1990.[43]

Drug Treatment Episodes: Does access to syringes, particularly in strategies that have an educational component, such as pharmacy-based or syringe exchange, lead to entrance into drug treatment programs? Do increased access programs act as bridges to treatment? In cities with comprehensive programs, the number of people in drug treatment has increased. For example, in Victoria, Australia, there has been a tenfold increase in the number of people on methadone maintenance between 1985 (150) and 1991 (1,558).[44] In Amsterdam, where increased syringe access strategies were implemented in 1984, the patient load of drug-free facilites doubled between 1983 and 1987.[45] It is impossible to say whether these increases are a result of syringe access programs, AIDS education campaigns, fear of HIV, or increased availability of drug treatment.

In the case of syringe exchange programs, it is a little simpler to evaluate how many program participants go into treatment. In the first 2 months of operation, 17 percent of the 242 clients enrolled in the New Haven Needle Exchange program requested help in entering drug treatment,[46] and 43 percent of methadone admissions over an 18-month period in Pierce County originated in the Tacoma syringe exchange program.[47]

Prevalence of HIV: Seroprevalence statistics are derived from different samples that may reflect very different behavior profiles. Interpreting HIV levels among program clients is problematic as well, because IDUs who know they are seropositive may become more dedicated in their exchange attendance; thus, exchange clients may appear to have a higher seroprevalence than do nonexchange clients. However, some differences in HIV among exchange clients have been documented. In Tacoma, 3 percent of exchange clients were positive compared to 8 percent among nonexchange clients.[48]

Perhaps most pertinent to measuring of HIV infection is not its prevalence within a population, but the incidence of new infections that outreach programs are designed to prevent. In Amsterdam, there has been a substantial decline in the incidence of HIV among new injectors.[49] Among the 200 active participants in the Swedish syringe exchanges, no new seroconversions have been reported in more than 4 years. Seroprevalence among IDUs in southern Sweden remains less than 2 percent.[50] There have been very few conversions among clients of the Central London exchange,[51] and no seroconversions among clients of the Liverpool exchange.[52]

Because participants in syringe access programs may be unwilling to participate in research activities, it can be difficult to assess the program's impact. A number of researchers have tried to use objective measures, such as testing syringes for HIV antibodies to determine the lower bounds of seroprevalence.[53] Syringe testing has been used in San Francisco to determine the lower bounds of seroprevalence among exchange clients, in New Haven to assess different prevalence patterns in syringes used in different venues, such as shooting galleries, and in New Zealand to establish the presence of HIV in the community and to determine geographic risk areas.[54]

Political Responses

Increasing access to injection equipment has been the strategy that most governments in countries with an IDU population have adopted in response to HIV among IDUs. These measures have been instituted in a variety of political climates. In some areas, the anticipated opposition to syringe access strategies never materialized. In other areas, political response has hampered syringe access, limited its coverage, or closed programs that were operating effectively.

There has been substantial debate in the United States about legal access to syringes. Currently, 11 states outlaw simple possession of a syringe without a prescription, and this law has had a chilling effect on the creation of syringe exchange programs. In Sweden, an estimated 3,000 injection drug users live in the province of Skåne (about 300 IDUs per 100,000 population), where a syringe distribution program was started in 1986 by the personnel of an infectious disease clinic. They acted without permission in starting distribution and after much political maneuvering, were permitted to continue in the cities of Lund and Malmö. Seroprevalence among IDUs in the province of Skåne in 1991 was estimated to be about 1 percent.[55] Among Stockholm drug injectors, it is estimated to be around 15 percent.[56] Here, too, there are complex reasons for the differences in seroprevalence, but the results are highly suggestive. Despite positive results of the program, in 1989, the Swedish parliament prohibited all needle exchange programs except for restricted projects in Skåne and 2 others in low-risk areas.[57]

Although the over-the-counter sale of syringes is legal in Brazil, police in Santos have shut down the syringe exchange program, claiming it posed a threat to the public safety.[58] The AIDS rate in Santos is the highest in South America (111/100,000), and nearly 50 percent of the cases are IDU related. In Montreal, on the other hand, the expected opposition to a syringe exchange program never materialized, with the exception of diabetics who felt the syringe exchange program should include them as clients as well.[59]

In Australia, the syringe regulations were lifted after much national debate, and a comprehensive plan for risk reduction and HIV prevention among IDUs was implemented in 1986–87. The program includes multiple modalities of drug treatment, access to syringes (the state of Victoria alone has more than 110 syringe exchange sites), pharmacy training, development of educational materials, and the involvement of active injection drug users in discussion at the policy-making level and in operation of various programs. Despite having high numbers per capita of injection drug users, the HIV infection rate among IDUs remains between 3 and 4 percent. The current fear is that the public will begin to question the expense of this comprehensive program because there is little evidence of HIV infection. The Australian national program is so successful at prevention that the political response may be to curtail it.

Conclusions and Critical Questions

Critical questions remain for policymakers in choosing syringe access strategies and in assessing their effectiveness.

What kind of coverage can a program provide? To what level must syringe access be increased in order to prevent epidemic spread? Evaluating various strategies can pose methodological and ethical problems, for only a randomized clinical trial would prove that syringe access schemes work; yet running that trial would mean denying access to syringes in the context of a fatal epidemic. Evaluating structural interventions, such as the impact of policy changes, is especially problematic. Looking at another area, it is important to consider the cost of various strategies. In countries where the price of a syringe is an important barrier both to the IDU and to the prevention program, which strategies make sense? What are appropriate strategies in developing countries with significant injection drug use–related HIV? Finally, it is difficult to untangle the impact of increased access strategies from the vital linkage to other services those strategies can provide for an underserved population. It may be that syringe access is only the first step in a spectrum of prevention activities, yet policy debate requires that its separate impact be assessed.

THE FEMALE CONDOM: A NEW OPTION FOR WOMEN

Laurie S. Liskin and Chuanchom Sakondhavat

Laurie S. Liskin is an associate with the Center for Communication Programs and an associate on the faculty of The Johns Hopkins University School of Hygiene and Public Health, Baltimore, Maryland; Dr. Chuanchom Sakondhavat is Associate Professor and Head of the Family Planning Unit in the Department of Obstetrics and Gynecology of Khon Kaen University, Thailand.

From the most developed to the least developed countries, women and their children are increasingly at risk from the HIV epidemic. In Zambia, 25 to 30 percent of women in prenatal care clinics are infected with HIV.[60] In Bangkok, as many as 50 percent of commercial sex workers carry HIV.[61] In New York City, AIDS is the leading cause of death in women in their twenties.[62] By the turn of the century, according to the World Health Organization, 6 to 8 million women and 10 million children worldwide will be infected with HIV.[63]

How can women protect themselves? At present, the options are few. Spermicides reduce the transmission of some sexually transmitted diseases (STDs), like gonorrhea and chlamydia, but they do not seem to be effective against HIV.[64] Good-quality latex condoms do prevent transmission of HIV and other STDs, but only if they are used. In most societies, however, men control the use of condoms, and women have too little power to influence their use. Thus, to a large extent, women's health and safety are often beyond their control.

This situation may be changing. Three new barrier methods under development will give women more power over contraception and disease prevention—a plastic sheath, a latex sheath, and a latex pouch.[65] These products promise a barrier method for women that is at least as safe and effective as the male condom. However, only one—the plastic sheath, better known as the plastic female condom—has been tested in diverse populations and is becoming available.

The Plastic Female Condom

The plastic female condom was first designed in the mid-1980s by a Danish gynecologist and his wife and developed by an international group of researchers and physicians. Combining features of a male condom and a diaphragm, it consists of a soft polyurethane sheath 17 centimeters long, with two flexible polyurethane rings. (See Figure 16.1.) The smaller ring lies inside the closed end of the sheath. It is inserted into the vagina and anchors the condom behind the pubic bone. The larger, outer ring lines the open end of the sheath and, after insertion, hangs outside the vagina.

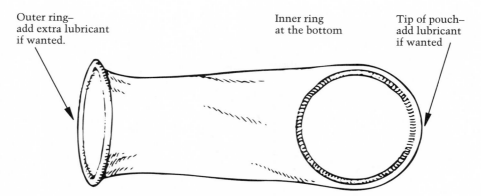

Outer ring–
add extra lubricant
if wanted.

Inner ring
at the bottom

Tip of pouch–
add lubricant
if wanted

Figure 16.1. Reality vaginal pouch (female condom) (Wisconsin Pharmacal Company, Inc.)

Since the mid-1980s, more than 1,700 women in 30 countries have used the female condom in more than 30,000 acts of intercourse.[66] A British manufacturing company (Chartex International) owns the patent on the device and will market it outside the United States and Canada under the brand name Femidom®. In North America, the female condom will be sold by the Wisconsin Pharmacal Company under the brand name Reality®.

A woman can insert the female condom as she would a diaphragm. Unlike the diaphragm, however, the inner ring of the condom comes in only one size and need not fit snugly over the cervix. The sheath lines the vaginal canal. During intercourse, the external outer end and ring cover the labia, preventing skin-to-skin contact with the base of the penis. The inner lining of the sheath is coated with a silicon-based lubricant. Women may add oil- or water-based lubricants on the outside of the sheath to facilitate insertion and on the inside to increase a natural feel during intercourse.

Protection against Infection and Pregnancy

Like its male counterpart, the new female condom promises to provide adequate but not complete protection against pregnancy and STDs. In laboratory studies and small feasibility trials, the female condom has proved to be an almost perfect barrier. But problems with improper use and breakage have emerged among larger and more diverse populations using the condom regularly.

Intact polyurethane is impermeable to sexually transmitted pathogens, including HIV. Using a laboratory model to simulate sexual intercourse—the same equipment used to test male condoms[67]—researchers report that the female condom completely prevented leakage of HIV and cytomegalovirus.[68] Additional laboratory studies, using liquid and gas diffusion methods, found that even particles smaller than the hepatitis B virus, one of the smallest known sexually transmitted viruses, do not leak through the platic membrane as long as it remains intact.[69] Female condoms retain their impermeability during intercourse. Among 521 condoms used for one act of intercourse and then tested with the standard waterburst test (American Society for Testing and Materials), less than 1 percent showed any leakage.[70]

The effectiveness of the female condom during day-to-day use is still undetermined. Family Health International and the Contraceptive Research and Development Program (CONRAD) are conducting trials in 9 centers in the United States, Mexico, and the Dominican Republic to clarify the issue. Preliminary results based on 168 women show a 6-month gross cumulative pregnancy rate of almost 13 per 100 women,[71] comparable to pregnancy rates for the male condom[72] and for other female barrier methods.[73] About one-quarter of these pregnancies were attributable to defects in a design feature of the product. Improper use or failure to use the female condom accounted for the rest.

As in most contraceptive trials, most of the pregnancies in the 9-center study occurred early, in the first 3 months of use. Pregnancy rates were almost twice as high among women in Latin American centers as in women from the United States. Although by no means conclusive, these preliminary results suggest that women in developing countries may have less success using the product than do women in developed countries.

The effectiveness of the female condom against sexually transmitted diseases has also been tested in a small field trial. After treatment for trichomonas and chlamydia, half of 104 women were given samples of the female condom and instructions on its use. None of the 20 women who used the product with every act of intercourse was reinfected with either disease, compared with 14 percent of the

50 nonusers. Among 34 women using the female condom intermittently, 15 percent were reinfected with trichomonas and 9 percent with chlamydia.[74]

Although polyurethane is tougher and more durable than latex, the female condom can still break during use. Problems with slippage and incorrect use have also been reported. Breakage rates typically range from 0 to 2.7 percent of female condoms used and up to 9 percent among Cameroonian commercial sex workers. By comparison, the rates for latex male condoms range from 0 to 12 percent.[75] Most of the female condoms broke during intercourse rather than during insertion and removal; breaks were equally divided between the sheath and at the outer ring.

Along with breakage, 2 other problems occur that increase the risk of sexually transmitted infection: the outer ring of the condom slips into the vagina during intercourse; and the penis misses the opening of the condom and enters the vagina next to the condom. More than one-third of the Cameroonian commercial sex workers experienced at least 1 of these problems with at least 1 client and attributed this to "rough sexual practices."[76] Other women report these problems much less frequently.

Acceptability

From a woman's perspective, the female condom offers many advantages. It can be obtained in clinics and pharmacies without a prescription or fitting from a health care professional. It is safe to use, with no vaginal side effects except infrequent labial itching and irritation.[77] With a little practice, most women easily learn how to insert and remove it. Both oil- and water-based lubricants can be used, a distinct advantage of polyurethane compared with latex condoms. And best of all, it gives women more control over their own protection.

But will women use it? Studies in diverse populations in both developed and developing countries and among women at low and high risk of HIV infection show mixed results. Overall, at least 50 percent or more women and their partners found the female condom acceptable and would be willing to use it again.[78] Nevertheless, reactions varied widely in different centers, and a significant proportion of women said the condom was uncomfortable and/or decreased sexual pleasure. The most enthusiastic endorsements came from commercial sex workers in Cameroon and from women who valued the product's effectiveness against STDs, suggesting that the condom will be used more for disease prevention than for contraception.

Design features of the condom, particularly the inner ring, caused the most problems. Up to a quarter of the women said they felt some physical discomfort from the female condom during intercourse.[79] In Thailand, a third of the commercial sex workers were so uncomfortable that they stopped using the condom. A second trial was conducted using a shorter, 15 cm sheath.[80] However, even with the shorter sheath, 80 percent of the women still said they felt discomfort during intercourse.[81] Men also had problems. One-fifth or more of the male partners reported discomfort, particularly from the penis pressing against the inner ring.[82] Some of these complaints may reflect the unfamiliarity of men and women with any vaginal method of contraception. For example, most of the Cameroonian commercial sex workers reported that they felt more comfortable with the female condom the longer they used it.[83]

Partly because of discomfort during intercourse, men and women in some studies reported that the female condom decreased their overall sexual satisfaction. Reactions varied widely, however, with many reporting no change and almost 10 percent of women reporting they enjoyed sex more,[84] possibly because of the extra friction as the outer ring rubs against the clitoris.

Some men and women had aesthetic objections to the condom, particularly its baggy appearance. Men complained about seeing the device hanging out of the vagina. And from 10 to 15 percent of women and their partners reported being bothered by noise during intercourse.[85]

Men's attitudes will likely play a large role in determining whether women will use the female condom, and their reactions are mixed. In developed countries, more than half of the men liked it. However, in the 2 studies that asked for a comparison, less than 40 percent preferred it to male condoms.[86] In developing countries, attitudes were more negative, both among cohabiting partners and among clients of commercial sex workers. In Thailand and Kenya, for example, many more men preferred the male condom to the female condom.[87] In Kenya, men's objections were the main reason 40 percent of the women chose to quit the study after the first 3 weeks.[88] In

Cameroon, more than 75 percent of the commercial sex workers said that some of their partners refused to have intercourse if the female condom was used, and more than half of these men also refused to wear a male condom instead.[89] As a result, and despite full awareness of the risks of STDs, 66 percent of the women had unprotected sex at least once during the 4 weeks of the study. It seems clear that men's objections to any kind of barrier method will continue to be a significant problem.

Marketing and Distribution

The female condom is already on the market in Switzerland. It may be available by late 1992 in several other European countries, and in 1993 in the United States. In early 1992, the Obstetrics and Gynecology Devices Panel of the United States Food and Drug Administration (FDA) recommended that the female condom be approved for marketing once the 9-center trial was completed and some other data were submitted. If the FDA grants final approval, women in the United States should be able to buy the condom in 1993. Depending on public sector pricing, the product may be provided by donor agencies to women in developing countries in 1993.

To reach potential users, the female condom will have to be promoted and widely distributed through the same channels as the male condom—over-the-counter commercial or social marketing retail sales, community-based distribution programs, and family planning, STD, and other health clinics. Ensuring availability to women at high risk of sexually transmitted disease is particularly important. Many of the newer social marketing programs for condoms in sub-Saharan Africa and the Caribbean aimed specifically at AIDS prevention are setting up commercial outlets in places where high-risk behavior is likely to occur, such as hotels, truck stops, and bars.[90] Such outlets should also sell the female condom.

Cost will be the major barrier. The plastic female condom will sell in the United States for $2 to $2.25 a piece, about 3 times the local price of male condoms. The United States Agency for International Development (USAID), which funded the 9-center trials, is negotiating with U.S. distributors for a substantially reduced public-sector price.[91] Even at half the retail price, however, the female condom will be too expensive for women in developing countries without substantial government and donor agency subsidies. Faced with limited budgets, USAID and other agencies may have to choose between expanding supplies of male condoms and providing female condoms.

Availability is only the first step in ensuring use. As a new kind of product, the female condom may not be accepted easily by women or by health care providers who will need information to promote the new method and to advise women accurately. Women will need culturally specific insertion instructions and information about the condom to understand its benefits, allay concerns about potential side effects, and ensure correct use. They also will need advice on convincing men to accept the product.

A pressing concern regarding counseling is possible reuse of the female condom, either with the same partner or with more than one partner. The female condom is intended for one use only. Nevertheless, a few of the women in clinical trials said they reused the same condom.[92] Because the female condom will be costly, it is likely that many women will want to use it more than once. This could pass on STDs unless they wash the condom carefully between uses. Also, it is not known whether multiple use increases the likelihood of breakage, putting both the woman and her partner at risk.

Conclusion

The female condom is a new and welcome addition to barrier methods for women. But like its male counterpart and other female barrier methods, it will not appeal to everyone. Given the design, the cost, and the objections of men, many women are likely to use the female condom primarily to prevent STDs and only then as a back-up method to the male condom.[93]

The plastic condom is the first generation of vaginal barrier methods designed specifically to prevent HIV transmission. Modifications are needed to make it more practical and more acceptable to all women, especially to those at highest risk of HIV infection. A product that men cannot see or feel is the ideal.[94] Short of that, a female condom with different-sized sheaths and inner rings and with a softer, more pliable inner ring should increase comfort and ease of use. An insertion applicator would also make the condom more attractive to women who prefer not to touch their genitals. Also important is the development of a product that is durable enough for multiple use.

In many parts of the world, men will probably have the final say on use of female condoms for some time to come. But because women can wear the product themselves, they may be more successful at negotiating its use than they are with male condoms.[95] By increasing the options available to women, the female condom offers new hope for HIV prevention. But providing technology is only the first step to action. Women need to know how to take advantage of this new technology. Efforts must begin now to help women gain the skills and the confidence to ensure that condoms—male or female—are used to safeguard their own health.

■ . . .

AN OVERVIEW OF INTERNATIONAL POLICIES FOR HIV PARTNER NOTIFICATION

Richard A. Keenlyside and Kathleen E. Toomey

Richard A. Keenlyside, M.D., is in the Academic Department of Genito-Urinary Medicine, University College and Middlesex School of Medicine, London; Kathleen E. Toomey, M.D., M.P.H., is in the Division of STD/HIV Prevention, National Center for Prevention Services, Centers for Disease Control, Atlanta, Georgia.

Partner notification, considered an essential component of sexually transmitted disease (STD) control programs in North America and Europe for more than 40 years, is the process of identifying sex partners of infected individuals and helping them receive curative or preventive STD treatment. As partner notification programs evolved to include notification for HIV infection, both sex and/or needle-sharing partners of HIV-infected people were offered risk reduction counseling as well as HIV testing and other services.

Using terminology adopted by public health groups worldwide,[96] partner notification for STDs (including HIV) can encompass 2 distinct approaches: patient referral or provider referral. All partner notification activities within STD/HIV prevention programs are based on some combination of these 2 approaches.

With patient referral, the HIV-infected person is encouraged to inform partners of their risk for infection, so that partners can seek appropriate medical services. Provider referral (previously called contact tracing) is a voluntary, confidential process in which health professionals obtain partner names and identifying information from an infected person, then notify the partners and help them to seek or obtain appropriate services.

With no curative therapy for HIV infection, the role of partner notification for HIV control has been controversial worldwide.[97] Concerns about the potential for discrimination of both index patients and identified partners have been weighed against the rights of exposed individuals to be informed of their risk for infection and the need to identify partners unaware of their risk for infection. Although the development of antiviral treatment and prophylactic antimicrobials has provided clear benefits for the early detection and treatment of HIV infection,[98] thereby reducing previous opposition to partner outreach, many countries lack the resources to provide these costly therapies and long-term care to individuals with HIV infection. Thus, the debate worldwide has continued to center on the role partner notification should play within HIV prevention programs relative to other preventive interventions.

The ability of any country to develop a formal HIV partner notification program has been influenced by a number of factors, including the organization and strength of services for STD diagnosis and treatment; the epidemiology of HIV infection in each country; the attitudes of health care professionals who must carry out partner notification in conjunction with other health care services; and the government structure for setting health policy. In most countries only a small proportion of STD cases—and presumably HIV cases—are seen in STD or other health department clinics. Treatment services are often fragmented and delivered by a variety of health care providers with limited skills in provider referral. Clinicians responsible for STD treatment and partner management, in general, have little support from organized HIV prevention programs and receive no special training for carrying out complex partner notification activities.

The experience of various countries with partner notification activities for HIV prevention is summarized in this article, with an emphasis on information available since the publication of the last comprehensive review on this topic.[99] The information in this section was obtained using country surveys developed by *AIDS in the World*. It was completed by personal interviews with selected health care providers and public health officials of individual countries and through a review of recently published articles and conference presentations.

Europe

The United Kingdom has a national network of 216 hospital-based genito-urinary medicine clinics that provide STD treatment as well as HIV counseling, testing, and partner notification by trained health advisers. Over 60 percent of the HIV cases from identified reporting sites in the United Kingdom during 1989–90 were from these STD clinics.[100] Although the majority of clinic staff agrees that patient referral should be encouraged, few providers working in the high HIV-prevalence areas of London support provider referral programs. They cite the lack of staff to carry out the notification activities and the potential for breach of confidentiality or alienation of clients. However, in other parts of the United Kingdom where HIV/AIDS case rates are lower, STD clinic staff routinely counsel index patients about partner notification and carry out provider referral.[101]

In Belgium, partner notification began as a pilot program at the Saint-Pierre Hospital in Brussels, supported by a grant from the Ministry of Health. Because 30 to 50 percent of all HIV infections reported in Belgium are among heterosexual adults, the program focused on identifying persons with heterosexual exposure who may be unaware of their risk for HIV infection.[102] Attending physicians offer partner notification counseling to any new patient seeking testing or care by the AIDS division; patient referral is encouraged and, additionally, provider referral is offered.[103] A social worker and a nurse with special partner notification training carry out the counseling, testing, and notification procedures. During an 18-month period starting in 1989, 296 heterosexual individuals were evaluated; 169 of them (57 percent) identified at least 1 partner. A total of 287 partners were reported; 175 of the 287 (61 percent) were located (one-third by provider referral, two-thirds by patient referral). The seroprevalence of HIV infection among the 165 partners who accepted testing was 33 percent.[104]

France, Spain, and Italy together account for more than 50 percent of total AIDS cases in Europe,[105] yet services for STD/HIV counseling, testing, and partner notification are not well developed. The high rates of injection drug use among AIDS patients in Spain and Italy, coupled with lack of support for partner notification by clinic staff, have limited the development of formal partner notification programs, even in high-risk clinic settings. Furthermore, the development of formal national policies in France, Spain, Italy, and Switzerland has been futher hampered by the decentralization of program responsibility. Consequently, the quality of services is variable and dependent on the support of regional administrations. For example, although Switzerland has one of the highest AIDS case rates in Europe, the Swiss government has little influence on policies for partner notification, because the decision-making authority for such public health activities lies with the cantons.

Provider referral has been used most extensively in the Scandinavian countries, which have comparatively low rates of HIV infection and a tradition of proactive outreach for STD control. In Sweden, where confidential provider referral for STD has been in place for more than 20 years, legislation requires health care providers to notify partners of STD patients; in 1985, this law was expanded to include HIV infection as an STD. (See Chapter 13, "Human Rights," for another perspective on the Swedish Experience.) Data from Sweden's national program have been used to assess the prevention impact of provider referral, as well as to study behavior change, transmission risk, and HIV incidence trends nationwide.[106]

In the national Swedish program, over an 18-month period in 1989–90, 365 HIV-infected persons reported 564 sex and needle-sharing partners; 26 percent of the index patients (including 33 percent of homosexual index patients) did not name a partner. Of the identified partners, 174 (31 percent) could not be located. Of the remaining 390 partners who received counseling, 350 had known test results; 127 partners (36 percent) were found to be infected. Only 53 (42 percent of all positives) were newly identified infections; 29 individuals (55 percent of those with new infections) were identified through provider referral. The estimated programmatic costs per newly diagnosed HIV infection was U.S.$700.[107]

The Directorate of Health of Norway actively encourages partner notification and has sent all physicians guidelines for carrying out the process.[108] In Oslo, partner notification has been incorporated into the AIDS prevention program since 1986; partners are sent a registered letter advising them to undergo HIV counseling and testing. Thirty-nine percent of partners presenting for testing were notified through provider referral. Overall, 37 percent of HIV partners were found to be infected, including 7 percent of partners found through provider referral. However, 30 of the 65 infected partners (46 percent) notified through provider referral were unaware of their risk for infection.[109]

In Iceland and Finland, patient referral is encouraged with less reliance on clinic staff to carry out provider referral. In Iceland, however, HIV-infected persons are obligated by law to name partners who subsequently must be tested for HIV. Extensive records in a central clinic in the capital can be used by staff to locate and notify sex partners.[110]

Compulsory notification of STDs was abandoned by Denmark in 1988. Although officially encouraged, partner notification remains the primary responsibility of individual physicians without formal involvement of other public health personnel. Greenland, with high rates of STDs and substance abuse among its indigenous peoples, presents a uniquely favorable environment for heterosexual HIV transmission. The first HIV infections, reported in 1985, prompted an aggressive control program that included mandatory AIDS reporting, reporting of both positive and negative HIV test results, and provider referral by district public health staff. By early 1992, 37 cases of HIV infection and 6 AIDS cases were reported from 6 generations of HIV contact investigations.[111]

The HIV epidemic began later in Central and Eastern Europe. None of the 8 countries in this region had reported domestic cases of AIDS before 1985, and since then, relatively few cases have been reported.[112] Early approaches to identifying cases and controlling HIV relied on widespread institutional testing (in STD clinics, prisons, and maternity hospitals), compulsory reporting of cases, and mandatory provider referral. For example, by January 1991, nearly 30 percent of the population of the former USSR and 54 percent of the population of Bulgaria had been tested through these screening programs, yielding 523 and 90 HIV infections, respectively. However, the iatrogenic transmission of HIV infection through poor sterilization practices and from infections with contaminated blood has emerged as a major cause of HIV transmission in some of these countries.

In the former USSR, provider referral is required by law for STDs, including HIV, with special attention given to wives and children and also to donors and recipients of blood transfusions. In general, patients will notify only their current partners, most often opting for provider referral rather than patient referral.

Government programs have identified chains of transmission. For example, 1 homosexual man was found to have infected 5 of his 22 sex partners; these partners, in turn, infected 4 women, who transmitted HIV to 2 of their children. Five other individuals were infected through blood transfusion from an infected partner, and one of the transfusion recipients transmitted HIV to her husband. This investigation identified 16 previously undiagnosed HIV infections.[113]

Similarly, a careful epidemiologic study in the former USSR, prompted by the discovery of an HIV-infected infant, uncovered a chain of heterosexual, vertical, and nosocomial transmission. In all, 197 children with iatrogenically acquired HIV infection were identified at 8 separate hospitals over a 6-month period.

In Romania, unscreened blood had been given extensively as *micro-injections* to malnourished children before HIV testing began in 1990. This practice resulted in more than 1,300 cases of HIV infection in children under 3 years of age, accounting for 94 percent of all the identified HIV cases in the country. By contrast, the pattern of HIV transmission in Yugoslavia and Poland is dominated by an unusually rapid spread among injection drug users, whereas in Bulgaria and Czechoslovakia, sexual transmission predominates. In Hungary, all persons with AIDS and HIV infection are reported, and regulations require that partners be screened if names are given.[114]

Whereas many of these countries, including the former USSR and Poland, have promoted provider referral, policymakers in some countries have begun to modify programs. For example, legislation will soon be introduced in Czechoslovakia to allow anonymous testing in the hope that clients will not be deterred from seeking HIV testing by having to reveal their names or the identity of partners.[115]

There are North-South and East-West differences in the prominence of partner notification in HIV control programs in Europe. Partner notification has been easier to implement in Scandinavia, where there is a low prevalence of infection and a small proportion of cases in drug users; a tradition of proactive programs for STD control with strong legislation; good access to treatment; and a generally positive attitude among health care providers. In the larger countries of Southern Europe and the Mediterranean, where these factors are not so recognizable, the evolution of partner notification has been very different. Here, the scale and complexity of the epidemic and the problems of putting into place basic prevention activities (e.g., health education and risk-reduction programs) have made partner notification a low priority in most countries.

In Western Europe, where the exposure groups are more heterogeneous, STD treatment services are accessible, but poorly coordinated in most countries (with the exception of the United Kingdom). Also, although health professionals are more aware of the issues, their concern about ethics and confidentiality seems to have dominated policymaking. Professional education and better coordination of STD control programs are needed before partner notification can be widely adopted.

Most countries in Eastern Europe, with few cases reported, have a history of coercive regulations for STD control. This prompted an aggressive approach to partner notification initially, but more recently, the lessons learned from programs in Western European countries have been recognized and acted on. Programs have adopted more voluntary and anonymous testing to improve compliance and avoid stigmatization of infected persons. As new programs are established in response to the growing epidemic, there is an opportunity to incorporate partner notification more appropriately.

Africa

In sub-Saharan Africa, HIV transmission occurs principally through heterosexual exposure and is closely linked to STDs. The control of STD has become a high priority, and patients are routinely encouraged to notify and refer partners. However, as the HIV epidemic escalated, the large number of cases made provider referral increasingly impractical. In Botswana, local health officials notified individuals who had been partners of infected blood donors or AIDS patients for the previous 3 years. The program was not successful because infected individuals often experienced discrimination, and patients were unwilling to identify extramarital partners.[116]

Of the 9 African and Middle Eastern countries responding to the *AIDS in the World* survey, only Côte d'Ivoire reports having a provider referral program for HIV infection at the present time. By contrast, Nigeria, Senegal, Tanzania, and Rwanda, as well as Côte d'Ivoire, report provider referral services for STDs.

Partner notification programs have not been a key part of STD or HIV programs in Africa. Cultural factors have inhibited the consistent use of patient referral within the (few) areas with established prevention programs. In theory, confidential provider referral for STDs, including HIV, might be feasible, even operating within these cultural constraints. However, due to the lack of resources available for health services and prevention—coupled with the sheer magnitude of the HIV epidemic—resource-intensive provider referral is not likely to become an integral component of HIV prevention programs in Africa.

Asia

Partner referral, used in prevention programs for STD control in Thailand for many years, was applied to HIV infection early in the epidemic. Index patients were almost exclusively female and male commercial sex workers, injection drug users, and prisoners identified through screening programs. Among 129 identified partners, 71 (55 percent) were foreigners. Only 25 of 58 Thai partners (43 percent) were notified and tested; 7 (28 percent) were found to be infected, compared to 80 percent for partners of STD patients notified through partner notification. The HIV epidemic has rapidly spread in Thailand among injection drug users and heterosexuals, and an estimated 400,000 persons nationwide are currently estimated to be HIV infected. Provider referral for HIV infection is not felt to be practical in Thailand given the current extent of the epidemic.

Provider referral for STDs has been routinely carried out in China. However, confidential provider referral for HIV has been difficult due to the common cultural practice of not directly informing a patient of serious personal illness. Instead, relatives or local leaders are usually told of the serious illness in others; when confidentiality for HIV is broken, the patient risks severe stigmatization. Public health groups are encouraging the development of confidential notification for HIV.[117]

In contrast, national law in Japan requires physicians to report AIDS cases and to inform patients about HIV infection. Although partner notification is encouraged in Japan, the survey reported that no formal provider referral program is in place. In exceptional circumstances, the name of the patient may be given to the prefectural governor if the physician suspects that a patient is transmitting HIV to others.[118]

The government of India reported provider referral programs for both STDs and HIV in response to the survey. However, these programs have been controversial and have had negative effects in some communities. It has been difficult to maintain confidentiality, and there are anecdotal reports that individuals have been identified in the media with dire consequences for themselves and their families— so much so that partner notification by providers has been actively discouraged in some areas.

Latin America and the Caribbean

The Caribbean countries have reported some of the highest rates for AIDS in the Americas, with an early rapid increase in cases and a later increase in cases among women due to heterosexual transmission.[119] Sexually transmitted diseases are also highly prevalent, and treatment programs have been established in Trinidad and Tobago, Jamaica, Barbados, Suriname, Guyana, and Belize. However, in many Caribbean countries, general practitioners outside the government programs may see many more STD cases than do hospital clinics.[120] Provider referral is commonly used for STDs and is recommended in regional guidelines for patient management, but has been approached more cautiously for HIV and is offered in a limited way in a few countries.

Both Haiti and St. Lucia reported in the *AIDS in the World* survey to have partner notification programs for both STDs and HIV. In Trinidad and Tobago, provider referral has not been officially encouraged because of fears of loss of confidentiality and stigmatization. However, the Ministry of Health recently gave permission to monitor contacts, and partner notification may now be pursued more vigorously by health care providers.[121]

In Jamaica, HIV/AIDS prevention was incorporated into the existing STD program while the prevalence of HIV infection was low. The names of all persons with HIV/AIDS infection are kept on a confidential register, and trained contact investigators from the program assist in notifying and counseling partners. In the mid-1980s, approximately 50 percent were found to be infected; by November 1991, 288 cases of AIDS and 800 HIV infections had been identified this way. However, public health workers have been diverted by increases in other STDs, especially syphilis, and more staff have been recruited to meet the extra demands of the HIV/AIDS program. The efficacy of the program is now under review, and the resource demands of the current partner notification policies are being evaluated.[122]

In Costa Rica, provider referral has been implemented for HIV/

AIDS cases, STD patients, prisoners, commercial sex workers, and blood donors using trained social workers from the Ministry of Health STD program. Early in the epidemic, 40 chains of transmission were investigated and 200 HIV-infected partners identified. These partners identified 1,500 additional partners, of whom 33 percent were investigated. However the cost per identified partner (approximately US$50) was high for a country with limited health care resources.[123]

The HIV control program in Cuba is controversial, based on mass screening of the population, mandatory contact tracing by Ministry of Health staff, seroepidemiological studies of all partners of infected persons, and indefinite quarantine of seropositive individuals.[124] As of January 1990, 309 of approximately 6.4 million HIV tests were positive; a high proportion of these involved Cubans returning from abroad. The Cuban program has raised many ethical, economic, and practical concerns, and the efficacy of this approach has not been established.[125]

Although in Mexico some public health jurisdictions offer provider referral for STDs and HIV, few areas presently offer these services. According to survey results, provider referral for HIV is generally not available in other Latin American countries, and no data are available from partner notification programs.

North America

In Canada, the 10 provinces and 2 territories are responsible for provision of health services (including public health functions) and are organized based on provincial legislation, regulation, and organization. In 7 of the 10 provinces (except for British Columbia, Alberta, and Quebec), reporting of HIV infection is required; in Quebec and Ontario, anonymous HIV testing is available. The resources invested in provider referral for HIV vary greatly from province to province and do not correlate with HIV reporting requirements.[126]

A review of partner notification for HIV as well as other STDs, was recently carried out by investigators at the University of Toronto and McMaster University. Based on a survey of 118 local health units, of which 103 (87.3 percent) responded, 74 percent of health units reported some partner notification activities, and 25 percent provided partner notification for more than half of HIV cases. The method of partner notification was distributed equally among provider referral, patient referral, or a combination of both. Physician cooperation in partner notification was reported to be poorer for HIV than for other STDs.[127]

In the United States, partner notification in some form has been required as a condition for receiving federal HIV prevention funds since 1988. At a minimum, patient referral is offered at publicly funded counseling and testing sites, and provider referral is offered by all states under certain circumstances.[128] Twenty-two states emphasize provider referral for clients accepting confidential HIV testing at STD clinics. Some states offer provider referral support for clients tested at primary care facilities, such as family planning or prenatal clinics. Some programs have limited partner notification to heterosexual clients, with an emphasis on women of reproductive age to prevent vertical HIV transmission.[129]

Although the cost of provider referral services is higher than the cost of community education efforts, state and local programs have demonstrated the effectiveness of these programs for locating partners who may not be aware of their risk for infection,[130] and who have consistently reported good patient compliance with the process.[131] The acceptance of provider referral by high-risk clients in the United States is encouraging, because recent studies have reported conflicting results for the success of patient referral alone among men who have sex with men.[132]

Several evaluations of provider referral are being carried out in the United States to assess the acceptance of provider referral and to identify populations that may benefit most from these programs. A randomized evaluation of partner notification in North Carolina found that provider referral was more effective than patient referral for reaching partners at risk.[133] Of the 74 clients agreeing to participate (out of 162 eligible clients), 39 were randomized to provider referral and 35 to patient referral. In the provider referral group, 78 of 157 partners (50 percent) were successfully notified compared with only 10 of 153 (7 percent) in the patient referral group. Of those notified through provider referral, 94 percent were not aware of their risk for HIV infection.

A multicenter evaluation currently is being conducted by the Centers for Disease Control at three STD clinic sites in Ft. Lauderdale and Tampa, Florida, and Paterson, New Jersey. Patients with HIV are randomized to 1 of 4 partner notification methods currently used in STD clinics in the United States: patient referral, patient referral with provider referral follow-up (contract referral), provider referral with clinic testing, and provider referral with field counseling and testing. Syphilis patients are similarly randomized to contract and provider referral strategies. This evaluation has already enrolled more than 1,000 clients and will assess the comparative efficacy as well as the cost and cost-effectiveness of provider referral and patient referral strategies for HIV and STD.[134] A similar evaluation of partner notification in drug treatment centers is being developed by the National Institute on Drug Abuse, in conjunction with the Centers for Disease Control, and will be implemented in the coming year. These evaluations will provide critical information to better focus partner outreach activities in HIV prevention programs in the United States.

Conclusions

Even though curative therapies are available for STDs, few countries report carrying out systematic partner notification for STDs, let alone HIV. Provider referral for STD has been reported to be successful in controlling focused outbreaks in limited areas; however, no systematic evaluation of its efficacy for endemic STDs has been undertaken.[135] Furthermore, cultural and resource constraints have limited widespread partner notification implementation. In much of the world, private providers rather than organized public health programs provide STD/HIV care. Partner notification activities are generally not monitored among these private sector clinicians and are carried out irregularly, if at all.

Partner notification for HIV infection can be conceptualized as targeted outreach to individuals at high risk for HIV infection—sex and/or needle-sharing partners of HIV-infected individuals. The long-term impact of partner notification on risk-reduction behavior may be even greater than that for other voluntary counseling and testing programs, because knowledge of personal exposure to HIV may motivate partners to sustain behavior changes.

The most developed programs for partner notification are in the industrialized countries, particularly Scandinavia and the United States, where provider referral for HIV has been integrated into some STD prevention programs. Among the less developed nations, especially in Africa, cultural and resource constraints have limited the implementation of organized partner notification programs.

The relative role partner notification programs will play within an HIV prevention program will be determined by the local epidemiology of HIV/STD, cultural variables affecting the acceptability of the process, existing HIV prevention activities, the availability of financial and personnel resources, and the structure of the health care delivery system.[136] Thus, no global template for an ideal partner notification program is possible.

However, several needs have been consistently identified by public health officials. Training programs on the management and referral of partners should be developed for health care professionals in a variety of patient care settings. With additional training, providers will have a better understanding of the objectives of partner notification and can develop the skills necessary to carry out both patient and provider referral counseling more effectively. Technical support is needed to develop such training programs and to initiate formal partner notification programs in both resource-rich and resource-poor settings.

Technical assistance is needed to develop meaningful quantitative and qualitative evaluations of partner notification, especially in resource-poor settings. Quantitative measures of program activity may include number of index persons identified; number of partners notified, counseled, and tested; and program costs. Qualitative program measures may include acceptability of the process, quality of counseling messages, and patient compliance with the process.[137] However, the exact evaluation measures chosen must reflect the nature of the individual programs.

In countries with well-developed provider referral programs, such as the Scandinavian countries and the United States, partner notification programs have successfully located many partners unaware of their risk for infection. Without notification, it is unlikely that these partners would have been tested for HIV, potentially gaining access to needed services early in the course of their infection. The potential for identifying partners as yet uninfected and unaware of their risk—to achieve primary prevention of HIV through risk-reduction behavior—is another compelling rationale for supporting partner notification outreach.

However, individuals with HIV/AIDS have experienced stigmatization in many countries. Thus, many providers are uneasy about carrying out partner notification themselves or endorsing widespread programs, fearing further discrimination against patients or partners. Providers have expressed the conflict they feel between their roles as counselors and patient advocates and their public health responsibilities for the prevention and control of STD/HIV.[138] Furthermore, the political discourse in many countries has polarized the debate around partner notification, linking provider referral with mandatory, coercive—even draconian—measures.[139] Mandatory partner-tracing programs, such as those in some Eastern European countries and in Cuba, have raised legitimate concerns about the potential for discrimination.

Recently, partner notification has received greater public acceptance by advocacy groups and clinical providers, in part due to the availability of improved prophylactic and antiviral therapies for HIV, as well as greater awareness of the potential public health benefits of the process. However, partner notification can only serve as a public health tool if the human rights of both index persons and their partners are protected. Only then, can voluntary, confidential partner notification serve appropriately as an adjunct to other HIV prevention, outreach, and education strategies.

■■■■■ .   .   .

AIDS IN THE MEDIA

Phyllida Brown

Phyllida Brown is a correspondent for *The New Scientist* in London.

If journalism is the first draft of history, future generations may remember the 1980s as much for the emergence of AIDS as for the collapse of communism or the faltering of apartheid. Worldwide, AIDS remained a top news story for the latter part of the 1980s, rivaling—and in many cases outlasting—wars, famine, civil disorder, and economic developments. This media fascination has endured into the 1990s, with AIDS becoming a media benchmark for evaluating the state of the world. In the parlance of journalists, AIDS has maintained its "newsworthiness" as a story because it combines the basic ele-

Table 16.3: Number of news items on AIDS compared with number on selected other subjects, 1991

Subject	Washington Post	Associated Press	BBC
AIDS[a]	554	436	270
Nelson Mandela	139	384	282
Mikhail Gorbachev	1,300	3,057	3,360
Saddam Hussein	1,615	2,454	7[b]
Breast cancer	103	49	1

Source: FT Profile Database.

a. Searching for articles on AIDS in an electronic database is complicated by the fact that the search will also identify articles containing the unrelated verb *aids* and the plural noun *aids*. In a sample analysis of 100 articles, roughly two-thirds of those identified by the search were found to be about the disease. The figures shown here have been adjusted accordingly to take this fact into acount. **Clearly, these figures are a guide only.**

b. There were 3,109 items mentioning the Gulf War.

ments of human existence—sex, life, and death—with scientific, social, cultural, and political issues.

Indeed, AIDS has become the first global health story. Like no other health story before it, AIDS spans all cultures and societies, in industrialized and developing countries alike. Yet for all its importance as a story, AIDS carries with it another obligation—thrusting onto the media the often unwanted and ambiguous role of educator for an audience that, by and large, relies on the press for nearly all it knows about AIDS. Thus, 10 years ito the AIDS pandemic, a number of questions can be posed about the media's role: What is the value of media coverage? Can it maintain its intensity? How have the media shaped the global response to the epidemic? Can the media educate people about AIDS? Are the lines between media objectivity and advocacy blurring? And most important, does media coverage matter?

The Role of Media Coverage

The reporting of AIDS has often been criticized,[140] but few critics challenge the media's importance in defining this disease and shaping society's response. Not only have news organizations helped to determine how and when AIDS has reached the public agenda;[141] but they are also the principal sources of information about AIDS for most people worldwide.[142]

This gives the media an enormous responsibility. If they inform their audiences accurately about HIV and how it is and is not transmitted, they can enable individuals to reduce their vulnerability to HIV—as well as the fear and discrimination that accopmany it. Conversely, if the media provide ambiguous or inaccurate information, they may contribute to placing people at increased risk of HIV infection.

AIDS Reporting in Context

AIDS has been called "the first media disease."[143] Although previous epidemics—particularly cholera and polio[144]—have attracted journalists' attention, this attention has tended to be more localized and coverage more limited. AIDS, by contrast, has triggered an unprecedented volume of media reports. Why?

The answers are complex, given the differing cultures in which AIDS has emerged. A cynical explanation is that AIDS, a disease that involves sex and death, provides journalists with all the ingredients for sensationalist copy. Another interpretation is that this disease, a major new threat to health in our time, has forced us to confront in ourselves, or resist confronting, the comfortable boundaries that define our own identity: gender, sexuality, nationality.[145]

Because of its unique nature, AIDS raises contested and dangerous issues. Journalists have responded by reporting AIDS with much greater intensity than other diseases. But they have also tended to report it within their own boundaries and prejudices.[146] Thus, AIDS first came into the news as a problem of "others"—gay men, foreigners, drug users—rather than as an urgent threat to all. A decade later, the picture is changing, but slowly.

Patterns in the Coverage of AIDS

Most analysts of media coverage have concentrated on the *content* of reporting.[147] They identify common themes that have recurred reliably over time and across cultures.

The theme of the infected *other* has been especially persistent.

Thus in the West, AIDS was first labeled the *gay plague*.[148] In many developing countries, the disease was seen as an exotic product of the distant, Western life-style. In Zimbabwe, journalists wrote more about AIDS in the United States than AIDS in Zimbabwe.[149] In Ghana, AIDS was described as a "white man's burden."[150] In Brazil, the media's portrayal of AIDS in the United States defined the disease as one of white, rich gay men. This meant, according to one analyst, that Brazilian society "responded to an imaginary model of AIDS and not to an epidemic with characteristics specific to its national culture and public health conditions."[151]

Once it became known in the West that HIV affected heterosexuals as well as homosexual men, many journalists in industrialized countries turned their attention to Africa. Theories about a supposed African origin for HIV received widespread coverage, and the media conveyed the impression that the whole African continent was synonymous with the disease.[152] These reactions, in turn, caused great offense among many Africans, triggering an epidemic of counterblame of the West.[153]

The media have repeatedly drawn distinctions between *innocent victims* of HIV, that is, infants and recipients of infected blood or blood products through health care, and other infected people who, by implication, are perceived as guilty of causing their own affliction. They, and not the virus, are seen as the principal threat to society.

Journalists have also consistently emphasized rare or bizarre ways in which HIV could be spread, rather than concentrating on the common modes of transmission. This tendency highlights one important potential conflict between the role of the journalist and that of the health educator. The journalist wants news about HIV; by definition, this may be different from the health educator's interest in explaining established risk factors.

Thus, the patients of a Florida dentist, who appear to have been infected in his office, have received massive coverage compared with the other one million HIV-infected people in the United States. In Zimbabwe, one analysis found stories about injection drug users to be more frequent than stories about blood screening or pregnancy, which, the authors argue, are "rather more relevant" in Zimbabwe.[154] *The News of the World*, a popular British tabloid Sunday paper with

Table 16.4: Number of items on AIDS compared with number of items on other selected diseases, *Washington Post*, 1984–1991

Subject	1984	1985	1986	1987	1988	1989	1990	1991
AIDS	110	290	332	717	665	546	514	554
Herpes	17	49	32	34	36	17	13	19
Breast cancer	24	52	56	76	73	84	96	103
Malaria	24	30	16	36	34	30	39	29

Source: FT Profile Database.

a circulation of 4.7 million, treated its readers to a rare feature on AIDS on the day that dying rock star Freddie Mercury announced he had the disease. Rather than discuss safer sex, the article tackled "peril at the dentist."

These, then, have been the common themes. But how has AIDS coverage evolved over time? Analysts in the United States and Europe identify three broad phases.[155] The hallmarks of reporting in the early years were ignorance, denial, and moral panic. The second phase, around 1987 and 1988, was characterized by energetic, even frenetic coverage, in which virtually any event or scientific development was seen as news. Reporters' knowledge of the subject was improving, but audiences were subjected to a roller-coaster of alternating optimism and despair, as claims of breakthrough mingled with apocalyptic projections.

The third phase, beginning around 1989, has seen a slight decline in the volume of reporting that nevertheless leaves AIDS higher on the public agenda than other health issues. (See Table 16.4.) In developing and industrialized countries alike, there is now a tendency to report AIDS as another running story in the policy arena. News organizations plan their reporting around prearranged events, such as the international AIDS conferences and World AIDS Day.

Although many journalists are now better informed, their cultural judgments still affect coverage. In 1991, for instance, the British press tried to explain the nation's gradually rising levels of heterosexual infection by blaming foreigners. At the VII International Conference on AIDS in Florence, Italy, in 1991, the parochial concerns of

Table 16.5: Volume of AIDS coverage in the science section *Jornal do Brasil*, January–February, 1987–1990

Period: January–February	Reports on AIDS in science section (%)
1987	25.0
1988	14.9
1989	9.3
1990	6.3

Source: Analysis by Brazilian journalist Sergio Adeodato, published in the *Boletim ABIA,* October 1990, provided by Silvia Ramos, Associaçïo Brasileira Interdisciplinar de AIDS (ABIA), Rio de Janeiro.

Washington dominated the coverage of a supposedly international meeting, while new science was trivialized and behavioral research ignored.

Ups and Downs in AIDS Reporting

Within each of these three broad phases, coverage has varied from month to month. News organizations have given AIDS saturation coverage only intermittently, usually when the disease looked less like a disease of others and more like a threat to the general audience. Thus, reporting has tended to be cyclical, with peaks of coverage interspersed with longer periods of routine, more reactive reporting. (See Tables 16.5 and 16.6.) For example, news peaked worldwide in 1985, when actor Rock Hudson sought treatment for AIDS and the disease first became real to most Americans, and again in late 1991, when basketball star Magic Johnson announced he was HIV infected. * Johnson made a huge media impact, not only in the United States but also in the developing world. Studies in the United States, Britain, and France suggest roughly the same patterns of peaks and quieter periods, with the same worries over the blood supply, infants, and heterosexual

*Dialog database of all major U.S. newspapers found 5,666 references to Magic Johnson between November 7, 1991 and January 9, 1992.

Table 16.6: Call attempts to the U.S. National AIDS Hotline, January–September 1991

Date/period	Number of call attempts	Concomitant events
January 10	10,730	America responds to AIDS public service announcement (PSA) aired on ABC during the "Doogie Howser, MD" program
February		Nothing significant
March 7	8,404	NBC news program "A Closer Look" airs a segment on teens and AIDS
March 11	10,089	CBS PSA featuring actress Michelle Lee with regard to support groups
April 9	10,341	HBO program "First Love Fatal Love"
April 20	8,896	HBO program rebroadcast of "First Love Fatal Love"
April 26	9,404	America responds to AIDS PSA aired
May 21	10,576	News story concerning the American Red Cross and the safety of organ transplants
May 28	10,567	American responds to AIDS PSA aired
June 10	10,847	HBO program "First Love Fatal Love"
June 22	12,286	Kimberly Bergalis, VII International Conference on AIDS featured in the news
June 25	10,876	Kimberly Bergalis, VII International Conference on AIDS featured in the news
June 26	11,170	Kimberly Bergalis, VII International Conference on AIDS featured in the news
July 16	13,413	CDC announcement of new health care worker guidelines
July 17	10,310	ABC "Good Morning America" news segment on HIV/AIDS
August 29	9,473	NBC news program "A Closer Look" airs a segment on HIV/AIDS
September 18	38,523	PBS broadcast of "In the Shadow of Love: A Teen AIDS Story"

Source: U.S. Centers for Disease Control, Atlanta, Georgia.

transmission.[156] In Senegal and South Africa, comparable cycles have been observed, based on interviews with journalists and delegates in Dakar, in 1991.

AIDS is certainly not unique in its cyclical coverage. The pattern appears to be a feature of the media's response to many policy stories and is known as the *issue attention cycle*.[157] For example, coverage of global warming has tended to rise and fall; each rise comes when the media find a new angle. With AIDS, as with other subjects, the cycle is driven by news values and the agenda of the media, rather than by actual trends. For example, published research into HIV has increased consistently, first sharply and now more slowly, ever since 1981. However, news coverage has been much more erratic. Similarly, the volume of reporting has not matched trends in the numbers of people affected by the pandemic.

Assessing the Impact of the News

It is more difficult to gauge the impact of media coverage on nations, communities, and individuals. Any such assessment is open to pitfalls. For example, it is naive to imagine that a homogeneous media acts on an equally homogeneous society. It is also dangerous to conclude that specific coverage is causally linked with specific policy changes, or that the process works in one direction only. Journalists' sources, such as politicians or officials, can manipulate them to cover an issue from a particular angle, thus helping to set the political agenda.[158] Scientists, too, can manipulate reporters who still tend to view their word as gospel. This may lead to so-called expert opinion being reported as fact or to minor developments being portrayed as major breakthroughs.

Perhaps because of such complicating factors, few researchers have attempted formally to measure the impact of AIDS coverage on policies. One analysis has argued that peaks in news coverage have stimulated shifts in policy in the United States. Only where news coverage has been at saturation level and reassurance has been outweighed by concern, the authors argue, has public opinion on AIDS shifted and has discussion in government moved forward. Thus, these coverage peaks, not the number of AIDS cases or a *critical* mass of scientific concern, have set AIDS on the agenda.[159] The same authors have shown that the number of bills about AIDS introduced into the

Number of Seconds (thousands)

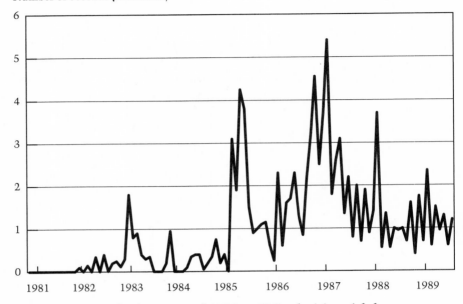

Figure 16.2. Seconds of coverage of AIDS on U.S. television nightly news, June 1981–December 1989.
Source: Vanderbilt University Television News Abstracts and Index, 1981–89, cited in D.C. Colby and T.E. Cook, "Epidemics and agendas: The politics of nightly news coverage of AIDS," *Journal of Health Politics, Policy, and Law* 16 (1991): 215-49.

U.S. Congress rose alongside the average number of seconds of media coverage of AIDS on nightly television news. In this study, the trend in the number of bills was "much closer to the irregular media attention than to the rise in cases or in medical attention." (See Figures 16.2 and 16.3.) An analysis of British coverage, however, suggests that the media have been "important, but not monolithic" in affecting public health policy on AIDS. For example, the right-wing press coverage on AIDS has attracted much criticism but has had relatively little effect on policy.[160]

Nevertheless, some peaks may have had a clear effect: the publicity surrounding Magic Johnson triggered a surge in demand for HIV tests in the United States and a consequent promise of more funds for testing.[161] The impact of other peaks, meanwhile, has been much less

Number of Bills

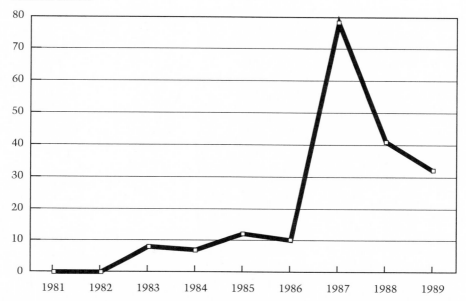

Figure 16.3. Number of bills on AIDS introduced into U.S. Congress, 1981–1989.
Source: SCORPIO Index, cited in D.C. Colby and T.E. Cook, "Epidemics and agendas: The politics of nightly news coverage of AIDS," *Journal of Health Politics, Policy, and Law* 16 (1991): 215-49.

obvious: despite the Rock Hudson furor, the U.S. government did not recognize AIDS as a national emergency. Recently, critical coverage of U.S. immigration and travel authorization policies on people with HIV has failed to shift the administration position.

Assessing the impact of news is, therefore, difficult—a problem that media sociologists recognized long before the emergence of AIDS. Their debate is excellently described elsewhere.[162] In summary, most consider that the media play a *part* in setting the agenda by stimulating discussion. News media can "tell the public what to think *about* if not exactly what to think."[163]

In the absence of better means to measure the media's effects, imperfect measures must be used. Developing countries have felt the alarming impact of media coverage about AIDS on their economies. In Kenya, for instance, the tourist industry is the second biggest source of foreign currency, employing some 85,000 people. Early in 1987, news reports in Britain said that two Kenyan resorts, Mombasa and Malindi, had been put out of bounds to British troops stationed in Manyuki because members of other British crews returning from leave in Mombasa had tested positive for HIV. One hotelier reported that 50 percent of his bookings had been canceled, and the hoteliers' association claimed widespread damage from the reports. A representative of the association begged the Kenyan government to take "urgent steps so as to stop these destructive headlines about Kenya."[164] In Haiti, too, adverse media attention has reportedly done lasting damage to the tourist industry.[165]

Governments forced to limit such damage may have been inhibited from giving AIDS vital publicity at a crucial early stage in the epidemic. As late as 1988, health ministers in some African countries were forced to spend time rebutting exaggerated reports by western journalists instead of building up their own AIDS programs.[166] In Thailand, however, when the government decided in the late 1980s to adopt an open, progressive attitude on AIDS, tourism overall was unaffected, despite the initial fears of the industry.[167]

Difficult as it may be to assess the effect of news on nations' policies, it is somewhat easier to see the impact on the public. One measure is the volume of calls to AIDS hotlines. For example, staff at the National AIDS Hotline in the United States know to expect *spikes* in the volume of calls after particular broadcasts and media coverage peaks. (See Figure 16.4.)

The volume of these calls indicates an overall impact but says little about individual understanding of the story. Small-scale studies have shed some light on this problem. For example, the Glasgow Media Group has surveyed the understanding of AIDS in the media among different audience groups.[168] The survey found that people were confused, for example, by the meaning of the term *body fluids,* which British newspapers used regularly in reference to HIV. Audiences were unsure whether this meant sexual fluids and blood, or other fluids such as urine or saliva. Such vague terms, the result of squeamishness on the part of editors, could contribute to making individuals more vulnerable to HIV infection. In Zambia in 1990, the public was similarly confused by news reports about the drug Kemron, thinking that the drug was a cure for AIDS.[169]

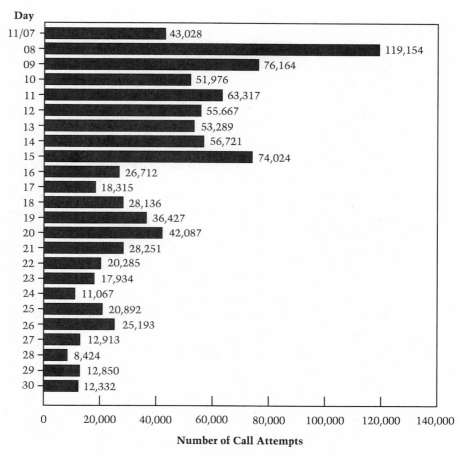

Figure 16.4. Calls to U.S. Centers for Disease Control National AIDS Hotline, November 7–30, 1991 (cumulative total: 915,158).
(Baseline for comparison: August 1–November 6, 1991, average daily call attempts=7,372.)

Looking to the Future

There is no sign that AIDS will stop being a media disease. But will it decline into the routine story that, say, cancer has become? Indications from the past would suggest that AIDS may remain unique, because of the cultural baggage that follows it everywhere. The frenzy of 1987 and 1988 has died down, but the same issues that made AIDS important to people in the 1980s will, it seems, continue to apply in the 1990s.

It is much more difficult to predict whether coverage will, or can, improve. In a few news organizations, particularly in the United States, specialized journalists are now covering the AIDS beat—with the result that coverage is better informed and is clearer in context. But others remain surprisingly slow to change. Critics have stressed the persistent failure of journalists to narrate AIDS from the viewpoint of those affected. They have also attacked reporters and editors for failing to realize that their audiences are diverse and concerned by AIDS. These criticisms are justified; nevertheless, the coverage of this disease has changed gear at least twice during the past decade and seems likely to do so again.

What should we expect of the media? Journalists can be highly effective communicators of information, but they are not health educators. Most do their utmost to get their facts right and to balance their accounts of events. According to interviews with journalists in Dakar in 1991 at the VI International Conference on AIDS in Africa, journalists in developing countries where the government may be the only source of information on AIDS often *do* function as health educators because they recognize that the priority is basic information. But where the media and their audiences have access to a range of sources, journalists can help to stimulate debate.

The response to AIDS in the next decade will be crucial. However media coverage changes in the future, the media will remain people's main source of information. If journalists accept their responsibility to get their facts right, and health educators accept the importance of news values, we may see a more accurate and socially useful account of AIDS in the 1990s.

AIDS AND MASS PERSUASION

Phyllis T. Piotrow, Rita C. Meyer, and Bernard A. Zulu

Phyllis T. Piotrow, Ph.D., and Rita C. Meyer are at the Center for Communication Programs, The Johns Hopkins University School of Hygiene and Public Health, Baltimore, Maryland; Bernard A. Zulu, M.A., is with Ben Zulu & Associates.

AIDS is the first international *mass media disease*. Throughout the world, most people have learned more about AIDS from radio, television, and the press than from personal contacts with health professionals.

In the United States, Western Europe, and Latin America, television is usually the major source of AIDS information.[170] In Asia and Africa, television reaches large cities, and radio reaches even remote villages and illiterate listeners with stories about AIDS.[171]

Although there has been considerable criticism of the media's coverage of AIDS,[172] virtually every treatment of AIDS in the mass media has in fact been a first. Whereas syphilis, gonorrhea, and other sexually transmitted diseases (STDs) remain, even today, relatively taboo as mass media topics, AIDS has been discussed extensively by the press, radio, and television. In the United States, AIDS was responsible for the first discussions of anal sex on television and, in many countries, for the first radio and television advertisements for condoms.[173]

News coverage of AIDS, however, has concentrated on new information released by scientists, on human interest stories, and on controversies rather than prevention messages. Journalists tend to focus on coverage that attracts large audiences. It is not surprising then that personalities and unique human interest stories (e.g., movie star Rock Hudson; basketball player Magic Johnson; teenager with hemophilia Ryan White, denied admission to school after contracting AIDS through a blood transfusion; and Kimberly Bergalis, infected by her dentist) became the focus of massive news coverage. As different media compete to release information that appears to be new or controversial, for example, origins of the disease, proposed new laws, and new treatments, relatively little press and broadcast space is devoted to detailed analysis or to the natural history of the disease, and even less to specific recommendations on how to avoid contracting HIV.[174]

Many countries have organized national information/education campaigns on AIDS, because efforts to curb the epidemic cannot rely solely on news media whose coverage of AIDS has been slow, erratic, and focused on new and unusual events. National campaigns are designed to alert people to the dangers of AIDS and to indicate what help is available and where it can be obtained. The campaigns vary greatly in their scope, sophistication, and use of mass media. The first generation of AIDS campaigns was generally designed in haste, preceded by very little audience research, and carried out primarily to alert the public. Yet a decade of experience with AIDS has taught important lessons in the use of mass media for AIDS education and prevention.[175] As second and third generation campaigns have begun to apply these lessons, the mass media are gradually becoming more effective channels for AIDS education. At the same time, however, government resources and political motivation for mass media education campaigns are becoming constrained. This section focuses primarily on educational campaigns using mass media to influence knowledge, attitudes, and behavior relevant to AIDS in various populations. It also summarizes the major lessons to be learned from the first decade of AIDS in the mass media.

Major Lessons Learned

1. People usually want to learn more about reproductive health, including AIDS, from mass media than policymakers are willing to tell them.

Experience in family planning promotion, condom social marketing, and AIDS prevention campaigns shows overwhelmingly that people expect to acquire information about reproductive health from mass media, especially radio and television, and that the great majority are not offended by such information. Demographic and health surveys in more than 22 countries during the late 1980s have shown, for example, that a median of almost 90 percent of married women of reproductive age approve of messages about family planning on radio and television.[176] Similarly, surveys, operations research studies, and impact evaluation of condom promotion in countries as varied as Barbados,[177] the Philippines,[178] Egypt,[179] Côte d'Ivoire,[180] and Colombia[181] find little or no public opposition to the promotion of specific family planning methods, including condoms. In Great Britain, for example, a survey showed that only 6 percent of adults were opposed to condom advertising on television, and 50 percent thought it was a good idea.[182]

Reluctant policymakers, however, have repeatedly kept public service announcements (PSAs) and other AIDS prevention materials from reaching the public. President Yoweri Museveni, for example, refused to allow condom promotion in Uganda because of fears of religious opposition.[183] An evaluation of 21 PSAs about AIDS from public health departments in Canada, Denmark, Norway, Sweden, the United Kingdom, and the United States revealed that 3 of the 5 spots considered most effective by 56 knowledgeable viewers had been rejected for general broadcast. The announcements judged least effective (because they were less factual, straightforward, and sincere) were broadcast much more frequently.[184] In virtually every country in the world, carefully designed materials have not been released because of opposition from politicians, broadcasters, or other gatekeepers who were afraid of arousing religious or other resistance. Where PSAs and materials have been allowed to reach the public, they have been subject to compromises in tone, language, and texture.

How can policymakers be persuaded to be bolder in using mass media for AIDS prevention campaigns? A special workshop to increase policymakers' understanding of the economic and social impact of AIDS persuaded Papua New Guinea policymakers to promote and support mass media AIDS educational efforts. Pretesting and evidence of audience approval is the approach that persuaded government health officials in Peru and Colombia to support condom promotion campaigns.[185] Findings from demographic and health surveys, showing that large majorities want clear and specific information, may reassure some policymakers. Also, private sector AIDS advocacy groups can bring pressure on government officials to counteract anticipated pressures from other sources.

2. Mass media AIDS materials influence behavior most when they are designed and developed for different segments of the audience, with the specific needs and concerns of those segments in mind.

Many of the early AIDS mass media programs for the general public were begun hurriedly, often skipping the preliminary research needed to generate materials that would be understood by the intended audience. In the United Kingdom, for example, injection drug users, the intended target of a campaign using posters and television spots, did not even perceive that the messages were aimed at them.[186] In Uganda, the first radio and print materials on AIDS were neither pretested with nor understood by rural audiences.[187]

In many countries, mass media have increased the public's awareness of AIDS, but have failed to influence their behavior. In Brazil, for example, 79 percent of survey respondents considered AIDS to be Brazil's most pressing health problem, 67 percent saw AIDS as a potential epidemic among the general population, and 84 percent thought that high-risk behavior included sexual contact with the opposite sex; yet only 14 percent reported changing to low-risk behaviors.[188]

Audience segmentation has always been crucial to successful commercial advertising. Social marketing programs show that audience segmentation is effective in AIDS prevention even where mass media are used. People who practice high-risk anal intercourse with multiple partners clearly require different messages than monogamous heterosexual couples. In Switzerland, for example, Hot Rubber condoms are specifically promoted for homosexual men, as are the thicker Doublex condoms in the Netherlands.[189] For heterosexual men, the messages are different. Prudence condoms in Zaire are sold to men as protection against both pregnancy and STDs.[190] In Colombia, condoms promoted to young men advise, "Keep being free. Use Tahiti condoms."[191]

Women are increasingly recognized as an especially vulnerable group requiring very different messages than men. Most women, even commercial sex workers, cannot control their sexual partners' use of condoms.[192] Surveys in Zaire, for example, show that women understand the risks of HIV infection when their husbands have other partners, but they do not know what actions to take. "*Que puis-je faire?*" (What can I do?) they ask.[193] Mass media campaigns for women might focus on initiating discussion of condoms and persuading their partners to use them, rather than on raising additional fears.

Mass media can also influence less educated audiences, provided the messages and materials are designed to meet their needs. A carefully designed campaign in the rural Philippines produced 14 changes in AIDS-related beliefs, the greatest changes having occurred among the less educated.[194]

3. In mass media AIDS promotion (as in all other types of communication), the first effort will attract more attention than will any subsequent efforts. Yet because of time pressure, the first effort is often not pretested and, therefore, not as effective as it could be.

The advertising slogan "You never get a second chance to make a first impression" applies to mass media AIDS education. The first advertisements, announcements, posters, spots, and other products usually attract a much larger audience than do subsequent efforts. In the United Kingdom, the first public announcement was a long statement printed in small type with no illustration. It was not tested beforehand. A test afterward showed that although 42 percent of the population had seen or read the announcement, only 25 percent had understood it. A second announcement, with simpler language and larger type, was understood by more people, but only 24 percent had read it.[195] Similarly, in Zimbabwe, U.S. and European materials were not tested before use in the first national awareness campaign in 1988. One undesired result that the spots fostered was the view that Africans with AIDS were homosexual.[196]

Mass media in Uganda offer both good and bad examples. Slogans and spots produced by the AIDS Control Program—one of the first national campaigns in Africa—were sometimes poorly understood or considered irrelevant. Many people did not understand the slogan "Zero grazing" (which means, in this context, stay with one partner).[197] Another frequently repeated spot, using drum beats to spread a sense of fear, did not appeal to young people who interpreted the drums as an appeal for abstinence.[198] Neither spot had been pretested. On the other hand, *It's Not Easy,* a feature film on AIDS, was developed cooperatively over a 3-year period with assistance from the Federation of Uganda Employers, Uganda TV, the Experiment in International Living/Uganda, AIDSCOM, and the United States Agency for International Development (USAID). As the first, full-length feature film on AIDS produced in Africa and based on local conditions, it was shown widely in Uganda and throughout Africa. Preliminary evaluation among 1,600 workers in 8 worksites revealed that those who had seen the film understood the message and intended to act on it (see Lesson 7).[199]

4. Mass media messages should evoke a positive emotional response and propose a practical, realistic course of action.

The primary reason for most public health campaigns is to avoid some type of sickness. Thus, fear is a common element in public health promotion. AIDS has been no exception. Yet much evidence from other fields, as well as from AIDS campaigns, indicates that although a little fear may prompt action, too much fear discourages it.[200] In Australia's first mass media AIDS campaign, appeals to fear worried people at low risk, but were largely ignored by those at highest risk. The Australian campaign used a frightening Grim Reaper image to portray AIDS as imminent death. The result was an increase of more than 100 percent in the number of lower-risk heterosexuals and blood transfusion recipients requesting HIV blood tests, but a decrease in clinical visits by higher-risk homosexual men. All callers showed a high level of general anxiety,[201] but the fear aroused by the Grim Reaper visuals was apparently so great that those at highest risk practiced denial and did not respond.

Sensational news coverage or poorly planned mass media efforts can actually set back AIDS prevention efforts. In Nigeria, for example, frightening and confusing information about AIDS in radio broadcasts, newspapers, and print material resulted in negative attitudes toward people with AIDS and unfounded fears about the risk of infection.[202]

In contrast, the AIDS campaign in Switzerland illustrates the value of positive approaches and practical suggestions. The campaign slogan "STOP AIDS" uses a rolled-up condom in place of the O in STOP. Imaginative and humorous posters showed a rolled-up condom shining like the moon over various Swiss cities. Later versions, developed after consultation with religious leaders, show the same scene with the condom replaced by a shining wedding ring. The emotional tone is glamour, romance, and fidelity. This lighthearted approach, shown nationwide in many media, had a positive impact in Switzerland in increasing condom use among young people (see Lesson 6).[203]

Fortunately, more mass media projects are beginning to use positive approaches. For example, projects under way in Mexico with homosexual men and in Dominica with heterosexual men and women present condom use as part of the happy, stylish, and modern way of life. In Mexico, homosexual men rejected the idea of a special, gay condom brand and strong AIDS prevention messages and overwhelmingly preferred messages portraying condoms as part of a healthy, active, happy way of life for *all* people.[204] In Dominica, a poster depicted condoms as a product used by fashionable men and women. Condom sales increased by as much as 70 percent at some outlets.[205]

5. Mass media stimulate discussion between partners and among members of the community. Mass media can help couples raise sensitive sexual topics.

When couples begin to talk about AIDS protection, they are taking a crucial step toward protecting themselves. Coverage in the mass media can both legitimate public discussion of AIDS and put the issue on the national policy agenda. It can also encourage private discussion of a sensitive topic, such as mutual protection from AIDS. In Mexico, for example, the campaign and controversy over the promotion of condoms started people talking about AIDS. One parents' group charged that condom promotion would lead to promiscuity. Another parents' group defended public AIDS education. The campaign and the controversy generated extensive news coverage, focused public attention on the AIDS epidemic, and made condoms a household word. In addition, the campaign was responsible for correcting some misconceptions about AIDS and increasing safer behavior among university students, homosexual men, and commercial sex workers.[206]

Mass media and popular theater can also provide model scenarios and dialogues that teach people how to talk to each other about safer sex. In Peru, a series of television spots used animated clay dolls to teach the public about condom use. The directors thought, no doubt correctly, that clay dolls sitting in bed talking about condoms would be better accepted than live actors simulating sexual activity.[207] In Zaire, a television miniseries, seen by two-thirds of the young couples targeted, showed a dramatic bedroom scene with a discussion of condoms.[208] In many places, including the United States, the Caribbean, and Africa, popular theater serves as an ice breaker to encourage people to talk about AIDS.[209] In Cameroon, a group of commercial sex workers tours the country in a popular play about AIDS. By playing out the issues that arise when condom use is negotiated between a commercial sex worker and client, the play, *Marriage to the Condom*, helps to convince audiences to adopt safer sexual practices. The humorous, explicit dialogue and the presence of condoms on stage desensitize the audience, facilitating group discussions of AIDS prevention and correct condom usage.[210] In the United States, parents who recalled seeing an AIDS television spot, hearing a radio spot, or, especially, reading an AIDS brochure were significantly more likely to have discussed AIDS with their children than were those who had not.[211]

Evidence from family planning programs shows that couples who discuss family planning are more likely to use contraception and to achieve their family planning goals than are those who do not.[212] Like family planning programs, AIDS programs need to encourage couples and families to talk about AIDS risks and AIDS prevention measures. Mass media can start the discussion.

6. Mass media can change behavior. Mass media messages that are linked to interpersonal communication channels are especially effective in encouraging people to act. Information from the mass media leads people to seek out additional facts, services, and supplies.

Mass media publicity about AIDS influences people to take actions they otherwise might not take. Cross-national comparisons, operations research projects, and evaluation of specific family planning media projects show that well-designed mass media projects encourage people to seek out more information and to use available reproductive health services.[213] This information search can be the first step in the gradual process of behavior change.

When mass media are linked to interpersonal communication channels, such as hotlines or health services, they tap the strengths of both media—the reach and influence of mass media and the two-way interaction of interpersonal communication. For example, following mass media publicity that included specific telephone numbers, calls to AIDS hotlines in the United States almost doubled from May 1990 (16,691) to July 1991 (32,482).[214] In Mexico City, calls increased more than tenfold.[215] Queries and attendance at clinics increase both with news coverage (as when basketball player Magic Johnson announced he was infected with HIV) and with campaign publicity that identifies specific sites. In Israel, for example, attendance at a major AIDS testing site increased 431 percent after the first major television program on AIDS.[216]

The link between mass media messages and condom sales is especially evident in social marketing programs. Condom sales tend to increase with advertising and decrease when advertising is cut back.[217] An analysis of 10 major social marketing programs found that condom sales were more closely linked with the extent of advertising than with any other factor, including price, cultural attitudes toward family planning, and level of national socioeconomic development.[218] In Switzerland, for example, condom sales doubled between 1986 and 1989.[219] In Pakistan, broadcast advertising of Sathi brand condoms began in 1990—only after the fourth year of sales, and only on radio and the private television channel. Nevertheless, sales jumped from an initial $20 million in the first year to $74 million in 1990.[220]

7. Entertainment and mass media present powerful AIDS prevention messages to broad audiences. Entertainment works because it is:
Personal: People share the joys, sorrows, and most intimate thoughts and feelings of the characters.
Popular: People choose to watch and listen for their own enjoyment.
Pervasive: People can find it everywhere.
Persuasive: People can see other people like themselves being rewarded for certain behavior and punished for other behavior.
Profitable: People are willing to pay for entertainment, so producers, actors, sponsors, distributors, and health personnel are willing to cooperate.

Music and drama about AIDS can evoke the emotional involvement necessary to trigger action. Audiences often identify with and imitate the characters and behavior depicted in dramas and songs. Thus, popular young singers can show adolescents how to say no gracefully to premarital sex.[221] Soap opera stars can offer role models that enhance the status of women and promote healthy behavior.[222] This approach is called *enter-educate*—entertainment that educates—and has been pioneered by the Johns Hopkins University Center for Communication Programs and its Population Communication Services project. Systematic research in countries as diverse as Mexico, Nigeria, Turkey, the Philippines, Uganda, and Zaire has demonstrated that enter-educate projects can influence sexual behavior.[223] Enter-educate approaches are now being applied to many AIDS prevention activities.

One of the first AIDS enter-educate products to be evaluated is the Ugandan AIDS film, *It's Not Easy.* The film demonstrates that, even without the promotion of specific products or services, an emotional human interest drama can influence the behavior of viewers. According to preliminary data from 1,600 men and women interviewed in their workplaces, those who had seen the film were more than twice as likely to have used condoms in the previous two months (18.4 percent) as were those who had not seen the film (7.7 percent).[224]

In Zaire, almost three-fourths of the viewers of a television miniseries reported that they intended to change their behavior as a result of the drama. The program dramatized the plight of a young married woman and the tragic impact of AIDS on her family. More than two-thirds of the intended audience, "young and prospective parents," watched each episode, could recount their plots, and retained the essential messages.[225] In Zambia, more than half of those questioned in a recall survey in the Copperbelt province had listened to a radio drama on AIDS, and more than two-thirds of those who had listened to the radio the night before had listened to the program. The majority of those who had listened wanted the program to be longer.[226] In the Philippines, a popular television soap opera aired an episode showing what happened to a businessman and his wife after he acquired HIV infection from a commercial sex worker. The number of visits to sexually transmitted disease clinics in Manila doubled during the week after the broadcast.[227]

The power of popular music is evident in a successful health education activity undertaken in Zaire. In 1987, shortly after the city of Zananga had diagnosed its first cases of AIDS, the Zairean singer Luwambo Makiadi broadcast an AIDS ballad that evoked emotions of abandonment and despair, identified high-risk groups, and recommended preventive behaviors. A survey in late 1987 of 1,054 randomly selected women in Zananga found that 93.8 percent had heard about AIDS, over 70 percent knew of four modes of transmission, and over 50 percent knew that a person could be infected without knowing it. More people mentioned the song as a source of information than any other mass media product.[228]

8. Mass media AIDS messages that are high quality, attractively packaged, and developed with commercial sector expertise and talent can compete with commercial programs for attention and airtime. Commercial sector professionals are often willing to donate talent and broadcast time to worthy causes, as long as high production standards are maintained.

In many countries, AIDS messages have to compete with sophisticated commercial programs and advertisements. Consequently,

AIDS messages in mass media need to be professionally and creatively packaged. AIDS and family planning programmers have found that when private-sector professionals—advertising agencies, television and radio producers, scriptwriters, and entertainers—are enlisted to develop top-quality products, social messages are more likely to be heard by the intended audience and supported by media broadcasters. Television and radio broadcasters were happy to give the songs and videos of Tatiana and Johnny in Latin America,[229] Lea and Menudo in the Philippines,[230] King Sunny and Onyeka in Nigeria,[231] and Luwambo Makiadi[232] and Empompo Loway[233] in Zaire many hours of free airtime because they liked the messages of sexual responsibility and because the songs and videos were of high quality and commercially competitive. Similarly, in Australia, many television stations did not charge fees for broadcasting AIDS messages.[234]

Many entertainers, especially those touched by the AIDS epidemic, willingly put their talents to work for AIDS prevention. When Zaire's most famous musician, Franco-Luwambo, released a song about AIDS in 1988, he encouraged other musicians to sing out. Three songs, created and produced with Zaire's top bands, were released over a 1-year period and were guaranteed daily airtime through agreements with the national and regional radio stations. The project also enlisted Zaire's best-loved professional radio/television drama group, the Troupe Nzoi, in a television AIDS drama series that promoted marital fidelity and condom use.[235] In the Netherlands, more than 30 famous people were willing to say "I use them" in an eye-catching multimedia campaign promoting condoms. In 3 months, 75 percent of the 14- to 45-year-olds surveyed had seen the campaign.[236]

Condom campaigns, as noted earlier, rely heavily on commercial marketing techniques to boost sales. The competition inherent in marketing helps improve the quality of the material. Condom promotion campaigns in Europe,[237] Asia,[238] the Near East,[239] and Latin America[240] have turned to private advertising agencies for promotion. Proyecto SIDA in Peru hired McCann Erikson Advertising Agency to package its first AIDS mass media campaign. The agency came up with an innovative television package using the claymation technique described in Lesson 5. New and attractive to Peruvian viewers, the spots corrected much misinformation about AIDS, according to pre- and post-assessments.[241]

In the case of the Ugandan AIDS film, the quality of the production enabled the film to reach beyond Africa to Asia, Latin America, and the United States. *It's Not Easy* reached 90 percent of the Ugandan workforce, and it has been widely distributed in Africa, is doing well in the Caribbean, and has been shown on broadcast television in the Philippines and on video in selected sites. Pre- and post-tests of *It's Not Easy* in the United States indicate that the film increases correct knowledge about AIDS, decreases misinformation about transmission, and increases the belief that talking about AIDS is good for a relationship.[242] *It's Not Easy* is an unusual case of a developing country's product being used to change attitudes and behavior in a developed country.[243]

9. Nongovernmental, private, and commercial organizations are more effective than are governments in developing AIDS educational materials and campaigns, including those for mass media.

This lesson, which is well documented in the experience of family planning programs, is increasingly evident in AIDS education. Nongovernmental organizations act more quickly, design more attractive materials, better meet the specific needs of distinct audiences, and are more innovative in production. A comparative review of U.S. print materials, for example, provided fairly objective and quantitative evidence that the private, community-based agencies, often targeting a specific segment of the population at risk, produced better material. The quality of the material was judged by such criteria as, How factual were the messages? How effectively did they hold audience attention? What specific actions were recommended? Did the materials address such key cues to action as personal vulnerability to AIDS or barriers to behavior change? The materials from the private sector consistently scored higher than did those from the public sector.[244]

Brazil provides good examples of bold private sector use of video for reproductive health issues, even in the absence of strong government policies. Private groups, such as GAPA (Support Group for the Prevention of AIDS), ABIA (the Brazilian Interdisciplinary AIDS Association), and the Gay Group, in various areas have assumed leadership at the local level in the content and format of educational materials. ABIA, for example, worked with the Union of Construction Workers to prepare an AIDS video. The video *Ze Cabro Macho* develops a humorous image of the typical macho construction worker who is protected on the job by his heavy boots and helmet and in private life by his ever-ready condom. Both the visual images and the flippant humor would be out of bounds for government.[245] As one observer notes, "There is no doubt that a complicated set of political forces has limited its freedom in a variety of ways."[246]

10. Continued support of mass media AIDS campaigns may depend on evaluations that document impact and on increased participation from the private commercial and entertainment sectors.

Mass media are expensive, with heavy production and promotion start-up costs. The first Australian AIDS television campaign in 1987 cost $3.4 million;[247] the United Kingdom campaign, more than $6 million.[248] Coming up with such funding is increasingly difficult. Already limited public health resources and political pressure from AIDS activists to support the increasing costs of AIDS treatment are reducing the funds available for general education. In Great Britain, for example, the national campaign is focusing on press advertising to save money.[249] In the Netherlands, the bold and innovative advertising campaign that used well-known public figures to promote condom use did not document specific results attributable to the campaign alone and now faces much reduced funding.[250]

Unfortunately, there have been few attempts to document the cost-effectiveness of mass media health promotion of any kind, including AIDS prevention campaigns. In family planning, 2 studies have looked at media costs and impact. In Turkey, a multimedia campaign cost about $0.04 to reach one woman of reproductive age and about $0.67 to gain one modern family planning user.[251] In Zimbabwe, a radio soap opera for men cost about $0.16 for each man reached and $2.41 for each new contraceptive user.[252] Even though only a small percentage of those exposed to mass media change their behavior immediately, so many people are reached that the effort is usually more cost-effective than are group talks or print materials. This type of evidence may be needed increasingly in the future to sustain policymakers' support for AIDS mass media educational programs.

The Future for AIDS and Mass Media

Clearly, the mass media are and will continue to be a major source of information about AIDS, even though more and more people unfortunately will have personal contact with the disease. National programs and mass media campaigns will continue to influence knowledge, attitudes, and behavior to the extent that they can segment the population and develop specific materials for different people at risk; use research and pretesting to identify relevant products, services, and behavior; link mass media efforts to community service centers and personal communication; convey positive and practical messages; and document the impact on intended audiences. Conversely, government support for continued multimedia campaigns is likely to diminish, to the extent that policymakers are hesitant; campaigns are neither well designed nor pretested; and clear results are not available. In its place, the nongovernmental, private, or commercial sector will probably play a much larger role in mass media AIDS education during the 1990s. Three important private sector elements may be:

- *Condom or other preventive product manufacturers, promoting brand-name products to segmented populations with immediate feedback and payback through increased sales.* These sales provide a steady source of revenue to support media costs and to purchase high-quality commercial advertising and marketing services. Although social scientists may continue to argue about the influence of mass media, commercial firms are in the best position to monitor this impact precisely through product sales and to influence policymakers through their economic power. Other providers of products and services, such as private physicians, family-planning organizations, and STD clinics, may also become more visible in the media as they are able to document the cost-effectiveness of mass media in attracting new clients and changing behavior. Other products, such as the female condom discussed earlier in this chapter, may also be publicized by the mass media.

- *Entertainment, reaching large audiences with a range of personal, emotional, tragic, or humorous material and representing a large and self-sustaining international industry.* To the extent that entertainers work with health and AIDS officials toward common goals, the material can be accurate, motivational, and useful to individuals and communities. High-quality materials using popular entertainers can have tremendous impact on public tastes, trends, and behavior relating to AIDS. The human interest and emotion of AIDS provides a rich basis for dramas, songs, and other entertainment.

- *Private-sector, nonprofit organizations that have the motivation may be able to generate the necessary support for more extensive use of mass media.* Especially on a local or regional level, such organizations as AIDS community service centers, local offices of international nongovernmental organizations, and family planning organizations will probably use mass media more often and more effectively in the 1990s to promote specific sites and services.

In short, the manufacturers of commercially viable preventive products (such as condoms), the entertainment industry, and the private, nonprofit sector have the strongest motivation to deal with AIDS issues in the mass media. Manufacturers and entertainers have economic resources and the promise of direct returns. Nonprofit agencies have strong social commitment and the ability to raise funds—although perhaps not so easily for prevention as for care. Thus, all three are likely to play a significant role in how the mass media address AIDS in the 1990s. All three, however, may focus more on local messages or on messages for special segments of the population rather than on national coverage. Whether governments—which undertook the first substantial mass media efforts—have the political will and the communication skills to continue to use mass media effectively for AIDS prevention remains to be seen. That will be a crucial challenge for government AIDS prevention programs in the 1990s.

▬▬▬▬ · · ·

THE ETHICAL DIMENSIONS OF HIV TESTING

Ronald Bayer

ald Bayer is Professor
ublic Health,
mbia University
ol of Public Health,
York, New York.

The development of a test in 1985 to detect HIV infection in individuals who showed no signs of disease was a watershed in the AIDS epidemic. It opened the way to protecting the blood supply and allowed the identification of people who, while apparently healthy, could transmit a lethal infection to their sex and needle-sharing partners, and, in the case of women, to their own offspring. It did not take long to understand that this technical advance had two aspects: it could make an immeasurable contribution to slowing the spread of a lethal epidemic, but it could also expose HIV-infected individuals to stigmatization, discrimination, and even the loss of freedom.

Since 1985, both aspects have been manifest as nations have sought to confront the challenge of AIDS. The test has been used as an adjunct to counseling and programs of mass education; as a tool for identifying those who could be the targets of discrimination; as a diagnostic device to detect infection in those who could benefit from early therapeutic intervention; and as an epidemiological tool to chart the prevalence and incidence of infection with HIV. In each of these instances, there have been conflicts between those ·concerned with protecting the rights of the infected and those whose proposals for protecting public health could involve overriding individual privacy. As the epidemic has matured, the nature of the controversies has changed, as have the alliances forged in the context of the epidemic's first years.

Testing as a Strategy for Behavioral Change

Since becoming available in mid-1985, the role of the HIV-antibody test in limiting the spread of HIV has been subject to intense dispute. First applied with relative lack of controversy on a mass scale to the screening of blood donations, the HIV test was viewed by many as a critical tool in public health attempts at behavior change, which is the foundation of AIDS prevention efforts. Advocates of widescale voluntary testing believed that knowledge of one's antibody status would be a crucial factor in motivating such change. For those found to be infected, the information would underscore the importance of adopting behaviors that would protect sexual and needle-sharing partners. For the uninfected, it was expected that the test results would make clear that behavioral change was essential to self-protection from lethal infection.

Those who opposed an emphasis on testing viewed its role very differently. Everybody engaged in unsafe behavior, they reasoned, had to modify their conduct regardless of HIV serological status. Because the message to those who tested positive and negative was the same, the test was superfluous at best and dangerous at worst. Being identified as seropositive could produce psychological stress and stigma, opening the way to discrimination in all realms of life. Opponents believed that in lieu of costly testing, campaigns of mass education should be undertaken.[253]

This controversy took shape at a time when there was little

empirical evidence to substantiate claims on either side.[254] As evidence accumulated that the radical changes that had occurred among gay men and the more modest changes among injection drug users were unrelated to testing, the focus of debate shifted to the role testing might play in targeting screening and counseling at those who had yet to modify their conduct. Additionally, there was considerable interest in the role testing might play in providing women with information that could be important for their reproductive choices.

Although national programs have placed different levels of emphasis on testing as the key element of a strategy for behavioral change, they have, to a striking degree, rejected mandatory testing. In general, national programs have recommended testing for those deemed to be at increased risk for infection. A few have also urged testing of the general population. A strong emphasis on testing characterized policies in Germany,[255] France,[256] and the United States,[257] where the prevalence of AIDS has made it a critical public health issue. General population testing has been urged at times in countries such as Sweden, Japan, Morocco, and the former Soviet Union, where levels of HIV infection are thought to be very low. A few nations stand out as having adopted programs that relegate testing to a marginal role. In the Netherlands, such a policy is a legacy of the epidemic's first years, when public health officials actually warned gay men about the dangers of taking the HIV test.[258]

Because mandatory mass screening has been rejected virtually everywhere, programs have had to develop strategies to persuade those targeted for testing that submitting to the HIV test would be beneficial and not entail grave personal risks. A serious concern about discrimination has compelled governments to recognize that protection of confidentiality is essential to the public health goal of limiting the spread of HIV infection. Nevertheless, the extent to which legislative or regulatory measures have been initiated to secure the privacy of HIV-related records has varied widely.[259] Even where formal protection exists, breaches of confidentiality have not been uncommon. Recognizing that individuals might be concerned about breaches of confidentiality, a number of nations have made provisions for anonymous testing.

Debate about the desirability of HIV testing and of anonymity underwent a significant transformation as the prospects for clinical intervention improved. Of course, this applied especially in those nations where resources would permit access to treatments that might be used before the onset of symptomatic conditions linked to HIV infection. The focus of the role of testing in those nations increasingly shifted to the contribution of the test to clinical management of HIV disease. In this context, the importance of anonymity was questioned: people who were infected needed to be evaluated by physicians, and in that context, confidentiality rather than anonymity was almost universally deemed to be the most appropriate protective standard.

Screening, Safety, and Discrimination

Because AIDS represented a novel and terrifying threat, and because the causative agent was not identified until several years after the first official case reports, it is not surprising that it provoked considerable social anxiety. In advanced industrialized societies, AIDS also represented the first major challenge of an infectious disease in almost a generation. In some instances, the urge to identify individuals who might pose a threat of transmission was intimately linked to the desire to segregate those who could transmit disease.

Early epidemiological studies revealed, however, that HIV/AIDS could not be casually transmitted, thus removing any scientific justification for mandatory screening and discrimination. In the United States, the Centers for Disease Control (CDC) played a crucial role in stanching the calls for such exclusion in schools,[260] the workplace,[261] housing, and public accommodation. On an international level, the Global Programme on AIDS of the World Health Organization played a similar role.[262]

Nevertheless, there are numerous examples of mandatory screening programs designed to identify HIV-infected people. The most extreme case is Cuba, which set out to screen the entire sexually active population so that individuals who were infected could be quarantined,[263] thereby creating a system of medical preventive detention.

But even in nations that rejected mass mandatory testing, some compulsory testing programs were adopted. For example, in the United States, Australia, Mexico, and Thailand, military recruits were subject to such testing. Prisoners were compulsorily tested in the Slovak Republic, in some states in the United States,[264] and in Australia.[265] Concern about contamination from abroad was reflected in policies that sought to screen immigrants, short-term travelers, foreign students, and, in some cases, students returning home from studies abroad.

Employees were at times subject to screening as well. In Sweden, for example, pilots working for Scandinavian Airlines System had to undergo a test because of concerns that neurological impairments linked to HIV infection might endanger passenger safety.[266] On the other hand, a number of nations outlawed mandatory screening of workers for HIV infection as an unwarranted invasion of privacy and in recognition of the fact that barring people from employment solely on the grounds of HIV infection would represent an unjustified act of discrimination. This was the case in the United States, despite the government's own decision to screen military recruits, and in France.[267] Denmark[268] and the Netherlands[269] ruled that mandatory employee testing and discrimination were in violation of public policy.

The strongest impetus for mandatory screening emerged within the context of health care, driven by concerns of health care workers that they might risk acquiring HIV infection from their patients. Pressure among physicians was especially prominent among surgeons who were often exposed to substantial quantities of their patients' blood. Such pressure, by and large, has been resisted by policymakers who argued that the adoption of universal blood and body fluid precautions would deal more effectively with the small but not insignificant risks involved. Yet in 1991, a national survey of physicians and nurses in the United States found that three-quarters supported the mandatory screening of preoperative patients.[270] The disparity between formal policy and the preferences of health care workers helps explain the persistence of reports from around the world of hospitalized patients being tested without their consent, regardless of law or policy. In the United States, unconsented testing has broad support among the general population, despite the forceful and articulate opposition of AIDS advocates and proponents of civil liberties.[271]

Nothing more forcefully demonstrates the fragility of policies against mandatory screening in the health care setting than the controversy in the United States in 1991 over whether HIV-infected surgeons and dentists should be barred from performing invasive procedures that involved a theoretical risk of HIV transmission to patients.

Although there had been some discussion of the issue in earlier years[272]—and indeed some local efforts to bar clinicians with AIDS from patient contact—it was the case of Kimberly Bergalis in Florida that crystallized the issue and precipitated a furious conflict.

Ms. Bergalis had apparently become infected with HIV after a tooth extraction by a dentist with AIDS.[273] Subsequently, four additional cases of HIV infection were traced to the same dental practice.[274] Suddenly, a matter of theoretical concern had become very real. Although the precise nature of the conditions under which HIV had been transmitted could not be determined, the case suggested to the general public that patients were vulnerable to their care givers' lethal infections. Public pressure for corrective action mounted.

The early phase of the debate threatened the alliance of forces that had steadfastly opposed discrimination against those with HIV infection and resisted calls to dilute the principle of voluntary testing. A number of bioethicists had argued that HIV-infected clinicians had a moral obligation to desist from performing invasive procedures altogether or to seek the patient's consent before undertaking interventions that could impose some risk of HIV transmission.[275] This position was a logical outgrowth of a central tenet of medical ethics as it had evolved over the past 2 decades—that patients had the right to determine the conditions under which they would be exposed to hazard. Although they never called for mandatory testing, the logic of the position adopted by some bioethicists led inevitably to the compulsory identification of individuals who could place their patients at risk.

The American Medical Association endorsed the argument for the exclusion of HIV-infected clinicians from the performance of high-risk procedures, although it explicitly rejected mandatory screening.[276] Surveys of public and professional opinion in the United States, however, indicated a willingness to take exclusion to its logical conclusion—mandatory identification of health care workers infected with HIV.[277] Ninety percent of the public endorsed such efforts, as did more than half of physicians and nurses. The executive director of the prestigious *New England Journal of Medicine* also endorsed mandatory screening of health care workers as well as of hospitalized patients.[278]

Against this tide of opinion, people committed to voluntary testing argued, from a public health perspective, that such efforts would be irrational given the extremely remote risks involved and the costs associated both with excluding HIV-infected clinicians from practice and with repeatedly screening health care workers.[279] Finally, they suggested that the mandatory screening of health care workers would inevitably lead to the mandatory testing of patients. Thus, to avoid the threat of an extremely remote event, the entire fabric of voluntary HIV testing would be torn apart.

Despite such concerns, and under extraordinary political pressure, the CDC issued recommendations in the summer of 1991 that would have required infected clinicians to withdraw from the performance of an undefined set of invasive procedures or to inform their patients about their infected state.[280] Although the CDC explicitly rejected compulsory screening, the logic of its position dictated such a course, a point recognized by the United States Congress, which moved with great speed to enforce the CDC guidelines and require screening if necessary. The ensuing imbroglio, driven by powerful resistance from professional medical groups, compelled the CDC to withdraw its initial recommendations, thus reopening the issue.

The entire debate was followed with varying degrees of attention in other economically advanced democratic nations, but none was willing to require mandatory screening of health care workers or the exclusion of those with HIV from clinical practice. In the Netherlands, which has resisted making testing a critical feature of its efforts to contain HIV, this debate was widely viewed as another example of U.S. excess.

Another challenge to voluntary HIV screening in the name of safety arose in late 1991. This involved not the threat of HIV transmission, but tuberculosis. For some years, it had been observed that the AIDS epidemic had contributed to the dramatic increase in the number of tuberculosis cases in nations where tuberculosis was no longer considered a serious challenge to public health. Because tuberculosis is an airborne disease, compulsory measures to identify people capable of its transmission have long been accepted as legitimate.

In the past, depending on epidemiological conditions, schoolchildren, hospitalized patients, prisoners, and immigrants have been subject to compulsory tuberculosis screening. When cases of active tuberculosis were discovered, it was deemed appropriate for a government to require the initiation of treatment and even quarantine. Thus, the model of tuberculosis control has stood in sharp contrast to the voluntaristic strategy for responding to HIV. The epidemiological linkage of AIDS and tuberculosis poses new challenges, given the radical distinction between the two strategies.

Many individuals with HIV infection do not respond to tuberculosis test antigens and, thus, have negative tests for tuberculosis even when they are infected. Because the standard screening test for tuberculosis often produces false negatives in the presence of HIV, it has been suggested that screening for tuberculosis should include screening for HIV. Yet if screening for tuberculosis is compulsory, can it remain voluntary for HIV? This issue will be especially important in hospitals, prisons, nursing homes, and other facilities where large numbers of individuals live or work in close proximity. Crucial to any such policy will be a careful determination of whether knowledge of HIV infection can make any contribution to the identification of those with tuberculosis. There are scientific reasons to doubt such a claim.

Clinical Screening

In the first years of the AIDS epidemic, the debate over the role of HIV testing took place at a time of relative therapeutic impotence. Against this background, strict conditions of consent to testing were imposed, and gay organizations—where they existed—tended to adopt an extremely cautious, when not explicitly hostile, attitude toward efforts to identify those infected with HIV.

With advances in the capacity of medicine to affect the onset of AIDS-related conditions, if not the ultimate course of the disease, and especially with the growing consensus that people who were infected, but still asymptomatic, should benefit from prophylactic therapy, the context of the policy debate shifted. In addition, the perspective of those caring for people with HIV disease underwent a dramatic shift, along with the attitude of groups that had previously viewed the HIV test as a threat to privacy. Increasingly, a new perspective on testing developed, especially in nations with the resources to provide early therapeutic intervention.

In the United States, for example, the CDC is considering whether to urge all hospitals to recommend HIV screening to patients, under conditions of informed consent.[281] The American Medical Association would go even further, loosening the stringent requirements for consent and giving physicians broad discretion to order testing based on their clinical judgment.[282] In a national survey, 44 percent of physicians and 57 percent of nurses stated that all hospitalized patients should be required to undergo HIV testing.[283]

These trends in the United States stand in sharp contrast to the views of medical ethicists who assert that the requirements of informed consent to medical intervention should extend to tests that are a prelude to such interventions.[284] Moreover, they have argued that the unique nature of the HIV test requires that specific consent to the test be preserved despite the fact that, as a general rule, blood testing as part of clinical practice has rarely required such standards.

Less is known about policy directions in other countries regarding HIV screening for broad clinical purposes, although reports from economically advanced democratic nations indicate little by way of a trend to testing or testing without consent. In one context, however, there has long been a striking emphasis on voluntary HIV testing in virtually all economically advanced nations, as well as in some less developed nations—pregnancy. This is true even in the Netherlands, where the public health authorities have been less enthusiastic about HIV testing than in any other economically advanced nation, and where there is also less enthusiasm for early therapeutic intervention with such drugs as AZT. Initially proposed as a way of providing women with information crucial to decisions about their reproductive options, such testing is increasingly viewed as a way of identifying women in need of early clinical intervention and babies who will require close clinical supervision. In the former Soviet Union, HIV testing in pregnancy was mandatory; in the United States, three-quarters of surveyed physicians and nurses have supported such compulsory screening.[285] In France, there has been renewed discussion of mandatory pregnancy testing, although such proposals were formally rejected when first proposed by the minister of health in 1988.

The interest in screening pregnant women is driven, in large measure, by concerns over the threat posed to their offspring. In this regard, it is necessary to consider the prospects for proposals to undertake routine or mandatory newborn testing. In the United States, a significant proportion of pediatricians have supported such testing. Nevertheless, proposals for such screening were typically rejected for three reasons. First, because all babies born to infected mothers carry maternal antibody, despite the fact that only 20 to 30 percent are infected with HIV, antibody testing was deemed insufficiently specific to be of clinical utility. Second, there was little evidence that presymptomatic infants would benefit from treatment and considerable ethical concern about using the drugs like AZT when almost three-quarters of antibody-positive newborns would prove to be uninfected. Finally, ethicists argued that newborn testing would effectively mean mandatory testing of women who had just given birth, a breach in the commitment to voluntary testing and an unwarranted invasion of privacy.

Advances in the identification of HIV infection in newborns through the polymerase chain reaction (PCR) technique,[286] as well as evidence that prophylaxis against pneumocystis carinii pneumonia can be effective in newborns with compromised immune systems,[287] have redrawn the clinical parameters within which newborn testing is being discussed. Inevitably, it will be necessary to confront anew the ethical question of whether the interests of the child (for early treatment) should take precedence over the privacy interests of the mother.

In nations where mandatory or routine screening of newborns for inborn conditions is standard practice, pressure will mount to include HIV screening with these other tests.[288] As of 1992, the American Academy of Pediatrics explicitly rejected mandatory newborn screening for HIV after a long and acrimonious discussion.[289] Yet in nations where no routine or mandatory screening of newborns occurs, the debate over policy may be quite different. In those nations, it will be necessary to resolve the question of whether early identification of infection in newborns is so crucial to their well-being that HIV testing should be treated as a unique case. But in any event, mothers considered at high risk of HIV infection will more likely be strongly encouraged to permit the screening of their newborns.

In large measure, the ethics of newborn screening will depend on whether the appropriate medical and social services are available to both the child and the mother. In the absence of such services, either voluntary or mandatory screening for clinical reasons would be unjustified. The tragic absence of crucial medical services in virtually all nonindustrialized nations where pediatric AIDS is a major problem means that in such countries, the clinical, public health, or ethical justification for screening asymptomatic newborns for HIV does not exist.

The importance of screening infants and adults for clinical reasons and the inducements many individuals will experience to undergo testing at the behest of their care givers underscore the significance of ensuring the confidentiality of HIV-related medical records and of creating protections against unwarranted acts of discrimination. A failure to protect people with HIV infection from invasions of privacy, from stigmatization, and from scientifically unjustified exclusionary practices will discourage people from seeking testing or will compel a choice between potential medical benefits and threats to social well-being.

Screening and Epidemiology

Soon after the development of the HIV antibody test, it became apparent that epidemiological studies based on AIDS cases alone would be insufficient. An understanding of the prevalence and incidence of HIV infection was considered necessary.[290] Because mandatory testing of the population at large was rejected as a public health strategy in virtually every country, epidemiologists had to develop a methodology that could approximate the level of infection in specific population groups as well as the general population. Studies based on voluntary testing would be insufficient because of the problem of selection and participation bias. The approach settled on was to undertake blinded or unlinked seroprevalence studies, in which blood samples drawn for purposes other than HIV screening would be stripped permanently of all personal identification and then tested for HIV.

In the United States, such studies provoked little controversy when first proposed, and it was widely accepted that individual consent was not required.[291] In Canada, a special national review panel examined the ethical and policy issues involved and came to a similar conclusion.[292] The Global Programme on AIDS of the World Health Organization also endorsed such studies as both epidemiologically useful and ethically sound.[293]

However, in some nations, blind testing provoked profound controversy. In Great Britain, a 2-year debate centered on questions of whether such studies entailed an unacceptable violation of privacy and of informed consent. There was additional concern over whether such studies would preclude physicians from informing those with HIV about their status, thereby entailing a breach of both the clinician's duty to inform patients about their medical conditions and the public health duty to inform individuals about the risk they could pose to others. Finally, in 1988, the British Department of Health reversed its opposition to blinded studies, but with the proviso that individuals who would be part of such studies be informed of the right to opt out. In the Netherlands, the debate was even more intense and more protracted. In 1992, there was some indication that such screening under carefully limited circumstances would be tolerated. In Denmark, the Ministry of Health has continued to reject proposals to undertake blinded studies in pregnant women.[294]

When there was little that could be done therapeutically for individuals who were infected but asymptomatic, the ethics of surveillance and the ethics of case finding were fundamentally distinct. It is still possible to argue that the conduct of blinded studies does not violate the obligation of physicians to inform their patients of critical diagnostic findings, because individuals can still be vigorously encouraged to seek confidential testing for clinical purposes. Nonetheless, improved clinical prospects will inevitably produce pressure to rethink the issue: the ethics of surveillance undertaken at a time of therapeutic impotence may not be appropriate in a period of enhanced therapeutic capability.

Conclusions

Although an analysis of national AIDS programs must pay close attention to the official policies on HIV screening, the ability of clinicians and private sector employers to evade formal policies makes it necessary to study how closely practice conforms to official policy.

For example, although Swedish policy dictates that the sexual contacts of individuals with HIV infection be tested, there is considerable evidence that physicians do not routinely require such screening.[295] Although policy in many states in the United States usually requires the specific informed consent of patients before HIV testing, there is considerable evidence that surreptitious testing in hospitals occurs.[296] Even in Denmark, which has consistently opposed compulsory screening, there are reports that physicians have undertaken unconsented testing.[297]

Discrepancies also exist between policy and action by governmental agencies. Thus, although Japanese law permits the authorities to screen foreigners entering the country,[298] they rarely do so, and the law is typically only applied to commercial sex workers. In Canada, the law permits screening of short-term visitors, although the government has rarely exercised this prerogative.[299]

Finally, even where the formalities of policy are adhered to, the explicit and implicit pressures applied may, for all practicable purposes, render informed consent a hollow formality.

In the first years of the AIDS epidemic, when so much attention focused on what governments would and would not do, it was natural for researchers to concentrate on monitoring formal policy decisions. But important as such efforts were, they must now be viewed as only a starting point. Careful empirical studies are now needed, based on a close analysis of institutional and individual behavior.

CHAPTER SEVENTEEN

· ·

Policy and Program Issues

■■■■■■■ · · ·

HIV/AIDS POLICY FOR PRISONS OR FOR PRISONERS?

Timothy W. Harding and Georgette Schaller

￼othy W. Harding is
￼fessor of Legal
￼dicine, University of
￼neva; Georgette
￼haller is a research
￼sistant at the Institute
￼Legal Medicine,
￼versity of Geneva.

What has gone wrong with HIV/AIDS policies in prisons? Regarded early in the epidemic as a test case for the application of coherent public health policies and for the respect of human rights under difficult circumstances, prisons have so far failed the test. A World Health Organization (WHO) report in September 1990 to the United Nations Congress on Crime Prevention and Treatment of Offenders referred to widescale violations of prisoners' rights. It placed the weight of its report, however, on the worldwide failure to introduce effective preventive measures in prisons. The hard-hitting report of the U.S. National Commission on AIDS and HIV in correctional facilities, published in March 1991, focused on the predicament of prisoners living with HIV/AIDS and called the situation "nothing if not cruel and unusual."[1]

Thus, despite clear recommendations made by international bodies in 1987/88, so-called prison sessions at international AIDS congresses, the development of imaginative educational programs for prison staff and prisoners, and the substantive policy change in some countries, the overall picture is bleak. Discrimination, breaches of medical confidentiality, and segregation remain widespread. Treatment programs for HIV-infected prisoners are inadequate. Tuberculosis is increasing in prison populations due to a high prevalence among HIV-infected inmates. No effective measures for preventing HIV transmission through injection drug use are applied in most countries. The specific needs of women prisoners and young prisoners have not received sufficient attention. Prison medical services in many developing countries are unable to respond to even the most basic needs posed by the HIV epidemic.

This section reviews the state of HIV/AIDS policies in prisons in 1992; it shows that deficiencies are due to:

- preexisting inadequacies in prison health care
- lack of independence of prison medical services
- adoption of policies that serve the needs of institutions rather than those of inmates

Defining the Problem

A 1983 study in New York State's prison population alerted public health authorities to the importance of injection drug use in the transmission of HIV.[2] Researchers were using prisons as a convenient location to sample drug users. At the time, little attention was given to the practical problems concerning AIDS prevention in prisons, to the dangers of discrimination and violation of ethical principles, and to the humanitarian issues raised by people suffering and dying of AIDS while incarcerated.

In the following years, researchers were mainly interested in carrying out further seroprevalence studies in prisons. With the exception of an initial study in French prisons, the studies have consistently shown higher rates of HIV infection than in the general population, at least in industrialized countries. Particularly high rates have been reported from countries in southern Europe, for example, 26 percent in Spain and 17 percent in Italy.[3] A series of reports prepared for the U.S. National Institute of Justice mapped the highly variable HIV prevalence rates in North America.

It quickly became apparent that the number of HIV-infected prisoners was closely related to the proportion of those injecting drugs prior to imprisonment and to the rate of HIV infection among injection drug users in the community. In many European countries, over 30 percent of prisoners were regular users of opiate drugs prior to imprisonment.[4] The U.S. National Commission on AIDS has stated succinctly: "By choosing mass imprisonment as the federal and state governments' response to the use of drugs, we have created a de facto policy of incarcerating more and more individuals with HIV infection."[5]

In some developing countries, significant rates of HIV infection among prisoners also occur, but the epidemiological significance is different. For example, the prevalence rates of 16 percent in a Zambian prison and the large number of prisoners developing AIDS in Tanzanian prisons[6] probably reflect high rates of HIV infection due to heterosexual transmission among young adults in the general population. In Brazil and Thailand, HIV transmission by both injection drug use and heterosexual spread in the community has contributed to a significant HIV/AIDS problem in prisons.

Most AIDS researchers have wrongly conceptualized prisons as a static reservoir. In fact, prisons house people temporarily, often for brief periods, sometimes repetitively, and these people have lives in the community before, after, and between prison sentences. Prison should, therefore, be regarded as an integral part of the community. The orientation of research and public health strategies changes significantly if this concept is accepted; for example, preparing prisoners for parole periods and release would then be seen as a major task for prevention.

In 1985, panic reactions among both staff and inmates about the risk of contracting AIDS resulted in prison disturbances in both Europe and North America. In response, a number of prison authorities developed information and education programs for staff and inmates, but at the same time, questionable practices were introduced in many countries. These practices included routine, mandatory HIV-antibody testing for prisoners, separate housing of HIV-infected prisoners, and restriction of access to workplaces and other activities. The HIV/AIDS pandemic revealed a longstanding weakness in public health activities in prisons: health authorities rarely had responsibility to provide either curative or preventive health care. Prison health had become divorced from mainstream medicine and public health, and prisoners were clearly receiving substandard health care.[7]

International Recommendations

The first response at an international level came from the Council of Europe, which commissioned a study on AIDS prevention and control measures in 17 European countries in 1986. The results showed that mandatory HIV-antibody testing was practiced in 4 countries and some form of segregation of HIV-infected prisoners in housing or work activities occurred in 7 countries. Condoms were available to prisoners in only 4 countries.[8] The Council of Europe subsequently adopted clear recommendations to end discriminatory practices and to make preventive measures available. The Parliamentary Assembly's Recommendation 1080 was particularly clear.[9] Its policy was based on:

- information to prison staff and prisoners
- voluntary HIV-antibody testing and counseling
- integration of HIV-infected prisoners into normal housing and work activities
- transfer of prisoners who have developed AIDS to a hospital, and early release on humanitarian grounds for prisoners with advanced illness
- making condoms available
- allowing, in the last resort, the distribution of clean syringes and needles to injection drug users in prison

In November 1987, a consultation on AIDS and prisons was organized by the World Health Organization. The resulting consensus statement reached conclusions similar to those of the Council of Europe, although the issue of transmission by injection drug use was not realistically addressed. The consultation did, however, take a position on several important points:

- the need to improve environmental hygiene and medical care in prisons
- the principle of equivalence of preventive measures and health care between prisons and the outside community
- the need to reexamine criminal policies with regard to drug users to reduce the number of drug users in prisons

Five years later, it must be concluded that the effect of these recommendations has been limited.

The Situation in 1992

HIV-Antibody Testing: Mandatory screening is still fairly widely practiced in prisons in the United States, although, paradoxically, mainly in areas of low HIV prevalence. Some states have recently abandoned such testing, whereas others limit screening to so-called risk groups: injection drug users, self-declared homosexuals, and commercial sex workers. In Europe, mandatory testing has now been abandoned in nearly all countries, and steps have been taken to reinforce the confidentiality of voluntary test results. The superficially attractive doctrine of communicating the results to prison administrators on a need-to-know basis is being recognized ever more widely as unrealistic. In England and Wales, the authorities are now committed to phasing out Viral Infectivity Restrictions by which prisoners with HIV infection had a red V.I.R. stamped prominently on their personal records.

Housing and Access to Workplaces: The debate about segregation and participation in work activities by HIV-infected prisoners has been complicated by two factors. The first is the assertion that such prisoners require a protective environment in their own interests involving freedom from harassment by other prisoners and improved hygienic conditions, medical care, and nutrition. Thus, in some countries (e.g., Ireland) units with better than average conditions have been built to house HIV-infected prisoners. The second factor is the desire to protect the general prison population from violent or sexually predatory HIV-infected prisoners.

Nevertheless, segregation is often practiced arbitrarily, a response resulting from the concern and prejudice of prison staff. Such policies are also applied in a haphazard and inconsistent manner. Thus, in England and Wales, HIV-infected prisoners are housed in special wings in some prisons, in hospital accommodations elsewhere, and in normal locations in other prisons; in Scotland, no such discrimination is practiced. The European Committee on the Prevention of Torture and Inhuman and Degrading Treatment condemned this segregation and the "impoverished environment" suffered by HIV-infected prisoners in the United Kingdom.[10]

Although segregation is also widely practiced in North American prisons, there has been progress elsewhere. Twenty-three out of 31 European prison systems and 4 out of 7 Australian states have clear "no segregation" and "normal housing policies" for HIV-infected prisoners. Yet in these systems, HIV-infected prisoners may still be restricted from working in kitchens. If this factor is included, only 16 out of 31 systems in Europe and 3 out of 7 states in Australia are truly nondiscriminatory.

Finally, the problems of violence and sexual exploitation in prison should be dealt with directly. These behaviors are often the result of overcrowded conditions, insufficient staff, and the lack of programs and activities. If some prisoners are violent or predatory, their actions may justify isolation or other disciplinary measures, regardless of HIV status.

Information and Education

There has been real progress in bringing information on AIDS and risk behaviors to prison staff and prisoners. This has been effective in reducing tensions and dispelling many irrational fears. Discussion groups, counseling sessions, brochures, and videos have been developed, in some instances with the active involvement of outside, nonofficial agencies. For example, Deutsche AIDS-Hilfe in Germany has produced a booklet and a video specifically for prisoners, and the Terrence Higgins Trust developed a brochure that is widely distributed in English and Welsh prisons.

However, weakness in education programs results from the lack of congruence between preventive measures in the community and those offered in prisons, along with the failure to address the humanitarian issues of prisoners with HIV disease. The movie filmed in New York City prisons, "A Bad Way to Die," while a striking example of education based on fear, showed that if AIDS was a bad way to die, it was a lot worse in prisons.

Medical Care

Some prisoners receive up-to-date, state-of-the-art specialized care for their HIV disease. Many do not. Expensive treatments may not be financed by prison services; many therapies, such as aerosolized pentamidine, are not available to inmates unless they are hospitalized. In many instances, overstretched prison medical facilities are unable to organize and maintain the necessary care.

Progress of HIV disease appears to be significantly faster in some prison systems than in the corresponding community.[11] Prisoners are often unable to gain access to experimental treatment protocols for HIV disease, and some patients already on research protocols have been withdrawn on entry to prison. The right of prisoners to participate in experimental therapeutic procedures with informed consent has been established, but many obstacles remain to securing real access to therapeutic trials. Prisoners are dependent on the initiative of the prison medical staff to make contact with research groups in specialized treatment facilities. Finally, when the disease takes its course, decisions about early release are taken erratically so that prisoners either die in prison or are released at a very late stage in their illness. The basic requirement to allow prisoners to die in dignity is not met.

Availability of Preventive Services

There has been some success in making condoms available to prisoners. In 1989, the French government reversed its earlier policy, which had prohibited condom distribution on the grounds that homosexuality was unlawful in public and that prisons were public places. Nevertheless, this argument still prevails elsewhere. Latest figures from the World Health Organization's network on HIV/AIDS in prison show that 23 out of the 52 systems sampled allow condom distribution inside prison. Furthermore, no country that has adopted condom distribution in prisons has reversed the policy. Yet finding the best distribution channels and encouraging condom use remain problems, even when the principle of availability is accepted. For example, in a 1991 study in Switzerland, the rate of condom distribution varied widely among individual prisons, despite general acceptance of the principle of availability. One successful strategy is to make condoms easily available in medical services and to stress condom use not only within prison, but also during parole periods and following release.

Progress on measures for preventing HIV transmission through injection drug use has been much slower. No prison system has authorized the distribution or exchange of clean syringes or needles. The Swiss Federal Bureau of Health is planning a pilot project in one prison, but elsewhere, there is strong resistance from prison authorities on the grounds of security risk (needles and syringes being used as weapons) and of conflict with institutional policies about illicit drug use. Even communities that have enthusiastically adopted wide-ranging *harm reduction* policies (e.g., Amsterdam) have not extended these policies to prisons. In addition, alternative harm reduction strategies have not generally been applied in prisons. Thus, although the best alternative seems to be distributing diluted sodium hypochlorite solutions (or bleach in powdered form in airtight sachets) with clear instructions on how cleaning works, this policy has been adopted by only 16 out of the 52 systems surveyed late in 1991. Finally, methadone maintenance in prisons may also be effective in reducing the risk of infection, and it is being adopted in some jails and a few long-term penitentiaries.

Women Prisoners

In most systems, women constitute fewer than 10 percent of the prison population. Many studies, however, show high rates of HIV infection among women prisoners, as well as alcohol and drug problems. Women prisoners have special needs in relation to both AIDS and their general health. These needs include gynecological examination and treatment; education on mother-child HIV transmission and safer sex; counseling for pregnant prisoners; availability of voluntary pregnancy termination or follow-up care during pregnancy; and care for children born to HIV-infected prisoners.

HIV Infection and Tuberculosis

An important association has been established in a number of prison systems between an increase in the incidence of active pulmonary tuberculosis and HIV infection. In addition, prisons are frequently poorly ventilated and overcrowded, creating a heightened risk of airborne transmission of tuberculosis to other prisoners (whether HIV-infected or not). This risk of airborne transmission of tuberculosis also exists for prison staff. The increasing incidence of active pulmonary tuberculosis among HIV-infected prisoners has been confirmed in prisons in France, Spain, Switzerland, and the United States. There is a likelihood that this association exists also in prisons in developing countries, where tuberculosis is endemic. In view of prison conditions—a closed environment with frequent overcrowding and lack of ventilation—the problem of infectious tuberculosis requires special attention. However, necessary measures are infrequently applied, due to a lack of coordination between prison medical services and community tuberculosis control services.

Conclusion

Is this brief review too pessimistic? Certainly, there are many examples of innovative and imaginative initiatives in the field of HIV/AIDS in prisons. These include a buddy system for HIV-infected prisoners in Edinburgh's Saughton prison; independent counselors from outside the prison who visit regularly in England and Germany; condoms and diluted bleach included in a pocket pharmacy distributed to all prisoners in a Zurich penitentiary; powdered bleach sachets available in prisons in the State of Victoria (Australia); well-produced videos on AIDS and hepatitis B in Canada; and a comprehensive tuberculosis control program in Spain's prisons. However, these isolated initiatives do not match the coverage and cohesion of comprehensive HIV/AIDS programs in the community, thus highlighting a larger and more general problem underscored by AIDS—health initiatives in prison are not integrated into community health care. As long as prison administrations remain responsible for health care, services will tend to be oriented toward the needs of institutions rather than people.

■■■■■   ·   ·   ·

LIVING WITH HIV/AIDS: A ROOM OF ONE'S OWN

Aart Hendriks

art Hendriks is a legal searcher attached to e Faculty of Law, iversity of Utrecht, the etherlands.

From Poland to Tanzania to the United States, discrimination against people living with AIDS or HIV often takes frightening dimensions: in Warsaw, an angry mob reportedly burned the home of a man with AIDS. In Dar es Salaam, a woman with AIDS was chased from her family compound, then abandoned and left to fend for herself. In New York, a man infected with HIV had to live without heating because repairmen refused to service his apartment.

Prejudice has marked the experience of people living with HIV from the onset of the epidemic. Some forms of discrimination, usually the most severe, have received widespread attention, for example, violence against people with HIV/AIDS or people suspected to be linked to the disease. Nevertheless, prejudice can also threaten the employment of persons with HIV/AIDS, their ability to obtain medical or dental treatment, or their right to attend school.

An equally important issue is adequate housing for people with HIV and AIDS. In a global housing market often characterized by shortages, evictions, and inadequate legal protection for tenants, people with AIDS suffer disproportionately. A recent survey in the United Kingdom commissioned by the AIDS and Housing Project revealed that 83 percent of people with HIV lived in unsuitable conditions.[12]

Why is meeting the housing needs of people with AIDS important? Granted, it is a valid strategy for care from a public health point of view. But in addition, housing is governed by law in many countries. More than 30 nations have incorporated provisions on housing into their constitutions.[13] Under such clauses, countries have an obligation to ensure housing to every citizen, irrespective of health status or the nature of the household. Affordability, accessibility, security of tenure, habitability, and availability are central to this right.[14]

The lack of adequate housing can have impacts beyond that of mere shelter. Experience in the AIDS epidemic is lending new force to Florence Nightingale's statement that the connection between health and dwellings of the population is one of the most important that exists. The implications of this statement are clear: adequate housing for a person with AIDS can mean the difference between quality of life, bare survival, or death.

Housing Needs of the HIV-Infected

At the community, national, and international levels, organizations are only beginning to grapple with this fundamental need, looking for comprehensive policies to bridge the gap between public housing and public health.

Ideally, programs designed for housing people with HIV/AIDS should fulfill three criteria. First, they should provide a sufficient number of places to live that are safe, clean, and adequate. This is of crucial importance given the strong evidence that substandard accommodation can lead to an accelerated decline in health status. Second, given the clear link between stress and the progression of AIDS, programs should include measures that minimize the concerns of HIV-infected persons for their physical safety, protect them from eviction, and guarantee the affordability and maintenance of the dwelling. Not surprisingly, people with AIDS, like people without AIDS or HIV infection, are better off in a familiar, comfortable environment, surrounded by family and friends, than in institutions. In addition, staying at home tends to be more economical for some individuals as well as for the health care system.[15] Lastly, programs should be flexible and capable of responding to changes in tenants' needs. Everyone should take note of one known social consequence of AIDS: people come forward and make their needs known if they are confident that their confidentiality will be protected.

Homelessness

Homelessness and substandard living are realities for a substantial number of the world's population. More than one billion people throughout the world lack adequate accommodation, and the number is rising steadily in both industrialized and developing countries.[16] In 1987, the Council of Europe reported that an estimated 10 million persons in Europe lacked adequate housing.

People already living under substandard conditions are least empowered to stop the spread of HIV.[17] Their general health is often poor. In New York, the homeless include at least 8,000 people with AIDS.[18] In Amsterdam, 80 percent of the homeless are reported to have problems with alcohol, drugs, or both, with obvious health consequences.[19] A study in San Francisco in 1991 found that homeless adults had a rate of HIV infection that was 10 times that of people with homes.[20]

AIDS also contributes substantially to homelessness around the world. From Zimbabwe to Brazil, HIV-infected people have been evicted from their homes, sometimes even by their own families. In Thailand, Spain, and Poland, people with HIV have been evicted by their landlords.[21] Other HIV-infected individuals may find it hard to keep and maintain their homes, or they may be forced out by persistent discrimination and harassment from both neighbors and landlords.

Many governments and community-based organizations have set up emergency programs for temporary and permanent placement of the homeless. Despite these efforts, homelessness continues to increase. In the United Kingdom, one of the few countries with a law providing citizens with the right to housing, the national housing charity Shelter reported 2 million homeless individuals in 1989, with homelessness having more than doubled during the 1980s.[22] Many other countries have also witnessed an enormous increase in homelessness in the last decade, paralleling the global economic recession.

International, National, and Community Group Responses

Some initiatives have been taken by international, national, and community-based organizations with respect to AIDS and housing.

The International Response: In 1989, the Council of Europe was the first intergovernmental organization to recommend action at the housing agency level, aimed at securing suitable housing for people with AIDS. In the European Community, the European Parliament and the Council of Ministers have stated explicitly that housing, as well as discrimination by housing associations and the eviction of HIV-infected tenants, deserves priority attention.[23]

In the United Nations, the World Health Organization (WHO) was the first to act on the issue in 1989. WHO stated that there was no public health rationale for restricting access to housing of HIV-infected individuals. Although WHO still has to formulate more specific plans, other UN initiatives may make progress in this area. The UN Committee on Economic, Social and Cultural Rights, for example, an expert body entrusted with monitoring progress and compliance with the International Covenant on Economic, Social and Cultural Rights, has adopted an aggressive attitude in judging its periodic country reports. When the United Kingdom appeared before this committee, government representatives were questioned at length about the human rights implications of both housing and HIV/AIDS policy.[24]

The UN Sub-Committee on the Prevention of Discrimination and Protection of Minorities may also play an important future role. One of its special rapporteurs responsible for reporting on HIV/AIDS-related discrimination outlined some of the housing problems in a 1989 note and a 1991 progress report. It is expected that the special rapporteur appointed in 1991, who is responsible for investigating forced evictions, will bring similar problems to light.

International housing advocacy groups have recently shown a strong interest in the problems encountered by people with HIV/AIDS. Representatives of Habitat International Coalition (HIC), which introduced the idea of having a special rapporteur on forced evictions at the UN, have expressed their willingness to work on developing HIV/AIDS and housing policies.

The National Response: AIDS and housing tend to be addressed by different agencies at the national level. Only a handful of countries have succeeded in integrating both large- and small-scale efforts. It is generally assumed that countries can best fulfill their public health and housing duties by working with provincial and local authorities, along with significant participation from community-based organizations. But unlike other areas of AIDS, local authorities often play a central role setting housing policies. In many countries, local authorities own or administer a considerable percentage of rental housing. Moreover, they often have the power to designate land use through zoning and other ordinances.

Very few countries have AIDS-specific housing legislation. In the United States, however, the Fair Housing Amendments Act (1988) gives people with disabilities, including HIV/AIDS, protection from discrimination in the private-housing sector. In November 1990, Congress also passed the National Affordable Housing Act, which specifically includes individuals with AIDS.

Housing legislation in most countries recognizes only persons with opportunistic diseases and/or disabilities. Consequently, people with asymptomatic HIV infection cannot fall back on these special housing provisions to secure their housing rights. The advantage of this approach is that HIV/AIDS is not singled out as a special disease. The disadvantage is that people with HIV/AIDS are not always given the priority they need. This approach also fails to address the issues of discrimination mentioned earlier.

Community-Based Organization Response: Service organizations were the first to respond to the housing needs of HIV-infected individuals. In 1988, London Lighthouse opened, offering an integrated-care approach for people with HIV; it has since served as a model for a low-threshold shelter. In France, the organization Aparts established a number of therapeutic apartments specifically designed for those with HIV/AIDS. The Foundation in Brussels and Jhr.mr. Schorerstichting in Amsterdam coordinate extensive buddy projects, making it possible for people to stay in their own homes.

In addition, locally run AIDS hospices have mushroomed around the world. These include the Coming Home Hospice in San Francisco; the Bailey-Boushay House in Seattle, Washington; Noah's Ark/Red Cross Foundation in Stockholm; and the more than 20 Monar hospices around Poland. There is also Caritas and similar organizations in Rome, Madrid, and Bilbao. Religious orders run shelters for the homeless with HIV in many Mediterranean and developing countries.

These community-based efforts frequently meet with local resistance. AIDS organizations around the world face the danger of attacks from neighbors, angry crowds, and hooligans—usually people acting out of fear and ignorance. The reigning attitude appears to be "Not in my backyard." In Poland, for example, the Monar clinic in the village of Gloskow closed in 1991 as a result of a neighborhood blockade. In Barcelona, efforts to set up an AIDS hospice failed after neighbors protested against the "SIDAtorium." In Rome, an AIDS hospice received arson threats. And in Amsterdam, AIDS service organizations and self-help groups have been systematically denied office facilities.[25]

It is unfortunate that while many individuals feel compassion for those infected with HIV, resistant attitudes impede the development of many humane housing alternatives. Failure to foster a universal realization that adequate housing is vital for people with HIV/AIDS has, therefore, become a metaphor for the global response to AIDS. The AIDS epidemic has been a story of individual successes, backed by a collective response that is sometimes courageous, but often sporadic and driven by fear. Failure to provide at least a modicum of adequate housing for people with AIDS and HIV represents a collective failure of will.

■   ·   ·   ·

AIDS SERVICE ORGANIZATIONS IN TRANSITION

Jeff O'Malley

Jeff O'Malley is Executive Director of the Global AIDS Policy Coalition, based at the Harvard School of Public Health, Boston, Massachusetts.

AIDS Service Organizations (ASOs), the principal institutional vehicles of volunteer, community-based AIDS prevention and care efforts, are now widely viewed as central components of an effective societal response to AIDS. These organizations are often quite small, staffed and supported by a remarkable variety of activists ranging from gay men to health ministers' wives to drug users to dedicated social workers. In many countries most profoundly affected by the pandemic, ASOs seem to be as ubiquitous as local chambers of commerce, the Boy Scouts, and rural women's organizations. Yet their future is unclear as the demographics of the pandemic touch new populations, as charismatic leaders burn out or die, and as societal needs for prevention, care, and social support outstrip volunteer efforts and modest fund-raising efforts. How did these groups emerge, and how have they evolved over the course of the pandemic? What functions do AIDS Service Organizations serve in the 1990s?

The Emergence of a Nongovernmental Response to AIDS

In September 1981, 40 men gathered in the apartment of New York writer Larry Kramer in order to *do something* about the new epidemic in their midst; that day, the Gay Men's Health Crisis was created. In the following 2 years, similar ASOs were formed in other major U.S. cities. Today, almost 16,000 U.S. groups are listed in the National AIDS Information Clearinghouse, many of them ASOs. The mushrooming of such groups across the United States is often attributed to a unique combination of American volunteer spirit and the history of community organizing among gay men.[26] Such analyses, however, may give too much credit to American culture and not enough to America's bad luck, epidemiologically speaking. Compassion, fear, and anger at indifference have accompanied the early stages of the pandemic everywhere, and in many different parts of the world they quickly led to a nongovernmental, volunteer-driven response to AIDS.

Indeed, by the middle of the 1980s, when governments began to move beyond ad hoc responses to planned interventions, there was already a truly international volunteer response, with substantial numbers of nongovernmental care and prevention programs already established in countries as diverse as Zimbabwe, Australia, Canada, and Mexico.* In contrast to the situation in the United States, most

---

*Unless otherwise noted, data cited in this section are drawn from an in-depth survey conducted by the Global AIDS Policy Coalition in 1992 of 25 of the world's first AIDS Service Organizations (ASOs) in 12 developing countries and nine industrialized countries (see Chapter 8, "National AIDS Programs"), as well as privileged communication with the founders or directors of some of the most important networks of ASOs: the International Council of AIDS Service Organizations, AIDES (France), the Canadian AIDS Society, the National Minority AIDS

of the popular response to the epidemic in developing countries was organized by preexisting nongovernmental organizations (NGOs), with ASOs emerging in significant numbers only in the late 1980s. However, it is interesting to note that the countries with the weakest overall NGO response to AIDS are not those with the lowest GNP per capita, but rather the countries that score most poorly on other indexes reflecting overall freedom levels, gender equality, literacy, and human development.[27]

This section focuses on AIDS service organizations (ASOs), or nongovernmental, nonprofit groups that work primarily with AIDS issues. The categorization of these groups as ASOs reflects real world dynamics, as many AIDS-specific groups have resisted attempts to be included in an undifferentiated manner with other NGOs working on AIDS, such as Red Cross societies and family planning groups. (For a description of other nongovernmental organizations working on AIDS, see Chapter 8.) Because the creation of new types of private, nonprofit organizations inevitably reflects at least some frustration with existing institutions, it is not surprising that organizers of the new AIDS-focused organizations often saw their groups as unique.

ASOs and Communities

Analyses of ASOs and their contributions almost inevitably refer to the advantages of prevention and care activities being community based.[28] In fact, very few NGOs of any kind would admit to *not* being community based, and the phrase obscures some real differences among organizations.

Although all ASOs surveyed have continuously drawn from some sort of unpaid volunteer base, that base grew much more rapidly in those groups working in industrialized countries. These early ASOs often helped coalesce a sense of community, even where it had not previously existed. This was not simply because of epidemiological

Council (United States), the Australian Federation of AIDS Organizations, and the Southern African Network of AIDS Service Organisations. We are indebted to Meena Thayu, Mia MacDonald, and Kim Humphrey for assistance in this effort. Nationwide data from Mexico, excluding specific reference to Colectivo Sol, are drawn from Adrian Figueroa, *Participación civil en la lucha contra el SIDA* (Mexico: Ford Foundation, 1990).

realities (HIV disease was recognized within some of these populations early in the epidemic), but because these groups were stigmatized by AIDS and forced to organize against an onslaught of institutional discrimination and pervasive prejudice.

ASOs working originally with gays, people with hemophilia, and expatriate Haitians uniformly saw care as part of their mission, pioneering buddy programs and home care. From the beginning of the epidemic, these organizations challenged governments and funders that saw prevention as an activity distinct from community development and support. These groups were also responsible for popularizing safer sex strategies, arguing for human rights promotion as an integral part of effective AIDS programs and providing treatment information in nonmedical contexts.

Just over half the ASOs surveyed were founded by a group of predominantly gay men, usually self-identified as white and middle class. The contribution of gay men and lesbians to creating an ASO movement is most notable in industrialized countries, but it was also relevant to the creation of ASOs in the developing world, particularly in Latin America and Southeast Asia, and even, in a discrete fashion, in at least three sub-Saharan African countries.

The notion of a community base is much more difficult to apply to those ASOs that responded to initially heterosexual transmission patterns. Almost all developing country ASOs surveyed were organized by women, usually with a health, social service, or academic background. The role of tight-knit religious communities, such as the Salvation Army, is notable especially in Africa, where preexisting NGOs were often the first to take up the challenges posed by AIDS. Regardless of the profile of the original activists, all the developing country groups shared an immediate challenge to reach beyond their own class, social network, religious affiliation, or gender.

Early ASOs with care and prevention missions oriented to heterosexuals (like many for injection drug users or commercial sex workers and their clients)* were formed to help *others*. One important

---

*Even though several European countries had drug user groups that were very important to the response to AIDS, there is little evidence that these groups were seen by large numbers of users as representative. More recently, some users and former users with HIV infection have been more successful at self-organizing,

consequence for prevention activities is that these groups often faced a formidable challenge in understanding the behaviors or social context that put particular individuals at risk, and then trying to support behavior change. Another challenge was that the consequences of HIV infection were less visible where morbidity and mortality were spread more widely. This undoubtedly also contributed to the fact that these ASOs drew on much smaller numbers of volunteers, however dedicated. Developing country ASOs pursued a wide variety of activities, but were much more likely than the more focused ASOs to participate in behavioral and epidemiological research, promote sexual abstinence as a prevention strategy, have links to institutional care providers, make use of mass media campaigns, and refer to the general public as a target audience.

There were a few high-profile exceptions to this pattern, including the well-documented The AIDS Support Organisation (TASO) in Uganda. Many people praise the pioneering efforts of TASO's founder, a woman whose husband had died of AIDS, and the small original group of volunteers. Although a number of prominent TASO activists are not HIV-antibody positive, TASO was created at about the same time as, and in many ways parallels, the PWA organizations catalyzed by Michael Callen's activities in the United States. With a strong initial emphasis on care and support, TASO was promoted as a self-help organization, helping to create a new community of families living with HIV. Ironically, TASO's early success at a focused and care-oriented approach resulted in external pressures to broaden its range of activities, even to the point where some funders saw TASO as a vehicle to prevent HIV infection from spreading further in the public at large.

ASOs and Governments

Overall, the founders of ASOs share a remarkable combination of being somewhat socially marginalized yet politically sophisticated, and well connected to sources of financial support within their com-

following, and in many cases directly emerging from, the People with AIDS (PWA) movement. Similarly, it is only recently that more than a few AIDS projects for sex workers have been self-initiated and organized, and we are aware of no such self-organization among clients of sex workers.

munities. The ability to raise funds locally or rely on volunteers was essential, as early financial links between ASOs and government tended to be weak. Only 14 percent of the ASOs surveyed received financial support from their local or national governments in their first year of operation, and the funding received was generally modest. Relationships between state or other official funders and ASOs often began with a great deal of mutual reticence; ASOs feared both real interference and a loss of credibility with their client and volunteer base, whereas many ministry of health officials and other funders expressed both skepticism and principled opposition to channeling public funds to private organizations.*

An exception was one of the first prominent ASOs in the Islamic world, the Casablanca-based Association de lutte contre le SIDA. It was created with the active encouragement of government officials who believed that only a nongovernmental group could deal effectively with the politically charged issues of sexual behavior and anonymous HIV-antibody testing. Most other ASOs surveyed indicated that the government either refused to address the concerns of the initial activists adequately or was incapable of addressing the challenges of HIV due to its alienation from groups affected or at risk. Seventy percent of industrialized-country respondents and 100 percent of developing-country groups indicated that some sort of broader political agenda has always been implicit in the groups' activities; industrialized-country groups frequently cited such issues as lesbian and gay liberation or expansion of universal health care, whereas developing-country ASOs mentioned expanding public participation in development, support of marginalized groups, such as sex workers, and gender politics.

Governmental structures and traditions have not only been affected *by* ASOs, but have also had a great deal of impact *on* ASOs. This is notable both in terms of ASO programs and the number of volunteer organizations created in response to the pandemic (some countries in Eastern Europe and Asia still have very few or none). The number of ASOs and the range of service they provide in a particular

---

*Over a 2-year period working for WHO/GPA with the responsibility of encouraging governments to fund ASOs and other NGOs, the author discussed these issues at great length with both ASOs and ministry officials around the world.

country can be seen as either a positive indicator of a decentralized, grassroots-based response to AIDS or a negative indicator of the failure of the state to adequately provide services and respond to community needs. When both are present, as in the United States with its virtual lack of national policy response to AIDS, a prolific and highly differentiated ASO response to AIDS can emerge.

In the industrialized world outside the United States, the widest range of focused services, advocacy activities, and community-specific prevention campaigns have arisen in countries with pragmatic and sectorally integrated policy development processes,* such as Canada, the Netherlands, and Australia. Countries with highly centralized administrations, such as France, were much more likely to be dominated by a few large ASOs claiming to serve many different communities. Countries like Italy and Belgium, identified as having biomedical AIDS policies, tend to have a variety of ASOs serving different communities, but the organizations are much less successful at building a national ASO movement or at accessing government funds to expand services.

Although political variations affect the number and foci of ASOs in different countries, virtually all ASOs in the age of triumphant liberal democracy and capitalism find themselves in a curious nether world between the government and the citizenry. Associação Brasileira Interdisciplinar de AIDS (ABIA) in Brazil, founded by Herbert Daniel whose background was revolutionary guerrilla warfare, may seem far removed from state-sponsored and nurtured organizations like Austria's AIDS-Hilfe. Nevertheless, both groups now act as organizers and advocates for the disenfranchised, while being taxpayer-financed, privatized delivery agents of functions and services most often viewed as within the purview of government.

Despite the wide variety of service programs delivered by ASOs, 95 percent of those surveyed indicated that, in their first year, general

---

*Typically, official responses are differentiated on the basis of the *process* of policy development (centralized, decentralized, or sectorally integrated) or the *driving force* of policy development. H. Moerkerk and P. Aggleton, "AIDS prevention strategies in Europe: A comparison and critical analysis," in *AIDS: Individual, Cultural and Policy Dimensions* (London: Falmer, 1990), describe "pragmatic," "political," "biomedical," and "emergent" responses.

public policy and advocacy work on such issues as sexual law reform and promoting governmental action on AIDS were included in their activities; 70 percent described such work as a major component of their initial program. An almost equal number, 82 percent, included community organizing and development work as part of their mandate, although in their first year of existence, they tended to see this as only a minor or adjunct activity.

Early examples of formalized government-community dialogue occurred at a municipal level in New York and San Francisco, and at a national level in the Netherlands, Australia, Zambia, and Zimbabwe. Nevertheless, the first AIDS activists felt that they were largely ignored and unsupported by governmental and intergovernmental authorities. Sometimes at the behest of WHO, which created a special liaison on NGOs, and sometimes on their own initiative, national governments began responding to activist pressure for representation on national planning and advisory committees. By June 1989, NGOs were represented on national AIDS committees or subcommittees in about 75 percent of 123 countries surveyed.[29] Anecdotal evidence suggests that the vast majority of ASOs welcomed this trend, although a few have remained adamant about retaining their independence and avoiding government bodies.

Recent Developments

Over the past 3 years, ASOs have not only dramatically increased their direct contacts with governments, but have also begun to build a series of informal and formal alliances and networks to achieve political goals. The primary benefits of both formal and informal networking cited by surveyed ASOs include accessing funds for AIDS programs; collective legitimization of specific policy goals, such as preventing human rights abuses; and influencing policies and programs of multilateral organizations, such as WHO and the United Nations Development Program (UNDP). ASOs from countries with recent histories of widespread political oppression also see international networking as providing the kind of visibility that makes government control of ASO activities more difficult.

This network building had been occurring from the beginning of the ASO movement, but it accelerated significantly in early 1989. In France, a new umbrella group was created to bring together community groups and governmental programs to share both funding and policy development responsibilities; by most accounts, however, the group has been more successful at representing France's activities abroad than at coordinating efforts domestically. In the United States, earlier efforts to create the National AIDS Network as a broad-based umbrella group floundered; but cooperative efforts in Washington-based advocacy solidified into the AIDS Action Council, a highly successful research and lobby group that broadened the profile of AIDS politics beyond the lesbian and gay movement. Internationally, the International Steering Committee for People with HIV and AIDS has helped to support the emergence of self-help groups in countries as diverse as Sierra Leone and India, and The International Council of AIDS Service Organizations (ICASO) is now supporting the formation of dynamic regional networks in Asia, Africa, Latin America, and Europe.

The general political notions of most groups when founded also began to evolve into more focused strategies by the late 1980s. In Vienna, a mostly European group of ASOs issued a statement challenging governments to overcome "structural impediments" to ASO efficacy, for example, laws that criminalized homosexuality or made sexually explicit education difficult. On a more international level, a small group of dedicated sex workers led by a dynamic Australian contingent managed to shift significantly the terms of reference of academic and programmatic approaches to the sex industry in many parts of the world, alternatively convincing and embarrassing program managers and funders into the position that sex workers deserved the same respect and support that many groups of gay men had achieved. In Canada, ASOs successfully pressured their government into introducing an emergency drug release program for experimental therapies. Zambian ASOs convinced their government to become the African pioneers of government funding for NGOs working on AIDS. In the United States, the success of ASOs in widening their political constituency and establishing formal lobbying programs was essential to the passage of two of that country's most important legislative responses to AIDS, the Ryan White Care Act and the Americans with Disabilities Act. Many activists in Chile's ASOs were involved in that country's democratization movement and were subsequently well placed to successfully encourage school-based AIDS education, despite some religious opposition.

The shift in attitudes since the early days of the epidemic is quite remarkable, with more than half of the ASOs surveyed having received some government funding by 1989. Indeed, the survey of well-established ASOs found steady *increases* in government support over the last few years, thus largely avoiding the extreme funding difficulties faced by newer organizations. Remarkably, two-thirds of surveyed ASOs report no significant pressure from funders regarding their program, and another 20 percent report mainly positive advice and useful technical support. Nevertheless, our survey found that more than 80 percent of respondents are concerned about the long-term financial viability of their organizations. Cuts in funding in 1992 to high-profile ASOs, like Deutsche AIDS-Hilfe, and the planned elimination in 1993 of WHO/GPA's NGO funding initiative indicate that their worries may be well founded.

An Evolving Program for an Evolving Pandemic

Most people involved with ASOs now recognize that although much has been accomplished through imagination, enthusiasm, and ad hoc crisis management, their organizations have to prepare for the long struggle ahead, as the pandemic and its impacts clearly are not going to be quickly overcome. Increasing numbers of gay-oriented groups are torn between growing needs in their own community and a sense of obligation to learn from other ASOs and to reach out to other vulnerable populations. (See Chapter 9, Box 9.14 on dehomosexualization.) In contrast, ASOs oriented to the general public have recognized the success of more focused organizations. They increasingly bring to their work a heightened interest in supporting peer-based education and care and a much stronger emphasis on acting as catalysts of community development and self-organization among marginal or vulnerable groups.

Several important dynamics have converged to change the ASO environment. Most significantly, perceptions and realities of the demographics of the pandemic have shifted. Heterosexual transmission is now recognized as much more of an issue in countries like France and the United States, and bisexual behavior is acknowledged to be widespread in many parts of the world. A dramatic epidemic has emerged in Thailand, and the potential for similar explosive situations is apparent in other countries. (See Chapters 2 and 14.) Thus, there has been an increasing pressure on ASOs based in narrow communities to reach out to populations newly recognized as vulnerable. These shifting epidemiological patterns are creating significant tensions within ASOs around the world, as it is widely recognized that the imperative of scaling-up initiatives directly conflicts with the two factors that have contributed most to ASO success: cost efficiency, based on community fundraising and use of volunteers, and program efficacy linked to the intimate connection between ASO workers and affected or targeted populations.

Another significant dynamic is the professionalization of ASOs. Although in the past it had been relatively easy to evaluate ASO success in providing care, emotional support, and welfare assistance to people with HIV, the efficacy of prevention efforts was uncertain at best. However, in the last few years, cohort studies and behavioral research began to demonstrate significant reductions in HIV incidence and risk behavior in several parts of the world, most strikingly among large, urbanized gay populations well served by ASOs. Although not always recognized by policymakers, ASO activists began to realize by the late 1980s that they had developed significant expertise in the prevention of HIV transmission and in unorthodox but effective techniques of community-based program planning and evaluation. Yet professionalization can be negative, as increasing cooperation between ASOs and governments has led to a situation in which certain leading organizations are well funded and well staffed but have become vulnerable to criticisms that they are part of a government-led AIDS establishment and less responsive to their original constituencies.

In the last few years, the number of groups working on AIDS has also proliferated, and three-quarters of the pioneering ASOs surveyed now find that they play an important role leading networks, coordinating multiagency collaborative projects, and providing education and training to other, newer organizations. Although the established ASOs place even more emphasis on their political role than in the past, they have moved from confrontation to cooperation and toward a bridging function between their governments and the newly emerging organizations and social movements. Indeed, none of the ASO respondents reported a deteriorating relationship with their national government; 84 percent reported improving collaboration.

These changes are reflected not only in the increasing acceptance of ASOs by funders and bureaucrats, but also in the increasing number of criticisms heard from the community. Among industrialized-country ASOs, 55 percent report that their most frequently heard complaint is that the organizations have become too bureaucratic, and nearly 30 percent indicate they are criticized for being either too gay identified or insufficiently diverse. Developing-country groups, on the other hand, are most often criticized for undermining public morality or cultural values, as they have begun to deemphasize the promotion of abstinence and skills training for prostitutes in favor of enthusiastic support for social marketing of condoms and self-organization of the marginalized.

The flow of government finance and membership on official committees have also led to other kinds of criticism from the communities. Pink Triangle in Kuala Lumpur, a group working primarily with gay Malaysians, has been criticized for refraining from provocative activities and for concentrating instead on building a good working relationship with their government, which still outlaws homosexuality. France has had a much more extreme situation; two Paris-based ASOs with strong connections to the governing Socialist Party have been accused by the gay press and activists from other ASOs of being more concerned with international public relations for France's AIDS efforts than with needed prevention or care activities. Gay Men's Health Crisis was roundly criticized for producing a sanitized, safe-sex video after it received government funding, although GMHC, like most other U.S. ASOs, has continued to receive only a very small proportion of total revenues from government grants, especially when compared to other industrialized-country groups.[30]

Such criticism is most prominent in the industrialized world, and especially the United States, where a substantial critical AIDS activist community outside of established ASOs has developed since 1987. It is relevant to note the importance of political environments that permit the constant creation of new volunteer organizations and movements as the pandemic's dynamics shift, as new needs emerge, and as other ASOs like those surveyed become more established. The enthusiasm and energy of new groups can create problems as well, such as the often-cited examples of ACT-UP groups alienating key political leaders. In Uganda, where the government and more established NGOs are pursuing a well-considered policy emphasizing community development and (nonfinancial) support for extended families in response to the increasing number of children without parents due to AIDS, as many as 60 different, new nongovernmental orphanages have been established, threatening to undermine efforts to support the vast majority of these children who will never be cared for in an institutional setting.

Into the Future

It is important to appreciate the complexity of social forces that have interacted over the last decade and contributed to the creation of today's ubiquitous ASOs. ASOs have demonstrated their ability to offer valuable services facilitating public participation, defending the right to privacy, decentralizing services, encouraging community control, promoting individual responsibility in health promotion, and acting as a bulwark against discrimination. Efficacy, of course, plays an important role. Vulnerability to HIV infection and its impact decreases where public health principles and human rights are respected. In addition, efficiency drives the support for ASOs, particularly as governments seek both to legitimize their HIV/AIDS programs and to reduce costs by privatizing implementation responsibilities.

Although the ideal outcome of these two potentially contradictory agendas is a cost-effective and effective response to AIDS, this is not inevitable. Most ASOs cherish their participation in official consultative bodies, but it is not clear that such participation provides real community input into policy development, as opposed to providing governments and multilateral organizations with the pretense of community consultation while reneging on public responsibilities to respond to the epidemic. The challenges to ASOs in the next few years are to recognize their strengths as well as their limitations and to demonstrate their efficacy in confronting a new, more differentiated and widespread pandemic. To accomplish this while maintaining efficient operations (as demanded by funders) and creating more sophisticated mechanisms to ensure responsiveness and legitimacy (as demanded by the communities ASOs reflect and serve) will not be an easy task.

━━━━━━━━━ . . .

SHIFTING PATTERNS IN INTERNATIONAL FINANCING FOR AIDS PROGRAMS

Anthony Klouda

:hony Klouda, M.D.,
he coordinator of the
)S Prevention Unit,
ernational Planned
renthood Federation,
idon.

"What is it that you cannot buy with money?"

AIDS programs in many developing countries are heavily dependent on external financial assistance and are, in turn, influenced by the structures, systems, and priorities of donors. This section is concerned with patterns of international financing undertaken by these donors— governmental, nongovernmental, and those within the United Nations system.

Governments everywhere were slow to respond to AIDS, and even slower in industrialized countries to develop comprehensive plans and programs. Nevertheless, when the official development assistance (ODA) agencies, such as the American USAID, the Norwegian NORAD, and the Swedish SIDA, did become involved, there was considerable unanimity among these agencies in their early support of the World Health Organization's Global Programme on AIDS (WHO/GPA), with its strategy of encouraging countries to establish national AIDS committees and national AIDS programs. (Encouraging specialized AIDS committees and programs could be seen as somewhat unusual for WHO, which typically stresses integrated approaches to health issues. For a description of the circumstances leading to the AIDS-focused approach, see Chapter 8.) For countries receiving development assistance, WHO/GPA agreed to act as a coordinating and funding mechanism, and it conditioned its financial support on each recipient country developing a plan, program, and staff committed to AIDS. Unfortunately, despite frequent reference to the interaction of AIDS and other development issues, governmental and intergovernmental cooperation agencies did not match their support for specialized AIDS programs with increased support for general health infrastructure and for comprehensive programs addressing the social and economic contexts that render people vulnerable to AIDS.

Not surprisingly, we are now witnessing a variety of responses from governmental development agencies:

- direct support of country AIDS programs
- a concern for improved support of nongovernmental organizations (NGOs—also known as Private Voluntary Organizations)
- support for a broader range of responses from individual UN agencies

Whereas most governmental and multilateral funding agencies have only recently begun to explore new strategies and patterns of funding, it should be remembered that many NGOs (whether acting as donors or working directly with communities) have continued to promote and maintain a variety of responses and patterns of funding. NGOs with a commitment to AIDS were typically quicker to respond to new circumstances and more willing to experiment with new approaches than were their governmental counterparts. However, few of the development-oriented groups have taken on HIV issues seriously, and these groups have often searched for quick and easy solutions, much like their governmental counterparts.

Therefore, we have arrived at a point at which there is little agreement concerning either the best ways of funding or the best approaches to programs. This section examines the current patterns of international financing of AIDS-related programs, the nature of the debates about funding, and how those patterns arose. The general conclusion is that although diversity is welcome, there is still:

- too much interest in developing (or imposing) programs that are *specific* to AIDS care or prevention
- too little commitment of support to the general infrastructures and the programs that concentrate on the key development issues, and for the empowerment of those at risk of ill-health in general, and of HIV infection in particular
- too little priority for AIDS, STDs, or sexuality on the agendas of development programs
- almost no increase in efforts to meet the needs of the poorest, the most vulnerable, the most isolated, or the least powerful

These problems are found within the major governments and donors as well as within many of the NGOs.

Pessimism or Optimism?

It is natural for people whose work is related to HIV and AIDS to be pessimistic when looking at the rapid progress of the pandemic and the extent of the personal and societal suffering caused by AIDS. It is also easy to be pessimistic about many of the decisions and actions made by people whose work relates to AIDS. When one looks at the decisions being taken by blood banks between 1984 and 1986 (the deliberate postponement of decisions concerning testing and screening); at the victim-blaming and neglect targeted at people most affected by this epidemic in most countries; at the feuding between scientific research bodies for prestige and financial gain; and at the quarrels between various groups affected by HIV to establish just who is the most politically correct and who should have the most funding; one sees the negative side of what many would prefer to be a noble and valiant cause.

One problem of this pessimism is that it often centers on AIDS alone, instead of on the context of health and other problems that face people throughout the world on a daily basis—issues that often concern them much more than the prospect of HIV infection. Because this context decides the extent of the epidemic, and because this context is not being addressed on a scale of any significance, it is hardly surprising that we must be pessimistic about the future of the various epidemics. But it would be folly to think that failure in curtailing the epidemics hangs solely on the lack of funding for AIDS-specific programs.

The factors that affect rapid change are extensive and complex. But unless the programs that aim to reduce transmission or improve care and social reaction try to change these factors, the chances of success are low.

- Although a particular technology may be *necessary* for success, it may not be *sufficient.* Any technology for prevention or care depends on a range of supporting factors that include transport, adequate roads, administration, management, the state of service structures, and the attitudes of the public, service providers, and politicians. Once these factors have been put in place, its use depends on whether people are truly in a position to make use of that technology.

- The successful provision of technologies from outside sources to reduce transmission or to provide care depends on adaptation to local situations and needs, but it must occur on a large-scale, widespread, and continuous basis. To date, most people have been concerned with showing that, *for a particular environment,* if sufficient resources are established then the technology is successful. Although there have been many attempts to alter the economies of poor countries so that they can afford to support all of the necessary technologies throughout the land on a continuous basis, externally imposed experiments have been overwhelmingly misguided and unsuccessful.

- The adoption of technologies and the changing of environments for the support of relevant behaviors depend on an essentially slow process that requires involvement of the targeted people in planning, implementing, and monitoring the action which they have chosen. This process gives people *access* to technologies, alters their situations to *enable* them to use them, and helps people *want* to use them. Although this process is faster for some groups of people who have control of their situations (and in such cases, the process can be greatly facilitated by such strategies as social marketing), for other groups their situations make the chances of change remote.

- There are a very large number of other priority situations that governments, communities, groups, and individuals have to address. For many people, some of these other situations are more immediately dangerous and life-threatening than is the threat of HIV infection. Unless the people affected are given a chance to address these problems, they are unlikely to take action in relation to HIV.

An understanding of these tensions and factors provides an essential background for a discussion of the current patterns of funding.

Evolution of Patterns of Funding

The Move to Coordination: By 1986, it was recognized that a series of epidemics of HIV transmission had been established in several parts of the globe. This recognition was mostly a result of the persuasive efforts of the

WHO's Special Programme on AIDS (later, the Global Programme on AIDS). A number of governmental donors agreed that more support should be given to WHO in order to help other governments recognize the nature of these epidemics and their seriousness and to coordinate and mobilize program and funding responses. At that time, there were serious abuses of national and human rights by researchers and others, and so it was felt that there should also be some element of control of AIDS-related activities in any country, in addition to a coordinating function. National AIDS Committees (NACs) were then rapidly established in most countries with the support of WHO/GPA, which provided guidance and helped coordinate and develop the various program components. (This occurred despite experience with the establishment of other national development committees, which had in general proved to be poor, e.g., the National Primary Health Care Committees.)

A method of country-level funding considered effective at that time was multi-bilateral funding, whereby donors would provide contributions through the local WHO office to an overall national plan drawn up by the country in question. This and other mechanisms are described in more detail in Chapter 12.

Varieties of Response: Since the introduction of international financing of AIDS programs by governments through WHO, a number of patterns of response to HIV have been established. Many of these responses were based on the experiences of communities and groups as they responded to AIDS in ways that they themselves developed. Some were organizational responses based on long experience of dealing with related problems. Many were informed by traditional public health thinking, with its strengths and limitations. Others were dependent merely on the prejudices or whims of program controllers. These patterns were certainly not new; they reflected traditional responses to a variety of situations that have long challenged development. The responses can be split roughly into the following six categories:

- Community response—where communities or groups of people have organized their own responses to the challenges posed by HIV or AIDS.
- Developmental responses—where people have responded by placing

the situation in which transmissions of HIV occur within a developmental context and have modified their developmental programs to address these situations.

- Interventionist responses—where organizations have developed programs that target individuals or situations only with specific relevance to the proximate problem of HIV transmission.
- Technical responses—where the programs are based on the provision of a simple technology (e.g., condoms, testing kits, medicines, information) without consideration of other factors.
- Legalistic responses—where governments have assumed that applying the law or developing new regulations would solve the problem.
- Ignoring responses—where people or organizations have refused to modify their programs or approaches in the belief either that HIV transmission has little to do with their program, or that it is not something that should be addressed.

New Priorities for Governmental and Intergovernmental Donors: In addition to the recognition of various possible responses, there have been a number of forces that have shifted governmental donors away from their initial support of the coordinating mechanism offered by WHO.

The first is the experience of the national AIDS control programs (NACPs), as outlined in Chapter 8. NACPs provided important technical guidance at first, but were often overwhelmed and lost focus as more and more communities, NGOs, and international organizations began participating in AIDS prevention and care efforts. Some NACPs emphasized a narrow medical approach, and many found it difficult to differentiate between useful coordination functions and counterproductive efforts to control all contributions. Politics and traditions made some slow to respond to changing circumstances; some were corrupt, and many unimaginative.

Second, after 5 years of support of WHO/GPA, many governmental donors claim to be impressed by the responses of some NGOs that mounted care and prevention efforts with relatively little in the way of resources. This parallels developments in many other areas of development assistance, where official donors increasingly seem to believe (somewhat uncritically) in the efficiency and efficacy of NGOs. There is anecdotal evidence that the same donors often feel that they have been giving large amounts of money toward national programs through WHO/GPA without much obvious effect on the various epidemics (whereas, in fact, funds available to WHO/GPA were modest in comparison to either ODA for other purposes or such factors as Third World debt repayment).

Third, the donors have been building up their expertise with regard to HIV/AIDS programming and have developed individual and divergent views regarding what constitutes effective action. As a result, many donors are turning toward direct funding of individual governmental programs using the bilateral route, promoting programs in which they are interested and can have control, and for which they can take credit. They have also begun to seek new ways of funding local NGO work.

This also reflects a move away from the general provision of funds for a large number of countries and toward the selection by particular donors of fewer countries in which they have a particular interest. This is evident in the large new programs funded by the USAID through Family Health International, and it has been justified largely by the need to focus resources. Little, however, is being said about the countries that will lose their ODA support.

At the same time, donors are seeking a clarification of the WHO/GPA role with regard to coordination and leadership. They are trying to ensure that a balanced approach to programs is established, using the expertise of a range of UN agencies—perhaps with multiple leadership for different program aspects. The work of some of these other UN agencies is itself becoming very interesting. The UNDP, UNICEF, and the World Bank are all mounting programs that are potentially of great relevance, although each is hampered by its agency's own institutional agendas and politics (UNICEF avoids condoms and controversial communities; the World Bank's loan programs are not seen as the champion of improved health infrastructure). If it succeeds at raising funds from donors, the UNDP wants to concentrate on the facilitation of multisectoral efforts in development programming, often with the involvement of ministries of planning or their equivalents. The World Bank is undertaking a series of in-depth analyses of various country situations.

As part of this general drive toward other programs, the Rockefeller Foundation is coordinating a search for ways of channeling funds to local NGOs in developing countries. This idea originated within USAID, but is now tentatively supported by a large number of donors. Work has started by sending groups of consultants to 5 countries for 2 to 3 weeks to assess the current state of NGO work in those countries, the extent to which some NGOs could support others, and the possibilities for establishing a funding and support structure in those countries. There is no clear idea of the mechanism that could be developed to sustain NGO development in the countries concerned, nor is it clear how criteria are to be established for what constitutes relevant work. While any initiative to improve support for NGOs must be welcomed, there are several concerns related to this initiative.

One of the most interesting aspects of the shifts in AIDS funding by governmental donors is that it may follow a similar shift in patterns of funding of Primary Health Care (PHC) programs. In PHC, it has increasingly been recognized that diversity is the key to success. This requires that a number of programs be mounted simultaneously, which reinforce one another but do not necessarily do the same thing, and are not necessarily coordinated by any particular body.

If donors are moving in this direction, the funding of a number of different types of programs through a range of organizations will be welcome. However, if there is a move to organizations that impose simplistic technological interventions in the hope they will provide a quick fix (as happened with some donors and multilateral organizations when funding PHC), then the likelihood of success against HIV infection will be reduced.

The NGO Experience

Many decisions about funding have centered on beliefs about the value of NGO programs. Many NGOs have particular agendas linked to their specialization in selected health or social fields, whereas others emphasize multisectoral support for general community developmental efforts. Some of these developmental NGOs have been trying consistently to promote the importance of other programs that are not specific to HIV in order to balance the AIDS-specific activities. This is because the situations that lead to transmission of HIV are essentially determined by social and economic development. However, the actual experience of NGOs in implementing programs—AIDS-specific or more general—illustrates a number of serious difficulties.

Success Breeds Distortion—The Uganda Experience: It is a well-known funding syndrome that success breeds distortion. The pattern generally is as follows. A local NGO works out a very good system of interaction and support with a group of people in a community. It seeks funds to maintain or expand its work. In the process, the funder and the NGO publicize the work—partly through local (or even international) meetings and workshops. The work of that NGO starts being quoted as a paradigm. The NGO is driven by this exposure to maintain that paradigm in a larger or more complex situation that can no longer be related to the original work. The NGO cannot modify that work, as donors are only interested in maintaining the original paradigm. More funds are poured into that paradigm until, ultimately, the paradigm is recognized to have distorted the development picture. Then attention shifts to the work done by another organization. And so the cycle continues.

TASO (The AIDS Support Organization) in Uganda may be in the throes of such a pattern. This is an organization that bravely and successfully set up a system of support for people with HIV in Uganda. It has now received so much funding that it is providing an excellent and comprehensive health and social support service for people with HIV. The problem is that only people with HIV can use the service. Unfortunately, there is almost no equivalent support service for people with other very serious health problems in Uganda. The Primary Health Care service, for example, could not begin to provide as comprehensive a system of support for individuals as that provided by TASO.

Although TASO has at least been supported adequately in this expansion, there are many NGOs that are most successful if left at a particular level; when they are led to expand, they are not given the support necessary to cope with the required management and administrative changes.

Larger Issues Ignored—The Malawi Experience: Currently, there is much stated concern about achieving a balance between what is called *prevention* and what is called *care* in relation to AIDS programs. The concept is good and promises a balance that has been sought for many years by several NGOs. The problem is the large element of ambiguity in the ostensible support proclaimed by the donors. This is seen in the evidence from Malawi.

In 1988, the Malawi government froze its contributions to the mission hospitals, which provide roughly half of all patient care in Malawi. This occurred at a time when AIDS was beginning to have a dramatic impact on hospitals. Today, AIDS-related conditions (including TB and cancers) account for approximately a third of all hospital beds. Hospitals have had to face an expanding problem with a continuously diminishing budget; the budget now stands at 40 percent of the 1988 level. When appeals were made to donors in 1990–91, the applications were universally turned down, on the basis that this would reduce pressure on the Malawi government to increase its own contributions.

Recently, two donors provided approximately $550,000 to Malawi mission hospitals for training schools, but no funds were provided for care. At the same time, Malawi is completing a very costly medical school—again supported by donors. Although these priorities may be regarded by some people as correct, they hardly square with a commitment to balancing care and prevention; they simply point to the fact that if the real situation is to change, then donors will have to inject massive amounts of money regularly to prop up the health and social service side of the equation.

Who Should Be Funded? The perennially difficult question is who should be chosen for support. There have never been any logical criteria in the funding world for choosing one project over another. Mostly, it depends on chance (the particular project has been stumbled on by one representative of the donor), which is then coupled with the current political correctness of the organization seeking funds. When funds are around, there is, of course, competition among organizations for those funds. In these competitions, the most eloquent, the ones with senior officials in high social circles, and the ones with the best knowledge of how to play the game are generally the ones who obtain the bulk of the funds.

Potential Impact

Impact on HIV Transmission: The central question is whether shifts in funding patterns by governmental donors will have any impact* on the pandemic, on care and social reaction,† as well as on other developmental work. So far, the evidence for impact on the overall epidemic is scanty. It is probable that some HIV transmission has been reduced in health care settings in rich countries (and in some of those in poorer countries) by adequate control of blood and instruments, and that some of the small-scale interventions with people in a range of groups have had an influence on some of the sexual or needle transmission for some of the time. It is also clear that funding of particular programs of hospital and community care has been beneficial and that there are many instances of shifts of attitude following educational programs. It has been shown that in large populations with adequate access to social services, with extensive employment, and with health services that have safe blood supplies and adequate treatment, the rate of spread of HIV is relatively low. (The word *populations* is crucial because although such factors may be present, they may not be usable by particular segments of the community.)

The critical factors in controlling the epidemic do not lie among people who can make choices, but rather among those who cannot—especially the poorest, least powerful, most vulnerable, and most isolated—those who are marginalized in various ways.

This conclusion is important and leads to the question of the

---

*The debate around the use of the term *impact* is complex. It is very unlikely that any particular program could have as a realistic objective a measurable impact on the epidemic. Instead, most programs would set objectives in relation to a particular situation or behavior, which are staged over adequate lengths of time and modifiable in the light of experience. It is unclear how anyone could demonstrate the extent to which particular interventions had an impact on an epidemic, but when there is a continuing epidemic, and huge amounts are being poured into a number of interventions, it is natural to ask whether the sum total of those interventions is meaningful in relation to the epidemic.

†Some would also argue that the levels of expenditure on AIDS programs should be achieved for other developmental programs on a permanent basis, but as this is unlikely for most countries, this argument will not be addressed further.

objectives behind the funding and development of programs related to AIDS prevention. Some of the implications for these objectives are:

- Current development programs working to empower people should also raise awareness about gender issues, sexuality, and STDs. These issues should similarly be raised in all education programs (school and otherwise).
- Current programs to strengthen health services should include components that ensure widespread access to STD recognition, diagnosis, and therapy, in addition to work on protocols for effective care of people with illness (including illness as a result of AIDS) at low cost at home.
- Groups that offer support for people with particular social or care problems (such as those with HIV) should be supported.

Impact on Other Programs: An examination of expenditure on health and social services in most developing countries reveals gross inattention, with the military and other sectors consuming huge portions of foreign aid and government expenditure. Yet within the health sector, the amount of funding for AIDS programs may distort a country's priorities, with money being shifted away from other programs, such as PHC. This argument can be made about all focused development assistance and can be countered by the claim that interest in AIDS helps to bring additional resources and attention to the health and social sector. Unfortunately, there is no consistent pattern, and accurate figures are hard to obtain, but undoubtedly, in some countries spending in other essential areas of health and social services is lagging considerably.

With a population of about 18 million, Uganda has a high prevalence of HIV infection and AIDS. The overall government expenditure on the health sector for the year 1988 was about $11.2 million. AIDS activities in the medium term plan (entirely borne by external donors) was $4.1 million in 1988, $11.1 million in 1989, $9.9 million in 1990, $4.55 million in 1991, and about $4.6 million in 1992. Furthermore, in 1992, the UNDP will be adding $18 million to the national AIDS program. USAID has added a further $10 million for earmarked projects over 5 years, which include support for TASO and for voluntary testing clinics. The Belgian government is giving $7 million for orphans. The UK Medical Research Council has given $3 million for the 5-year prospective study of 10,000 people in the Masaka district. There will be a further $5 million for vaccine trials and redevelopment at Mulago hospital provided by the African Development Bank. Many other donors are adding to this considerable expenditure. In contrast, other health and social services are deteriorating badly in the context of massive debt and declining global ODA.

Nepal has a population of about 15 million but currently has a very low prevalence of HIV infection and AIDS. In 1988, its total health expenditure was $27.4 million. The three-year medium term AIDS Control Programme for 1989–91 envisaged an average annual expenditure of $660,000.

Neither of these scenarios takes into account nongovernmental expenditure, but it is easy to appreciate the enormous imbalance in the case of Uganda, where the overall health care system, undermined by years of war and underfunding, now lacks not only appropriate financial support but also absorptive capacity.

Unless the infrastructure for service provision is present throughout a country, then specific programs for HIV or AIDS will have little chance of success. There is a need for roads, staff, buildings, and a whole range of material resources (such as drugs for treatment of STDs and care of the various conditions in AIDS), in addition to the requirements to prevent and treat other common illness—all of which are often forgotten in the development of specific programs.*

A Question of Balance

Thus, it is vital to widen the agenda beyond areas that are specific to AIDS (such as research, epidemiology, therapies, immunization, information) with those that are nonspecific (including most efforts at social development). If the set of issues that surround AIDS can be integrated to embrace other development programs, then there is little need for the directive coordination envisaged in the mid-1980s. In-

---

*A depressing side effect of the distorting funds is the impact on morale in other sectors that cannot find the funds for the things they need. Further, the subsidies received by many individuals with country posts in AIDS work leads to an imbalance of power with those who may be more senior, but who now have less financial clout.

stead, a new pattern of mutually supportive interaction should be developed. Of course, this depends on adequate funding and political support for these parallel social development efforts, a serious and daunting challenge in an era of declining international aid levels and increasing emphasis on privatization and structural adjustment.

Many people working in AIDS-focused programs oppose such arguments. They claim that the challenges posed by transmission of HIV have forced us to look anew at the problems of development and the approaches to solving them. But although innovations are occurring in the AIDS programs themselves, there is no evidence of this having an impact on overall development approaches, and to date, no one has proposed any strategies that differ from those already known.[31]

There is also a claim that current development programs have no answer. There is much truth in this, but few agencies (apart from some NGOs) have bothered to test this argument by modifying development programs in a suitable way. The argument requires that the compass of development activities has to be enlarged. For too long, some development programs have restricted themselves to promoting a rather narrow range of interests and have not been concerned with AIDS. (See the "ignoring" response discussed earlier.) An example is seen in PHC programs. Many programs that have contented themselves with merely providing a service should now address critically what they are doing about the development of the people they serve.

It is also true that few development programs have successfully answered the problems of the poorest, most oppressed, least powerful, most isolated, and most vulnerable. However, very little money has been put into ensuring consistent long-term efforts with such groups, or more important, with the political and social environments that control those groups.

If coordination is required, it must ensure that these kinds of changes take place throughout the spectrum of development programs. Some coordination of this kind is possible at the level of bilateral and multilateral donors because of the power they wield.

Conclusions

It is important to remember that some local efforts have been successful in helping people to challenge and change their situations. There have been many successful examples of programs that have altered people's attitudes toward HIV/AIDS, STDs, and sexuality: such programs are an essential component of strategies to deal with the epidemic of social reaction.

However, for the poorest, weakest, least powerful, and most vulnerable, their situations will continue to put them at risk generally—HIV infection being added to a long list. A fear is that when vaccines and adequate therapies are discovered and made available to the wealthier countries and people, the suffering and situations of those most vulnerable will be forgotten.

The experience of development organizations is that the most successful development programs are often low key, low cost, and grass roots. Such efforts need to be multiplied extensively. Most current AIDS expenditure is not like that, and although the necessary expenditure on the provision of services and on biomedical aspects must continue, perhaps the governmental donors are, in a somewhat peculiar way, trying to reestablish the necessary balance in the development process. HIV and AIDS are with us far beyond the short term. We all have to adjust to that fact and put mechanisms in place to cope with it.

▬▬▬   ·   ·   ·

INTERNATIONAL SUPPORT FOR AIDS PREVENTION AND CONTROL

Margaret Phillips

..rgaret Phillips is a
..alth economist who has
..rked with several
..ganizations involved in
..DS control and
..evention activities
..cluding the World
..nk, USAID, WHO, and
..ICEF).

The international response to the AIDS pandemic has been marked from the start by a diversity of approaches. This section describes the approaches of the larger organizations to illustrate some of the complexity of the international response to HIV/AIDS.* Table 17.1 summarizes their activities.

USAID

Since it started AIDS work in 1986, the United States Agency for International Development (USAID) has spent more than $236 mil-

---

*Information for this section was drawn from cited documents and communication with individuals at each organization.

Table 17.1: Focus on five international AIDS agencies: A review by *AIDS in the World*, 1992

Executing agency	Type of agency	Year AIDS activities initiated	Budgets since beginning of program through 1991 (millions $US)	Countries supported
USAID	Official development assistance agency	1986	$236	74 in all regions
Official Dutch Government Assistance Program	Official development assistance agency	1987	$22.7	Rwanda, Tanzania, Zambia
Norwegian Red Cross	Nongovernmental organization	1985	$5	Rwanda, Kenya, Trinidad and Tobago, and others
UNESCO	United Nations specialized agency	1987	Not Available	Various, including Africa and Pacific and Caribbean islands
World Bank	International development lending organization	1986	$55.8	20+ countries, mostly in Africa, but also Brazil and Indonesia

lion on AIDS through 1991, making it the largest program of its kind in the world.[32] The USAID program has grown consistently, with estimated annual spending in 1991 reaching over $76 million. Forty-three percent of USAID AIDS resources have gone to the World Health Organization's Global Programme on AIDS (WHO/GPA), making USAID the single largest contributor to GPA, providing roughly 25 percent of its total budget.

Of the remaining money, the majority is directed at sub-Saharan Africa, which received 44 percent of USAID bilateral funding in 1990, followed by Latin America with 26 percent. Asia and the Middle East together receive less than 10 percent. Interregional funding accounted for the remainder.

USAID has supported 650 projects in 74 developing countries in all regions of the world. Most of its resources are directed at countries where the current prevalence of HIV or the potential for transmission of HIV is considered high. A country must have favorable diplomatic relations with the United States to qualify for USAID support, and although countries must first seek assistance, the agency now encourages them to request assistance and helps them apply.

USAID disburses its bilateral support in several ways. The AIDS Technical Support Project, established in 1987, controls 65 percent of the funds, including both the central USAID budget and the sums that USAID's country offices (Missions) contribute when they *buy into* the project. (Mission buy-ins account for nearly 39% of the total project expenditure, reflecting the value that missions attach to AIDS activities.) In recent years, several projects were nestled within the AIDS Technical Support Project, the two largest being AIDSCOM and the AIDSTECH, which together accounted for 72 percent of resources in 1990. AIDSCOM ($24.4 million from 1987 to 1992) has helped organizations apply communication and behavioral sciences to AIDS and has assisted in developing institutional capacities for health communication efforts. AIDSTECH ($41 million from 1987 to 1992) has had a broader goal, namely to strengthen national AIDS prevention programs. AIDSTECH has operated in 45 countries, conducting behavioral and epidemiological research and developing programs to prevent the sexual transmission of AIDS and to improve the safety of blood supplies.*

Nongovernmental organizations, private voluntary organizations, and other community organizations play an important role in im-

---

*An internal review has led to a proposal both to substantially expand and to redirect activities in the AIDS Technical Support Project when the current contracts finish in 1992/93. The additional $260 million *mega-grant* for AIDS represents the biggest public health action in the history of USAID. Not only is the new program much larger than originally conceived, but it also will be more focused than before with fewer priority countries and fewer activities. Prevention will concentrate almost exclusively on sexual transmission (promoting reduction in the number of sexual partners and the use of condoms), putting to one side interventions designed to reduce transmission through blood and drug injection.

plementing USAID's bilateral AIDS program. Thirty-two percent of bilateral funding in 1990 went to these organizations to support community prevention activities. USAID attempts to avoid depending too much on ministries of health as implementing agencies for AIDS programs, arguing that AIDS efforts need to extend beyond the normal scope of such ministries.

USAID has established 3 special programs to encourage both international and country-based NGOs to become involved in AIDS activities. The HIV/AIDS Prevention in Africa Program has made awards averaging $1.2 million a year to 9 projects in 7 countries for community-based prevention programs. Second, USAID provides support for the National Council for International Health (NCIH) based in Washington, D.C., which encourages NGOs based in the United States to develop AIDS projects in their overseas operations. Finally, an NGO small-grants program awarded grants worth a total of $1.7 million in 1989–1990.

Because the effectiveness of funding strategies is hard to evaluate, USAID spreads its support among a variety of agencies. However, it is much more explicit in what it wants programs to do—focus on prevention of infection, particularly through sexual transmission.

USAID seems to create sustainable programs that the recipient countries will eventually be able to continue funding themselves. Many development agencies have the same goal, which is a healthy reaction to earlier approaches that invested heavily in capital and technology, thus burdening developing countries with major and usually unaffordable recurrent expenditures. Financial self-sufficiency, however, is not a realistic short- or medium-term objective for many countries severely affected by AIDS. Self-reliance in terms of management, planning, and implementation, however, is feasible, and USAID is planning to develop management training in the future. As in the past, USAID relies heavily on U.S.-based consulting groups for the planning, monitoring, and evaluation of its projects.

The Official Dutch Government Assistance Program

The Dutch government was one of the first supporters of overseas AIDS programs. The Dutch have channeled more than 95 percent of their international AIDS resources through WHO/GPA, on the assumption that this is the most efficient way to coordinate international efforts. For the past 5 years, they have contributed an average of about $3.2 million annually to GPA, principally as unrestricted multilateral support.

Bilateral funding, however, is likely to increase in the future. The Dutch have argued strongly that AIDS prevention and control activities should be incorporated into existing health care structures at as early a stage as possible. Partly for this reason, their bilateral programs have focused on developing countries with which they have already established strong relationships in the field of health care. Rwanda (AIDS prevention), Tanzania (epidemiological and behavioral research and HIV screening), and Zambia (AIDS program coordinator) are 3 countries that have benefited from Dutch bilateral support for AIDS.

The Dutch recognize that their approach neglects many developing countries with a significant AIDS problem. They hope to address this need by channeling support through NGOs based in those developing countries.

Rather than identifying specific aspects of AIDS work that they are prepared to fund, the Dutch use the developing country's national AIDS program to guide Dutch-supported AIDS activities. Human rights are also an important factor; projects that jeopardize the rights of people with AIDS would be rejected, although such a situation has not yet arisen.

The Dutch government provides additional support for the international AIDS effort by contributing to the Netherlands Organization for International Development. This group directs its attention broadly toward social and economic development. Their AIDS activities, mainly in the form of conferences and networks, have concentrated on women's and human rights issues.

The Norwegian Red Cross

Red Cross Societies in Nordic countries were among the first to become active in international support for AIDS activities. They had already established an AIDS task force by 1986, even before the League of Red Cross and Red Crescent Societies had formulated an AIDS policy. Within this group of active societies, the Norwegian group has been particularly dynamic. It was the first to become involved in AIDS work internationally, paving the way for other NGOs to embark on similar programs, and it played an important role in encouraging the involvement of the Norwegian government in international AIDS work.

In 1985, the Norwegian Red Cross Society (NRCS) took the unconventional step of asking all its sister societies in Africa whether they would be interested in collaborating in the prevention of HIV infection.[33] Rwanda alone responded. Working jointly, the two Red Cross Societies developed health education materials for the general population, health professionals, and teachers, distributed them nationwide, and held seminars. The following year, the Norwegian Red Cross supported the Kenyan and Ugandan Red Cross in an information dissemination project. And in 1987, it provided blood-testing equipment for Red Cross centers in Zambia and Haiti.

The NRCS has an open policy toward collaboration: any country where the local Red Cross Society is interested in establishing collaborative efforts is eligible, provided the country is willing to supply adequate information and resources. In some cases, additional criteria are applied. For example, the NRCS agreed to fund projects in Panama, Uruguay, and Chile as long as the messages were *sex positive,* and the projects collaborated with groups already working with AIDS, especially gay groups, who were recognized as being better informed about the issues than the Red Cross Societies, particularly in the early years of the epidemic.

The NRCS has focused on incorporating AIDS messages into existing Red Cross teaching programs and on teaching Red Cross workers and volunteers about AIDS. It has tended to support broadly based campaigns with a special emphasis on children. In general, the NRCS has not directly targeted risk-prone groups, such as commercial sex workers, out of a concern that this might victimize them.

From 1985 to 1990, the NRCS spent $3.6 million on AIDS, 64 percent of which was directed bilaterally to Red Cross organizations in developing countries. Bilateral arrangements are always made with that country's national Red Cross organization, nor with any governmental body. Overestimation of the capacity of national Red Cross societies to manage AIDS programs has sometimes led to problems in program implementation.

The NRCS also supports AIDS activities multilaterally through the former League of Red Cross and Red Crescent Societies (now the International Federation of Red Cross and Red Crescent Societies), providing 46 percent of all of the League's funds for AIDS programs. Funding channeled through the League has paid for regional health delegates, whose responsibilities include AIDS, and has supported national Red Cross societies and regional training programs for a variety of activities. The results have been mixed. Several specific country-level projects initiated recently in Latin America have not been judged particularly worthwhile, whereas support for society member involvement in various seminars and workshops has been considered valuable. WHO sees the Federation as a leader among NGOs, particularly in their blood supply activities and programs for educating youth.

The NRCS has extended its financial support for AIDS work beyond its contributions to the Red Cross by channeling funds to two independent information groups: the Appropriate Health Resources and Technologies Action Group (AHRTAG), with their publication *AIDS Action*, and the Panos Institute, an international organization that has published a series of important books and newspaper articles and has held media workshops on AIDS, with a focus on developing countries.

Despite its relatively modest financial investment in AIDS work, the NRCS is widely acknowledged as having assumed a leading role in recognizing and supporting emerging needs. Its activities often anticipated government efforts and served to lead the way or initiate action when governments were unwilling or unable to do so.

While impressive in its performance overall, the NRCS has also exhibited some weaknesses in planning, management, and evaluation. A recent external evaluation points out that the initial goal of the NRCS, namely to alert the public and decision makers to the nature and significance of the AIDS pandemic, has been more or less completed and suggests that it should now turn more attention to education, counseling, and home care. The evaluation further recommends that more attention be paid to planning and evaluation and to ensuring that its expectations of sister organizations are realistic.

UNESCO

The United Nations Educational, Scientific and Cultural Organization's AIDS prevention programs were established in 1987 to concentrate largely on educating children through schools. UNESCO reasons that school-aged children are either sexually active or about to become so, that values and knowledge conveyed in schools can have a considerable impact on their lives, and that those who do not attend school are often in contact with those who do.[34]

UNESCO has adopted two principle strategies in its AIDS work. The first is to collect and analyze educational materials designed for school-age youth in different regions of the world. These materials—including more than 1,000 publications, 120 videos and films, and 300 posters—and their analyses are available to teachers and educational institutions through the AIDS School Education Resource Center in Paris, which is part of a network of documentation units concentrating on AIDS prevention. The organization focuses on Africa because of the severity of the AIDS problem and because Africa is a priority for UNESCO's operations in general.

The second broad strategy is to test innovative educational approaches through pilot projects in various countries, including Ethiopia, Fiji and other Pacific Islands, Sierra Leone, Mauritius, Tanzania, Jamaica, and Venezuela. Once tried and tested in real classroom settings, the materials are assessed and revised and their use extended to the national level. A sample of approaches includes peer tutoring, either between children or teachers; education of adults by children; and participatory activities, such as plays and songs. Teacher training, workshops on educational material design, and active soliciting of community support are other features of UNESCO's projects.

In addition to its activities in the field of education, UNESCO supports AIDS control activities within its Natural Science Sector through groups studying the pathology of AIDS and exploring possibilities for vaccines and treatment. In the Social Science Sector, UNESCO established a joint program with WHO in 1990 on the social implications of AIDS. One of their major activities has been the Venice Appeal launched in June 1991, designed to alert the international community of the need to strengthen collaboration in activities against AIDS. UNESCO intends to use the extra-budgetary funds raised through this appeal for action to strengthen national AIDS programs in the least developed countries, especially in Africa; development of education, training, and research; and assistance to some 10 million children who, by the year 2000, will have become orphans as a result of AIDS.

UNESCO is sensitive to human rights issues and speaks out in defense of the rights of people with AIDS and HIV. Together with WHO, UNESCO boycotted a 1990 congress in Bangkok, demanding that Thailand change its legislation, which was seen to discriminate against travelers infected with HIV.

The World Bank

The World Bank is unique for three reasons: the size of its financial resources (the amount it lends for population, health, nutrition, and related activities each year—$1.6 billion in 1991—is by far the largest financial commitment of its kind); its broad-based and multisectoral involvement; and its emphasis on economic concerns.[35]

The World Bank began its support for AIDS in 1986 with the inclusion of $150,000 for blood screening in Niger as part of a much larger health sector loan. Total Bank lending for AIDS from financial year 1986 to 1991 has now reached more than $55 million and has involved more than 20 countries, 57 percent of which are in Africa. Most of the projects have involved some of the following elements: information/education/communication (IEC); blood screening; and epidemiological research.

Although the Bank does have certain goals for the types of projects it wants to support, it does not, in contrast to many donors, set aside money for AIDS from which interested countries can draw. The project profile is very much a function of independent negotiations at the country level. The result is that the Bank's AIDS program is comprised of a rather disparate collection of projects, most of which are part of broad-based health sector projects.

In addition to its country loans, the Bank has also donated $1 million in each of the last 3 years to support research activities on AIDS coordinated by WHO, and has undertaken health sector reviews and assessments that have, in many cases, paid particular attention to the AIDS problem. For example, a major study of AIDS has been conducted in Tanzania to look beyond the health sector to problems of employment, savings, and exports. It has explored cost-effective interventions and the process for selecting these interventions according to the epidemiological and institutional characteristics of districts in Tanzania. This project represents a very different, more economi-

cally rigorous, much lengthier, and more expensive approach to identifying suitable interventions than adopted by many other agencies.

The Bank has no explicit high-level policy on AIDS (nor on any
other specific disease). The Bank now expects most of its missions,
and certainly those in the health sector, to address explicitly the issue
of AIDS and to identify opportunities for support. The closest the Bank
has come to developing AIDS policy was its internal review of the
implementation of AIDS activities in Africa, conducted in mid-1991.
It found that because AIDS was being defined as an isolated issue in
the health sector, insufficient attention was being paid to it by other
sectors, and opportunities for collaboration were being missed. The
review also suggested that more attention needed to be given to
countries with a low prevalence of HIV infection but a high prevalence
of sexually transmitted diseases, because these were countries where
future AIDS epidemics were otherwise inevitable. The review proposed a variety of mechanisms for ensuring that AIDS receives appropriate priority from the Bank.

One distinctive feature of the World Bank is that it lends money
and is not a grant-making organization. Regular loans usually have a
maturity of 15 to 20 years, including a 3- to 5-year grace period, and
an interest rate of about 7.5 percent. For countries with GNP per
capita below about $800, there are special soft loans that involve a
30- to 50-year payback period, with 10 years grace and a service charge
of 0.75 percent per year. Most of the Bank's support for AIDS has been
to countries that qualify for soft loans. Until recently, other countries
have been unwilling to borrow money for AIDS prevention and control because grant money has been available from other sources. However, this situation is changing as demand for assistance begins to
outstrip supply, and the Bank expects that requests for loans will
become more common.

Given the size and breadth of its activities and its considerable
influence over finance and planning ministries, it is not surprising
that the Bank has been seen as a potentially useful partner in efforts
to control AIDS. Rather than be uncomfortable with economic arguments, for example, the Bank demands them. Even so, in contrast to
its approach in other sectors, where a country must show an acceptable internal rate of return before loans are approved, the Bank does
not employ strict economic criteria in health or other social sectors.
Yet some of the characteristics that make the Bank a potentially

powerful ally also contribute to its image as unwieldy, insensitive, and even dictatorial. Finally, although other agencies have acknowledged the financial power and influence of the Bank, they are less convinced of its noneconomic technical capacities. The Bank is a relative newcomer to the health sector, having begun its direct lending for health in the early 1980s.

Conclusions

Official development agencies (ODAs) appear increasingly reluctant to channel resources through government institutions in which they have invested for decades with limited success. One route for possibly avoiding some of these pitfalls is support for local NGOs, an option that many donors are now exploring more intensely.

Not all organizations have evaluated their overall program of AIDS activities, and those that have done so have not always elected to expose themselves to external scrutiny. Yet an objective assessment of overall progress and impact is clearly necessary. Several agencies lack well-defined discrete AIDS policies, which makes the task of evaluation both more difficult and more necessary.

A focus on prevention characterizes the efforts of all of the organizations described here. This can be justified on a variety of grounds, including the current lack of any cure. Nevertheless, more attention should now be paid to treatment. If seen to include a package of medical, psychological, and social support together with educational messages designed to discourage further transmission, treatment is one of the important responsibilities of health services.

Most donors provide a substantial proportion of their funding bilaterally and have adopted some kind of criteria for deciding which countries they will support in AIDS work. Although these criteria are often designed to direct resources to where they are most needed or most likely to be well used, political factors also intrude, and there seems to be no reason the net result will be the optimum distribution of donor AIDS money.

More resources may become available from the ODAs under review, but probably under increasingly stringent conditions. ODAs need to establish and maintain contact with one another to ensure that scarce resources are used wisely. Also, they need to respond sensitively to the wishes of recipient countries and avoid blindly imposing their own agendas.

AZT: GLARING GLOBAL INEQUITY

This section is based on a survey done by Sean Hosein of the Community AIDS Treatment Information Exchange, Toronto, Canada, in collaboration with the editors of *AIDS in the World*.

Five years after the introduction of AZT (azidothymidine, formerly known as zidovudine), there are clear signs of growing inequity in access to this antiviral drug, both within affluent countries and for the developing world. (AZT was first marketed in 1987 by the pharmaceutical manufacturer Burroughs Wellcome. The drug is sold under the brand name Retrovir®. AZT inhibits the viral enzyme reverse transcriptase and also terminates DNA chain synthesis.) This treatment equity gap is most apparent with AZT, but it also exists for other simpler and often less expensive drugs used in the prevention and treatment of AIDS-related opportunistic infections. Thus, today, millions of people with HIV infection cannot benefit from treatment with AZT (or other drugs) because of their socioeconomic status, lack of access to care, or simply because they live in poor communities or countries. As the number of people with HIV/AIDS increases dramatically over the coming decade, this inequity will grow rapidly from a gap to a chasm. (Although our concern here is with the provision of HIV/AIDS treatments, it is important to acknowledge equity gaps in basic medical services and treatments both in developing countries and in segments of the industrialized world. It is, however, beyond the scope of this discussion to address these gaps.)

Thus, the restricted availability of AZT epitomizes inequity in health care: the drug is a well-established treatment capable of extending life and improving the well-being of people with AIDS or HIV infection.[36] Years after its release, AZT is not universally available in affluent countries and even less so in the developing world, although such a goal could be achieved. AZT can be produced in sufficient quantities to satisfy demand; innovative approaches could be developed to reduce the cost of the drug to make it affordable by all.

The Cost of AZT Treatment

Burroughs Wellcome currently sells Retrovir® to the wholesaler at $120.19 per one hundred 100mg capsules.[37] At wholesale price, one year of standard AZT treatment (500 mg/day) would cost $2,190. Since its introduction in 1987, the price of Retrovir® has been reduced twice, each time by 20 percent. Along with these price reductions, accepted use of lower doses has also substantially reduced the overall cost of treatment. Although Wellcome states that the wholesale price of AZT is similar in most countries, it would not disclose actual production costs.

In February 1991, the American Public Health Association added its voice to the protests of activist groups, stating that "in the case of AZT, the company [Wellcome] did not incur the costs of research and development as it was not the first to synthesize the drug, nor to test its effectiveness against HIV and its safety on individuals; and that . . . after being given the exclusive right to manufacture and market AZT, Burroughs Wellcome Company had reportedly made $100 million in profits on AZT in one year."[38] Although efforts are underway to reduce further the cost of AZT and other HIV/AIDS drugs and to create mechanisms that would enable governments to control prices, the current affordability of this drug to society must be examined critically.

A survey conducted by *AIDS in the World* in late 1991 found that the estimated annual cost of AZT varies from $2,000 to $4,500 per patient. (See Figure 17.1 and Table 17.2.) The annual cost of AZT for one person as a percentage of 1989 Gross National Product (GNP) per capita ranged from 14 percent in the United States and 22 percent in Australia, to 85 percent in Brazil, 93 percent in South Africa, and 168 percent in Argentina. If AZT were available in sub-Saharan Africa, its price would represent from 158 percent of per capita GNP in Botswana to 500 percent or more in Rwanda, Uganda, and many other countries (the rates for Botswana, Uganda, and Rwanda are based on average estimated AZT costs of $3,000 per year). Although per capita GNP represents only an average, it is safe to assume that, for most people in the developing world who are HIV infected, AZT is impossibly expensive.

Retrovir® is supplied free of charge to people enrolled in clinical trials sponsored by Wellcome;[39] of the estimated 20,000 people enrolled in such trials, the vast majority are in North America, Europe, and Australia/New Zealand. Though treatment programs are underway in some developing countries, such as Kenya, Uganda, Zambia, Zaire, Mexico, and Thailand, these limited trials represent only a

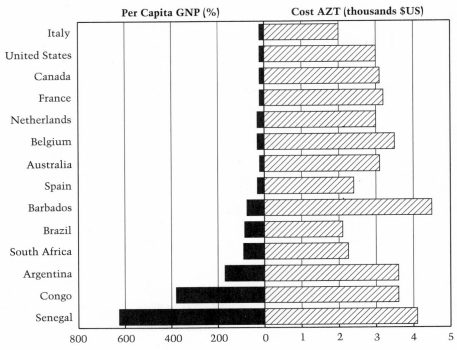

Figure 17.1. Cost of one year course of AZT, and as a percentage of per capita GNP, 1989.
Source: AIDS in the World survey, 1992.

fraction of all AZT protocols. Furthermore, enrolling in a trial is not equivalent to receiving specialized AIDS-specific medical care. Results from a 15-country survey by *AIDS in the World* indicated that, apart from persons participating in research protocols, the high cost of AZT leads some people with HIV/AIDS and/or clinicians to self-prescribe or undermedicate. The contribution of erratic or inadequate administration on the potential emergence and spread of AZT-resistant strains of HIV is not known. Finally, when one considers that the total health expenditure represents only 5 to 10 percent of GNP in industrialized countries and less than 2 percent in developing countries, the gap between resources and AIDS treatment needs grows even wider.

Who Pays for AZT?

Despite the fact that AZT is available in most industrialized countries, its accessibility depends on social security and health insurance systems and the degree to which governments are willing to allocate public funds for those people who either cannot enter or have fallen out of these systems. Thus, in Western Europe and countries like Australia, New Zealand, Japan, and Canada, where social security and health insurance schemes are extensive, most people have access to AZT. In these countries, the cost of AZT is usually covered by health insurance plans, provided predominantly by public and private sectors (e.g., the United Kingdom, Switzerland, New Zealand, Denmark, Canada, and Italy), or funded through employment-linked mandatory health insurance schemes subsidized by the government (e.g., France, Germany, and Australia).

In general, people in industrialized countries who do not have access to AZT are poor, marginalized, or aliens with uncertain resident status. Women represent a particularly vulnerable group: gender inequity compounds socioeconomic inequity. For example, a study conducted in public hospital clinics and community-based AIDS organizations in 9 U.S. cities between 1988 and 1989 investigated access to AZT among 880 people with AIDS or symptomatic HIV infection.[40] Even though this study used the presence of certain clinical signs of HIV infection and AIDS rather than CD4 count as criteria for prescribing AZT, it found that traditionally disadvantaged groups were less frequently referred for AZT treatment. Those most often overlooked were women, blacks, the uninsured, and injection drug users.

Increasingly, when formal channels fail to meet the demand for AZT and other therapies, informal, underground procurement and distribution systems arise, seeking to make available both approved and unapproved drugs.[41] Though these systems meet a need, they raise issues of product quality, safety, cost, and continuity in supply.

In 1991, the National Commission on AIDS in the United States estimated that 29 percent of people with AIDS were uninsured, even though some received care through such health programs as the Veterans Health Administration, the Public Health Service, or other institutions.[42] Even in countries such as France, where AZT is provided free of charge to people not covered by health insurance or medical

Table 17.2: Access to AZT in 15 countries

Country	Who prescribes AZT?	Medical criteria for AZT	CD4 count for AZT (per µl)	Does PWA/M.D. adjust dose?	% who adjust dose
Industrialized countries					
Australia	Select M.D.s	CD4 only	<500	NA	NA
Belgium	Select M.D.s	CD4/other guidelines	<500	No	—
Canada	GPs	CD4 only	<500	NA	NA
France	M.D.s in select hospitals	CD4 only	<350	Yes	1
Italy	M.D.s in select hospitals	CD4/CDC guidelines	<500	No	—
Netherlands	Select M.D.s	M.D.s judge[b]/CD4	<400	No	—
South Africa[c]	Select M.D.s	M.D.s judge[b]	<400	Yes	20
Spain	M.D.s in select hospitals	CD4 only	<500	No	—
United States	GPs	CD4 only	<500	Yes	NA
Developing countries					
Argentina	NA	M.D.s judge[b]	<500	Yes	20–30
Barbados	M.D.s in any hospital	M.D.s judge[b]	NA	Yes	75
Brazil	Select M.D.s	CD4/clinical signs	<400	Yes	NA
Congo	Select M.D.s	CD4/CDC guidelines	NA	Yes	25–50
Senegal	Select M.D.s	CD4 only	<200	Yes	NA
Thailand	M.D.s in any hospital	CD4/CDC guidelines	NA	Yes	10–15

Note: M.D. = doctor; PWA = person with AIDS; pub. = public; priv. = private; NA = not applicable; govt. = government; — = information not available; NSS = national social security; GPs = general practitioners; CDC = U.S. Centers for Disease Control; PI = private medical insurance.

Who pays for AZT?	Cost of AZT ($US)	Where CD4 tests available	Cost of CD4 test in pub./ priv. lab ($US)	Who pays for CD4 test?	Problems of access
Govt./pub.	3,121	Many sites	40	Govt./ pub.	Lack of labs/other support Few M.D.s to treat PWAs Awareness
NSS	3,500	Many sites	13	Govt./ pub.	Cost
Govt./pub.	3,100	Many sites	84	Govt./ pub.	None
NSS	3,200	Many sites	NA	Govt./ pub.	NA
NSS	2,000	Many sites	30	Govt./ pub.	Few M.D.s to treat PWAs Awareness
PI/govt./ pub.	3,000	Many sites	100	Govt./ pub./PI	Other
PWA	2,293	Few sites	71	Govt./ pub./PI	Cost Lack of labs/other support
NSS	2,431	Many sites	100	Govt./ pub.	Few M.D.s to treat PWAs Awareness
All sources	3,000	Many sites	100–150	Many sources	Cost Awareness
PWA/NSS	3,650	Many sites	45–215	PWA/govt./ pub.	Cost
PWA	4,526	—	—	NA	Cost Lack of labs/other support
PWA/govt./pub.	2,160	Few sites	35–109	PWA/govt./ pub.	Cost
PWA	3,640	—	—	NA	Cost
PWA/PI	4,048	Few sites	NA	Research	Cost
PWA	NA	Few sites	20–80	PWA	Cost Lack of labs/other support

a. Cost is based on actual costs provided by each country surveyed.
b. Referral for AZT treatment based on the doctor's judgment.
c. Of the countries surveyed, South Africa was the only one in which AZT was not licensed.

assistance plans, eligibility is based on biological criteria that require tests whose cost can create another barrier to AZT access. Furthermore, the cost of hospital care, biomedical follow-up, or essential drugs is still often borne by the individual. Thus, even in publicly funded systems that have made a determined effort to provide full access to AZT, inequity in the services that precede or support the provision of this drug remains. In developing countries, particularly those most severely affected by the HIV/AIDS pandemic, health insurance programs cover only a small proportion of the population, such as civil servants, military personnel, miners, or other large-scale industrial employees. Even these groups are not provided with such drugs as AZT or others used to treat cancer. Only a small number of privileged people—high-ranking officials and wealthy citizens—can benefit from treatment overseas.

Wellcome declined to provide figures on the total production and sales of Retrovir® or its world distribution patterns. It has stated, however, that it "has created capacity with its factory investments to meet current levels of demand. As demand increases, [it] will be able to expand this capacity and maintain supplies."[43] In 1991, Wellcome's worldwide sales of Retrovir® were reported to be worth approximately $305 million.[44] Assuming an average daily treatment dose of 500 mg, this represents about 140,000 treatment-years, which would have been enough to cover the needs in both the industrialized and developing countries in 1991 should the care services have been fully accessible.

Access to Supportive Health Care Services

To implement an effective and safe AZT regimen requires periodic monitoring of T cell lymphocyte counts and medical follow-up. In all countries surveyed by *AIDS in the World*, the minimum criterion for prescribing AZT was a CD4 count at or below 500. Such a laboratory test, however, requires sophisticated equipment and laboratory technician skills common mainly in affluent countries.

The estimated cost of a CD4 count was approximately $100 to $150 in the United States, $20 to $80 in Thailand, $70 in South Africa, $13 in Belgium, $30 in Italy, $80 in Canada, and between $45 to $215 in Argentina. In Spain and Australia, the test costs $40 and $100, respectively, in private laboratories, although certain government facilities provide it at no cost.

In industrialized countries, the CD4 test is a technique used in better-equipped facilities or designated AIDS centers. When unavailable, referral systems to other facilities exist. In contrast, developing countries, especially those in sub-Saharan Africa, have little or no means of making laboratory services accessible to the many people who need them. In most developing countries, the stage has not been set for AZT to be effectively and safely administered to people with AIDS, outside of a few specialized hospitals, even if it were available.

The Cost of Equity

The experience with AZT not only points to inequalities in the developing world, but also underscores how richer countries are not immune from the same problems. In industrialized countries, where the majority of new drugs are developed and manufactured, access to these drugs is limited by issues of licensing and affordability. In the United States, the HIV/AIDS epidemic has prompted an acceleration of the regulatory process of the Food and Drug Administration (FDA). Activists have played a role both in accelerating this process and exercising pressure on drug manufacturers and governments to lower the price of drugs.[45] Internationally, there is growing cooperation among regulatory bodies in the United States, Canada, Japan, and the European Community to harmonize regulatory procedures and standards. But such efforts will depend largely on the willingness of each country to modify its own regulatory system.[46] This applies particularly to the United States, where regulatory procedures and standards are considered the most stringent and where most of the new HIV/AIDS drugs and vaccine candidates are being developed.

Governments and activists must apply further pressure to lower the cost of AIDS drugs. Even if prices fall, the relative cost of AZT must also be compared with the cost of drugs in general. Excluding the cost of medical and laboratory services, which varies, providing AZT to the 2.8 million projected adult cases of AIDS that will occur in the world between 1992 and 1995, in addition to people who have already undertaken treatment, would require between $1.5 billion and $3 billion annually. This impressive total is less than 2 percent of the $174 to $186 billion annual value of the 1990 world pharmaceutical market;[47] it is also less than 0.4 percent of the $824 billion in annual global health expenditures; and it is certainly less than the $923 billion spent in 1990 on the military.[48] Thus, there is a theoretical possibility of achieving equity on AZT if the national and international political commitment existed.

On the global scale, AZT inequity underscores the impact of political choices on economic and social development. In developing countries, it is generally assumed that the degree of access to quality care is determined by the finite amount of resources available to the health sector. Accordingly, the debate tends to revolve around the allocation of meager resources to competing health priorities rather than the more politically loaded issue of the share of national and international resources designated to the health and social sectors. As the HIV/AIDS pandemic extends its reach globally, the need to advance the fundamental, universal right of all people to health is the most vital and paramount concern.

．　．　．

GUIDANCE ON COUNSELING: A REVIEW

David Miller

David Miller, Department of Public Health Medicine and Epidemiology, University Hospital and Medical School, Nottingham, England

Counseling in HIV infection and disease has been a controversial issue. Both preventive and supportive counseling exist largely because the groups directly affected demanded that it be so. In most countries, HIV counseling programs and services were established from within communities primarily affected by HIV, well in advance (often many years) of official initiatives. More recently, debate has continued among health planners about how counseling can best be defined and what it can realistically accomplish.

There is a startling dearth of acceptable data on the efficacy of counseling. In practice, counseling has, at times uneasily, combined the roles of health education and provision of HIV information. These roles were first developed in the context of HIV-antibody testing, where counseling has been advocated as ethically desirable, and more recently as an integral part of prevention programs in many countries.

The concept of counseling is novel to some cultures. For example, there is no precise term for HIV counseling in the French, Arabic, or Japanese languages. Establishing the notion of HIV/AIDS counseling has required a major international effort, initiated by the World Health Organization (WHO)—an effort that, by its very nature, raised concerns about the imposition of a so-called western notion of care on nonwestern peoples. As a result, the appropriateness and role of counseling as a critical component of epidemic management have been consistently misunderstood. Furthermore, counseling strategies and programs have frequently not been given the chance to develop their potential.

Surprisingly, the reasons people seek counseling have rarely been studied or well documented. Counseling was established in response to the observed psychosocial consequences following from a diagnosis of HIV disease—for those affected directly and indirectly. However, more recent information from people about what they want from counseling—and how their counseling needs may be changing—is hard to find.

Nevertheless, the well-documented psychosocial impact of HIV is compelling and has led to wide acceptance of counseling as an ethically necessary part of information provision, both before and after HIV-antibody testing. As such, counseling is an important part of prevention, particularly when health education can also be provided, to encourage and empower individuals to negotiate low HIV-risk behavior. Similarly, counseling has a crucial supportive function, sometimes requiring clinical psychosocial management skills. Counseling, therefore, has functions that place it in close collaboration with health education and medical management, while to some degree it is an extension and a mediator of both.

Although the precise needs for counseling are not clearly characterized, more is known about what counseling users expect of the process. This includes confidentiality, accessibility, a nonjudgmental perspective from the counselor, time, consistency in approach to individuals' needs, accurate information, and a supportive attitude. Meeting these requirements requires heavy investment in personnel and training. For many countries, the cost of counseling added to already overburdened health care systems virtually ensures that little will be done, despite the recognition of the need and its potential (though unproven) benefits.

Who Can Provide Counseling?

This question is clearly related to how counseling is perceived and defined in each culture. In many countries, the multiplicity of claims on the counselor's role has perpetuated confusion over the aim and place of counseling. Also, because HIV/AIDS counseling is frequently perceived as being a professional health worker activity, it often lies beyond the competence of governments to provide sufficient professional counselors to meet all the needs.

Yet in many cultures, while HIV counseling has not been formally defined, the role of counselor has been established for generations under other names. Health workers, ranging from primary health care staff to traditional midwives and healers, are a common source of expertise and local knowledge that, with appropriate training and low technology resources, may form a vital work force of HIV/AIDS counselors. Volunteers from affected communities may also have the understanding, sensitivity, credibility, accessibility, and motivation—with necessary information and acceptance from formal health care services—to provide counseling in pre- and post-test HIV situations. Indeed, volunteers from communities most directly affected were often the first to develop those HIV/AIDS counseling initiatives on which many programs are now founded. Involving the community has many advantages. For example, the credibility associated with HIV care and prevention within local communities may save much time in establishing a program.

In many developing countries, most counseling, except perhaps that provided before a test, is currently provided by AIDS service organizations (ASOs). ASOs include organizations staffed by unpaid peers, nongovernmental organizations (NGOs), and church workers.

Training is vital in HIV/AIDS counseling. The information given must be accurate. Counseling also frequently involves the application of clinical skills. Further, counselors need to know of companion services and be able to liaise effectively with them.

In HIV/AIDS, counseling structures separate from preexisting health care structures have often been criticized on the grounds of cost. There is, however, another point to consider: incorporating counseling into health care may also help ensure that standards of professionalism are maintained. Furthermore, with appropriate training, health professionals may then be in a position to recruit, train, supervise, and monitor volunteers to provide counseling at the community level.

Is HIV Counseling Effective?

How much does counseling reduce the psychological and social impact of HIV disease? What is the relative public health benefit of counseling? Are there viable alternatives to counseling? No one can answer these questions with certainty, as the available evidence is primarily anecdotal. This is surely one of the greatest weaknesses of HIV counseling, and societies cannot be expected to keep paying for an activity for which there is no proof of efficacy. Clear evidence would require models of HIV counseling that incorporate various definitions of aims and roles, and ways of achieving them—and the models are still lacking.

None of these problems are new; but their resolution is essential if the role of counseling is to be sustained and improved. Steps to improve this situation include:

1. Clients seeking counseling should be asked what outcomes they expect, where they would prefer to receive counseling, from whom, and why. Needs of clients should be characterized in specific settings as soon as possible.
2. There is a need to identify and establish models of effective community-based counseling. Potentially replicable models do exist; for example, in Uganda, community-based counseling efforts have shaped the national management of HIV. It is also important that information be shared about those services that were based initially on western models and were successfully adapted and refined to meet local needs.
3. How efficacy is assessed needs to be reviewed and, perhaps, redefined. Studies of efficacy should not be burdened with unrealistic methodological requirements.

Further Developments in HIV/AIDS Counseling

Counseling associated with early medical intervention is not relevant for much of the world's population.

- More work needs to be done on counseling for blood donors; blood donation presents a major opportunity for prevention counseling and linkage with primary health care and other community care structures.
- Counseling to support the empowerment of women, particularly on negotiation of safer sex, requires urgent attention.
- There is an ongoing need to counsel health care workers on testing. Experienced staff are a critical resource that requires nurturing and support.

Conclusion

Counseling must not become another lost opportunity in HIV management. Counseling need not be expensive if it is based on available resources within existing structures. If HIV counseling is to gain the strength it needs, it urgently requires renewed leadership; a new, clearer perception of counseling requires work from within the discipline.

CHAPTER EIGHTEEN

. . . .

The Next Epidemic

Laurie Garrett

Laurie Garrett is a
science and medical
writer for *Newsday*,
based in New York.

In the 1960s, the world mounted a campaign against smallpox, eliminating the disease from the planet. With victory in sight, Surgeon
General William H. Stewart in 1969 told the U.S. Congress that it
was time to "close the book on infectious diseases," declare the war
against pestilence won, and shift national resources to such chronic
problems as cancer and heart disease. Even as he spoke, a new pestilence—AIDS—was brewing that would in 25 years claim more lives
than had smallpox in the previous decades of the twentieth century.

Congress shifted funds, closing virtually every tropical and infectious disease outpost run by the U.S. Military and Public Health
Service. Only the Centers for Disease Control (CDC) in Atlanta,
Georgia, the U.S. Army's biological research center at Fort Detrick,
Maryland, the Navy Medical Research Unit programs in Egypt, Indonesia, and the Philippines, and some overseas army programs survived
the budget slashes of the early 1970s.

Although the World Health Organization (WHO) and the Pan
American Health Organization (PAHO) maintained their outposts in
developing countries through this period, funding declined for such
projects, particularly from the United States. Young scientists got the
message that fields such as medical entomology, parasitology, and
host pathology were not the paths to rewarding, productive careers.
Funding of most programs at universities was terminated and the large
majority of support for tropical disease research became controlled by
the U.S. military and the U.S. Agency for International Development.

It did not take long for nature to show the medical world the folly of its arrogance. From the reservoir of viral infections came a series of diseases, some of which may not have existed before, others that had jumped ecologic niches or geography. Since the discovery of human retroviruses and the advent of the AIDS pandemic, scientists have debated whether the danger of newly emerging viruses is merely an outgrowth of enhanced technologies of detection or the result of environmental and other pressures encouraging viruses to cross into new niches, mutate, or both. From a microbial point of view, the global village of the 1990s is minuscule. Never has it been so obvious that poor health care and disease surveillance in one corner of the planet can imperil every person on earth, rich, as well as poor.

"The ravaging epidemic of acquired immune deficiency syndrome has shocked the world," wrote Nobel Laureate Joshua Lederberg in the *Journal of the American Medical Association* in 1988. "It is still not comprehended widely that it is a natural, almost predictable phenomenon. We will face similar catastrophes again, and will be ever more confounded in dealing with them, if we do not come to grips with the realities of the place of our species in nature."[1]

■■■■ . . .

A BRIEF HISTORY OF RECENT VIRAL EPIDEMICS

HIV is but one of a long series of microbes that have recently surfaced, and will be followed by more. An analysis of the history of viral discovery over the past decades shows clearly the roots of our unpreparedness for HIV, and provides a warning that much needs to be done if we are to avoid being caught off-guard again by the next, possibly even more virulent, viral pandemic.

In the last 40 years, numerous infectious viruses have been discovered. (See Tables 18.1, 18.2, and 18.3.) Most have undoubtedly existed for centuries, escaping detection because the viruses co-existed successfully with hosts, producing symptoms that were not previously recognized as being caused by infectious agents.[2]

Improvements in viral detection technology, particularly the invention of the polymerase chain reaction (PCR) method, have opened up new frontiers in human biology, showing the links between previously unnoticed slow viral infections and diseases whose cause had

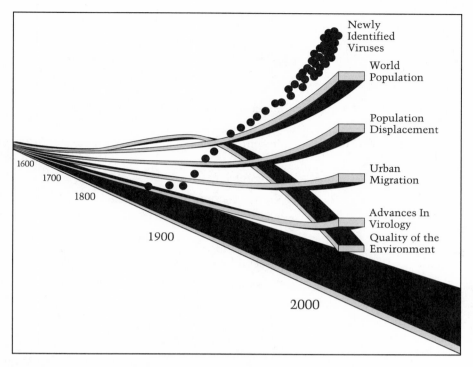

Figure 18.1. The emergence of new viruses in the Global Village.

been unknown.[3,4] As study of the relationship between viruses and neurological disorders or cancer advances, the list of diseases caused by slow viruses will expand.

Of greater concern is the movement of viruses across biological niches or vast geographic regions. In the 1980s, mosquitoes capable of carrying the hemorrhagic strain of dengue fever found their way from Southeast Asia to Brazil in shipments of used tires.[5] The dengue vector is now taking hold in the Caribbean, and isolated outbreaks have been reported in several states in the United States. Mosquitoes and other insect vectors are readily moving into new niches all over the world due to a variety of environmental pressures, such as construction of tracts of suburban homes along old growth forest land.[6] There is now concern that global warming will move tropical vectors

Table 18.1: Newly recognized viral agents (origins unknown)

Agent	Target	Vector/mode of transmission	Year of outbreak or discovery	Source
Omsk hemorrhagic fever	Human	Rodent/wild mammal/tick	1945	J. Casals et al. (1970) *Journal of Infectious Diseases* 122:437
Chikunga virus	Human	Monkey/mosquito	1952	C. M. Robinson (1955) *Trans. R. Soc. Trop. Med. Hyg.* 49:28
O'nyong Nyong	Human	Mosquito	1959	H. Shore (1961) *Trans. R. Soc. Trop. Med. Hyg.* 55:361
Epstein-Barr virus (EBV)	Human	Semen/blood	1963	M. A. Epstein & Y. M. Barr (1964) *Lancet* 1:252
Feline leukemia virus	Feline	Blood	1966	W. F. Jarrett (1966) *Proc. Roy. Soc. Med.* 59:661
Marburg	Human	Blood/Ugandan green monkey	1967	J. S. S. Gear et al. (1975) *British Medical Journal* 4:489
Human parvovirus B-19	Human	Nosocomial	1975	Y. E. Cossart et al. (1975) *Lancet* 1:72 and L. Bell (1989) *New England Journal of Medicine* 321:485
Rocio encephalitis	Human	Mosquito	1975	T. P. Monath (1987) *Textbook of Pediatric Infection* Vol II:1445
Delta virus (HDV)	Human	Blood/semen	1976	H. L. Sanger et al. (1976) *Proceedings of the National Academy of Sciences* 73:3852
Ebola virus	Human	Monkey/blood	1976	*Bull. WHO* (1978) 56:247
HTLV-1	Human	Blood/semen	1980	R. Gallo (1985) *Cancer Res.* 45:4524s
HIV-1	Human	Blood/semen	1981	F. Barré-Sinoussi et al. (1983) *Science* 220:868
HTLV-II	Human	Blood/semen	1982	V. Kalyanaraman et al. (1982) *Science* 218:571
Ochelbo disease	Human	Mosquito	1982	D. K. Lvov et al. (1988) *American Journal of Tropical Medicine and Hygiene* 39:607
Necrotic hepatitis	Rabbit	Blood	1984	"Emerging Viruses: The Evolution of Viruses and Viral Diseases" NIH 1989

Table 18.1 (cont.): Newly recognized viral agents (origins unknown)

Agent	Target	Vector/mode of transmission	Year of outbreak or discovery	Source
HIV-2	Human	Blood/semen	1985	F. Clavel et al. (1986) *Science* 233:343
SIVmac	Macaque	Blood/semen	1985	M. D. Daniel et al. (1985) *Science* 228:1201
SIVagm	African green monkey	Blood/semen	1985	P. Kanki et al. (1985) *Science* 230:951
HHV-6	Human	Blood/semen	1986	S. Salahuddin et al. (1986) *Science* 234:956
SIVsmm	Sooty Mangabey	Blood/semen	1986	P. N. Fultz et al. (1986) *Proceedings of the National Academy of Sciences* 83:5286
FIV	Feline	Blood/semen	1987	J. E. Barlough et al. (1991) *Acquired Immune Deficiency Syndromes* 4:219
Hepatitis C	Human	Blood	1989	Choo et al. (1990) *British Medical Bulletin* 46:423
Human pestivirus	Human	Fecal	1989	*Medical World News* (1989) June 26:36
SIVmnd	Mandrill	Blood/semen	1989	H. Tsujimoto et al. (1989) *Nature* 341:539
Borna virus	Human	?	1990	S. Vandewoude et al. (1990) *Science* 11/29/90
Hepatitis E	Human	Fecal	1990	Reyes et al. (1990) *Science* 247:1335
HHV-7	Human	Blood (?)	1990	N. Fenki et al. (1990) *Proceedings of the National Academy of Sciences* 87:748
Crimean-Congo hemorrhagic fever	Human	Tick/livestock/ blood	?	H. Hoogstraal (1979) *J. Med. Ent.* 15:307

Table 18.2: Old viruses found in new locales or using a new mode of transmission

Agent	Target	Vector/mode of transmission	Year of outbreak or discovery	Source
Dengue fever Asia	Human	Mosquito	1943	G. F. Lumley and F. H. Taylor "Dengue" Service Publication, Sch. of Public Health, Tropical Med. #3, Australia
Kyasanur forest disease	Human	Tick/monkey	1957	M. A. Sreenivasan et al. (1986) *Trans. R. Soc. Trop. Med. Hyg.* 80:810
Argentine hemorrhagic fever (Junin virus)	Human	Field mouse	1958	J. I. Maiztegui et al. (1979) *Lancet* 2:1216
Oropuche fever	Human	Midge	1959	F. P. Pinhiero et al. (1981) *Am. J. Trop. Med. Hyg.* 30:149
Bolivian hemorrhagic fever (Machupo)	Human	Field mouse	1964	C. R. Howard & P. R. Young (1984) *Trans. R. Soc. Trop. Med. Hyg.* 78:299
Lassa fever	Human	Rodent/blood/urine	1969	J. Frame et al. (1970) *Am. J. Trop. Med. Hyg.* 19:670
Venezuelan equine ence-phalitis	Human	Horse/mosquito/rodent	1969	R. E. Shope in *Virology* (1985) Raven Press, pp. 931–53
Human-monkey pox	Human	Squirrel/monkey	1970	"Emerging Viruses: The Evolution of Viruses & Viral Diseases" (1989) NIH
Herpesvirus Simiae	Human	Monkey	1973	*Morbidity Mortality Weekly Report* (1987) 36:380
Rift Valley fever	Human	Livestock/mosquito	1977	*WHO Bull.* No. 63 (1982)
Canine parvovirus (CPV)	Dog	Fecal/blood	1978	"Emerging Viruses: The Evolution of Viruses & Viral Diseases" NIH (1989)
Sindbis virus	Human	Bird/mosquito	1982	A. Espmark & B. Niklasson (1984) *Am. J. Trop. Med. Hyg.* 33:1203
Seoul Hantaan	Human	Rodent	1985	J. LeDuc et al. (1986) *WHO Bull.* 64:139

Table 18.2 (cont.): Old viruses found in new locales or using a new mode of transmission

Agent	Target	Vector/mode of transmission	Year of outbreak or discovery	Source
Samoan hemorrhagic conjunctivitis (Coxsackievirus A24)	Human	Fecal/hygiene	1986	L. Sawyer et al. (1989) *American Journal of Epidemiology* 130:1187
Morbillivirus	Lake Baikal seal	Blood	1987	R. Dietz and C. T. Ansen (1989) *Nature* 338:627
Morbillivirus	North Sea harbor seal	Blood	1988	S. Kennedy et al. (1988) *Nature* 335:404
Dengue fever Americas	Human	Mosquito	1988	*Morbidity Mortality Weekly Report* 39:741 (1990)
Phocine distemper virus	Seal	Blood	1988	J. Harwood (1988) *New Scientist* 2/18/88:38
Manipur rotavirus	Human	Fecal/oral	1989	S. K. Ghosh and T. N. Naik (1989) *Archives of Virology* 105:119
California Bunyamwera	Human	Mosquito	1989	G. L. Campbell et al. (1989) Am. Soc. of Trop. Med. Hyg. Honolulu Conference
St. Louis encephalitis	Human	Mosquito	1990	*Morbidity Mortality Weekly Report* (1990) 39:756
Morbillivirus	Dolphin	Blood	1990	M. Domingo et al. (1990) *Nature* 348:21
Hemorrhagic fever with renal syndrome	Human	Vole	1990	J. Pilaski et al. (1991) *Lancet* 337:111
Morbillivirus	Monk seal	Blood	1991	J. Harwood (1988) *New Scientist* 2/18/88:38
Type D retrovirus	Human	Monkey	1991	R. J. Ford et al. (1991) *Journal of Virology* (Nov.)

Table 18.3: Mutated viruses with enhanced virulence, host range, or transmission

Agent	Target	Vector/mode of transmission	Year of outbreak or discovery	Source
Paralytic poliomyelitis	Human	Fecal	1894	F. Fenner et al. (1974) *The Biology of Animal Viruses* Academic Press, pp. 638–39
Influenza	Human	Respiratory	1917	A. Greenough & J. A. Davis (1983) *Lancet* 1:922
Seal influenza	Seal	Bird dropping	1980	"Emerging Viruses: The Evolution of Viruses and Viral Diseases" NIH (1989)
Chicken influenza	Chicken	Duck/turkey	1983	"Emerging Viruses: The Evolution of Viruses and Viral Diseases" NIH (1989)
Semliki forest virus	Mouse	Blood	1985	A. D. T. Barrett et al. (1986) *J. Gen. Virol.* 67:1727
Yellow fever Nigeria	Human	Mosquito	1988	M. E. Ballinger & B. R. Miller (1989) Am. Soc. of Trop. Med. Hyg. Honolulu Conference
Feline rotavirus	Human	Fecal	1989	T. Nakagomi & O. Nakagomi (1989) *J. Virol.* 63:1431

into now-temperate zones, taking such viruses as dengue and a variety of encephalitis agents into new latitudes.[7]

Hantaan viruses, a family of rodent-borne hemorrhagic viruses, members of which caused severe, often lethal disease in allied forces in Korea, have now been found virtually worldwide. Although the viruses found in diverse parts of the world are not the same ones as those causing severe disease, they probably were spread from Asia in part by infected rodents on ships.

Since 1987 hundreds of dolphins have been found dead along European beaches, victims of the combined effects of high levels of immune system-depressing polychlorinated biphenyls and a newly detected strain of morbillivirus, similar to canine distemper virus.[8,9]

HOW HUMANS HELP VIRUSES SPREAD

"Most 'emerging viruses' are not really new, but represent existing agents that acquire new significance, such as new hosts," according to Rockefeller University's Dr. Stephen Morse. "Viruses like dengue or Hantaan may move into new territory. Conditions that allow the introduction of previously restricted viruses into new host populations are therefore of prime importance. Such conditions may be more prevalent now."[10] Among the conditions Morse listed are rapid means of travel, co-evolution of arthropod vectors and their dispersal, and global environmental changes that may expand climates favorable for some diseases.

This is good news for viruses, but not for human beings. For example, in 1976 an isolated group of hospital workers in Zaire were "wiped out wholesale," according to retired CDC scientist Dr. Karl Johnson, as victims of a previously unknown agent later named ebola virus. Mortality among ebola-infected individuals exceeded 90 percent, Johnson said, and the real question was whether we had run into a strain that could literally wipe out the world's population.

As it turned out, ebola transmission was contained in the remote Zairean region—after which it was named—through standard public health measures. But Johnson warned that if something like ebola appeared that could be dispersed in the air, it would be "the most lethal possibility"[11] he could imagine.

These concerns were highlighted in 1990 following two outbreaks of ebola-like viral infection in primate facilities in the United States.[12,13] When research monkeys began to die from what appeared to be an airborne-transmitted filovirus, the State of New York unilaterally put a halt to primate importations through its facilities. Because the majority of all animals imported to the United States are housed temporarily at John F. Kennedy Airport in New York, this effectively halted the influx of animals destined for facilities nationwide. Fortunately, the ebola strain that had originated in the Philippines turned out to be incapable of producing disease in human beings; its host range being limited to monkeys.

But the specter of an ebola event in New York City equivalent to the original 1976 outbreak in Zaire was ominous. Had a dangerous strain of filovirus been involved, the numbers of primarily and secondarily exposed people at J.F.K. Airport alone would have been staggering. Naturally, any virus that is spreading at an airport is bound to find itself off to landing strips all over the world, carried by unwitting human vectors.

Human beings not only travel freely, but also interact intimately with other people in distant lands. Sexually transmitted diseases do not remain confined to the red-light districts of a single town, nation, or continent; witness the current global epidemics of AIDS, chlamydia, syphilis, human papillomavirus, herpes simplex type II, and antibiotic-resistant gonorrhea.

The HIV epidemic pointed out the need to screen exported blood products and human organs for viral contamination, revealing that numerous other viruses are spread through such means, such as hepatitis C,[14,15] HTLV-1 and HTLV-2,[16] and HHV-6.[17] In countries that permit individuals to sell their organs and blood, lax surgical and transfusion procedures have led to the spread of hepatitis B and HIV both domestically and to nations of export.

Despite the generally sedentary behavior of injection drug users, viruses spread easily inside these communities and from one drug-using population to another. HTLV-1 and HTLV-2, only discovered in 1980 and 1982 respectively, have spread among injection drug users in the United States.[18,19] The startling rapidity of the spread of HIV-1 in Thailand is due in part to injection use of heroin.[20] Hepatitis viruses types B, C, and delta can all be transmitted through injection drug use. It seems prudent to assume that any blood-borne virus can be transmitted through shared needles and injection equipment and that viruses that can readily infect injection drug users can move around the globe.

Human movement and population expansion are creating environmental pressures, particularly in impoverished areas, that encourage viruses to be transmitted and emerge in new areas. The most dramatic case is urbanization, which accelerated in the latter third of the 20th century as people migrated from rural areas and birth rates soared in the world's largest cities. In 1970, only a quarter of the developing world lived in cities. By 2010, the figure will reach nearly half, according to 1987 United Nations estimates.[21]

As cities swell, their basic public health facilities struggle to meet the challenge, or start to fail altogether. The United Nations also estimated that at least half the world's urban population currently live in shanties and slums without safe drinking water and that a third have no collection facilities for disposal of solid waste. In 1990 WHO estimated that children living in such communities are 40 times more likely to die of preventable diseases before age 5 than are their rural counterparts.[22] The lack of sewage treatment is undoubtedly the source of endemic hepatitis A, enteroviruses, and rotaviruses.

ARE VIRUSES ADAPTING FASTER?

The role of mutation and selection is less certain, though some cases of viral recombination in this century have led to the appearance of more virulent strains of viruses capable of infecting different hosts (see Table 18.3). Dozens of human influenza pandemics that have clearly arisen when a virus mutates in a local area and is then spread around the world by human travelers and in some cases by birds can be added to the list.

Many scientists believe that HIV-1 and HIV-2 are mutations from the simian immunodeficiency virus (SIV) species, and genomic comparisons certainly suggest that the known HIVs are cousins, if not descendants, of SIVs.[23] Similar assumptions are made about the evolution of HTLVs from STLVs.[24]

The sudden appearance of lethal viruses in a given population always tempts researchers to conclude that the microbe itself is new, but this may not be so. Ebola virus, for example, could have caused disease in Africa previously, but it escaped the attention of outsiders. However, it is not unusual for insects, particularly mosquitoes, to feed on several animals or people, thereby becoming infected with two or more viral strains simultaneously. When this occurs, the strains can recombine to make viruses that are even more lethal.[25-28]

Therapeutic drugs themselves could be creating new dangers. Retired Harvard University tropical disease expert and Nobel Laureate Thomas Weller has warned that widespread use of antiviral drugs could place selection pressure on RNA viruses at least as efficient as that placed on bacteria by inappropriate antibiotic use.[29] Certainly, antiviral drug use selects for HIV strains that are resistant to AZT, ddC, and ddI. Nobel Laureate Howard Temin from the University of Wisconsin warned, "If we now apply strong selection to the HIV population in the form of successful use of chemicals and/or vaccines, then there would be a strong selective advantage to HIV mutants . . . thus, successful biomedical intervention would probably cause a difference in the HIV population at large."[30] Even in the absence of such selection pressure, HIV is known to have a high rate of genetic mutation.[31] And further, according to Temin, there are viruses that mutate more frequently than does HIV, using similar splicing and deletion strategies.

——— · · ·

HOW SERIOUS IS THE MUTATION PROBLEM?

A variety of approaches have been used to determine how frequently viruses undergo the changes that lead to mutation, but the results do not yield clear answers. John Holland, of the University of California, San Diego, looked at guanine substitutions in RNA from vesicular stomatitis virus. The substitutions are very frequent, but how many substitutions does it take to create a new virus?[32] Holland says, "it seems reasonable to expect that 'new' RNA (and DNA) viruses will emerge occasionally, but that their nature and timing will generally be difficult to predict."[33]

Nature and timing are just what are needed to be able to predict. The problems were highlighted when Dr. Russell Doolittle and his University of California at San Diego colleagues used computerized sequence analysis to study 9 different retroviruses (including HIV and HTLV-1 and 2).[34] Not surprisingly, they concluded that all of these viruses have descended from a common ancestor in the not too distant past. But they add, "Given the episodic nature of viral change, however, it is difficult to gauge how recent [this] may be."[35]

Worse yet, any successful RNA seems to have the ability to recombine quickly. James and Ellen Strauss of the California Institute of Technology have concluded that all RNA viruses need to maintain a high rate of recombination in order to adapt to hosts and escape the attention of the immune system.[36] They have warned, "The continued divergence of RNA viruses poses a clear threat to our physical well being. . . . We now recognize that RNA viruses will continue to evolve rapidly as they have over the millennia. As the recent epidemic of AIDS makes clear, new pathogens can and will arrive."[37]

Two recently published studies give some support for this possibility. The first, reported from the University of California at San Francisco laboratory of Jay Levy, shows that simultaneously infecting human peripheral blood cells in vitro with both HIV-1 and HIV-2 results in new viruses that carry sequences of both parent strains. The researchers warned that the data suggest a process that could take place in infected people and "give rise to HIV strains with expanded cellular host range and conceivably new biological properties."[38] Similar results are reported out of Case Western Reserve University, where both in vitro and in vivo studies of cells superinfected with Chicken Herpes Virus (Marek Disease Virus) and a retrovirus (Reticuloendotheliosis Virus) result in recombination and the production of a progeny that contains sequences of both the herpes and retrovirus parent strains.[39] Of course, such experiments are not conclusive; they serve mainly to raise questions and to stimulate thinking and field investigation.

But, when added to previous evidence that co-infection of cells with HIV-1 and cytomegalovirus can produce offspring with a wider HIV host range, it seems urgent to establish whether HIV-positive people who are simultaneously infected with other retroviruses (HTLV-1 and HTLV-2) are producing new HIV strains—even species— with enhanced host ranges or biologic capabilities.

▬▬▬▬   .   .   .

THE NEXT EPIDEMIC: ARE WE PREPARED?

The world was caught off guard by the immunodeficiency virus; will it be better equipped to handle the next emerging virus? Lederberg has concluded that the answer is a resounding "No." He has joined colleagues in calling for the creation of a $150 million tropical disease surveillance center dedicated to monitoring the appearance of emerging viruses.

Dr. Donald Henderson, former Dean of the Johns Hopkins School of Hygiene and Public Health, thinks something even more ambitious is needed—a global surveillance network of 15 medical research centers in tropical countries. Some advocate creation of an international system of surveillance and vaccine production, akin to the system that has identified newly emerging influenza strains every year for more than 3 decades, stimulating the production and distribution of proper vaccines before strains become pandemic. But in these times of global economic recession, disease surveillance and vector control programs are facing cutbacks, rather than expansion.

In December 1989, the annual meeting of the American Society of Tropical Medicine and Hygiene (ASTMH) created a scenario in which an unknown virus appeared in a tropical underdeveloped area that was in a state of war. As the scenario was played out by representatives of the U.S. military, the National Institutes of Health, the Centers for Disease Control, WHO, and other leading public health agencies, it became painfully obvious that the human beings were going to lose the war if the virus could be transmitted as an aerosol, dispersed in the air.

The entire field of tropical medicine is handicapped by a lack of facilities, experts, and training programs. Basic equipment, such as airtight portable containment facilities for research and treatment of lethal airborne viruses, is sadly lacking. Of the roughly 1,000 members of the ASTMH, for example, the majority are retired or approaching retirement age. The current global outbreak of multiple drug–resistant tuberculosis has again revealed an acute generation gap—this time in mycobacteria research—with only a limited number of trained personnel and a handful of laboratories currently capable of studying the organisms.

"The situation has gotten so bad that doctors graduate from medical school without having a single course in parasitology," said Dr. Jacob Frenkel of the University of Kansas School of Medicine at the 1989 meeting. "Last year a former Peace Corps volunteer died in Washington, D.C., of malaria. He died because doctors misdiagnosed it as the flu." U.S. disease surveillance is based on physicians, he added, and few doctors have been trained to spot tropical diseases.[40]

The same meeting heard Dr. William Reeves, professor emeritus from the University of California at Berkeley and one of the world's experts on disease-carrying insect control, say: "You could take any disease as a model—ebola, malaria, whatever—and it would reveal the same thing. We aren't ready. Where are the people? The expertise? The equipment?"[41]

Even where expertise exists, there often is a failure to appreciate that newly emerging viruses will likely first take hold in the most impoverished areas: communities in frontier areas distant from health services, or urban ghettoes. These communities have, as a rule, the least medical help and the fewest number of professionals trained to identify new disease outbreaks.

The key to global surveillance lies in developing a strong medical infrastructure throughout Africa, Asia, and South America, according to Joseph McCormick, the CDC's ebola expert. But this requires a level of North-South financial and political cooperation that does not currently exist, including open dialogue on global health and a clear willingness on the part of wealthy nations to subsidize improvements in the social and environmental conditions that promote the spread of disease in developing countries. "I still think that the responsibility ought to be more long-term in these countries, looking every day for the unusual. Industrialized countries cannot wait for new viruses to reach their own shores," said McCormick, adding that they must give aggressive support to the development of surveillance and public health infrastructures in the developing world. "Look at the AIDS situation. If we had spotted that disease when the first cases appeared, imagine how different the situation could be today."[42]

Afterword

This first edition of *AIDS in the World* has sought to describe many dimensions of the HIV/AIDS pandemic, including its course, global impact, and the response to its challenges.

From a global perspective, there are two main findings: the pandemic is expanding worldwide, and the national and international response is lagging behind. The pace of the pandemic is fast outgrowing the pace of the response, and the gap is widening rapidly and dangerously. (See Figure A.1.) In the several years that followed the initial recognition of AIDS in 1981, the pandemic was proceeding while the response was quite limited, involving a constellation of community-based groups and a few governments. The world mobilization against AIDS, starting in 1986–1987, created enough momentum to begin narrowing the gap between the pandemic and the response, drawing from scientific progress a fast-growing understanding of the epidemiology of HIV/AIDS, its behavioral determinants, and its deep social and cultural roots. In the early 1990s, the pandemic continues to accelerate and expand, while the response reaches a plateau or even declines. The time has clearly come for a new vision, for a revitalized mobilization, and for directions and approaches that will be capable of stemming the HIV/AIDS pandemic.

There is a danger that these conclusions may sound as if the commitment of many thousands of people around the world has not made a difference; yet nothing could be further from the truth. It is essential, for our common future, that we not shrink from sounding

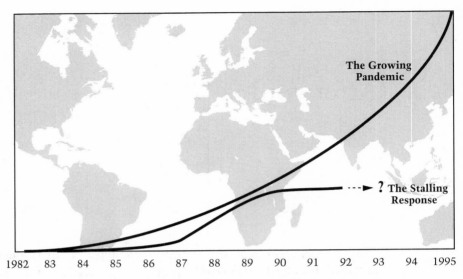

Figure A.1. The growing HIV/AIDS pandemic and the stalling response.

the alarm, even if the message is grim. Neither denial nor complacency will help us as we seek ways to prevent infection and care for those affected.

We pay homage here—and throughout the book—to the leadership, innovation, and courage of people who have challenged the status quo when it was unacceptable, and who have dedicated their lives to helping others. We believe that their work—as individuals and in communities—will ultimately provide the energy, ideas, and inspiration to control the pandemic and its impact.

The Global AIDS Policy Coalition plans to produce a new edition of *AIDS in the World* each year. In future years, the book will build on the foundation established in this edition, in two ways. First, we will focus on a series of selected themes to track the progress and evolution of the pandemic, the response, and vulnerability to further spread. Our intent will be to help the reader to develop and sustain a clear global picture, year to year.

Second, we will continue to identify critical emerging issues for special emphasis. The pandemic and the response are dynamic and volatile, and new information, trends, hopes, and fears will merit targeted attention each year.

These themes and issues may include analysis of areas of policy uncertainty and implications of the future development of the pandemic, as well as an examination of basic health and social issues critical for progress in HIV/AIDS prevention and care. Among the issues to be examined in the next edition of *AIDS in the World* are:

- What interventions can successfully prevent HIV infection through sexual, injection drug use, perinatal, or blood-borne transmission? *AIDS in the World* will highlight not only demonstrated successes, but also critical shortcomings in research and evaluation methodologies that make it difficult to reach conclusions about intervention efficacy.
- What are the implications, constraints, and advantages of integrating HIV/AIDS interventions with different kinds of STD and/or primary health care programs?
- What will be the future demands on health and social service systems?
- What is the political economy of the manufacture, distribution, and availability of diagnostic tests, therapeutic drugs, and vaccines?
- How do sexuality, the status of women, and gender relations impact on AIDS and health?
- How are the roles of individuals, community organizations, and governments evolving in relation to funding and provision of health services, defining people's needs, and developing health policy and societal leadership to address health issues?

We will continue to try—through the powerful tool of information—to lay the groundwork for individual and collective action. Our goal is to contribute to the prevention and control of AIDS by promoting and strengthening individual capacity for informed advocacy. As individuals we are linked to the whole; how to connect the individual and the global, the personal and universal—this is the destiny and special challenge of our time.

International Guidelines
Appendixes
Reference Notes
About the Editors
Acknowledgments
Index

International Guidelines

section is based on
mation provided by
Appropriate Health
ources and
nologies Action
p (AHRTAG) in
on and was
ared with the
tance of Christopher
e, AHRTAG's AIDS
mation Officer.

The global response to HIV/AIDS has unleashed a torrent of words—sometimes words of warning, sometimes words of practical advice, and often, words that are difficult to comprehend. From a small stream at the start, these words have become a growth industry of guidelines. At first, their production was largely limited to local, nongovernmental organizations (NGOs), based in industrialized countries—AIDS was not considered an international or global problem until the mid- to late 1980s. Since the start of the second half of the last decade, however, that scenario has changed: governments, the World Health Organization (WHO), and other intergovernmental organizations and international NGOs have produced documents covering a wide range of HIV/AIDS subjects: scientific and social, programmatic and pragmatic. The development of these guidelines was rapid during the latter part of the first decade of AIDS. Now, as we enter the second decade, it is time to ask how useful these guidelines have been.

To address this question, some 30 agencies and individuals working in the field of HIV/AIDS around the world were surveyed by the Appropriate Health Resources and Technologies Action Group (AHRTAG) at the behest of *AIDS in the World*. The goal was to provide an inventory of the most relevant international guidelines produced to date and to identify any major gaps. To obtain data covering the period 1985–1991, AHRTAG sought a list of international guidelines that provided policy direction or managerial or technical guidance at the global or regional level, or that were published or released by international organizations. The survey excluded national policy documents, national adaptations of international documents, and directives published by agencies concerning their own internal AIDS policies.

Several questions are worth asking about the list of international guidelines produced: What is their value? How well have they "aged" since being written—are they still relevant, accurate, consistent, and useful? Is there a need for follow-up and updating? What should be done to broaden, refine, or improve their scope? (The list of guidelines pending publication is long, with some unpublished guidelines—particularly in the case of WHO—referring to meetings and consultations held more than 2 years ago.) Rather than being a comprehensive analysis of all international guidelines, this review sought to answer these questions for the guidelines on counseling (see the section "Guidelines under the Microscope: Counseling").

It is clear from the survey that the coming years will require intense efforts to meet the need for relevant and timely international guidelines. Human rights, sexual health, the problems of sex workers and the realities of the sex industry, condom social marketing programs, community health and development, care for orphans, and psychosocial research were all identified by the panel of experts as subjects pleading for more attention. Like most curves measuring the rate of response to the epidemic of HIV/AIDS, the guideline curve is losing its upward trajectory. Fatigue and recession are shrinking international will and resources. The challenges of the 1990s will be to update what already exists and to develop new guidelines to meet the need for the best and most current information.

Guidelines for Action

What is the specific task of international guidelines? International guidelines must encourage a consistent and coordinated approach to a particular issue. They must also suggest a framework for action, outline policy options, and offer possibilities for cooperation in areas in which such requirements may be difficult to meet. How and to what extent have international guidelines met the challenge?

In the context of HIV/AIDS, guidelines have been elaborated on topics ranging from sterilization and disinfection techniques to the correct use of condoms—subjects whose difficulties are more formidable when the international range and scope of ability to provide such services are considered. Of course, guidelines have their limitations. They are not usually intended as complete and comprehensive blueprints, but as reference points from which action plans and decision-making strategies can be developed. For this reason, guidelines must be presented in a way that encourages creative and appropriate adaptation at the local level.

Who produces international guidelines? The list of internationally relevant guidelines shows that the bulk have been produced by WHO and other United Nations agencies, followed by governments and nongovernmental organizations. Authorship is important; the perceived authority and prestige of the producing agency influences heavily the extent to which guidelines will be accepted and used. This may also partially explain the tendency among many groups and individuals not to question guideline content.

Where no previous information exists, guidelines often set standards. In some cases, guidelines intended only as a general framework have been accepted and implemented as policy. When universal guidelines fail to consider what is realistic at the local level, they are usually ignored. Thus, these various uses and interpretations of guidelines highlight the need to evaluate their application and effectiveness. Surprisingly, until now, very little systematic review has taken place.

Types of Guidelines

There are essentially two types of guidelines: those outlining standard procedures (requiring little adaptation to the local environment), and those providing a broad framework for action (requiring more extensive adaptation). Examples of guidelines that encourage standard procedures include: HIV-infection control in hospital and clinical settings, treatment of opportunistic infections (with local adaptation based on drug/resource availability), technical aspects of HIV antibody testing methodologies, definition of safer sex, and instructions for proper condom use. Guidelines providing a broad framework for action include those on counseling (including pre- and post-HIV test and AIDS clinical counseling), appropriate uses of and ethics surrounding HIV testing, condom promotion techniques, health education and prevention, and monitoring and evaluation methodologies.

Certain issues require both procedural and broad framework approaches. Guidelines for HIV testing, for example, involve both the technical aspects of HIV testing in the laboratory (standard procedures) and appropriate screening and testing strategies, including ethical and human rights aspects.

Guideline Development

To be useful and effective, guidelines should be developed with a number of goals in mind. These goals include considering the extent to which the proposed guidelines are to be universal, defining the intended audience, and consulting with them to identify what information is needed. The intended audience should also be reviewed in the final draft to ensure that information is relevant and clear. Complaints are still raised that guidelines are developed solely by so-called academic or research experts rather than by persons working in the field. Those who develop guidelines should also consider the perceptions and priorities of the people most often affected—including those with HIV/AIDS—and, when possible, invite them to join in guideline production. In addition, limitations and the context in which guidelines were developed should be noted, and other information, reading, and practical advice on where to find more information should be listed.

GUIDELINES UNDER THE MICROSCOPE: COUNSELING

Prepared by David Miller, Department of Public Health Medicine and Epidemiology, University Hospital and Medical School, Nottingham, England

Counseling in the context of HIV has a history of controversy—about its most appropriate definitions and hence its aims, about who should most often provide counseling, and about its usefulness for prevention of HIV transmission and/or support of those affected by HIV.

The concept of counseling as an integral element of pandemic management is new and therefore untried. Accordingly, it has been important to develop counseling guidelines and training materials. The development of guidelines and training materials also serves the important function of legitimizing this new concept.

To assess the effectiveness of some of the information currently available, 4 specialist HIV/AIDS counselors were provided with 3 sets of materials providing guidance on counseling and counseling training. Materials reviewed included "Counselling and AIDS," by D. Stone and N. Kaleeba, in *The Handbook for AIDS Prevention in Africa,* ed. P. Lamptey and P. Piot (Durham, N.C.: Family Health International, 1990); *Counselling Skills—A Training Manual* by R. Woolfe (Edinburgh: Scottish Health Education Group, 1989); and *WHO AIDS Series 8: Guidelines for Counselling about HIV Infection and Disease* (Geneva: WHO, 1990). The reviewers were: Gary Lloyd, Institute for Research and Training in HIV/AIDS Counseling, School of Social Work, Tulane University; Yvonne Sliep, St. Luke's Hospital,

Chilema, Malawi; and Brigid Willmore and Elizabeth Matenga, AIDS Counseling Trust, Harare, Zimbabwe.

All reviewers made criticisms of the specific works under review: use of language that was too confusing (in Stone and Kaleeba) or too specialized (in Woolfe). There was much uniformity in suggestions about how to improve *all* published guidance and training material on HIV counseling. In particular, reviewers agreed on the need to specify target audiences, to ensure greater cultural specificity and local awareness, to give much more attention to the *process* of counseling (how to *do* it and how to *implement* it), to include more case studies and issues reflecting developing world cultures, and to identify the skill levels of the intended readership.

Cultural Specificity

Guidance must be culturally relevant. The reviewers suggested that even though the models of counseling reviewed are based on Western experiences, guidance for developing countries should include examples emerging from the developing country context.

This is an important issue. For too long, the Western basis of HIV counseling has been a target for critics, who assume that Western models reflect inadequately the reality of counseling needs in the developing world. The reviewers (three of whom are based in developing countries) did not reject the models presented; they simply questioned the extent to which these models have been adapted successfully to local cultures and circumstances. Indeed, as one reviewer suggested, piloting guidelines and training materials in the targeted setting with target audiences is an essential step in ensuring that the guidance is going to be relevant in practice.

The Counseling Process

Advice was lacking on the implementation of counseling. Reviewers commented that the materials presupposed knowledge about HIV counseling—a vital flaw in documents for health professionals who, perhaps without prior experience or training in HIV counseling, are charged with the design and implementation of counseling services.

Guidance is also required for the development of HIV/AIDS counseling programs. Health planners, trainers, and providers need information on establishing and maintaining counseling activities and on how to assess costs and efficacy.

The implications of counseling for linkage with other community initiatives should be stressed. Methods for encouraging and maintaining such linkage should be addressed and clarified.

Reviewers also highlighted the need for clear guidance on the identification and training of possible counselors. None of the publications provided detailed coverage on monitoring and evaluation procedures—vital if their usefulness is to be established for health program managers.

Successful models for counseling in community, home-based, and clinic settings are now available. Future guidance on counseling should be more locally case- and model-driven.

Bibliography of International Guidelines for HIV/AIDS*

This bibliography lists guidelines considered to be internationally relevant. Twenty-seven resource and information centers around the world were surveyed. The selection criteria required that guidelines provide policy direction or managerial/technical guidance at the global or regional level, with publication after 1985 by organizations including international NGOs, United Nations agencies, and regional

---

*The following organizations participated and assisted in compiling this bibliography: AIDS Coordination Bureau, Royal Tropical Institute, the Netherlands; AIDS Education and Health Promotion Materials Exchange Centre for Asia and the Pacific (AIDSED), Thailand; AIDS Info Doc Schweiz, Switzerland; AIDSTECH/Family Health International, United States; American Foundation for AIDS Research (AmFAR), United States; Canadian Public Health Association, Canada; Centre Régional d'Information et de Prévention du SIDA (CRIPS), France; Centro Regional de Intercambio, Documentación e Información sobre el SIDA (CONASIDA), Mexico; Deutsche AIDS Hilfe, Germany; International Federation of Red Cross and Red Crescent Societies, Switzerland; International Labour Office, Switzerland; International Planned Parenthood Federation (IPPF), United Kingdom; National AIDS Clearinghouse, United States; National HIV Prevention Information Service, United Kingdom; South Pacific Commission Information Centre for the Prevention of AIDS and STDs, New Caledonia; UK NGO AIDS Consortium, United Kingdom; United Nations Children's Fund (UNICEF), United States; United Nations Population Fund, United States; and World Council of Churches/Christian Medical Commission, Switzerland.

bodies.* *Excluded* from selection were national policy documents, adaptations of international documents intended to reflect country policies, and directives published by agencies concerning their own internal policies related to AIDS.

Epidemiology

Current and future dimensions of the HIV/AIDS pandemic: A capsule study. WHO, 1991. WHO/GPA/RES/FI/91.4.

Manual de vigilancia epidemiológica VIH/SIDA (HIV/AIDS epidemiological surveillance manual). Instituto Nacional de Diagnóstico y Referencia Epidemiológicas, 1990. Available in Spanish only from CRIDIS, Comercio y Administración 13–2, Col. Copilco Universidad, CP 04360 Mexico D.F., Mexico.

Report on the informal consultation on developing an epidemiologically based strategy for control of AIDS/HIV in Asia, New Delhi, 6–8 June 1988 (15 pages). WHO, 1989.

Policy and Program Management

AIDS: Need for policy in the workplace. H. C. Jain. International Labour Organisation, CH-1211 Geneva 22, Switzerland, 1989.

AIDS: Policies and programs for the workplace. K. C. Brown and J. G. Turner. International Labour Organisation, CH-1211 Geneva 22, Switzerland, 1989.

AIDS and human rights: An international perspective. M. Breum and A. Hendriks. International Labour Office, International Labour Organisation, CH-1211 Geneva 22, Switzerland, 1988.

AIDS and the workplace. Paris: 25–26 April 1990. UNESCO, 7 Place de Fontenoy, 75700 Paris, France, 1990.

AIDS and the workplace: A practical approach. G. Tillet. International Labour Organisation, CH-1211 Geneva 22, Switzerland, 1989.

"AIDS and the workplace: Some policy pointers from international labour standards." *International Labour Review* 128(1) (1989):29–45. International Labour Office, International Labour Organisation, CH-1211 Geneva 22, Switzerland, 1989.

AIDS book: Information for workers. International Labour Organisation, CH-1211 Geneva 22, Switzerland; Service Employees International Union, Washington, D.C., 1989.

AIDS, discrimination and employment law. B. W. Napier. International Labour Organisation. CH-1211 Geneva 22, Switzerland, 1989.

---

*The World Health Organization (WHO) has issued the great majority of publications surveyed in the following pages. WHO publications are generally available from Distribution and Sales, WHO, 1211 Geneva 27, Switzerland. Materials are free unless the price is quoted. WHO regional offices may also stock and distribute these publications.

AIDS funding: A guide to foundations and charitable organizations (175 pages). 2d ed. The Foundation Center, 79 Fifth Avenue, New York, NY 10003, U.S.A., 1991.

AIDS in the workplace: Resource material. International Labour Organisation, CH-1211 Geneva 22, Switzerland; Bureau of National Affairs, Washington, D.C., 1989.

Aportes de la ética y el derecho al estudio del SIDA (Contributions of ethics and law to the study of HIV). Pan American Health Organization, Washington, D.C., 1990.

Avoidance of discrimination in relation to HIV-infected people and people with AIDS: The forty-first World Health Assembly adopted resolution WHA 41.24 on 13 May 1988. WHO, 1988.

Consensus statement from consultation on partner notification for preventing HIV transmission, Geneva, 11–13 January 1989. WHO, 1989. WHO/GPA/INF/89.3.

Consensus statement from the first international meeting of AIDS Service organisations, Vienna, 28 February–3 March 1989. WHO, 1989.

Consultation on AIDS and the workplace. GPA: Statement from the consultation on AIDS and the workplace, Geneva, 27–29 June 1988. WHO, 1988.

Consultation on nursing and HIV infection, Geneva, 7–9 March 1988. WHO, 1988.

Double jeopardy: Threat to life and human rights. Discrimination against persons with AIDS: A survey of AIDS as an international human rights issue and of international efforts to combat discrimination against persons with AIDS. R. Cohen and L. S. Wiseberg. International Labour Organisation, CH-1211 Geneva 22, Switzerland, 1990.

Guide concernant le SIDA et les premiers secours sur le lieu de travail (Guidelines for AIDS and first aid in the workplace). League of Red Cross and Red Crescent Societies, Federation of Red Cross and Red Crescent Societies, Switzerland, 1990. Available in English and French. Price: SwF6.00.

Guidelines for the development of a national AIDS prevention and control programme (iv + 27 pages). WHO, 1988. Price: SwF8.00 (5.60 in developing countries).

Guidelines for nursing management of people infected with human immunodeficiency virus (HIV) (iv + 42 pages). WHO, 1988. Price: SwF9.00 (6.30 in developing countries).

The handbook for AIDS prevention in Africa. P. Lamptey and P. Piot. Family Health International, P.O. Box 13950, Research Triangle Park, Durham, NC 27709, U.S.A., 1990. Available in French and English. Price: U.S.$28.00 (includes postage).

HIV testing and quality control: A guide for laboratory personnel. N. Constantine et al. Family Health International, P.O. Box 13950, Research Triangle Park, Durham, NC 27709, U.S.A., 1991.

How to plan a project and apply for funds. AIDS Action, issue 12. AHRTAG, 1

London Bridge Street, London SE1 9SG, U.K. Free in developing countries (subscription £10.00/U.S.$20.00 elsewhere), in English, French, Spanish, and Portuguese.

Human rights: Report of an international consultation on AIDS and human rights, Geneva, 26–28 July 1989. United Nations, 1989.

"International Organization for Migration seminar on migration medicine: AIDS, travel and migration: Legal and human rights aspects." K. Tomasevski. *International Migration* 29(1) (1990):33–48. International Labour Organisation, CH-1211 Geneva 22, Switzerland.

Inventory of nongovernmental organizations working on AIDS in countries that receive development cooperation or assistance. WHO, 1990. WHO/GPA/DIR/90.5.

Managing AIDS in the workplace. S. B. Puckett and A. R. Emery. International Labour Organisation, CH-1211 Geneva 22, Switzerland, 1988.

Le Manifeste de Montréal: Declaration of the universal rights and needs of people living with HIV disease. AIDS Action Now, 517 College St., Suite 324, Toronto, Ontario M6G 1A8, Canada, 1989.

Monitoring of national AIDS prevention and control programmes: Guiding principles (iii + 71 pages). WHO, 1989. Price: SwF8.00 (5.60 in developing countries).

Nutritional guidelines for people with HIV. AIDS Letter no. 17 (Feb./March 1990). Royal Society of Medicine Services Ltd., 1 Wimpole Street, London W1M 8AE, U.K. Subscription £12.00 per year.

Population and human rights: Proceedings of the Expert Group Meeting on Population and Human Rights, 3–6 April 1989. UN Department of International and Social Affairs Expert Group Meeting on Population and Human Rights, International Labour Organisation, CH-1211 Geneva 22, Switzerland, 1989.

Report of the consultation on AIDS and the workplace. National AIDS Clearinghouse, Canada, 1988.

Report of the consultation on AIDS and the workplace, Geneva, 27–29 June 1988. WHO, 1988. WHO/GPA/DIR/88.4.

Report of the consultation on partner notification for preventing HIV transmission, Geneva, 11–13 January 1989. WHO, 1989.

Report of the Global Commission on AIDS first meeting, Geneva, 29–31 March 1989. WHO, 1989.

Report of an informal consultation on national AIDS programme reviews, Geneva, 11–13 October 1989. WHO, 1989.

Resolution WHA42.34 of the forty-second World Health Assembly: Non-governmental organisations and the global strategy for prevention and control of AIDS, Geneva, 19 May 1989. WHO, 1989.

Screening and testing in AIDS prevention and control programmes. WHO, 1988. WHO/SPA/INF/88.1.

Screening workers: An examination and analysis of practice and public policy.

P. A. Greenfield et al. International Labour Organisation, CH-1211 Geneva 22, Switzerland, 1989.

Sentinel surveillance for HIV infection: A method to monitor HIV infection trends in population groups. G. Slutkin et al. WHO, 1988. WHO/GPA/DIR/88.8.

SIDA et milieu de travail: Données médicales, juridiques et éthiques (AIDS and the workplace: medical, legal and ethical facts). H. Seillan and D. Berra. International Labour Organisation, CH-1211 Geneva 22, Switzerland, 1990.

Simple approaches to evaluation. AIDS Action, issue 16. AHRTAG, 1 London Bridge Street, London SE1 9SG, U.K. Free in developing countries (subscription £10.00/U.S.$20.00 elsewhere), in English, French, Spanish, and Portuguese.

Social aspects of AIDS prevention and control programmes. WHO, 1988.

Solidarity against AIDS. Special issue, *IDRC Reports* 18 (2) (April 1989). International Research Development Centre, P.O. Box 8500, Ottawa, Canada.

Special issue on AIDS prevention: Strategies for behavior change—slowing the spread of AIDS. Network 12 (1) (June 1991). Family Health International, P.O. Box 13950, Research Triangle Park, Durham, NC 27709, U.S.A.

Statement from the consultation on AIDS and the workplace. National AIDS Clearinghouse, Canada, 1988.

Statement on screening of international travelers for infection with HIV. WHO, 1988. WHO/GPA/INF/88.3.

Tabular information on legal instruments dealing with AIDS and HIV infection. Part 1: *all countries and jurisdictions, including the USA (other than state legislation).* WHO, 1989.

The third epidemic: Repercussions of the fear of AIDS (320 pages). Panos, 9 White Lion Street, London NI 9PD, U.K., 1990. Price: £5.95.

Trade unionists and AIDS: Report of TUC seminar on AIDS. International Labour Organisation, CH-1211 Geneva 22, Switzerland, 1988.

The United Kingdom Declaration of the Rights of People with HIV and AIDS (16 pages), UK Declaration Working Group, National AIDS Trust, 1991. Available from NAT, Room 1403, Euston Tower, 286 Euston Road, London NW1 3DN, U.K.

Unlinked anonymous screening for the public health surveillance of HIV infections: Proposed international guidelines. WHO, 1989. GPA/SFI/89.3.

Use of HIV surveillance data in national AIDS control programmes: A review of current data use with recommendations for strengthening future use. WHO, 1990. WHO/GPA/SFI/90.1.

Workplace privacy: Employee testing, surveillance, wrongful discharge, and other areas of vulnerability. I. M. Shepard et al. International Labour Organisation, CH-1211 Geneva 22, Switzerland, 1989.

Information, Education, Communication

Action for youth: AIDS training manual. League of Red Cross and Red Crescent Societies. Federation of Red Cross and Red Crescent Societies, P.O. Box 372,

CH-1211 Geneva 19, Switzerland, 1990. Available in English, Spanish, French, and Arabic. Price: SwF20.00.

AIDS Education: Lessons from international health. Academy for Educational Development, 1255 23rd St. N.W., Washington, DC 20037, U.S.A., 1988.

AIDS health promotion: Guide for planning (39 pages). WHO, 1988. GPA/HPR/88.1.

AIDS prevention education: Towards a UNESCO plan of action and intervention. Clearinghouse on Development Communications, 1815 N. Fort Meyer Drive, 6th Floor, Arlington, VA 22209, U.S.A., 1987.

AIDS prevention through health promotion: Facing sensitive issues. WHO, 1991.

Broadcasters' questions and answers on AIDS. WHO, 1989.

Developing materials for culture groups. G. Smallwood. Pergamon Press, Maxwell House, Fairview Park, Elmsford, NY 10523, U.S.A., 1988.

Extending the role of AIDS hotlines in AIDS prevention programs in developed and developing countries. Academy for Educational Development, 1255 23rd St. N.W., Washington, DC 20037, U.S.A., 1989.

Guide to planning health promotion for AIDS prevention and control (iv + 71 pages). WHO, 1989. Price: SwF14.00 (9.80 in developing countries).

Guide to planning health promotion for AIDS prevention and control. WHO, 1990.

Learning about AIDS: A manual for pastors and teachers. WCC AIDS Working Group. World Council of Churches/Christian Medical Commission, Geneva, Switzerland, 1989.

Learning AIDS (270 pages). 2d ed. American Foundation for AIDS Research, 733 Third Avenue, 12th Floor, New York, NY 10036–8901, U.S.A., 1989. Tel.: (212) 682–7440 or (212) 682–9812. Price: U.S.$24.95.

Spreading the word: AIDS media pack. League of Red Cross and Red Crescent Societies. Federation of Red Cross and Red Crescent Societies, P.O. Box 372, CH-1211 Geneva 19, Switzerland, 1990. Available in English, Spanish, French, and Arabic.

Understanding AIDS: Training exercises for developing countries. J. Hubley. Leeds Polytechnic, Leeds, U.K., 1988.

What is AIDS? A manual for health workers. World Council of Churches/Christian Medical Commission, Geneva, Switzerland, 1989. Available in English, French, Spanish, Portuguese, and Kiswahili.

Working towards understanding. A workplace training pack including a set of 60 slides. League of Red Cross and Red Crescent Societies. Federation of Red Cross and Red Crescent Societies, P.O. Box 372, CH-1211 Geneva 19, Switzerland. Available in English, Spanish, French, and Arabic. Price: SwF80.00

Blood/Laboratory/Medical

Biosafety guidelines for diagnostic and research laboratories working with HIV (iv + 28 pages). WHO, 1991. Price: SwF8.00 (5.60 in developing countries).

Blood transfusion guidelines for international travellers. WHO, 1988.

A code of practice for sterilisation of instruments and control of cross infection

(58 pages). ISBN 0-7279-0274-1. British Medical Association, P.O. Box 295, Tavistock Square, London WC1H 9JP, U.K., 1989.

Common fungal infections in HIV disease. AIDS Action, issue 12. AHRTAG, 1 London Bridge Street, London SE1 9SG, U.K. Available in English, French, Spanish, and Portuguese. Free in developing countries (subscription £10.00/ U.S.$20.00 elsewhere).

Commonsense and sensitivity (ethical guidelines). *AIDS Action,* issue 14. AHRTAG, 1 London Bridge Street, London SE1 9SG, U.K. Available in English, French, Spanish, and Portuguese. Free in developing countries (subscription £10.00/U.S.$20.00 elsewhere).

Consultation on criteria for international testing of candidate HIV vaccines. WHO, 1989.

Decontamination of instruments and appliances used in the vagina. U.K. Department of Health, 1988. EL(88) (MB)/210. Available from Health Publications Unit, No. 2 Site, Heywood, Lancs OL10 2PZ, U.K.

Diarrhoea and AIDS. AIDS Action, issue 7. AHRTAG, 1 London Bridge Street, London SE1 9SG, U.K. Available in English, French, Spanish, and Portuguese. Free in developing countries (subscription £10.00/U.S.$20.00 elsewhere).

Genital ulcer disease. AIDS Action, issue 6. AHRTAG, 1 London Bridge Street, London SE1 9SG, U.K. Available in English, French, Spanish, and Portuguese. Free in developing countries (subscription £10.00/U.S.$20.00 elsewhere).

Global Blood Safety Initiative: Consensus statement on accelerated strategies to reduce the risk of transmission of HIV by blood transfusion, Geneva, 20–22 March 1989. WHO, 1989.

Global Blood Safety Initiative: Essential blood components, plasma derivatives and substitutes, Geneva, 20–22 March 1989. WHO, 1989.

Global Blood Safety Initiative: Minimum targets for blood transfusion services, Geneva, 20–22 March 1989. WHO, 1989. WHO/GPA/INF/89.14.

Guidance for clinical health care workers: Protection against infection with HIV and hepatitis viruses: Recommendations of the expert advisory group on AIDS. UN Department of Health, 1990. International Labour Organisation, CH-1211 Geneva 22, Switzerland.

Guidelines for treatment of acute blood loss. WHO, 1988. WHO/GPA/INF/88.5.

Guidelines on sterilisation and disinfection. AIDS Letter no. 16 (Dec. 1989/Jan. 1990). Royal Society of Medicine Services Ltd., 1 Wimpole Street, London W1M 8AE, U.K. Subscription £12.00 per year.

Guidelines on sterilisation and disinfection methods effective against human immunodeficiency virus (HIV) (iv + 11 pages). 2d ed. WHO, 1989. Price: SwF4.00 (2.80 in developing countries).

HIV: The causative agents of AIDS and related conditions. Advisory Committee on Dangerous Pathogens, 1990. HMSO (Her Majesty's Stationery Office), P.O. Box 276, London SW8 5DT, U.K.

HIV and the nervous system. AIDS Action, issue 11. AHRTAG, 1 London Bridge Street, London SE1 9SG, U.K. Available in English, French, Spanish, and

Portuguese. Free in developing countries (subscription £10.00/U.S.$20.00 elsewhere).

Immunisation against infectious disease (181 pages). 1990. HMSO, P.O. Box 276, London SW8 5DT, U.K. Price: £4.00.

Operational characteristics of commercially available assays to determine antibodies to HIV-1, Geneva, March 1989. WHO, 1989. WHO/BMR/89.4.

Operational characteristics of commercially available assays to determine antibodies to HIV-1 and/or HIV-2 in human sera (report 2), Geneva, April 1990. WHO, 1990. WHO/BMR/90.1.

Oral signs of AIDS. AIDS Action, issue 8. AHRTAG, 1 London Bridge Street, London SE1 9SG, U.K. Available in English, French, Spanish, and Portuguese. Free in developing countries (subscription £10.00/U.S.$20.00 elsewhere).

Pneumocystis carinii pneumonia and tuberculosis. AIDS Action, issue 5. AHRTAG, 1 London Bridge Street, London SE1 9SG, U.K. Available in English, French, Spanish, and Portuguese. Free in developing countries (subscription £10.00/U.S.$20.00 elsewhere).

La pratique transfusionelle en milieu isolé: Prévention de la transmission du VIH (Practical blood transfusion guidelines: Prevention of HIV transmission) (26 pages). Médecins sans Frontières, France. Available in French only.

Report of a technical advisory meeting on research on AIDS and tuberculosis, 2–4 August 1988. WHO, 1988. WHO/GPA/BMR/89.3.

Report of a WHO consultation on traditional medicine and AIDS: Clinical evaluation of traditional medicines and natural products, Geneva, 26–28 September 1990. WHO, 1990. WHO/TRM/GPA/90.2.

Report of a WHO informal consultation on animal models for HIV infection and AIDS, Geneva, 28–30 March 1988. WHO, 1988.

Report of a WHO informal consultation on preclinical and clinical aspects of the use of immunomodulators in HIV infection, Geneva, 3–5 April 1989. WHO, 1989. WHO/GPA/BMR/89.6.

Report of a WHO informal consultation on traditional medicine and AIDS: In vitro screening for anti-HIV activity, Geneva, 6–8 February 1989. WHO, 1989.

Report of a WHO meeting on criteria for the evaluation and standardization of diagnostic tests for the detection of HIV antibody, Stockholm, December 1987. WHO, 1988.

Report of the consultation on AIDS and traditional medicine: Prospects for involving traditional health practitioners, Francistown, Botswana, 23–27 July 1990. WHO, 1990. WHO/TRM/GPA/90.1.

Report of the consultation on neuropsychiatric aspects of HIV infection. Global Programme on AIDS, Geneva, 14–17 March 1988. WHO, 1988. WHO/GPA/DIR/88.1.

Report of the Global Blood Safety Initiative meeting, Geneva, 16–17 May 1988. WHO, 1988.

Report of the meeting on HIV-2 diagnostics and priority areas for HIV-2 epide-

miological research, Geneva, 14–16 February 1989. WHO, 1989. WHO/GPA/ ESR/89.3.

Report of the meeting on strategies for the evaluation and implementation of laboratory diagnosis of HIV infection, Geneva, 31 August–2 September 1988. WHO, 1988. WHO/GPA/BMR/89.2.

Report of the second consultation on the neuropsychiatric aspects of HIV-1 infection, Geneva, 11–13 January 1990. WHO, 1990. WHO/GPA/MNH/90.1.

Skin conditions common to people with HIV infection/AIDS. AIDS Action, issue 10. AHRTAG, 1 London Bridge Street, London SE1 9SG, U.K. Available in English, French, Spanish, and Portuguese. Free in developing countries (subscription £10.00/U.S.$20.00 elsewhere).

Statement from the consultation on criteria for international testing of candidate HIV vaccines, Geneva, 27 February–2 March 1989. WHO, 1989. WHO/GPA/I NF/89.8.

Statement on AIDS and tuberculosis. WHO, 1989.

Sexual Behavior

A basic guide to safer sex. AIDS Action, issue 4. AHRTAG, 1 London Bridge Street, London SE1 9SG, U.K. Available in English, French, Spanish, and Portuguese. Free in developing countries (subscription £10.00/U.S.$20.00 elsewhere).

A code of practice for the safe use and disposal of sharps (64 pages). ISBN 0-7279-0294-6. British Medical Association, P.O. Box 295, Tavistock Square, London WC1H 9JP, U.K., 1990.

Consensus statement from the consultation on global strategies for coordination of AIDS and STD control programmes, Geneva, 11–13 July 1990. WHO, 1990. WHO/GPA/INF/90.2.

Consensus statement from the consultation on HIV epidemiology and prostitution, Geneva, 3–6 July 1989. WHO, 1989. WHO/GPA/ INF/89.11.

Consensus statement from the consultation on sexually transmitted diseases as risk factors for HIV transmission, Geneva, 4–6 January 1989. WHO, 1989. WHO/GPA/INF/89.1.

Handbook on sexually transmitted diseases. Australian Government Publishing Service, 1990. National Health and Medical Research Council of Australia, Alexander Building, Phillip, Australia.

How to sell safer sex (preventive education in the sex industry). *AIDS Action,* issue 15. AHRTAG, 1 London Bridge Street, London SE1 9SG, U.K. Available in English, French, Spanish, and Portuguese. Free in developing countries (subscription £10.00/U.S.$20.00 elsewhere).

Management of patients with sexually transmitted diseases. WHO, 1991. WHO Technical Report Series no. 810.

Prevention of sexual transmission of human immunodeficiency virus (iv + 28 pages). WHO, 1990. Price: SwF8.00 (5.60 in developing countries).

Promoting safer sex: Prevention of sexual transmission of AIDS and other STDs.

Proceedings of an international workshop, May 1989. M. Paalman. Falmer Press, Taylor and Francis, Inc., 1900 Frost Road, Suite 101, Bristol, PA 19007, U.S.A., 1990.

Promoting sexual health: The second international workshop on preventing the sexual transmission of HIV and other STDs, Cambridge, 24–27 March 1991. Health Education Authority, 1991. British Medical Association Foundation for AIDS, BMA House, Tavistock Square, London WC1H 9JP, U.K.

Safer sex guidelines: A resource document for educators and counsellors. Canadian AIDS Society, 1101–1170 Laurier West, Ottawa, Ontario K1P 5V5, Canada, 1989. Also available in French.

Sexuality in sub-Saharan Africa: An annotated bibliography. T. G. Barton. Family Health International, P.O. Box 13950, Research Triangle Park, Durham, NC 27709, U.S.A., 1991.

Sexually transmitted diseases: Guidelines for management. AIDS Action, issue 13. AHRTAG, 1 London Bridge Street, London SE1 9SG, U.K. Available in English, French, Spanish, and Portuguese. Free in developing countries (subscription £10.00/U.S.$20.00 elsewhere).

Statements by the WHO collaborating centres on AIDS: Heterosexual transmission of HIV, and HIV and certain common social situations. WHO, 1989. WHO/GPA/INF/89.5.

STD control as an AIDS prevention strategy. Special issue, Network 12 (4) (1992). Family Health International, P.O. Box 13950, Research Triangle Park, Durham, NC 27709, U.S.A.

Injection Drug Use

AIDS among drug abusers in Europe: Report on a WHO consultation, Stockholm, 7–9 October 1986. WHO, European Office, 1986.

AIDS and drug misuse, Part 1 (108 pages). Advisory Council on the Misuse of Drugs, 1988. ISBN 0-11-321134-1. HMSO, P.O. Box 276, London SW8 5DT, U.K. Price: £6.50.

AIDS and drug misuse. Part 2. (98 pages). Advisory Council on the Misuse of Drugs, 1989. ISBN 0-11-321207-0. HMSO, P.O. Box 276, London SW8 5DT, U.K. Price: £6.30.

Report of the meeting on HIV infection and drug injecting intervention strategies, Geneva, 18–20 January 1988. WHO, 1989. WHO/GPA/ SBR/89.1.

Summary of presentation on drug use and AIDS, Fifth International Conference on AIDS, 4–9 June 1989, Montreal. D. Wohlfeiler. WHO, 1989.

Counseling

AIDS: A guide to clinical counselling. R. Miller and R. Bor. Science Press, London, U.K., 1988.

AIDS: Some guidelines for pastoral care. Board for Social Responsibility, 1986. Church House Publishing, London, U.K.

The AIDS Handbook: A Guide to the understanding of AIDS and HIV. J. Hubley. Macmillan, London, U.K., 1990.

AIDS resource kit. Medical Assistance Programs International, P.O. Box 50, Brunswick, GA 31521–0050, U.S.A., 1988.

AIDS resource kit: Discussion guide. Medical Assistance Programs International, P.O. Box 50, Brunswick, GA 31521–0050, U.S.A., 1988.

Counselling after HIV testing. G. Ornelas Hall. Pergamon Press, Maxwell House, Fairview Park, Elmsford, NY 10523, U.S.A., 1988.

Counselling before HIV testing. B. Harris. Pergamon Press, Maxwell House, Fairview Park, Elmsford, NY 10523, U.S.A., 1988.

Counselling of persons with AIDS. D. Miller. Pergamon Press, Maxwell House, Fairview Park, Elmsford, NY 10523, U.S.A., 1988.

Guidelines for counselling about HIV infection and disease (v + 48 pages). WHO, 1990. Price: SwF11.00 (7.70 in developing countries).

A guide to HIV/AIDS pastoral counselling. WCC AIDS Working Group, World Council of Churches/Christian Medical Commission, 150 Route de Ferney, Geneva, Switzerland, 1990.

Health workers, the community and AIDS. M. O. Ngandu. Pergamon Press, Maxwell House, Fairview Park, Elmsford, NY 10523, U.S.A., 1988.

HIV counselling: A psychosocial guide for care-givers. Canadian Haemophilia Society, 1450 City Councillors, Suite 840, Montreal, Quebec H3A 2E6, Canada, 1990.

L'intervention face au SIDA: Un guide pratique pour accueillir, informer, conseiller et accompagner les personnes infectées par le VIH (Social action guide against AIDS: A practical guide to support people infected with HIV). B. Cohen et al. ARCAT-SIDA, 1991. CRIPS, 3/5 rue de Ridder, 75014 Paris, France. Available in French only.

Prevention counselling: Integrating concepts and techniques in all AIDS prevention strategies. D. Stone et al. Academy for Educational Development, AIDSCOM Project, 1255 23rd St. N.W., Washington, DC 20037, U.S.A., 1989.

Report from consultation on psychosocial research needs in HIV infection and AIDS, Geneva, 25–28 May 1987. WHO, 1989.

Responding to AIDS. L. Heise. W. W. Norton and Co., 500 Fifth Avenue, New York, NY 10110, U.S.A., 1989.

Talking AIDS: A guide for community work. G. Gordon and T. Klouda. 1988. IPPF, U.K. Available in English, Spanish, Portuguese, French, and Arabic. Price: £2.00/U.S.$4.00 (includes postage).

What to tell someone who has AIDS. AIDS Action, issue 4. AHRTAG, 1 London Bridge Street, London SE1 9SG, U.K. Available in English, French, Spanish, and Portuguese. Free in developing countries (subscription £10.00/U.S.$20.00 elsewhere).

Working with uncertainty. P. Gordon. 1990. UK Family Planning Association, 27–35 Mortimer Street, London W1N 7RJ, U.K. Available in English only. Price: £12.99.

AIDS/HIV infection: A reference guide for nursing professionals. J. H. Flaskerud. W. B. Saunders, London, U.K., 1989.

AIDS management: An integrated approach. (Zambia) Strategies for Hope Series, no 3. Available from TALC, P.O. Box 49, St. Albans, Herts AL1 4AX, U.K. Price: £1.50 each (plus postage).

The AIDS manual: A guide for health care administrators. Ed. J. A. DeHovitz and T. J. Altimont. National Health Publishing, 99 Painters Mill Road, Owings Mills, MD 21117, U.S.A., 1988.

AIDS orphans: A community perspective from Tanzania. Strategies for Hope Series, no 5. Available from TALC, P.O. Box 49, St. Albans, Herts AL1 4AX, U.K. Price: £1.50 each (plus postage).

The caring community: Coping with AIDS in urban Uganda. Strategies for Hope Series, no 6. Available from TALC, P.O. Box 49, St. Albans, Herts AL1 4AX, U.K. Price: £1.50 each (plus postage).

From fear to hope: AIDS care and prevention at Chikankata Hospital, Zambia. Strategies for Hope Series, no 1. Available from TALC, P.O. Box 49, St. Albans, Herts AL1 4AX, U.K. Price: £1.50 each (plus postage).

Guidance for clinical care workers: Protection against infections with HIV and hepatitis viruses (52 pages). Expert Advisory Group on AIDS, 1990. HMSO, London.

Guidelines on AIDS and first aid in the workplace (iii + 12 pages). WHO, 1990. Price: SwF4.00 (2.80 in developing countries).

HIV testing and quality control: A guide for laboratory personnel (165 pages). Family Health International (FHI), P.O. Box 13950, Research Triangle Park, Durham, NC 27709, U.S.A., 1991. Price: U.S.$10.00 (includes postage).

El laboratorista frente el SIDA (The laboratory technician faced with AIDS). CONASIDA, 1989. CRIDIS, Comercio y Administración 13–2, Col. Copilco Universidad, CP 04360 Mexico D.F., Mexico. Available in Spanish only.

Living positively with AIDS: The AIDS Support Organisation (TASO), Uganda. Strategies for Hope Series, no 2. Available from TALC, P.O. Box 49, St. Albans, Herts AL1 4AX, U.K. Price: £1.50 each (plus postage).

El medico frente el SIDA (The doctor faced with AIDS). CONASIDA, 1989. CRIDIS, Comercio y Administración 13–2, Col. Copilco Universidad, CP 04360 Mexico D.F., Mexico. Available in Spanish only.

Meeting AIDS with compassion: AIDS care and prevention in Agomanya, Ghana. Strategies for Hope Series, no 4. Available from TALC, P.O. Box 49, St. Albans, Herts AL1 4AX, U.K. Price: £1.50 each (plus postage).

El odontólogo frente el SIDA (The dentist faced with AIDS). CONASIDA, 1989. CRIDIS, Comercio y Administración 13–2, Col. Copilco Universidad, CP 04360 Mexico D.F., Mexico. Available in Spanish only.

Report of second WCC international consultation on AIDS and pastoral care, Moshi, Tanzania, December 1988. World Council of Churches/Christian Commission, 150 Route de Ferney, Geneva, Switzerland.

Women

Report of the consultation with international women's NGOs on AIDS prevention and care, Geneva, 21–22 December 1989. WHO, 1989. WHO/GPA/ DIR/91.3.

Report of the meeting on research priorities relating to women and HIV/AIDS, Geneva, 19–20 November 1990. WHO, 1990. WHO/GPA/ DIR/91.2.

Statement from the consultation on breastfeeding, breastmilk and HIV, Geneva, 23–25 June 1987. WHO, 1987.

Triple jeopardy: Women and AIDS. (104 pages). Panos, 9 White Lion Street, London N1 9PD, U.K., 1990. Price: £6.95.

Women and AIDS in the developing countries (report of the conference). UK NGO AIDS Consortium, U.K., 1991. Price: £2.50.

Reproductive Health

AIDS in the third world. Ed. D. Wulf. *International Family Planning Perspectives* 13 (3) (September 1987). Alan Guttmacher Institute, 111 Fifth Avenue, New York, NY 10003, U.S.A.

AIDS prevention: Guidelines for mother and child health/family planning programme managers, 1: AIDS and family planning. WHO, 1990. WHO/MCH/ GPA/90.1.

AIDS prevention: Guidelines for mother and child health/family planning programme managers, 1: AIDS and maternal and child health. WHO, 1990. WHO/MCH/GPA/90.2.

The health of mothers and children in the context of HIV/AIDS, November 1989. WHO, 1989. WHO/GPA/INF/89.19.

International conference on the implications of AIDS for mothers and children: Technical statements and selected presentations, Paris, 27–30 November 1989. WHO, 1989.

IPPF Medical Bulletin: Statement on contraception for clients who are HIV positive (4 pages). International Planned Parenthood Federation (IPPF), P.O. Box 759, Inner Circle, Regents Park, London NW1 4LQ, U.K., 1991.

Preventing a crisis: AIDS and family planning. G. Gordon and T. Klouda. International Planned Parenthood Federation (IPPF), P.O. Box 759, Inner Circle, Regents Park, London NW1 4LQ, U.K., 1990. Available in English, Spanish, Portuguese, French, and Arabic. Price: £4.00/U.S.$8.00 (includes postage).

Youth/Children

Children orphaned by AIDS: A call for action by NGOs. National Council for International Health, U.S.A., 1991. Price: U.S.$5.00.

Joint WHO/UNICEF statement on early immunisation for HIV infected children, Geneva, January 1989. WHO, 1989. WHO/GPA/ INF/89.6.

Knowing where to start (working with street youth). *AIDS Action,* issue 11. AHRTAG, 1 London Bridge Street, London SE1 9SG, U.K. Available in English, French, Spanish, and Portuguese. Free in developing countries (subscription £10.00/U.S.$20.00 elsewhere).

Statement from the consultation on human immunodeficiency virus (HIV) and routine child immunisation, Geneva, 12–13 August 1989. WHO, 1987.

Others

Aboriginal AIDS resource directory. National AIDS Clearinghouse, Canadian Public Health Association, 1565 Carling Avenue, Suite 400, Ottawa, Ontario K1Z 8R1, Canada, 1991.

Action kit: How to create, plan and organise a World AIDS Day. WHO, 1990.

Action kit for World AIDS Day, 1 December 1990, and National HIV and AIDS Awareness Day, 3 December 1990. American Association for World Health, 2001 S St. N.W., Suite 530, Washington, DC 20009, U.S.A., 1990.

AIDS: Profile of an epidemic. Pan American Health Organization, AIDS Program, 525 23rd St. N.W., Washington, DC 20037, U.S.A., 1989.

AIDS Action. Quarterly newsletter on AIDS prevention and control worldwide. Available from AHRTAG, 1 London Bridge Street, London SE1 9SG, U.K. Available in English, French, Spanish, and Portuguese (Brazilian and African versions). Free in developing countries (subscription £10.00/U.S.$20.00 elsewhere).

AIDS, NGOs, and private sector initiatives: NCIH Conference, 23–27 June, Arlington [Virginia]. National Council for International Health, 1701 K St. N.W., Suite 600, Washington, DC 20006, U.S.A., 1991.

Blaming others: Prejudice, race and worldwide AIDS (168 pages). R. Sabatier. Panos/New Society Publishers, 1988. Price: U.S.$9.95.

Consensus statement from the consultation on AIDS and seafarers, Geneva, 5–6 October 1989. WHO, 1989. WHO/GPA/INF/89.21.

Consensus statement from the consultation on AIDS and sports, Geneva, 16 January 1989. WHO, 1989. WHO/GPA/INF/89.2.

Directory of European funders of HIV/AIDS projects in developing countries (includes guidelines on applying for funds). UK NGO AIDS Consortium, Fenner Brockway House, 37–39 Great Guildford Street, London SE1 0ES, U.K., 1991. Free in developing countries, £10.00 to others.

Information to undertakers: Infectious diseases. UK Department of Health, 1988. PL/CMO/88.7. Available from Health Publications Unit, No. 2 Site, Heywood, Lancs OL10 2PZ, U.K.

Meeting with non-governmental organisations on co-ordinating AIDS related activities, 10 May 1988. UN Economic and Social Council, UN Plaza, New York, NY 10017, U.S.A., 1988.

Panos Dossier: AIDS and the third world. R. Sabatier and M. Foreman. New Society Publishers/West, P.O. Box 582, Santa Cruz, CA 95061, U.S.A., 1989.

"Seminar on migration medicine." D. Kuntz. *International Migration* 35 (1990):13–21. International Labour Organisation, CH-1211 Geneva 22, Switzerland.

Statement from the consultation on prevention and control of AIDS in prisons, Geneva, 16–18 November 1987. WHO, 1987. WHO/ SPA/INF/87.14.

Documents in Preparation

Blood donor counseling guidelines for HIV and other transmitted transfusion infections. Available late 1992 from International Federation of Red Cross and Red Crescent Societies, and World Health Organization, Geneva, Switzerland.

Education in sexual health. Norwegian Red Cross Society. Available in English, French, and Spanish, summer 1992, from AHRTAG, 1 London Bridge Street, London SE1 9SG, U.K., and the International Federation of Red Cross and Red Crescent Societies, P.O. Box 372, CH-1211 Geneva 19, Switzerland.

The handbook for AIDS prevention in the Caribbean. P. Lamptey et al. Available summer 1992 from Family Health International, P.O. Box 13950, Research Triangle Park, Durham, NC 27709, U.S.A. Estimated price: $15.00 (domestic), U.S.$28.00 (overseas).

HIV/AIDS and overseas employment: A guide for employers. Originally produced in March 1989; currently under revision and expected to be available in 1992 from UK NGO AIDS Consortium, Fenner Brockway House, 37–39 Great Guildford Street, London SE1 0ES, U.K.

HIV infection, tissue banks and organ donation. UK Department of Health. Available late 1992 from Health Publications Unit, No. 2 Site, Heywood, Lancs OL10 2PZ, U.K.

Training for families in home care for people with AIDS. Norwegian Red Cross Society. Available in English, French, and Spanish, summer 1992, from AHRTAG, U.K., and the International Federation of Red Cross and Red Crescent Societies, Switzerland.

Women and AIDS handbook. Available late 1992 from AHRTAG, 1 London Bridge Street, London SE1 9SG, U.K.

Documents in Preparation by WHO

AIDS prevention: What MCH/FP service providers need to know.

Application for collaborative research projects, sections A and B.

Bench level laboratory workshop training manual for HIV screening assays.

Clinical management guidelines for HIV infection in adults.

Field guidelines for HIV sentinel surveillance.

First meeting of joint WHO/IFPM working groups on development, testing and utilisation of drugs and vaccines for HIV infection and HIV-related diseases, Geneva, 3 October 1991.

Guidelines for monitoring HIV infection in populations & WHO/UNESCO guide for school health education to prevent AIDS and other sexually transmitted diseases (merging of two technical documents for an AIDS series publication).

Guidelines for preventing occupational transmission in a health care setting.

Lessons from family planning and their application to AIDS prevention & male involvement programs in family planning: Lessons learned and implications for AIDS prevention (merging of two documents).

Monograph on home care programmes in Africa.

Physician's handbook on AIDS in Africa (renamed *A manual for physicians*).

Policy guidelines for school health education to prevent AIDS and sexually transmitted diseases.

Preparatory technical working group on virology and immunology. International conference on the implications of AIDS for mothers and children, Paris, 24–25 November 1989.

Proposed operational procedures for the GPA research steering committee.

Report of a WHO technical working group on criteria for laboratory characterisation of HIV isolates, 11–12 December 1989.

Report of a pilot study on an alternative approach to confirming anti-HIV reactivity.

Report of conferences on AIDS and the workplace, Paris, 25–26 April 1990.

Report of a technical working group on criteria for the identification, assessment and strengthening of potential field sites for the evaluation of HIV candidate vaccines, 12–14 November 1990.

Report of a technical working group (no. 3) on the epidemiology of HIV-1 infection in mothers and children, 25–26 September 1989.

Report of the first meeting of the steering committee on clinical research and drug development, 3–4 June 1991.

Report of the first meeting of the steering committee on diagnostics, Geneva, 22–23 May 1991.

Report of the first meeting of the steering committee on epidemiological research, surveillance and forecasting, Geneva, 28–29 May 1991.

Report of the first meeting of the steering committee on vaccine development, Geneva, 2–3 May 1991.

Report of the HIV-2 collaborating group meeting, Abidjan, 14–16 March 1990.

Report of the informal consultation on guiding principles for the conduct of international collaborative AIDS research.

Report of the technical working group on HIV and pregnancy, Geneva, 26–27 October 1989.

Report of the WHO technical working group on research needs in diagnostics and treatment for paediatric AIDS.

Review of six HIV/AIDS home care programmes in Uganda and Zambia.

Scientific meeting on factors for progression to AIDS: Intracellular pathogenic mechanisms offering opportunities for therapeutic intervention, 18 February 1991.

Statement and report from the WHO technical working group on standardisation of polymerase chain reaction (PCT) for HIV diagnosis and AIDS research.

Technical working group on psychosocial issues of mothers and children with HIV/AIDS, Geneva, 11–12 October 1989.

Technical working group on the impact of HIV/AIDS on families, 11–12 October 1989.

Technical workshops on monoclonal antibodies for the characterisation of HIV-1, Bethesda, Maryland, 6–7 November 1989.

. . . .

Distribution of Countries by Geographic Area of Affinity (GAA)

GAA 1 North America	GAA 2 Western Europe	GAA 3 Oceania	GAA 4 Latin America
Canada	Andorra	American Samoa	Argentina
United States	Austria	Australia	Belize
	Belgium	Cook Islands	Bolivia
	Cyprus	Federated States	Brazil
	Denmark	of Micronesia	Chile
	Finland	Fiji	Columbia
	France	French Polynesia	Costa Rica
	Germany	Guam	Ecuador
	Greece	Kiribati	El Salvador
	Iceland	Mariana Islands	French
	Ireland	Marshall Islands	Guiana
	Italy	Nauru	Guatemala
	Liechtenstein	New Caledonia	Guyana
	Luxembourg	New Zealand	Honduras
	Malta	Niue	Mexico
	Monaco	Palau	Nicaragua
	Netherlands	Papua New Guinea	Panama
	Norway	Samoa	Paraguay
	Portugal	Solomon Islands	Peru
	San Marino	Tokelau	Suriname
	Spain	Tonga	Uruguay
	Sweden	Tuvalu	Venezuela
	Switzerland	Vanuatu	
	United Kingdom	Wallis and Futuna	
	Vatican City		

GAA 5
Sub-Saharan Africa

Angola	Malawi
Benin	Mali
Botswana	Mauritania
Burkina Faso	Mauritius
Burundi	Mozambique
Cameroon	Namibia
Cape Verde	Niger
Central African Rep.	Nigeria
Chad	Reunion
Comoros	Rwanda
Congo	São Tomé and Príncipe
Côte d'Ivoire	Senegal
Djibouti	Seychelles
Equatorial Guinea	Sierra Leone
Ethiopia	Somalia
Gabon	South Africa
Gambia	Sudan
Ghana	Swaziland
Guinea	Tanzania
Guinea-Bissau	Togo
Kenya	Uganda
Lesotho	Zaire
Liberia	Zambia
Madagascar	Zimbabwe

GAA 6
Caribbean

Anguilla
Antigua and Barbuda
Bahamas
Barbados
Bermuda
British Virgin Islands
Cayman Islands
Cuba
Dominica
Dominican Republic
Grenada
Guadeloupe
Haiti
Jamaica
Martinique
Montserrat
Netherlands Antilles
St. Kitts and Nevis
St. Lucia
St. Vincent
Trinidad and Tobago
Turks and Caicos Islands

GAA 7 Eastern Europe	GAA 8 South East Mediterranean	GAA 9 North East Asia	GAA 10 Southeast Asia
Albania	Afghanistan	Bhutan	Bangladesh
Bulgaria	Algeria	Cambodia	Brunei
Czechoslovakia	Bahrain	China	Burma
Hungary	Egypt	Hong Kong	India
Poland	Iran	Korea, DPR	Indonesia
Romania	Iraq	Korea, Republic of	Malaysia
Commonwealth	Israel	Japan	Maldives
of Independent	Jordan	Laos	Nepal
States	Kuwait	Macao	Philippines
Yugoslavia	Lebanon	Mongolia	Singapore
	Libya	Vietnam	Sri Lanka
	Morocco		Thailand
	Oman		
	Pakistan		
	Qatar		
	Saudi Arabia		
	Syria		
	Tunisia		
	Turkey		
	United Arab Emirates		
	Yemen		

. . . .

Methods for the Estimation of the Number of HIV Infections, AIDS Cases, and Deaths in the World, January 1, 1992, and Projections to 1995 and the Year 2000

In order to estimate the number of HIV-infected persons and people with AIDS as of January 1, 1992, and also to proceed with projections through 1995, *AIDS in the World* used Epimodel. This model is based on a specific survival distribution, as described by Chin and Lwanga, and permits the reconstruction of the epidemic curve since the beginning of the pandemic.* The application of this model requires several important parameters: in particular, the year of assumed wide spread of HIV infection; a point prevalence of HIV for a particular year; the location of this year on the HIV epidemic curve; and the shape of the epidemic curve.

   To define these parameters, three types and sources of information were used: results from HIV seroprevalence surveys conducted in 1988–1990, the number of AIDS cases reported by countries to WHO through 1991, and information obtained from an expert panel through a modified Delphi survey. Figure 2.2A is a diagrammatic representation of the process; the underlying assumptions are described below.

Method

Analysis of Seroprevalence Survey Results, 1988–1990: Results from seroprevalance surveys were obtained through the U.S. Bureau of the Census,

---

*J. Chin and S. K. Lwanga, "Estimation and projection of adult AIDS cases: A simple epidemiological model," *Bulletin of the World Health Organization* 69(4) (1991):399–406.

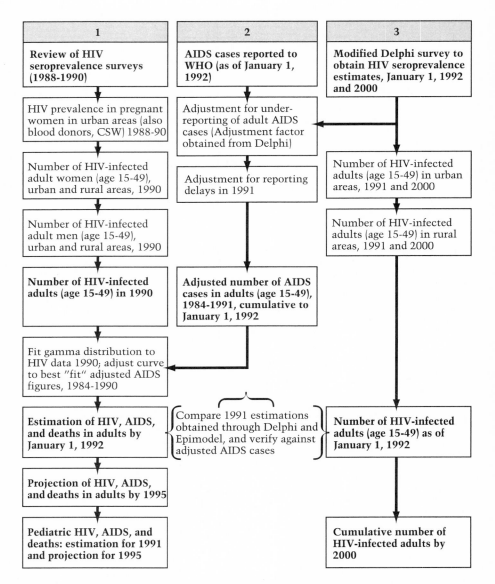

1	2	3
Review of HIV seroprevalence surveys (1988-1990)	**AIDS cases reported to WHO (as of January 1, 1992)**	**Modified Delphi survey to obtain HIV seroprevalence estimates, January 1, 1992 and 2000**
HIV prevalence in pregnant women in urban areas (also blood donors, CSW) 1988-90	Adjustment for under-reporting of adult AIDS cases (Adjustment factor obtained from Delphi)	
Number of HIV-infected adult women (age 15-49), urban and rural areas, 1990	Adjustment for reporting delays in 1991	Number of HIV-infected adults (age 15-49) in urban areas, 1991 and 2000
Number of HIV-infected adult men (age 15-49), urban and rural areas, 1990		Number of HIV-infected adults (age 15-49) in rural areas, 1991 and 2000
Number of HIV-infected adults (age 15-49) in 1990	**Adjusted number of AIDS cases in adults (age 15-49), 1984-1991, cumulative to January 1, 1992**	
Fit gamma distribution to HIV data 1990; adjust curve to best "fit" adjusted AIDS figures, 1984-1990	Compare 1991 estimations obtained through Delphi and Epimodel, and verify against adjusted AIDS cases	
Estimation of HIV, AIDS, and deaths in adults by January 1, 1992		**Number of HIV-infected adults (age 15-49) as of January 1, 1992**
Projection of HIV, AIDS, and deaths in adults by 1995		
Pediatric HIV, AIDS, and deaths: estimation for 1991 and projection for 1995		**Cumulative number of HIV-infected adults by 2000**

Figure 2.2A. Three approaches used concurrently in estimating the global numbers of HIV infections, AIDS cases, and AIDS-related deaths in adults and children, for the years 1991, 1995, and 2000.
Source: AIDS in the World, 1992.

the WHO European Center for the Epidemiological Monitoring of AIDS, the U.S. Centers for Disease Control, the Pan American Health Organization (PAHO/WHO), and from multiple inquiries with experts in various countries. These survey results were then reviewed, country by country, for each Geographic Area of Affinity (GAA). To reflect the recent status of the epidemic, and at the same time amass sufficient data for a worldwide analysis, studies conducted from 1988 onward were considered. In the absence of general population studies, seroprevalence estimates in pregnant women were considered to be most indicative of HIV prevalence in women between the ages of 15 and 49 years.

When such studies were not available for a particular country, the HIV prevalence in blood donors was substituted. A series of comparisons between prevalence estimates in pregnant women and in blood donors had shown that the former could be used as a surrogate for the latter. Prevalence estimates were derived from these studies, wherever possible separately for women and men. To calculate the prevalence of HIV when information was available for one gender only, male-to-female ratios were estimated and applied for each GAA and included among the assumptions.

Only a few seroprevalence studies, however, provided rates for rural populations. In such instances, the ratio of the HIV prevalence in urban and rural areas was built into the assumptions.

In a number of countries, estimates for both pregnant women and blood donors were unavailable; however, seroprevalence surveys had been carried out among commercial sex workers. When this occurred, an assumption was made that a particular range of seroprevalence in commercial sex workers would correspond to a broad range of seroprevalence in the urban adult population. A fuller representation of the above assumption is presented and discussed in Chapter 2.

In other countries, particularly among those assumed to have a low prevalence of HIV infection, no HIV seroprevalence survey results were available. In such situations, plausible ranges of prevalence—always deliberately conservative—were chosen. These figures were either based on expert information or estimated by analogy to neighboring countries that shared similar health, social, and economic epidemiological characteristics.

Reported AIDS Cases: The adjustment of the model applied to the HIV prevalence data required an estimation of the number of AIDS cases that occurred at a particular point during the pandemic. The number of AIDS cases reported to WHO was available, but because it is affected by both reporting delay (late reporting of cases) and underreporting (incomplete reporting of cases), these reports did not accurately reflect the true picture of the pandemic (see Box 3.1, "Reporting AIDS to WHO"). Based on a review of past reporting patterns from countries to WHO, reporting delays could be adjusted. A survey of a panel of experts (Delphi survey) provided a correction factor for underreporting in each GAA.

Modified Delphi Survey: The Survey, which relied on the opinion of an expert panel, was undertaken with the following objectives: (1) to obtain adjustment factors for the underreporting of AIDS; (2) to obtain HIV prevalence estimates for each GAA in 1991 (and a projection for the year 2000); and (3) to estimate the contribution of different modes of HIV transmission to the pandemic in 1991 (and in the year 2000). Twenty-two HIV/AIDS experts participated in this survey.* (See Box 2.4 on the Delphi approach.)

A detailed analysis of the survey results is presented below.

Adjustment for underreporting of AIDS cases: For each of the 10 GAAs, respondents were invited to provide an estimate of reporting

---

AIDS in the World would like to thank the following respondents to the Delphi Survey for their cooperation: Anthony Adams, Department of Health, Housing, and Community Services, Australia; Michael Adler, University College and Middlesex School of Medicine, United Kingdom; Uwe Brinkmann, Harvard School of Public Health, United States; Euclides Castilho, Ministério da Saúde, Brazil; Roy Chan, Action for AIDS Singapore (AFA), Singapore; Peter Drotman, Centers for Disease Control (CDC), United States; Josef Estermann, Federal Office of Public Health, Switzerland; Donato Greco, Istituto Superiore di Sanità, Italy; Jakob K. John, Christian Medical College, India; Ann Marie Kimball, Washington Department of Health, United States; Samuel Okware, Ministry of Health, Uganda; Jean William Pape, Institut National de Laboratoire et de Recherches, Haiti; Vadim Pokrovsky, Russia (Union) AIDS Center, Russia; Thomas Quinn, Johns Hopkins Hospital, United States; Martin Schechter, University of British Columbia, Canada; David Sokal, Family Health International (FHI), United States; and Peter Way, Center for International Research, United States. Five respondents requested that their names be withheld.

efficiency. Because it was assumed that reporting efficiency varied over time, respondents were asked to provide 2 correction factors: one for the period 1985–1987, the other for 1988–1990. These figures were expressed as ranges, expressing high and low reporting efficiency. Applying the given ranges to the number of cases reported to WHO as of January 1, 1992, adjusted annual and cumulative numbers of adult AIDS cases through 1991 were adjusted for each GAA and for the world.

Because there are considerable reporting delays in the international notification system, a further adjustment was made for the number of AIDS cases that would have occurred in 1990 and 1991 but had not been reported to WHO by January 1, 1992.

Expert panel's estimate of HIV prevalence for the years 1991 and 2000: The survey provided a range of HIV seroprevalence estimates for the adult population (ages 15–49) at the end of 1991. These estimates were calculated separately for urban and rural populations and for each of the 10 GAAs. When applied to the 1991 adult population, the number of HIV-infected adults alive at the end of that year was estimated between 6.6 and 21.3 million. The cumulative number of adult infections estimated through the application of Epimodel (5.9 to 11.8 million) fell within this range. As the latter method was considered more precise, its results were used in further analysis and projections.

An estimate was also obtained from the expert panel for the year 2000. This and other elements of the Delphi Survey are discussed later, in the context of short- and medium-term projections.

Application of a Type II Epidemiological Model: Epimodel: The estimated number of people with HIV infection in 1990, as derived from the above review of seroprevalence surveys and the number of AIDS cases (now adjusted for underreporting and reporting delay), provided two reference points for further analysis. Then, by adding year of widespread HIV to the above reference points and by adjusting the model parameters, several epidemiological curves could be produced for each GAA and for the world.

The application of the model assumes the existence of annual progression rates from HIV infection to AIDS, which are applied to

Table 2.2A: Correction factors for the adjustment of reported AIDS

GAA	1985–1987 reporting		1988–1990 reporting	
	Low	High	Low	High
1 North America	1.25	1.00	1.25	1.00
2 Western Europe	1.30	1.00	1.30	1.00
3 Oceania	1.25	1.00	1.25	1.00
4 Latin America	5.90	2.70	4.80	2.50
5 Sub-Saharan Africa	15.00	5.00	7.15	2.90
6 Caribbean	4.80	2.50	2.40	1.70
7 Eastern Europe	1.65	1.25	1.25	1.00
8 South East Mediterranean	20.00	5.00	4.80	2.50
9 North East Asia	5.00	2.50	5.00	2.50
10 Southeast Asia	4.80	2.50	4.00	2.20

annual cohorts of HIV-infected adults moving along the continuum from HIV infection to AIDS and death. Model parameters were set to ensure a best approximation to the temporal curve of AIDS-adjusted cases. The model then provided the number of HIV infections that were estimated to have occurred annually and cumulatively in adults each year between the beginning of the pandemic and the end of 1991.

Basic Assumptions for Calculations and Models

1. Correction Factors for Reported AIDS Cases Derived from Delphi Survey

    a. Correction factors apply to two distinct 3-year periods: 1985–1987 and 1988–1990.

    b. High and low estimates were developed for each GAA and for each time period.

    c. Correction factors are multiplied by the number of cases reported to WHO to obtain the adjusted number of AIDS cases estimated to have occurred during the reporting periods.

    d. The correction factors for underreporting in 1988–1990 also apply

Table 2.2B: Gender and urban/rural ratios, HIV infected adults age 15–49, 1991

GAA	HIV gender ratio male:female	HIV urban/rural ratio urban:rural
1 North America	8.5:1	3.2:1[a]
2 Western Europe	5.0:1	5.0:1
3 Oceania	7.0:1	3.3:1
4 Latin America	4.0:1	2.3:1
5 Sub-Saharan Africa	1.0:1	3.6:1
6 Caribbean	1.5:1	3.6:1
7 Eastern Europe	10.0:1	3.2:1
8 South East Mediterranean	5.0:1	12.0:1
9 North East Asia	5.0:1	5.0:1
10 Southeast Asia	2.0:1	6.0:1

a. Applies only to certain metropolitan areas.

to cases reported in 1991. Furthermore, because as of January 1, 1992, the reporting of AIDS cases for the year 1991 is incomplete, adjustment is needed for reporting delays.

2. Calculation of the Number of HIV Infections from Serosurvey Data

a. Seroprevalence data from surveys conducted between 1988 and 1990 provide a conservative estimate of the seroprevalence rates in 1990.

b. Seroprevalence data from studies in pregnant women are valid surrogates for seroprevalence in the adult women population in the same countries.

c. Estimates of seroprevalence in blood donors and commercial sex workers (CSWs) can be used in fixed ratios to approximate the HIV prevalence in the urban, adult population where seroprevalence in pregnant women is unavailable.

d. The proportion of urban population in the total population is the same for males and females.

Table 2.2C: Sources of HIV prevalence data for each GAA

GAA	Source
1 North America	United States: CDC family of serosurveys Canada: Estimate from national expert, based on published and unpublished data Abstracts from International Conference on AIDS, Florence, Italy, 1991
2 Western Europe	WHO European Centre for the Epidemiological Monitoring of AIDS, Saint Maurice, France • Published survey results and abstracts presented at International AIDS Conferences
3 Oceania	Australian HIV surveillance report, January 1992 Published survey results for other countries
4 Latin America	PAHO/WHO for the numbers of HIV infected for some countries (AIDS/HIV/STD Annual Surveillance Report, 1990) U.S. Bureau of the Census Survey data in other countries
5 Sub-Saharan Africa	Seroprevalence surveys, through the U.S. Bureau of Census for 36 of the 50 countries Estimated rates for 14 sub-Saharan countries where no survey results available
6 Caribbean	Same as GAA 4
7 Eastern Europe	Same as GAA 2
8 South East Mediterranean	Survey results for half of the countries In other countries, *AIDS in the World* applied range of HIV prevalence in adult women in urban areas: low: 0.001%; high: 0.01%
9 North East Asia	Survey results for Japan Conference on AIDS in Asia and the Pacific, Canberra, 1990 Few representative survey data available for China: *AIDS in the World* applied range of HIV prevalence in adult women in urban areas: low: 0.001%; high: 0.005%.
10 Southeast Asia	Thailand and India: from surveys Australian HIV surveillance report, January 1992 For countries where no survey results available: *AIDS in the World* applied range of HIV prevalence in women in urban areas: low: 0.001%; high: 0.01%

Table 2.2D: Estimating HIV prevalence rates in adult women based on rates in commercial sex workers

Range of HIV prevalence in commercial sex workers (%)	Assumed corresponding range of HIV prevalence in adult women, age 15–49, urban areas (%)	
	Low	High
0	0	0
0–0.99	0.0075	0.01
1–2.49	0.1	0.25
2.5–4.99	0.25	0.5
5–7.49	0.5	0.75
7.5–9.99	0.75	1.0
10–24.99	1.0	2.5
25 and over	2.5	5.0

e. The proportion of urban population in the total population for 1990 (from UN Population data) applies also to 1991.

f. In GAAs, HIV prevalence differs by gender and urban/rural regions, as shown in Table 2.2B.

g. The population growth rate for 1985 to 1990 also applies through 1991.

h. HIV-2 occurs at significant levels only in West Africa.

Table 2.2C shows the sources of HIV prevalence data for each GAA. Table 2.2D shows the method applied to estimate HIV prevalence rates in adult women in urban areas for those countries where only rates in commercial sex workers were available.

When rates of HIV prevalence were not available, either from pregnant women or from blood donors, rates obtained from commercial sex worker surveys were applied in order to determine, by extrapolation, the range of HIV seroprevalence in adult women (Table 2.2D). The correlation between seroprevalence in pregnant women and in commercial sex workers was examined by the U.S. Bureau of the Census research team as one of their contributions to Chapter 2.

Table 2.2E: Start of widespread HIV in each GAA

GAA	Year of wide spread
1 North America	1978
2 Western Europe	1978
3 Oceania	1979
4 Latin America	1978–79
5 Sub-Saharan Africa	1977–78
6 Caribbean	1979
7 Eastern Europe	1982–83
8 South East Mediterranean	1982
9 North East Asia	1982–84
10 Southeast Asia	1983–84

Table 2.2F: Interval between diagnosis of AIDS and death

Interval	Percentage of adults dying, by year, after AIDS diagnosis		Percentage of children dying, by year, after AIDS diagnosis	
	Industrialized countries	Developing countries	Industrialized countries	Developing countries
Year 1	55	90	95	95
Year 2	75	95	99	99
Year 3	90	98	99	99

Table 2.2G: Age-specific fertility rates, by GAA

GAA	Age-specific fertility rates					
	15–19	*20–24*	*25–29*	*30–34*	*35–39*	*40–44*
1 North America	3.8	9.2	11.4	7.2	2.0	1.0
2 Western Europe	1.6	8.5	12.2	6.3	1.9	0.8
3 Oceania	4.0	10.5	14.5	7.8	2.5	0.5
4 Latin America	10.1	22.4	21.8	16.8	12.0	6.4
5 Sub-Saharan Africa	15.1	28.5	28.9	26.2	20.5	12.6
6 Caribbean	10.7	21.6	20.9	14.4	9.8	5.1
7 Eastern Europe	4.9	17.4	11.3	5.1	2.1	0.9
8 South East Mediterranean	6.1	20.9	25.7	21.9	14.9	7.2
9 North East Asia	6.2	16.8	16.7	12.2	7.5	3.2
10 Southeast Asia	6.2	16.8	16.7	12.2	7.5	3.2

Sources: World Population Monitoring 1989 Special Report: The Population Situation in the Least Developed Countries, Population Studies, no. 113 (New York: United Nations, 1990); and F. Arnold and A. K. Blanc, "Fertility levels and trends," Demographic and Health Surveys, Comparative Studies, no. 2, Institute for Resource Development/Macro Systems, Inc., Columbia, Md., October 1990.

3. Modeling the AIDS/HIV Numbers beyond 1991

a. A gamma distribution is adequate in all GAAs.

b. The same progression rates from HIV infection to AIDS apply to all GAAs.

c. The HIV point prevalences in 1990 are valid (as derived under the set of assumptions in Section 2, above).

d. The models fit closely the corrected number of AIDS case numbers (derived under the set of assumptions in Section 1, above), assuming less reporting delay in the years 1987–1989 than in 1985–86 and, in industrialized countries, in 1990.

e. The years of wide spread of HIV in different GAAs were as shown in Table 2.2E

f. The age distribution of women infected with HIV derived from Table 2.2B applies.

Table 2.2H: Estimate of the rate of reporting of AIDS cases in the world in the periods 1985–1987 and 1988–1990[a]

GAA	1985–1987 (%)	1988–1990 (%)
1 North America	81–100	71–91
2 Western Europe	77–97	77–97
3 Oceania	81–100	81–100
4 Latin America	17–37	21–40
5 Sub-Saharan Africa	7–20	14–34
6 Caribbean	21–40	41–60
7 Eastern Europe	61–80	81–100
8 South East Mediterranean	5–20	21–40
9 North East Asia	20–40	20–40
10 Southeast Asia	21–40	25–45

a. In areas with more than one respondent, percentages have been averaged to obtain the listed ranges.

g. Specific fertility rates were obtained from UN Demographic and Health Surveys and World Population Monitoring, 1989–90. These rates apply to all scenarios.

h. The rate of transmission of HIV from mother to child is 30 percent.

i. The rates at which AIDS evolves to death in industrialized and developing countries are as shown in Table 2.2F.

Analysis of the Results of the Consensus Survey (Modified Delphi Survey), March 1992

Estimates of the Rates of Adult AIDS Reporting

Question 1 invited respondents to estimate the rate of AIDS reporting for two periods: 1985–1987 and 1988–1990. Table 2.2H summarizes the results.

Questions 2 and 3 invited respondents to estimate the proportion of HIV-infected persons, age 15–49, in urban and rural areas, of their country or region, respectively, through the end of 1991. Questions 4

Table 2.2I: Cumulative number of reported and adjusted AIDS cases through 1991

GAA	1990 population (thousands)	WHO reported AIDS:[a]	WHO estimated AIDS:[a]	AIW/Delphi adjusted[a] Low	High
1 North America	275,745	208,089	260,000	237,000	298,500
2 Western Europe	435,312	58,370	85,000	67,000	84,500
3 Oceania	26,199	3,175	5,000	3,500	4,500
4 Latin America	414,205	36,997	145,000[b]	116,000	225,500
5 Sub-Saharan Africa	526,748	128,818	970,000	581,000	1,464,000
6 Caribbean	33,562	7,859		13,000	20,000
7 Eastern Europe	412,571	2,053		2,500	3,000
8 SE Mediterranean	376,466	457		1,500	4,000
9 North East Asia	1,416,200	469		1,500	3,000
10 Southeast Asia	1,370,952	349	10,000	1,000	2,000
Total	5,287,960	446,636	1,475,000	1,024,000	2,109,000

a. As of January 1, 1992.
b. Includes the Caribbean.

Table 2.2J: Mean estimated HIV point prevalence rates for adults age 15–49 in urban and rural areas as of 1991 and 2000 (%)

GAA	Urban 1991 Low	High	Rural 1991 Low	High	Urban 2000 Low	High	Rural 2000 Low	High
1 North America	0.70[a]	3.00[a]	0.05	1.10	1.20[a]	3.65[a]	0.05	1.70
2 Western Europe	0.15	0.283	0.007	0.083	0.47	0.883	0.19	0.40
3 Oceania	0.10	0.20	0.03	0.06	0.10	0.20	0.03	0.06
4 Latin America	0.04	0.843	0.0007	0.067	0.713	3.373	0.035	0.671
5 Sub-Saharan Africa	4.30	7.30	0.90	2.58	8.50	12.50	2.45	3.80
6 Caribbean	1.00	20.00	0.50	5.00	2.00	30.00	2.00	10.00
7 Eastern Europe	0.0005	0.003	0.0001	0.001	0.001	0.01	0.0005	0.003
8 SE Mediterranean	0.10	0.50	0.0001	0.05	0.50	2.00	0.10	0.25
9 North East Asia	0.0001	0.0025	0.0001	0.001	0.001	0.10	0.0001	0.0025
10 Southeast Asia	0.09	0.29	0.01	0.06	3.00	6.38	0.30	3.93

a. Rates applicable to certain large metropolitan areas only.

Table 2.2K: Mean estimates of percentage of HIV infection by mode of transmission for adults age 15–49 at the end of 1991 and 2000

GAA	End of 1991					End of 2000				
	Het	*Hom*	*Bloo*	*IDU*	*Oth*	*Het*	*Hom*	*Bloo*	*IDU*	*Oth*
1 North America	9	56	3	27	5	15	43	<1	35	7
2 Western Europe	14	47	2	33	4	26	36	<1	34	3
3 Oceania	6	87	2	3	2	8	85	0	5	2
4 Latin America	24	54	6	11	5	40	30	3	20	7
5 Sub-Saharan Africa	93	<1	4	<1	1	95	<1	2	<1	1
6 Caribbean	75	10	5	9	1	82	3	3	11	1
7 Eastern Europe	10	80	2	5	3	30	30	<1	39	1
8 SE Mediterranean	20	35	18	22	5	48	20	6	20	6
9 North East Asia	50	20	10	20	0	75	10	5	10	0
10 Southeast Asia	70	8	6	14	2	80	3	3	11	3

Note: Het = heterosexual; Hom = homosexual; Bloo = blood transfusion and blood products; IDU = injection drug use; Oth = other and unidentified modes of transmission.

and 5 asked respondents to predict the proportion of HIV-infected persons, age 15–49, in urban and rural areas, respectively, of their country or region through the end of the year 2000. Table 2.2J summarizes the results.
Table 2.2J

Question 6 asked respondents to estimate the proportional contribution of various modes of HIV to infections that they estimated to be present among adults age 15–49 in their country or region at the end of 1991 and at the end of year 2000. Table 2.2K summarizes the results.

. . . .

Summary Tables of Estimations of HIV and AIDS for 1992 and Projections through 1995 and 2000

This appendix summarizes estimations and projections that were presented from a methodological standpoint in Appendix 2.2. In this appendix, the reference date for 1992 estimations is January 1, 1992, which covers the period from the beginning of the pandemic through 1991. Projections for 1995 correspond to the period through 1995 (therefore with a reference date as of January 1, 1996). Projections for the year 2000 have a reference date as of January 1, 2001.

Table 2.3A: Estimates of adult HIV infections, 1990 and as of January 1, 1992 (cumulative numbers)

GAA	WHO estimate, 1990	WHO estimate as of January 1, 1992	AIW estimates for 1990[a]		AIW estimates as of January 1, 1992[b]	
			Low	High	Low	High
1 North America	1,000,000	1,000,000	674,000	865,000	949,000	**1,167,000**
2 Western Europe	500,000	500,000	430,000	535,000	577,000	**718,000**
3 Oceania	30,000	30,000	13,000	22,000	18,000	**28,000**
4 Latin America	1,000,000	>1,000,000	355,000	752,000	477,000	**995,000**
5 Sub-Saharan Africa	6,000,000	>6,000,000	2,701,000	5,385,000	3,576,000	**7,803,000**
6 Caribbean			81,000	235,000	108,000	**310,000**
7 Eastern Europe	20,000	20,000	13,000	21,000	16,000	**27,000**
8 SE Mediterranean	30,000	30,000	15,000	27,000	20,000	**35,000**
9 North East Asia	20,000	20,000	12,000	31,000	16,000	**41,000**
10 Southeast Asia	500,000	>1,000,000	101,000	509,000	145,000	**675,000**
Total	9,100,000	>10,000,000	4,395,000	8,382,000	5,902,000	**11,799,000**

a. Based on a review of seroprevalence surveys.
b. Estimated by applying a model to seroprevalence survey results in 1990.

Best estimate

Table 2.3B: Projections of adult HIV infections, 1995–2000 (cumulative numbers)

GAA	WHO estimates, 1995	WHO estimates, 2000	AIW estimates, 1995		Delphi estimates for 2000[a]	
			Low	High	Low	High
1 North America			1,164,000	**1,495,000**	1,811,000	8,150,000
2 Western Europe			954,000	**1,186,000**	1,188,000	2,331,000
3 Oceania			22,000	**40,000**	22,000	45,000
4 Latin America			675,000	**1,407,000**	1,599,000	8,554,000
5 Sub-Saharan Africa			5,083,000	**11,449,000**	20,778,000	33,609,000
6 Caribbean			149,000	**474,000**	536,000	6,962,000
7 Eastern Europe			19,000	**44,000**	>2,000	>20,000
8 SE Mediterranean			31,000	**59,000**	893,000	3,532,000
9 North East Asia			30,000	**80,000**	>6,000	486,000
10 Southeast Asia			343,000	**1,220,000**	11,277,000	45,059,000
Total	15–20 million	30–40 million	8,470,000	**17,454,000**	>38,112,000	>108,748,000

a. Based on modeling the Delphi estimated point prevalence in 2000.

Best estimate

Table 2.3C: Estimates of adult women with HIV as of January 1, 1992 (cumulative numbers)

GAA	AIW estimates as of Jan. 1, 1992	
	Low	High
1 North America	104,500	128,500
2 Western Europe	98,000	122,000
3 Oceania	2,000	3,500
4 Latin America	95,500	199,000
5 Sub-Saharan Africa	1,788,000	3,901,500
6 Caribbean	43,000	124,000
7 Eastern Europe	1,500	2,500
8 SE Mediterranean	3,500	6,000
9 North East Asia	3,000	7,000
10 Southeast Asia	48,000	223,000
Total	2,187,000	4,717,000
		Best estimate

Table 2.3D: Adult AIDS cases as of January 1, 1992 (cumulative numbers)

GAA	Reported to WHO	Estimated by WHO[a]	AIW adjusted[a,b]		AIW estimates[c]	
			Low	High	Low	High
1 North America	208,089	260,000	237,000	298,500	256,000	257,500
2 Western Europe	58,370	85,000	67,000	84,500	79,500	99,000
3 Oceania	3,175	5,000	3,500	4,500	4,500	4,500
4 Latin America	36,997	145,000	116,000	225,500	91,000	173,000
5 Sub-Saharan Africa	128,818	970,000	581,000	1,464,000	602,000	1,367,000
6 Caribbean	7,859		13,000	20,000	19,000	43,000
7 Eastern Europe	2,053		2,500	3,000	2,000	2,500
8 SE Mediterranean	457		1,500	4,000	2,000	3,500
9 North East Asia	469		1,500	3,000	1,500	3,500
10 Southeast Asia	349	10,000	1,000	2,000	7,000	65,000
Total	446,636	1,475,000	1,024,000	2,109,000	1,064,500	2,018,500
						Best estimate

a. WHO estimates are made for broader geographic areas than *AIDS in the World's* GAAs. In WHO estimates, the Caribbean is combined with Latin America; Eastern Europe with Western Europe; some countries in the South East Mediterranean are included in Western Europe, others in Africa, yet others in Asia; North East Asia is combined with Southeast Asia, under a region called Asia.
b. Adjusted based on correcting factors for reporting delays (*AIW*) and for underreporting (Delphi).
c. Model estimates, based on modeling the adjusted AIDS incidence curve.

Table 2.3E: Projected adult AIDS cases, 1995–2000 (cumulative numbers)

GAA	WHO estimate, 1995[a]	WHO estimate, 2000	AIW estimates, 1995 Low	AIW estimates, 1995 High	AIW *Delphi* estimates, 2000[a,b] Low	AIW *Delphi* estimates, 2000[a,b] High
1 North America	800,000		471,000	534,000	671,000	3,603,000
2 Western Europe			225,000	279,500	268,000	536,500
3 Oceania			8,500	11,500	10,500	20,500
4 Latin America	445,000		206,500	417,500	175,000	1,883,000
5 Sub-Saharan Africa	2,500,000		1,483,500	3,277,500	5,505,000	10,583,000
6 Caribbean	67,500		45,500	121,000	156,000	2,505,000
7 Eastern Europe			6,000	9,500	>500	>3,000
8 SE Mediterranean			7,000	12,500	150,000	711,500
9 North East Asia			5,500	14,500	>1,000	51,000
10 Southeast Asia	250,000		45,000	240,500	1,051,000	4,111,000
Total	4,062,500	10,000,000	2,503,500	4,918,000	7,988,000	24,007,500

Best estimate

a. For 1995, WHO estimates are made for broader geographic regions than *AIDS in the World*'s GAAs. In this table, WHO estimates for North America, Western Europe, and Oceania are shown under *North America*. North East Asia, Southeast Asia, and part of the South East Mediterranean are included by WHO in a region called Asia. The corresponding estimate is shown here under Southeast Asia. WHO does not provide specific estimates for 1995 for Eastern Europe or for countries in the South East Mediterranean not included in Asia. For the year 2,000, WHO does not provide a regional breakdown.

b. Based on modeling the Delphi-estimated HIV point prevalence in 2000.

Table 2.3F: *AIDS in the World* estimates of adult deaths from HIV/AIDS as of January 1, 1992, and 1995 (cumulative numbers)

GAA		Deaths as of January 1, 1992		Deaths as of 1995	
		Low	High	Low	High
1	North America	219,000	**214,500**	426,000	**475,500**
2	Western Europe	63,000	**78,500**	191,500	**238,000**
3	Oceania	3,500	**3,500**	7,500	**10,000**
4	Latin America	87,500	**166,000**	201,000	**406,000**
5	Sub-Saharan Africa	577,000	**1,312,000**	1,441,000	**3,184,000**
6	Caribbean	18,500	**41,000**	44,500	**117,000**
7	Eastern Europe	1,500	**2,000**	5,500	**7,500**
8	SE Mediterranean	1,500	**2,500**	5,500	**10,500**
9	North East Asia	1,000	**3,500**	5,000	**14,000**
10	Southeast Asia	6,500	**61,500**	43,000	**231,000**
	Total	979,000	**1,885,000**	2,370,500	**4,693,500**
			Best estimate		**Best estimate**

Table 2.3G: *AIDS in the World* estimates of pediatric HIV infections as of January 1, 1992, and 1995 (cumulative numbers)

GAA	Estimated pediatric HIV infections as of January 1, 1992		Estimated pediatric HIV infections as of 1995	
	Low	High	Low	High
1 North America	15,000	16,000	24,500	29,000
2 Western Europe	6,500	8,000	15,500	19,500
3 Oceania	500	500	500	1,000
4 Latin America	20,500	40,500	41,000	84,000
5 Sub-Saharan Africa	434,500	969,500	920,000	2,030,500
6 Caribbean	6,500	16,000	13,500	37,500
7 Eastern Europe	100	200	500	500
8 SE Mediterranean	500	1,000	1,500	3,000
9 North East Asia	500	750	1,000	2,000
10 Southeast Asia	3,500	24,000	15,000	72,500
Total	488,100	1,076,450	1,033,000	2,279,500
		Best estimate		**Best estimate**

Table 2.3H: *AIDS in the World* **estimates of pediatric AIDS cases as of January 1, 1992, and 1995 (cumulative numbers)**

GAA	Estimated pediatric AIDS cases as of January 1, 1992		Estimated pediatric AIDS cases as of 1995	
	Low	High	Low	High
1 North America	9,000	**9,000**	18,500	**21,000**
2 Western Europe	3,000	**4,000**	9,500	**12,000**
3 Oceania	200	**200**	400	**500**
4 Latin America	11,500	**21,500**	28,000	**56,000**
5 Sub-Saharan Africa	226,500	**520,500**	605,000	**1,338,500**
6 Caribbean	3,500	**8,000**	9,000	**23,500**
7 Eastern Europe	100	**100**	200	**300**
8 SE Mediterranean	200	**400**	900	**1,500**
9 North East Asia	100	**300**	400	**1,100**
10 Southeast Asia	900	**9,500**	7,000	**40,500**
Total	255,000	**573,500**	678,900	**1,494,900**
		Best estimate		**Best estimate**

Table 2.3I: *AIDS in the World* estimates of pediatric deaths from HIV/AIDS as of January 1, 1992, and 1995 (cumulative numbers)

GAA	Estimated pediatric deaths as of January 1, 1992		Estimated pediatric deaths as of 1995	
	Low	High	Low	High
1 North America	9,000	**9,000**	18,500	**20,500**
2 Western Europe	3,000	**4,000**	9,500	**12,000**
3 Oceania	200	**200**	400	**500**
4 Latin America	11,000	**21,000**	27,500	**55,000**
5 Sub-Saharan Africa	222,000	**511,000**	597,000	**1,320,500**
6 Caribbean	3,500	**7,500**	9,000	**23,000**
7 Eastern Europe	100	**100**	200	**300**
8 SE Mediterranean	200	**400**	800	**1,500**
9 North East Asia	100	**300**	400	**1,100**
10 Southeast Asia	900	**9,000**	7,000	**40,000**
Total	250,000	**562,500**	670,300	**1,474,400**
		Best estimate		**Best estimate**

· ·

Reported AIDS Cases in Countries by Geographic Area of Affinity (GAA), 1979–January 1, 1992

GAA	1979–1984	1985	1986	1987	1988	1989	1990	1991[a]	Cumulative cases as of Jan. 1, 1992[b]
1 North America									
Canada	259	357	579	876	1,007	1,133	867	270	5,348
United States	10,546	11,315	18,423	27,464	33,297	37,556	36,658	38,382	213,641[c]
Area total	10,805	11,672	19,002	28,340	34,304	38,689	37,525	38,652	218,989
2 Western Europe									
Andorra	0	0	0	0	0	0	0	0	0
Austria	16	23	21	87	104	139	152	165	707[d]
Belgium	109	67	74	121	138	159	184	194	1,046
Cyprus	0	0	5	3	2	3	7	0	20
Denmark	36	37	69	100	126	172	196	211	947[d]
Finland	6	4	7	8	17	17	18	23	100
France	367	564	1,218	2,188	2,976	3,631	3,857	3,035	17,836
Germany	203	319	586	1,075	1,357	1,633	1,263	1,097	7,533
Greece	6	7	22	53	82	107	135	116	559
Iceland	0	1	3	1	5	3	3	6	22
Ireland	6	5	6	20	37	50	55	62	241
Italy	44	196	452	1,036	1,741	2,413	2,977	2,750	11,609
Liechtenstein	0	0	0	0	0	0	0	0	0
Luxembourg	0	3	3	3	4	11	9	12	45
Malta	1	1	3	2	7	0	1	7	22

GAA	1979–1984	1985	1986	1987	1988	1989	1990	1991[a]	Cumulative cases as of Jan. 1, 1992[b]
Monaco	0	0	0	0	1	2	2	2	7
Netherlands	55	66	137	242	322	385	405	405	2,017[d]
Norway	6	15	21	35	25	43	54	53	252[d]
Portugal	4	29	32	70	114	167	205	195	816[d]
San Marino	0	0	0	0	0	1	0	0	1
Spain	65	158	437	974	1,992	2,618	2,811	2,500	11,555
Sweden	18	32	55	79	86	131	119	125	645
Switzerland	51	75	163	257	423	511	459	289	2,228
United Kingdom	258	234	461	663	863	1,007	1,111	854	5,451
Vatican City	0	0	0	0	0	0	0	0	0
Area total	1,251	1,836	3,775	7,017	10,422	13,203	14,023	12,132	63,659

3 Oceania

GAA	1979–1984	1985	1986	1987	1988	1989	1990	1991[a]	Cumulative cases as of Jan. 1, 1992[b]
American Samoa	0	0	0	0	0	0	0	0	0
Australia	53	122	226	371	522	568	591	684	3,137[d]
Cook Islands	0	0	0	0	0	0	0	0	0
Fed. St. Micronesia	0	0	0	0	0	0	0	2	2
Fiji	0	0	0	0	0	3	0	0	3
French Polynesia	0	0	0	1	0	7	8	11	27
Guam									10
Kiribati	0	0	0	0	0	0	0	0	0
Mariana Islands	0	0	0	0	0	0	0	0	0
Marshall Islands	0	0	0	0	0	0	0	2	2
Nauru	0	0	0	0	0	0	0	0	0
New Caledonia	0	0	0	0	2	0	12	4	18
New Zealand	8	12	18	33	45	69	61	28	274
Niue	0	0	0	0	0	0	0	0	0
Palau	0	0	0	0	0	0	0	0	0

GAA	1979–1984	1985	1986	1987	1988	1989	1990	1991[a]	Cumulative cases as of Jan. 1, 1992[b]
Papua New Guinea	0	0	0	2	9	5	13	8	37
Samoa	0	0	0	0	0	0	0	1	1
Solomon Islands	0	0	0	0	0	0	0	0	0
Tokelau	0	0	0	0	0	0	0	0	0
Tonga	0	0	0	1	0	0	1	0	2
Tuvalu	0	0	0	0	0	0	0	0	0
Vanuatu	0	0	0	0	0	0	0	0	0
Wallis and Futuna	0	0	0	0	0	0	0	0	0
Area total	61	134	244	408	578	652	686	750	3,513
4 Latin America									
Argentina	14	28	31	72	169	229	377	378	1,298
Belize	0	0	0	4	5	2	0	1	12
Bolivia	0	1	2	3	10	2	7	16	41
Brazil	158	481	945	2,162	3,580	4,516	4,421	6,320	22,583
Chile	5	6	18	40	53	65	68	245	500
Colombia	0	0	61	181	263	330	450	904	2,189
Costa Rica	6	3	11	23	52	56	81	83	315
Ecuador	0	0	15	19	25	15	53	28	155
El Salvador	0	1	6	16	48	94	118	40	323
French Guiana	0	0	31	62	20	37	82	0	232
Guatemala	0	0	16	12	18	18	78	94	236
Guyana	0	0	0	10	34	40	61	60	205
Honduras	0	5	12	102	184	231	513	548	1,595
Mexico	121	220	452	1,027	1,411	900	1,776	3,166	9,073
Nicaragua	0	0	0	0	2	2	7	13	24

(continued)

GAA	1979–1984	1985	1986	1987	1988	1989	1990	1991[a]	Cumulative cases as of Jan. 1, 1992[b]
Panama	0	0	26	30	61	75	57	79	328
Paraguay	0	0	2	5	4	3	12	10	36
Peru	5	4	3	60	68	117	141	143	541
Suriname	1	1	2	5	4	35	35	16	99
Uruguay	0	0	7	7	20	32	82	97	245
Venezuela	16	20	55	132	268	326	244	512	1,573
Area total	326	770	1,695	3,972	6,299	7,125	8,663	12,753	41,603
5 Sub-Saharan Africa									
Angola	0	3	6	32	63	0	0	317	421
Benin	0	1	2	6	18	57	50	51	185
Botswana	0	1	10	25	22	29	91	99	277
Burkina Faso	0	0	10	21	394	481	72	0	978
Burundi	0	0	269	652	1,054	809	521	0	3,305
Cameroon	0	0	21	20	33	60	61	234	429
Cape Verde	0	1	1	16	0	10	4	0	32
Central African Rep.	0	0	0	108	622	432	702	0	1,864
Chad	0	0	2	2	7	10	38	71	130
Comoros	0	0	0	0	1	0	1	0	2
Congo	0	0	250	1,000	330	360	465	0	2,405
Côte d'Ivoire	0	2	118	404	1,193	1,930	3,189	1,461	8,297
Djibouti	0	0	0	0	1	6	51	107	165
Equatorial Guinea	0	0	0	0	1	2	2	4	9
Ethiopia	0	0	2	17	62	283	796	658	1,818
Gabon	0	0	13	4	10	24	66	0	117
Gambia	0	0	11	16	30	21	46	56	180[c]
Ghana	0	0	26	35	266	899	1,011	615	2,852
Guinea	0	0	0	4	29	49	138	118	338

GAA	1979–1984	1985	1986	1987	1988	1989	1990	1991[a]	Cumulative cases as of Jan. 1, 1992[b]
Guinea-Bissau	0	0	0	0	0	123	34	0	157
Kenya	0	10	264	1,223	2,817	4,825	0	0	9,139
Lesotho	0	0	1	1	3	6	0	33	44
Liberia	0	0	2	0	0	3	0	19	24
Madagascar	0	0	0	0	0	0	0	2	2
Malawi	0	72	72	858	3,034	3,812	4,226	0	12,074
Mali	0	1	5	23	99	106	104	0	338
Mauritania	0	0	0	0	5	6	5	10	26
Mauritius	0	0	0	1	1	2	1	4	9
Mozambique	0	0	1	3	23	37	98	126	288
Namibia	0	0	4	15	43	127	122	0	311
Niger	0	0	0	18	24	38	213	204	497
Nigeria	0	0	0	10	3	35	36	0	84
Reunion	0	0	0	3	10	34	2	0	49
Rwanda	83	161	501	236	299	1,005	2,204	2,089	6,578
São Tomé and Príncipe	0	0	0	0	1	1	0	4	6
Senegal	0	0	6	60	115	126	118	223	648
Seychelles	0	0	0	0	0	0	0	0	0
Sierra Leone	0	0	0	2	13	12	7	6	40
Somalia	0	0	0	1	4	3	5	0	13
South Africa	15	9	34	48	94	176	304	339	1,019
Sudan	0	0	1	1	64	122	130	182	500
Swaziland	0	0	0	1	2	7	18	43	71
Tanzania	109	295	1,121	2,931	4,824	4,822	7,073	6,221	27,396
Togo	0	0	0	2	15	39	44	0	100
Uganda	0	21	126	3,477	3,625	6,029	8,441	8,471	30,190

GAA	1979–1984	1985	1986	1987	1988	1989	1990	1991[a]	Cumulative cases as of Jan. 1, 1992[b]
Zaire	0	0	440	1,988	3,501	6,408	2,425	0	14,762
Zambia	0	1	240	468	985	1,115	1,393	1,600	5,802
Zimbabwe	0	0	0	119	202	1,281	4,362	4,587	10,551
Area total	207	578	3,559	13,851	23,942	35,762	38,669	27,954	114,522
6 Caribbean									
Anguilla	0	0	0	0	1	2	1	0	4
Antigua and Barbuda	0	0	0	0	3	0	0	3	6
Bahamas									835
Barbados	2	9	21	24	15	40	81	58	250
Bermuda	0	0	42	33	17	30	25	44	191
British Virgin Islands	0	0	0	0	0	1	1	2	4
Cayman Islands	0	0	0	2	2	0	2	4	10
Cuba	0	0	0	27	24	12	10	22	95
Dominica	0	0	0	5	1	2	4	0	12
Dominican Republic	9	40	67	294	292	499	284	89	1,574
Grenada	0	0	2	5	9	0	3	10	29
Guadeloupe	14	6	27	41	47	54	6	0	195
Haiti	443	110	242	477	731	453	630	0	3,086
Jamaica	2	4	5	32	30	66	62	34	235
Martinique	3	6	16	23	30	51	38	14	181
Montserrat									1
Netherlands Antilles									77
St. Kitts-Nevis									33
St. Lucia	0	0	0	6	5	5	2	22	40
St. Vincent	0	0	3	4	6	6	7	9	35

GAA	1979–1984	1985	1986	1987	1988	1989	1990	1991[a]	Cumulative cases as of Jan. 1, 1992[b]
Trinidad and Tobago	27	45	79	85	160	167	173	235	971
Turks and Caicos Is.	0	0	0	4	1	2	1	13	21
Area total	500	220	504	1,062	1,374	1,390	1,330	559	7,885
7 Eastern Europe									
Albania	0	0	0	0	0	0	0	0	0
Bulgaria	0	0	0	1	1	5	2	4	13
Czechoslovakia	0	1	6	2	3	7	5	2	26
Hungary	0	0	1	7	9	15	17	33	82
Poland	0	0	1	2	2	24	21	37	87
Romania	0	5	2	5	13	277	1,042	360	1,704[d]
Russian Federation	0	0	1	3	3	23	23	17	70
Yugoslavia	0	2	6	18	39	44	70	75	254
Area total	0	8	17	38	70	395	1,180	528	2,236
8 South East Mediterranean									
Afghanistan	0	0	0	0	0	0	0	0	0
Algeria	0	0	3	5	5	32	0	47	92
Bahrain	0	0	0	0	0	0	0	0	0
Egypt	0	0	2	3	6	9	7	12	39
Iran	0	0	0	1	3	5	10	25	44
Iraq	0	0	0	0	0	0	0	7	7
Israel	16	10	19	17	22	30	32	23	169
Jordan	0	0	1	3	1	5	1	6	17
Kuwait	0	0	1	0	0	0	0	5	6
Lebanon	0	0	8	0	4	4	8	5	29

GAA	1979–1984	1985	1986	1987	1988	1989	1990	1991[a]	Cumulative cases as of Jan. 1, 1992[b]
Libya	0	0	0	0	0	0	1	6	7
Morocco	0	0	1	9	13	20	27	28	98
Oman	0	0	1	5	6	4	7	1	24
Pakistan	0	0	0	3	3	7	1	4	18
Qatar	0	1	7	8	5	2	0	8	31
Saudi Arabia	0	0	0	14	4	7	7	8	40
Syria	0	0	0	4	1	4	0	8	17
Tunisia	0	1	4	14	17	14	27	28	105
Turkey	2	1	9	9	12	11	18	0	62[d]
United Arab Emirates	0	0	0	0	0	8	0	0	8
Yemen	0	0	0	0	0	0	0	0	0
Area total	18	13	56	95	102	162	146	221	813
9 North East Asia									
Bhutan	0	0	0	0	0	0	0	0	0
Cambodia	0	0	0	0	0	0	0	0	0
China	0	1	0	2	0	0	2	1	6
Hong Kong	0	3	0	6	7	16	12	5	49
Japan	0	11	14	34	31	92	189	82	453
Korea, D.P.R.	0	0	0	0	0	0	0	0	0
Korea, Rep.	0	0	0	1	3	1	2	1	8
Laos	0	0	0	0	0	0	0	0	0
Macao	0	0	0	0	0	0	0	1	1
Mongolia	0	0	0	0	0	0	0	0	0[d]
Vietnam	0	0	0	0	0	0	0	0	0
Area total	0	15	14	43	41	109	205	90	517

GAA	1979–1984	1985	1986	1987	1988	1989	1990	1991[a]	Cumulative cases as of Jan. 1, 1992[b]
10 Southeast Asia									
Bangladesh	0	0	0	0	0	0	1	0	1
Brunei	0	0	0	0	0	1	0	1	2
Burma	0	0	0	0	0	0	0	0	0
India	0	0	5	4	19	12	17	45	102
Indonesia	0	0	0	1	2	3	6	9	21
Malaysia	0	0	1	1	4	6	12	4	28
Maldives	0	0	0	0	0	0	0	0	0
Nepal	0	0	0	0	2	0	2	1	5
Philippines	1	2	6	9	10	7	11	7	53
Singapore	0	0	1	3	6	5	8	7	30
Sri Lanka	0	0	0	1	1	3	3	2	10
Thailand	1	1	0	7	5	29	54	82	179
Area total	2	3	13	26	49	66	114	158	431

Sources: For all GAAs except Western and Eastern Europe: World Health Organization, *Weekly Epidemiological Record* 67 (14) (1992):97–104; for Western and Eastern Europe: *AIDS surveillance in Europe,* European Center for the Epidemiological Monitoring of AIDS, Saint-Maurice, France, 1992.

a. Because of reporting delays, data for 1991 are incomplete.

b. Because several countries did not report AIDS cases annually until 1991, the annual totals for each GAA may differ from the cumulative number of reported AIDS cases as of January 1, 1992.

c. Reported through February 29, 1992.

d. Reported through January 31, 1992.

APPENDIX 6.1

. . . .

Assumptions Used in the World Bank Model to Project the Demographic Impact of AIDS in a Hypothetical African Country

The model used to project the demographic impact of AIDS was developed by Rodolfo Bulatao at the World Bank and has been detailed elsewhere. Only a brief description of the model and the selected parameter values are given here.

The model has two parts: an epidemiological model that simulates the spread of HIV, and a demographic model that incorporates AIDS mortality into a population projection. The demographic model is a standard cohort component model that projects an initial age-sex structure with a given set of age-specific vital rates. The demographic model can be used independently of the epidemiological model to generate population projections.

The epidemiological model is a numerical simulation of the spread of HIV, progression from HIV to AIDS, and from AIDS to death. Starting with an initial level of HIV seroprevalence, the model allows the virus to spread sexually, through injections and transfusions, and vertically from mother to child. For sexual transmission, the population may be divided into a maximum of 10 subgroups, varying by sexual behavior (e.g., the number of partners, the number of sexual acts per partner). Given some initial assumptions about the proportion infected with HIV in a particular year, the number of those sexually infected in each subsequent year is calculated subgroup by subgroup. In its basic form, the calculation of the number of HIV seroconversions (O) in one year (t) in a given subgroup (s) of one sexual orientation group (r) is given by

$$O_{rst} = M_{rs,t\text{-}1} \, P_{t\text{-}1} \, [[1 - (1 - O_I)(1 - O_T)\{1 - R_{r,t\text{-}1}[1 - (1 - T_r)^{Sr}]\}^{Frs}]]$$

Table 6.1A: Assumptions used in projection of the demographic impact of AIDS

Transmission probability

From male to female, per sexual contact	0.003
From female to male, per sexual contact	0.001
Genital ulcer effect on transmission	50.0
Condom use effect on transmission	
Perinatal transmission	0.33
Transfusion with infected blood	0.99
Injection with infected needle	

Disease progression

Adults, from infection to AIDS	Logistic, median of 10 years
Adults, from AIDS to death	Logistic, median of 1 year
Children, from birth to AIDS	Logistic, median of 1 year
Children, from AIDS to death	Logistic, median of 1 year

Behavioral characteristics

Condom use	2 percent of sex acts protected
Number of sexual partners, high-risk females	120 per year
Number of sexual partners, low-risk females	1 per year
Number of sexual partners, high-risk males	50 per year
Number of sexual partners, low-risk males	1 per year
Condom-genital ulcers association	0.75

Source: World Bank model for hypothetical country.

where M is the number of HIV seronegatives in the subgroup, P is the likelihood of adult survival from mortality unrelated to HIV, R is the proportion of potential sexual contacts, or agents, who are infective, T is the likelihood of transmission to group r through sexual contact, S is an average number for sex acts per partner, and F is the annual number of new partners. (Different values of F and S are the main factors distinguishing sexual orientation subgroups.) Infection with HIV through needles and blood accounts for the terms O_I and O_T. The adult population is divided into crosscutting subgroups for number of annual injections and number of annual transfusions, with the bulk of adults typically assumed to be in zero-frequency subgroups. The probability of infection (O_I or O_T) in each subgroup is then a function of the proportion of agents (needles or blood) infected, the likelihood of transmission through a single exposure to an infected agent, and the frequency of such exposure, through injections or transfusions, for the particular subgroup.

The proportion of agents *(R)* infective to subgroup s is the weighted proportion across all other subgroups with which subgroup s has sexual contact who are asymptomatic but HIV-seropositive (A). The weights used are the frequencies (F) with which these other subgroups take new sexual partners. The asymptomatic seropositives (A) in a given subgroup are calculated by summing up all those infected in previous years and subtracting those expected to progress to AIDS or to die from other causes. Progression from infection with HIV to the onset of AIDS and from AIDS to death is determined by logistic functions.

The model allows for various complications that affect the transmission process, such as the presence of genital ulcers and the extent of condom use. Membership in sexual activity subgroups may be varied, as may mixing among the subgroups.

Assumptions for parameter values in the projection of a hypothetical country were selected from those recommended by the UN/WHO modeling workshop as well as from a preliminary working group on demographic impact of AIDS at Family Health International. Table 6.1A lists the values used for some of the key parameters.

. . . .

Characteristics of Countries Invited to Participate in *AIDS in the World* National AIDS Program Survey

GAA and country	Responded to survey	Central/ federal govern- ment[a]	1990 population (x 1,000)[b]	Ranking on Human Develop- ment Index[c]	Cumulative adjusted no. of AIDS cases, 1991[d]	% of population covered	% of AIDS cases covered
North America							
Canada	Yes	Federal	26,521	High	5,246		
United States	Yes	Federal	249,224	High	202,843		
Total			275,745		208,089	100	100
Western Europe							
France	Yes	Central	56,138	High	17,038		
Germany	Yes	Federal	77,573	High	7,172		
Italy	Yes	Central	57,061	High	10,900		
Netherlands	Yes	Central	14,951	High	1,911		
Norway	Yes	Central	4,212	High	244		
Sweden	Yes	Central	8,444	High	635		
Switzerland	Yes	Federal	6,609	High	2,147		
United Kingdom	Yes	Federal	57,237	High	5,209		
Total			282,225		45,256	65	75
Oceania							
Australia	Yes	Federal	16,873	High	2,813	64	89
Latin America							
Argentina	Yes	Central	32,322	High	2,553		
Brazil	No	Federal	150,368	Middle	53,038		
Colombia	Yes	Central	32,978	Middle	3,756		
Mexico	Yes	Central	88,598	High	21,958		
Total			304,266		81,305	73	87

GAA and country	Responded to survey	Central/federal govern-ment[a]	1990 population (x 1,000)[b]	Ranking on Human Develop-ment Index[c]	Cumulative adjusted no. of AIDS cases, 1991[d]	% of population covered	% of AIDS cases covered
Sub-Saharan Africa							
Cameroon	Yes	Central	11,833	Low	1,346		
Congo	Yes	Central	2,271	Low	9,646		
Côte D'Ivoire	Yes	Central	11,997	Low	25,473		
Ethiopia	Yes	Central	49,240	Low	4,549		
Guinea-Bissau	No	Central	964	Low	462		
Nigeria	Yes	Federal	108,542	Low	268		
Rwanda	Yes	Central	7,237	Low	16,683		
Senegal	Yes	Central	7,327	Low	1,759		
Tanzania	Yes	Federal	27,318	Low	89,288		
Uganda	Yes	Central	18,794	Low	71,319		
Zaire	No	Central	35,568	Low	48,402		
Zambia	Yes	Central	8,452	Low	15,249		
Zimbabwe	No	Central	9,709	Low	22,033		
Total			299,252		306,477	57	74
Caribbean							
Haiti	Yes	Central	6,513	Low	5,545		
St. Lucia	Yes	Central	150	Middle	65		
Trinidad and Tobago	Yes	Central	1,281	High	1,466		
Total			7,944		7,076	24	53
Eastern Europe							
Czech Republic[e]	Yes	Central	10,000		27[e]		
Poland	Yes	Central	8,423	High	79		
Slovak Republic	Yes	Central	5,000		—[e]		
USSR[f]	Yes	Federal	288,595	High	67		
Total			342,018		173	83	8
South East Mediterranean							
Egypt	Yes	Central	52,426	Low	88		
Morocco	Yes	Central	25,061	Low	250		
Pakistan	Yes	Central	122,626	Low	50		
Total			200,113		388	53	28
North East Asia							
China	Yes	Federal	1,139,060	Middle	15		
Japan	Yes	Central	123,460	High	1,013		

GAA and country	Responded to survey	Central/ federal govern- ment[a]	1990 population (x 1,000)[b]	Ranking on Human Develop- ment Index[c]	Cumulative adjusted no. of AIDS cases, 1991[d]	% of population covered	% of AIDS cases covered
Korea	No	Central	42,793	High	0		
Total			1,262,520		1,028	89	88
Southeast Asia							
India	Yes	Federal	853,094	Low	191		
Singapore	No	Central	2,723	High	68		
Thailand	Yes	Central	55,702	Middle	265		
Total			911,519		524	66	67
Survey total			3,902,475		653,129		
World total			5,287,960		798,685	74	82

a. The survey collected information from centralized and federal governments. As defined for purposes of this survey, in a federal political system or a federation of states, regional diversity exists alongside nationally unified programs. Thus, different constitutional powers are distributed to both the national and regional levels, providing the individual regions with some degree of independence. Though realizing the existence of these distinct levels, because of time, resource, and access constraints *AIDS in the World* surveyed only the federal governments. Because individual states within one country were not surveyed, the data are not totally representative of the country. (This federal division probably had the greatest effect on the funding and budgetary reports.) For a central political system, which maintains one body of laws and one budget for the entire country, the issue of diffuse powers, laws, and funding allocation does not arise.

b. Population figures were provided by the United Nations Population Division, 1990.

c. The Human Development Index, a statistical measure of human development created by the United Nations Development Program, attempts to quantify countries' socioeconomic progress. To reflect sustainable progress, the index combines several indicators such as GNP, literacy rate, and average years of schooling. Of course, the concept of human development is much broader than this measurement, and "it can not capture all the dimensions of human choices. It is a national average that conceals important differences in the regional, local, ethnic, and personal distributions of human development indicators" (UNDP Report, 1991, pp. 15–16). However, the index is a start to understanding beyond per capita GNP.

d. The cumulative number of AIDS cases reflects cases reported to the World Health Organization as of December 31, 1990. Because of different reporting systems worldwide, adjustments have been made to correct for underreporting and reporting delays. The lower of these estimates are presented here.

e. The cumulative number of AIDS cases is not reported separately for the Czech and Slovak Republics. The 27 cases represent the number of cases for both republics.

f. When the survey was initially carried out in 1991, the then USSR responded through the Central Center in Moscow, which provided information for the Union's 1990–91 activities. For the Czech and Slovak Republics, however, dual inquiries had to be made. Thus, information for the Commonwealth of Independent States (previously the USSR) is presented as one entity, while most of the data on the Czech and Slovak Republics are presented separately.

APPENDIX 8.2

. . . .

Program Profile Summary of *AIDS in the World* Survey of 38 National AIDS Programs, 1992

A questionnaire was sent to national AIDS program managers in 38 countries, and follow-up inquiries were made with other appropriate respondents in those countries. Below is a selection of questions included in the questionnaire. Responses to these questions and to others not listed here are recompiled throughout AIDS in the World. *The method applied to the National AIDS Program Survey (NAPS) is presented in further detail in Box 8.3. Because all the countries surveyed have national AIDS programs (NAPs), the "yes" answers to Question 1 are not included in the table.*

Question	Response		
1. Is there a national AIDS program?	Yes 1	No 2	N/A (skip to 6)
2. If so, in what year was the first national AIDS program created?	_____		
3. Is the AIDS program separate from or integrated with the program for sexually transmitted diseases (STDs)?	Separate	Integrated	Partial N/A
4. Has the head of government or head of state ever addressed the public on AIDS?	Yes 1	No 2	
5. What was the approximate date of the head of government's/state's first address on AIDS?	Year of address _____		
Funding			
6. Program management	__% of funds		
7. Prevention of sexual transmission (information, education, and communication ([IEC], condoms, STDs, voluntary testing], injection drug use, control of blood and blood products, prevention of mother-to-child transmission, providing care	__% of funds		

| 8. Research | ___ % of funds |
| 9. Other (specify) | ___ % of funds |

	Yes	No
10. Has NAP ever been evaluated?	1	2

If Yes:

	Yes	No
11. By national organization?	1	2
12. By international organization?	1	2
13. Is HIV reporting mandatory?	1	2
14. Is there an HIV sentinel sureveillance system?	1	2

Is HIV testing required for:

	Yes	No
15. Blood donors	1	2
16. Military recruits	1	2
17. Immigrants	1	2
18. Commercial sex workers	1	2
19. Prisoners	1	2
20. Pregnant women	1	2
21. Country's own students	1	2

	Every-where	Only in large cities	Only in the capital city	No-where
22. Foreign students	1	2	3	4
23. Is voluntary testing offered?	1	2	3	4

Is voluntary testing recommended for:

	Yes	No
24. General population	1	2
25. Pregnant women	1	2
26. Commercial sex workers	1	2

Is voluntary testing:

	Always	Sometimes	Rarely	Never
	1	2	3	4
27. Anonymous	1	2	3	4
28. Not anonymous, but confidential	1	2	3	4
29. Are test results reported as part of the notification system?	1	2	3	4

Is counseling provided to those found:

	Always	Sometimes	Rarely	Never
	1	2	3	4
30. HIV seropositive	1	2	3	4
31. HIV seronegative	1	2	3	4
32. What proportion of persons receiving voluntary HIV testing also receive counseling?	0–25% 1	26–50% 2	51–75% 3	76–100% 4

Availability of diagnostic facilities for HIV in the country:

	Widely	In few places	None
	1	2	3
33. In the cities	1	2	3
34. In rural areas	1	2	3

	<50%	51–99%	100%
35. What proportion of the demand for diagnostic kits are met by suppliers?	<50% 1	51–99% 2	100% 3

36. 1990 country population per 1000 ——

37. Number of AIDS cases as of April 1992, WHO Report ——

38. Year AIDS case first diagnosed ——

	Centers for Disease Control	Bangui	PAHO/ WHO	Other (specify)	Left to clinician's judgment	Unknown
39. Which case definition of AIDS is most commonly used for surveillance purposes in country?	1	2	3	4	5	6

GAA and country	Year national AIDS program (NAP) created (2)	Is NAP separate from or integrated with STD program? (3)	Did head of state ever address public on AIDS? (Yes = 1, No = 2) (4)	If yes, year of first address (5)
North America				
Canada	1983	Integrated	1	1987
United States	1981	Integrated	1	1990
Western Europe				
France	1989	Separate	1	1989
Germany	1985	Separate	1	1984
Italy	1987	Partially int.	1	1990
Netherlands	1987	Partially int.	1	N/A
Norway	1986	Separate	1	1986
Sweden	1986	Partially int.	1	1986
Switzerland	1985	Separate	1	N/A
United Kingdom	1985	Integrated	1	1990
Oceania				
Australia	1984	Integrated	1	1985
Latin America				
Argentina	1985	Integrated	1	1991
Colombia	1988	Integrated	2	DNA
Mexico	1986	Separate	1	1984
Sub-Saharan Africa				
Cameroon	1987	No answer	2	DNA
Congo	1987	Integrated	1	1987
Côte d'Ivoire	1987	Partially int.	2	DNA
Ethiopia	1986	Integrated	2	DNA
Nigeria	1986	Integrated	2	1991
Rwanda	1987	No answer	1	1987
Senegal	1987	Integrated	1	1989
Tanzania	1988	Integrated	1	1985
Uganda	1986	Integrated	1	1986
Zambia	1988	Separate	1	1986
Caribbean				
Haiti	1987	Partially int.	2	DNA
St. Lucia	1987	Integrated	2	DNA
Trinidad and Tobago	1987	Partially int.	2	DNA
Eastern Europe				
Czech Republic	1989	Separate	2	DNA
Poland	1988	Partially int.	2	DNA
Slovak Republic	1989	Separate	1	1990
USSR	1991	Separate	2	DNA
South East Mediterranean				
Egypt	1986	Partially int.	2	DNA
Morocco	1986	Integrated	2	DNA
Pakistan	1988	No answer	2	DNA
North East Asia				
China	1986	Partially int.	1	1986
Japan	1987	Separate	1	1987
Southeast Asia				
India	1987	Separate	2	DNA
Thailand	1988	Partially int.	1	1989

Note: N/A = information not available; DNA = does not apply.

Funds allocated to program management (%) (6)	Funds allocated to STD, IDU, blood, care, mother-child (%) (7)	Funds allocated to AIDS research (%) (8)	Funds allocated to other programs (%) (9)	Has NAP been evaluated? (Yes = 1, No = 2) (10)
11	N/A	37	21	2
N/A	N/A	27	42	2
2	84	15	N/A	1
N/A	N/A	N/A	N/A	1
N/A	N/A	5	1	2
N/A	N/A	N/A	N/A	1
N/A	N/A	N/A	N/A	2
4	N/A	1	4	1
N/A	N/A	33	7	1
N/A	N/A	8	N/A	1
2	N/A	7	0	1
N/A	N/A	3	11	1
4	N/A	2	2	N/A
4	57	5	33	1
12	N/A	2	11	1
N/A	N/A	N/A	N/A	1
22	N/A	N/A	11	1
9	N/A	N/A	48	1
15	65	5	15	N/A
N/A	N/A	N/A	N/A	1
22	N/A	3	N/A	1
37	N/A	8	N/A	1
20	N/A	N/A	20	1
N/A	N/A	N/A	N/A	1
N/A	N/A	N/A	N/A	1
N/A	77	8	N/A	1
N/A	N/A	N/A	N/A	1
0	55	5	40	2
N/A	N/A	N/A	N/A	2
N/A	N/A	N/A	N/A	1
N/A	N/A	N/A	N/A	2
20	70	0	10	2
10	90	0	0	2
15	N/A	N/A	17	2
15	57	15	13	2
2	16	62	20	1
6	N/A	N/A	50	2
4	N/A	3	46	1

GAA and country	Was evaluation done only by national groups? (Yes = 1, No = 2) (11)	Evaluated by international groups? (Yes = 1, No = 2) (12)	Is HIV reporting mandatory? (Yes = 1, No = 2) (13)	Is there HIV sentinel surveillance system? (Yes = 1, No = 2) (14)
North America				
Canada	DNA	DNA	1	2
United States	DNA	DNA	N/A	N/A
Western Europe				
France	1	2	2	1
Germany	1	2	N/A	N/A
Italy	DNA	DNA	2	1
Netherlands	1	2	2	2
Norway	DNA	DNA	1	2
Sweden	1	2	1	1
Switzerland	DNA	1	1	1
United Kingdom	1	2	2	1
Oceania				
Australia	1	1	1	1
Latin America				
Argentina	1	1	2	2
Colombia	N/A	N/A	N/A	N/A
Mexico	N/A	1	N/A	N/A
Sub-Saharan Africa				
Cameroon	N/A	1	1	1
Congo	1	1	N/A	N/A
Côte d'Ivoire	N/A	1	2	1
Ethiopia	1	2	2	1
Nigeria	N/A	N/A	N/A	N/A
Rwanda	1	2	1	1
Senegal	N/A	2	1	1
Tanzania	N/A	1	N/A	N/A
Uganda	1	1	2	1
Zambia	N/A	1	N/A	N/A
Caribbean				
Haiti	1	2	2	2
St. Lucia	N/A	2	1	2
Trinidad and Tobago	1	1	2	2
Eastern Europe				
Czech Republic	DNA	DNA	1	1
Poland	DNA	DNA	N/A	N/A
Slovak Republic	1	1	1	2
USSR	DNA	DNA	1	2
South East Mediterranean				
Egypt	DNA	DNA	N/A	N/A
Morocco	DNA	DNA	1	2
Pakistan	DNA	DNA	N/A	N/A
North East Asia				
China	DNA	DNA	N/A	N/A
Japan	1	1	2	1
Southeast Asia				
India	DNA	DNA	2	1
Thailand	N/A	1	N/A	N/A

Is HIV test required for blood donors? (Yes = 1, No = 2) (15)	Is HIV test required for military? (Yes = 1, No = 1) (16)	Is HIV test required for immigrants? (Yes = 1, No = 2) (17)	Is HIV test required for commercial sex workers? (Yes = 1, No = 2) (18)	Is HIV test required for prisoners? (Yes = 1, No = 2) (19)
1	2	2	2	2
1	1	1	2	2
1	2	2	2	2
1	2	2	2	2
1	2	2	2	2
1	2	2	2	2
1	2	2	2	2
1	2	2	2	2
1	2	2	2	2
1	2	2	2	2
1	1	1	2	1
1	2	1	2	2
1	1	2	2	2
1	1	2	1	1
1	2	2	2	2
1	2	2	2	2
1	2	2	2	2
1	2	2	2	2
1	2	2	2	2
1	1	2	2	2
1	1	2	1	2
1	2	2	2	2
1	2	2	2	2
1	2	2	2	2
1	1	1	2	2
1	2	2	2	2
1	2	2	2	2
1	2	1	2	2
1	2	2	2	2
1	2	2	2	1
1	2	1	2	1
1	2	1	2	1
1	1	2	2	2
1	2	2	2	2
1	2	1	1	1
1	2	2	2	2
1	2	2	2	2
1	1	2	2	2

GAA and country	Is HIV test required for pregnant women? (Yes = 1, No = 2) (20)	Is HIV test required for own students coming from abroad? (Yes = 1, No = 2) (21)	Is HIV test required for foreign students entering country? (Yes = 1, No = 2) (22)	Where is there voluntary testing? (Everywhere = 1, Large cities = 2, Capital = 3, Nowhere = 4) (23)
North America				
Canada	2	2	2	1
United States	2	2	2	1
Western Europe				
France	2	2	2	1
Germany	2	2	2	1
Italy	2	2	2	1
Netherlands	2	2	2	2
Norway	2	2	2	1
Sweden	2	2	2	1
Switzerland	2	2	2	1
United Kingdom	2	2	2	1
Oceania				
Australia	2	2	2	1
Latin America				
Argentina	2	2	2	2
Colombia	2	2	2	2
Mexico	2	2	2	2
Sub-Saharan Africa				
Cameroon	2	2	2	4
Congo	2	2	2	2
Côte d'Ivoire	2	2	2	2
Ethiopia	2	2	2	4
Nigeria	2	2	2	2
Rwanda	2	2	2	2
Senegal	2	2	2	2
Tanzania	2	2	2	2
Uganda	2	1	2	2
Zambia	2	2	2	4
Caribbean				
Haiti	2	2	2	N/A
St. Lucia	2	2	2	2
Trinidad and Tobago	2	2	2	2
Eastern Europe				
Czech Republic	2	2	2	2
Poland	2	2	1	1
Slovak Republic	2	2	1	1
USSR	1	1	1	1
South East Mediterranean				
Egypt	2	2	1	3
Morocco	2	2	2	2
Pakistan	2	2	2	2
North East Asia				
China	2	1	1	2
Japan	2	2	2	1
Southeast Asia				
India	2	2	1	2
Thailand	2	2	2	1

Is voluntary testing recommended for general population? (Yes = 1, No = 2) (24)	Is voluntary testing recommended for pregnant women? (Yes = 1, No = 2) (25)	Is voluntary testing recommended for sex workers? (Yes = 1, No = 2) (26)	Is voluntary testing anonymous? (Always = 1, Sometimes = 2, Rarely = 3, Never = 4) (27)	Is voluntary testing anonymous but not confidential? (Always = 1, Sometimes = 2, Rarely = 3, Never = 4) (28)
2	2	2	2	1
1	1	1	2	2
1	1	1	1	1
N/A	1	1	1	1
2	1	N/A	3	1
2	2	2	4	1
2	1	1	2	1
1	1	1	2	1
2	1	2	1	2
2	1	1	2	1
2	2	1	3	1
2	1	1	4	1
N/A	N/A	N/A	N/A	N/A
2	2	1	1	2
2	2	2	4	1
1	1	1	3	2
1	1	1	1	1
2	2	2	N/A	N/A
2	2	1	2	2
1	1	N/A	1	2
2	1	1	1	N/A
2	1	2	N/A	1
1	1	1	1	N/A
N/A	N/A	N/A	N/A	N/A
2	2	2	N/A	1
1	2	1	2	1
2	2	1	4	1
2	2	1	2	1
2	2	1	3	1
N/A	1	1	2	2
1	1	1	2	2
2	1	1	N/A	1
1	1	1	2	2
1	1	1	2	2
2	2	1	2	1
1	1	1	1	4
1	1	1	2	1
1	1	1	1	N/A

GAA and country	Is test result part of notification? (Always = 1, Sometimes = 2, Rarely = 3, Never = 4) (29)	Is counseling provided for those found HIV positive? (Always = 1, Sometimes = 2, Rarely = 3, Never = 4) (30)	Is counseling provided for those found HIV negative? (Always = 1, Sometimes = 2, Rarely = 3, Never = 4) (31)	% who receive voluntary HIV testing and thus receive counseling (32)
North America				
Canada	2	2	2	4
United States	1	1	1	4
Western Europe				
France	4	2	2	N/A
Germany	1	1	1	4
Italy	2	1	2	4
Netherlands	4	1	1	4
Norway	1	1	2	2
Sweden	1	1	2	1
Switzerland	1	1	2	3
United Kingdom	1	1	1	N/A
Oceania				
Australia	1	1	2	2
Latin America				
Argentina	2	1	1	4
Colombia	N/A	N/A	N/A	3
Mexico	1	1	1	4
Sub-Saharan Africa				
Cameroon	4	2	4	1
Congo	2	3	3	1
Côte d'Ivoire	1	1	1	1
Ethiopia	1	1	4	4
Nigeria	1	2	2	1
Rwanda	3	1	1	N/A
Senegal	1	1	3	1
Tanzania	1	1	1	4
Uganda	4	1	1	3
Zambia	N/A	1	2	1
Caribbean				
Haiti	2	2	3	1
St. Lucia	1	1	2	2
Trinidad and Tobago	N/A	1	1	4
Eastern Europe				
Czech Republic	1	1	2	4
Poland	1	1	2	4
Slovak Republic	1	1	4	4
USSR	1	1	3	1
South East Mediterranean				
Egypt	1	1	1	4
Morocco	2	2	3	1
Pakistan	2	1	1	4
North East Asia				
China	1	2	2	2
Japan	1	1	2	N/A
Southeast Asia				
India	2	2	4	1
Thailand	4	1	2	3

Diagnostic clinics available for HIV in cities (Widely = 1, In few places = 2, Not available = 3) (33)	Diagnostic clinics available for HIV in rural areas (Widely = 1, In few places = 2, No clinics = 3) (34)	Demand for diagnostic kits met by suppliers (Less than 50% = 1, 51–99% = 2, 100% = 3) (35)	Country's 1991 population (x 1,000) (36)
1	1	3	26,752
1	1	3	251,213
1	1	3	56,331
1	1	3	78,925
1	1	3	57,047
1	1	3	15,044
1	1	3	4,226
1	1	3	8,461
1	1	3	6,633
1	1	3	57,366
1	4	3	17,093
1	4	3	32,719
1	4	3	33,600
1	4	3	90,445
1	2	2	12,191
1	N/A	2	2,341
2	2	2	12,411
1	2	1	50,470
1	2	2	111,846
2	2	1	7,462
1	2	2	7,518
2	2	1	28,231
1	1	1	19,427
1	1	N/A	8,740
2	4	1	6,641
1	2	3	153
2	4	3	1,300
1	2	2	15,701
1	4	3	38,666
1	1	3	
1	1	3	290,807
1	2	3	53,609
2	4	3	25,670
2	4	1	126,504
1	2	1	1,124,783
1	1	3	123,984
1	4	3	869,875
1	1	3	56,523

GAA and country	AIDS cases reported to WHO as of April 1992 (37)	Year first AIDS case diagnosed (38)	AIDS case definition most commonly used (CDC = 1, Bangui = 2, PAHO/WHO = 3, Other = 4, Medical judgment = 5, Unknown = 6) (39)
North America			
Canada	5,348	1983	1
United States	213,641	1981	1
Western Europe			
France	17,836	1979	1
Germany	7,533	1979	1
Italy	11,609	1982	1
Netherlands	2,017	1982	1
Norway	252	1983	1
Sweden	645	1982	1
Switzerland	2,228	1980	3
United Kingdom	5,451	1981	1
Oceania			
Australia	3,147	1986	1
Latin America			
Argentina	1,298	1983	1
Colombia	2,189	1985	1
Mexico	9,073	1983	1
Sub-Saharan Africa			
Cameroon	429	1986	6
Congo	2,405	1986	1
Côte d'Ivoire	8,297	1986	2
Ethiopia	1,818	1987	3
Nigeria	84	1988	2
Rwanda	6,518	1986	2
Senegal	648	1987	3
Tanzania	27,396	1986	2
Uganda	30,190	1986	2
Zambia	5,802	1985	2
Caribbean			
Haiti	3,086	1983	4
St. Lucia	40	1984	3
Trinidad and Tobago	971	1983	4
Eastern Europe			
Czech Republic	26	1980	3
Poland	87	1986	1
Slovak Republic		1980	1
USSR	70	1987	4
South East Mediterranean			
Egypt	39	1987	1
Morocco	98	1988	3
Pakistan	18	1988	4
North East Asia			
China	6	1986	3
Japan	453	1983	4
Southeast Asia			
India	102	1986	3
Thailand	179	1986	1

Mini-Survey of National AIDS Program (NAP) Managers, February 1992

	Initial government response						
Country	Year 1st AIDS case reported in country	Year govt. 1st acknowl- edged AIDS in public address	Year medium- term AIDS program started	Year national AIDS program established	Location of program in ministry of health	National AIDS advisory committee (NAC)	Year NAC created
Cameroon	1985	1986	1987	1987	+	+	1987
Canada	1979	1981	1986	1986	+	+	1983
Chile	1984	1984	1990	1984	+	+	1988
Congo	1983	1985	1988	1987	+	+	1985
Ethiopia	1986	1985	1987	1987	+	+	1987
Fiji	1989	1989	1989	1989	+[b]	+	1987
Ireland	1982	1985	1985	1987	+	+	1988
Jamaica	1982	1982	1988	1985	+	+	1988
New Zealand	1984	1984	1992	1983	+	+	1988
Nigeria	1986	1986	1989	1986	+	+	1989
Papua New Guinea	1987	1987	1989	1989	+	+	1988
Philippines	1986	1987	1988	1988	+	+	1988
Tanzania	1983	1985	1987	1988	+	+	1990
Uganda	1983	1986	1987	1987	+	+	1987

Note: In this and the following tables, + = yes; − = no; — = information not provided.

a. Deputy minister of health.

b. Ministry of Health/Ministry of Environment.

c. Pressures from ministry of health, other governmental sectors, NGOs, or international organizations to restructure.

d. G = good; FG = fairly good; VG = very good.

Country	National AIDS advisory committee (NAC) answerable to:			Composition of NAC		
	Minister of health	Prime minister	Head of state	Female or male chairperson	No. of members	No. of female members
Cameroon	+			M	22	5
Canada	+			M	16	5
Chile	+[a]			F	12	7
Congo	+			M	40	12
Ethiopia	+			M	11	2
Fiji	+			M	22	5
Ireland	+			F	22	7
Jamaica	+			M	50	25
New Zealand	+			F	25	7
Nigeria	+			M	15	5
Papua New Guinea	+			M	19	3
Philippines	+			M	9	4
Tanzania		+		M	20	2
Uganda			+	M	20	<5

Country	NGOs represented?	No. of times met in last 12 months	NAC restructured?	Reasons for restructuring		
				Need to involve more sectors	Need for women's participation	Need for more visibility
Cameroon	+	0	+	+		
Canada	+	4	+	+		+
Chile	−	—	+	+	+	+
Congo	+	>2	+	+	+	+
Ethiopia	+	12	+	+		
Fiji	+	6	+	+	+	+
Ireland	+	>2	+	+	+	+
Jamaica	+	>2	−			
New Zealand	+	3	−			
Nigeria	+	>2	+	+	+	+
Papua New Guinea	+	>2	+	+		+
Philippines	−	>2	+	+		+
Tanzania	+	>2	+	+	+	+
Uganda	+	>2	+	+		+

| Country | Reasons for restructuring | | Year present NAP manager appointed | Has NAP manager changed? | Has other key staff changed? | Program now centralized? |
	Need for decentralization	Need for integration				
Cameroon	+		1991	+	−	
Canada	+	+	1991	+	−	
Chile	+	+	1987	+	+	
Congo	+	+	1987	−	−	+
Ethiopia	+		1991	+	+	
Fiji	+	+	1989	−	−	+
Ireland	+	+	1991	−	+	+
Jamaica			1986	−	+	
New Zealand			1988	−	−	+
Nigeria	+	+	1991	+	−	
Papua New Guinea	+	+	1989	−	−	
Philippines	+	+	1988	+	−	±
Tanzania	+	+	1991	+	+	
Uganda	+	+	1990	+	−	+

Note: ± = restructuring in progress.

Country	Year of decentralization	Pressures exerted?[c]	Year NGO collaboration with govt. began	Govt. NGO relations[c]	% of govt. funds to NGOs	Have main sources of funds changed?
Cameroon	1991	−	1990	G	<5	−
Canada	1988	+	1982	FG	15	−
Chile	1987	+	1987	VG	50	−
Congo		−	1990	G	5	−
Ethiopia	1991	+	1987	FG	10	−
Fiji		+	1989	FG	10	−
Ireland		+	1988	FG	20	−
Jamaica	1982	+	1982	G	20	−
New Zealand		−	1988	VG	90	−
Nigeria	1991	+	1989	VG	5	−
Papua New Guinea	1987	−	1989	G	10	−
Philippines		−	1987	G	15	−
Tanzania	1989	−	1988	VG	25	−
Uganda		−	1987	VG	15	+

Global AIDS Strategy Donor and Recipient Countries, 1986–1991[a]

Donor country	Recipient country	Donor country	Recipient country
Australia	Regional support—East Asia		Belize
	Regional support—Oceania		Brazil
	Regional support—sub-Saharan Africa		Chile
			Guyana
	Mauritius		Peru
Belgium	Chad		Bangladesh
			Papua New Guinea
Canada	Regional support—Caribbean		Thailand
	Antigua and Barbuda		Angola
	Barbados		Kenya
	Dominica		Lesotho
	Dominican Republic		Mozambique
	Grenada		Nigeria
	Haiti		Swaziland
	Jamaica		Tanzania
	St. Kitts and Nevis		Uganda
	St. Lucia		Zambia
	St. Vincent and the Grenadines		Zimbabwe
	Trinidad and Tobago		Regional support—sub-Saharan Africa
	Turks and Caicos Islands	Denmark	Kenya
			Malawi
			Mozambique
			Rwanda

a. Includes bilateral and multi/bi assistance

Donor country	Recipient country
	Tanzania
	Uganda
	Zambia
	Zimbabwe
Finland	Kenya
	Pakistan
France	Congo
	Mozambique
	Senegal
	Zaire
	Zimbabwe
	Regional support—sub-Saharan Africa
	Thailand
Germany	Benin
	Burkina Faso
	Burundi
	Cameroon
	Central African Republic
	Congo
	Côte d'Ivoire
	Ghana
	Madagascar
	Malawi
	Namibia
	Rwanda
	Tanzania
	Togo
	Uganda
	Zaire
	Brazil
	Jamaica
	St. Lucia
	Trinidad and Tobago
	Thailand

Donor country	Recipient country
Italy	Regional support—South America
	Regional support—North Africa
Japan	Côte d'Ivoire
	Thailand
Netherlands	Rwanda
	Zambia
	Bulgaria
	Czechoslovakia
	Hungary
	Poland
	Yugoslavia
Norway	Angola
	Benin
	Botswana
	Chad
	Kenya
	Mozambique
	Namibia
	Senegal
	Tanzania
	Uganda
	Zambia
	Zimbabwe
	Nicaragua
	Sudan
	Indonesia
	Nepal
Spain	Equatorial Guinea
Sweden	LDCs—unspecified
	Ethiopia
	Guinea-Bissau
	Kenya
	Lesotho
	Mozambique

Donor country	Recipient country
	Namibia
	Tanzania
	Uganda
	Zimbabwe
	Bolivia
	Peru
	India
	Nepal
	Vietnam
	Regional support—Caribbean
Switzerland	LDCs—unspecified
United Kingdom	Botswana
	Gambia
	Ghana
	Kenya
	Lesotho
	Malawi
	Swaziland
	Tanzania
	Uganda
	Zambia
	Zimbabwe
	Anguilla
	British Virgin Islands
	Montserrat
	Turks and Caicos Islands
	Regional support—Caribbean
	Romania
USSR	Albania
	Bulgaria
	Czechoslovakia
	Hungary
	Poland
	Romania
United States	Belize
	Bolivia

Donor country	Recipient country
	Brazil
	Chile
	Colombia
	Costa Rica
	Dominican Republic
	Ecuador
	El Salvador
	Guatemala
	Haiti
	Honduras
	Jamaica
	Mexico
	Peru
	Turks and Caicos Islands
	Regional support—Eastern Caribbean
	Regional support—West Indies
	Botswana
	Burkina Faso
	Burundi
	Cameroon
	Central African Republic
	Congo
	Côte d'Ivoire
	Gambia
	Ghana
	Kenya
	Malawi
	Mali
	Mauritania
	Mozambique
	Niger
	Nigeria
	Rwanda
	Senegal
	South Africa
	Swaziland
	Tanzania

Donor country	Recipient country	Donor country	Recipient country
	Togo		Regional support—South Pacific
	Uganda		
	Zaire		Egypt
	Zambia		Morocco
	Zimbabwe		Philippines
	Indonesia		Yemen
	Thailand		

Sources: Correspondence from OECD to *AIDS in the World* (October 18, 1991); Support program on AIDS for Developing Countries; Federal Republic of Germany, Ministry of Economic Cooperation (1991); *HIV Infection and AIDS—A Report to Congress on the USAID Program for Prevention and Control* (May 1991), U.S. Agency for International Development; Correspondence from the Canadian International Development Agency—Cumulative List—AIDS Control projects (September, 1991); Correspondence from WHO, Regional Office for Europe (November 15, 1991); WHO-GPA summary data—Donor Contributions for Specified Countries from 1987 to 30 June 1991 (updated July 31, 1991).

Reference Notes

2. HIV

1. Centers for Disease Control, "HIV prevalence estimates and AIDS case projections for the United States: Report based on a workshop," *Morbidity and Mortality Weekly Report* 39(RR-16)(1990):1–31.

2. S.-E. Ekeid, World Health Organization, personal communication.

3. P. Piot, F. A. Plummer, M. A. Rey, et al., "Retrospective seroepidemiology of AIDS virus infection in Nairobi populations," *Journal of Infectious Diseases* 133(6)(1987):1108–12.

4. M. Tyndall, P. Odhiambo, and A. R. Ronald, The increasing seroprevalence of HIV-1 in males with other STDs in Nairobi, Kenya, presented at the VII International Conference on AIDS, Florence, Italy, June 1991.

5. A. M. Kimball, R. Gonzalez, R. Caleron, et al., The AIDS pandemic in the Americas: Using surveillance information to reinforce national control programs, presented at ibid.

6. R. Doorly, A. Kadio, K. Brattegaard, et al., Trends in HIV-1 and HIV-2 infections in Abidjan, Côte d'Ivoire, 1987–1990, presented at ibid.

7. G. Duarte, M. M. Mussi-Pinhata, M. C. C. Feres, et al., The ascendent pattern of seropositivity for HIV antibody and the risk factors associated with HIV transmission in parturients cared for at a school hospital in Brazil, presented at ibid.

8. Piot et al., "Retrospective seroepidemiology."

9. N. Temmerman, G. Naithn, J. G. Ndinya-Achola, et al., HIV-1 and syphilis infection in pregnant women in Nairobi, Kenya, presented at the VI International Conference on AIDS, Dakar, Senegal, December 1991.

10. K. Mokwa, V. Batter, F. Behets, et al., Prevalence of sexually transmitted diseases in childbearing women in Kinshasa, Zaire, associated with HIV infection, presented at the VII International Conference on AIDS, Florence, Italy, June 1991.

11. E. Metelus-Chalumeau, P. Larco, and G. Poumerol, Four years (April 1986–June 1990) of epidemiological trends of HIV infection among blood donors in Port-au-Prince, Haiti, presented at ibid.

12. D. Des Jarlais, K. Choopanya, J. Wenston, et al., Risk reduction and stabilization of HIV seroprevalence among drug injectors in New York City and Bangkok, Thailand, presented at ibid.

13. World Health Organization Global Programme on AIDS, HIV/AIDS in countries of Central and Eastern Europe: Epidemiology, prevention and control, Report of GPA/EURO (Copenhagen, 24 July 1991).

14. Ibid.

15. S. D. R. Green, N. Nganga, M. Nganzi, et al., Seroprevalence of HIV-1 and HIV-2 infection in pregnancy in rural Zaire, presented at the V International Conference on AIDS in Africa, Kinshasa, Zaire, October 1990.

16. S. N. Benoit, G. M. Gershy-Damet, A. Coulibaly, et al., "Seroprevalence of HIV infections in the general population of the Côte d'Ivoire, West Africa," *Journal of Acquired Immune Deficiency Syndromes* 3(1990):1193.

17. A. Cabello, M. Cabral, E. Vera, et al., The risk of sexually acquired HIV infection in Paraguay, presented at the VII International AIDS Conference, Florence, Italy, June 1991.

18. M. Melbye, J. Misfeldt, J. Olsen, and G. Schou, AIDS and HIV epidemiology in Eskimos, presented at ibid.

19. National Center in HIV Epidemiology and Clinical Research, *Australian HIV Surveillance Report* 8 Suppl. 1(January 1992).

20. T. O. Harry, W. Gashau, O. Ekenna, et al., Growing threat of HIV infection in a low prevalence area, presented at the V International Conference on AIDS in Africa, Kinshasa, Zaire, October 1990.

21. Ibid.

22. L. P. Deodhar and U. M. Tendolkar, "Genital ulcers and HIV antibody," *Lancet* 336(8707)(1989):112.

23. H. Rubsamen-Waigmann, A. Prutzner, C. Scholz, et al., Spread of HIV-2 in India, presented at the VII International Conference on AIDS, Florence, Italy, June, 1991.

24. P. Ramachandran, "Sentinel surveillance for HIV infection," *CARC Calling* 4(1991):25.

25. S. Sankari, S. Solomon, et al., Trends of HIV infection in antenatal/infertility clinics—an ominous sign, presented at the VII International Conference on AIDS, Florence, Italy, June 1991.

26. G. G. Bhava, U. D. Wagle, S. P. Tripathi, et al., HIV serosurveillance in promiscuous females of Bombay, India, presented at the VI International Conference on AIDS, San Francisco, U.S., June 1990.

27. Thailand Ministry of Public Health, National Sentinel Seroprevalence Survey, August 1991 (unpublished tables).

28. Ibid.

29. T. C. Quinn, J. P. Narain, and R. K. Zacarias, "AIDS in the Americas: A public health priority of the region," *AIDS* 4(1990):709.

30. Mexican Ministry of Health, *Boletin Mensual SIDA/ETS* 4(1990):1017.

31. T. A. Kellogg, M. J. Wilson, G. F. Lemp, et al., Prevalence of HIV-1 among homosexual and bisexual men in the San Francisco Bay Area: Evidence of infection among young gay men, presented at the VII International AIDS Conference, Florence, Italy, June 1991.

32. L. Solomon, J. Astemborski, D. Warren, et al., Differences in risk factors for seroconversion among female and male IVDUs, presented at ibid.

33. Dr. K. Holmes, personal communication, October 1991.

34. Centers for Disease Control, "Update: Acquired immunodeficiency syndrome—United States, 1981–1990," *Morbidity and Mortality Weekly Report* 40(1991):358–69.

35. Centers for Disease Control, "Acquired immunodeficiency syndrome—Dade County, Florida, 1981–1990," *Morbidity and Mortality Weekly Report* 40(1991):489–93.

36. J. Kengeya-Kayondo, A. Amaana, W. Naamara, et al., Anti-HIV seroprevalence in adult rural populations of Uganda and its implications for preventive strategies, presented at the V International Conference on AIDS, Montreal, Canada, June 1989.

37. S. W. Berkley, W. Naamara, S. Okware, et al., The epidemiology of AIDS and HIV infection in women in Uganda, presented at the IV International Conference on AIDS and Associated Cancers in Africa, Marseilles, France, October 1989.

38. W. Naamara, Official release of the National Serosurvey for human immunodeficiency virus (HIV) in Uganda (AIDS Control Programme, Ministry of Health, Kampala, Uganda, 1990).

39. C. Bizimungu, A. Ntilivamunda, M. Tahimana, et al., "Nationwide community-based serological survey of HIV-1 and other human retrovirus infections," *Lancet* 1(8644)(1989):941–43.

40. A. Sangare, G. Leonard, G. Gershy-Damet, et al., Epidemiology of HIV-1 and HIV-2 Virus in Ivory Coast during the period 1986–1989, presented at the IV International Conference on AIDS and Associated Cancers in Africa, Marseilles, France, October 1989.

41. S. Benoit, G. Gershy-Damet, A. Coulibaly, et al., "Seroprevalence of HIV infection in the general population of the Côte d'Ivoire, West Africa," *Journal of Acquired Immune Deficiency Syndromes* 3(12)(1990):1193–96.

42. G. Gershy-Damet, K. Koffi, B. Soro, et al., "Seroepidemiological survey of HIV-1 and HIV-2 infections in the five regions of Ivory Coast," *AIDS* 5(4)(1991):462–63.

43. N. Padian, "Prostitute women and AIDS: Epidemiology," *AIDS* 2(6)(1988):413–19.

44. A. Larson, "Social context of HIV transmission in Africa: Historical and cultural basis of East and Central African sexual relations," *Review of Infectious Diseases* 11(1989):916–31.

45. H. Hethcote and J. Yorke, *Gonorrhea Transmission Dynamics and Control*, Lecture Notes in Biomathematics, no. 56 (New York: Springer-Verlag, 1984).

46. World Health Organization (WHO), *Current and Future Dimensions of the HIV/AIDS Pandemic: A Capsule Summary*. Global Programme on AIDS, WHO/GPA/SFI/90.2, Rev. 1 (Geneva, 1990).

47. J. N. Wasserheit, "Epidemiological synergy: Inter-relationships between

HIV infection and other STDs," in *AIDS and Women's Reproductive Health*, ed. L. Chen, J. Sepúlveda Amor, and S. J. Segal (New York: Plenum Press, 1992).

48. M. Carael, M. Carballo, B. Ferry, et al., Prevalence of high-risk sexual behaviors in some African countries: Evidence from recent surveys, presented at the VII International Conference on AIDS, Florence, Italy, June 1991.

49. B. Torrey, M. Mulligan, and P. Way, Blood donors and AIDS in Africa: The gift relationship revisited, U.S. Bureau of the Census, Center for International Research, Staff paper no. 53 (1990).

50. S. Berkley, W. Naamara, S. Okware, et al., "AIDS and HIV infection in Uganda—Are more women infected than men?" *AIDS* 12(1990):1237–42.

51. U.S. Department of Health Services, Public Health Services, Centers for Disease Control, National HIV seroprevalence surveys—Summary of results (1989).

52. U.S. Department of Health Services, Centers for Disease Control, U.S. Public Health Service national HIV serosurveillance through 1990 (in press).

53. U.S. Department of Health and Human Service, Public Health Service, National Center for Infectious Diseases, Division of HIV/AIDS, HIV/AIDS surveillance, year-end edition (January 1992).

54. Institut de Médecine et d'Epidémiologie Africaine, Centre Collaborateur de l'OMS, European Center for the Epidemiological Monitoring of AIDS, AIDS surveillance in Europe, quarterly report no. 32 (1991).

55. Australian National Centre in HIV Epidemiology and Clinical Research, *Australian HIV Surveillance Report* 8 Suppl. 1(January 1992).

56. Pan American Health Organization (PAHO), Regional Office of the World Health Organization, 1990 AIDS/HIV/STD surveillance report.

57. P. Piot, B. M. Kapita, J. B. O. Were, et al., "The first decade and challenge for the 1990s," *AIDS* 5 (suppl. 1)(1991):S1–5.

58. J. Chin, "The epidemiology and projected mortality of AIDS," in *Disease and Mortality in Sub-Saharan Africa*, ed. R. Feachem and D. T. Jamison (World Bank, in press).

59. K. M. De Cock, F. Brun-Vézinet, and B. Soro, "HIV-1 and HIV-2 Infections and AIDS in West Africa," *AIDS* 5 Suppl. 1(1991):S21–28.

60. PAHO, 1990 AIDS/HIV/STD surveillance report.

61. WHO Global Programme on AIDS, HIV/AIDS in countries of Central and Eastern Europe.

62. U. K. Brinkmann, "Features of the AIDS epidemic in Thailand," Department of Population and International Health, Harvard School of Public Health, Working Paper no. 2 (Boston, U.S., 1992).

63. Directorate General of Health Services, Government of India, National AIDS Control Programme, India: Country scenario (1991).

4. Interactions of HIV and Other Diseases

1. R. J. Biggar, W. Burnett, J. Miki, and P. Nasca, "Cancer among New York men at risk of acquired immunodeficiency syndrome," *International Journal of Cancer* 43(1989):979–85.

2. C. S. Rabkin, R. J. Biggar, and J. W. Horm, "Increasing incidence of cancers associated with the human immunodeficiency virus epidemic," *International Journal of Cancer* 47(1991):692–96.

3. R. J. Biggar, J. W. Horm, J. F. Fraumeni, Jr., et al., "The incidence of Kaposi's sarcoma in the United States and Puerto Rico, 1973–1981," *Journal of the National Cancer Institute* 73(1984):89–94.

4. Rabkin et al., "Increasing incidence of cancers."

5. Ibid.

6. J. Casabona, M. Melbye, and R. J. Biggar, "Kaposi's sarcoma and non–Hodgkin's lymphoma in European AIDS cases: No excess risk of Kaposi's sarcoma in Mediterranean countries," *International Journal of Cancer* 47(1991):49–53.

7. V. Beral, T. A. Peterman, R. L. Berkelman, and H. W. Jaffe, "Kaposi's sarcoma among persons with AIDS: A sexually transmitted infection," *Lancet* 335(1990):123–28.

8. R. J. Biggar, "The AIDS problem in Africa," *Lancet* 1(1986):79–83.

9. Beral et al., "Kaposi's sarcoma."

10. R. J. Biggar and the International Registry of Seroconverters, "AIDS incubation in 1981 HIV-seroconverters from different exposure groups," *AIDS* 4(1990):1059–66.

11. D. W. Northfelt, J. O. Kahn, and P. A. Volberding, "Treatment of Kaposi's sarcoma," *Haematology and Oncology Clinics of North America* 5(1991):297–309.

12. L. A. G. Ries, B. F. Hankey, B. A. Miller, et al., *Cancer Statistics Review 1973–88*, NIH Pub. no. 2789 (Washington, D.C.: National Cancer Institute, 1991).

13. Casabona et al., "Kaposi's sarcoma and non-Hodgkin's lymphoma."

14. V. Beral, T. Peterman, R. Berkelman, and H. Jaffe, "AIDS-associated non–Hodgkin's lymphoma," *Lancet* 337(1991):805–09.

15. R. J. Biggar, "Cancer in acquired immunodeficiency syndrome: An epidemiological assessment," *Seminars in Oncology* 17(1990):251–60.

16. Rabkin et al., "Increasing incidence of cancers."

17. M. H. Gail, J. M. Pluda, C. S. Rabkin, et al., "Projections of the incidence of non-Hodgkin's lymphoma related to acquired immunodeficiency syndrome," *Journal of the National Cancer Institute* 83(1991):695–701.

18. Rabkin et al., "Increasing incidence of cancers."

19. Gail et al., "Projections of the incidence of non-Hodgkin's lymphoma."

20. Biggar et al., "Cancer among New York men."

21. Beral et al., "AIDS-associated non-Hodgkin's lymphoma."

22. S. E. Krown, "Treatment of AIDS-associated malignancy," *Cancer Detection and Prevention* 14(1990):405–09.

23. Biggar et al., "Cancer among New York men."

24. Rabkin et al., "Increasing incidence of cancers."

25. R. J. Biggar, P. L. Gigase, M. Melbye, et al., "ELISA HTLV retrovirus antibody reactivity associated with malaria and immune complexes in healthy Africans," *Lancet* 2(1985):520–23.

26. D. J. Volsky, Y. T. Wu, M. Stevenson, et al., "Antibodies to HTLV-III/

LAV in Venezuelan patients with acute malarial infections," *New England Journal of Medicine* 314(1986):647–48.

27. Biggar, "The AIDS problem in Africa."

28. R. J. Biggar, "Possible nonspecific associations between malaria and HTLV-III/LAV," *New England Journal of Medicine* 315(1986):457–58.

29. A. E. Greenberg, C. A. Schable, A. J. Sulzer, et al., "Evaluation of serological cross-reactivity between antibodies to *Plasmodium* and HTLV-III/LAV," *Lancet* 2(1986):247–49.

30. P. Nguyen-Dinh, A. E. Greenberg, J. M. Mann, et al., "Absence of association between *Plasmodium falciparum* malaria and human immunodeficiency virus infection in children in Kinshasa, Zaire," *Bulletin of the World Health Organization* 65(1987):607–13.

31. P. Nguyen-Dinh, A. E. Greenberg, R. W. Ryder, et al., Absence of association between HIV seropositivity and *Plasmodium falciparum* malaria in Kinshasa, Zaire, presented at the III International Conference on AIDS, Washington, D.C., 1987.

32. P. Nguyen-Dinh, A. E. Greenberg, R. L. Colebunders, et al., HIV infection, AIDS, and *Plasmodium falciparum* malaria in an adult emergency ward population in Kinshasa, Zaire, presented at the 36th Annual Meeting of the American Society of Tropical Medicine and Hygiene, Los Angeles, Calif., November 1987.

33. A. E. Greenberg, P. Nguyen-Dinh, J. M. Mann, et al., "The association between malaria, blood transfusions, and HIV seropositivity in a pediatric population in Kinshasa, Zaire," *Journal of the American Medical Association* 259(1988):545–49.

34. N. Shaffer, K. Hedberg, F. Davachi, et al., "Trends and risk factors for HIV-1 seropositivity among outpatient children, Kinshasa, Zaire," *AIDS* 4(1990):1231–36.

35. O. O. Simooya, R. M. Mwendapole, S. Siziya, and A. F. Fleming, "Relation between falciparum malaria and HIV seropositivity in Ndola, Zambia," *British Medical Journal* 297(1988):30–31.

36. R. J. Leaver, Z. Haile, and D. A. K. Watters, "HIV and cerebral malaria," *Transactions of the Royal Society of Tropical Medicine and Hygiene* 84(1990):201.

37. O. Muller and R. Moser, "The clinical and parasitological presentation of *Plasmodium falciparum* malaria in Uganda is unaffected by HIV-1 infection," *Transactions of the Royal Society of Tropical Medicine and Hygiene* 84(1990): 336–38.

38. S. Allen, P. Van de Perre, A. Serufilira, et al., "Human immunodeficiency virus and malaria in a representative sample of childbearing women in Kigali, Rwanda," *Journal of Infectious Diseases* 164(1991):67–71.

39. Nguyen-Dinh et al., HIV infection, AIDS, and *Plasmodium falciparum* malaria.

40. Simooya et al., "Relation between falciparum malaria and HIV seropositivity."

41. F. Wabwire-Mangen, C. J. Shiff, D. Vlahov, et al., "Immunological effects

of HIV-1 infection on the humoral response to malaria in an African population," *American Journal of Tropical Medicine and Hygiene* 41(1989):504–11.

42. M. Troye-Blomberg and P. Perlmann, "T cell functions in *Plasmodium falciparum* and other malarias," *Progress in Allergy* 41(1988):253–87.

43. M. Ho and H. K. Webster, "Immunology of human malaria: A cellular perspective," *Parasite Immunology* 11(1989):105–16.

44. Nguyen-Dinh et al., Absence of association.

45. Simooya et al., "Relation between falciparum malaria and HIV seropositivity."

46. Muller and Moser, "The clinical and parasitological presentation."

47. Allen et al., "Human immunodeficiency virus."

48. Shaffer et al., "Trends and risk factors."

49. Muller and Moser, "The clinical and parasitological presentation."

50. R. Colebunders, Y. Bahwe, W. Nekwei, et al., "Incidence of malaria and efficacy of oral quinine in patients recently infected with human immunodeficiency virus in Kinshasa, Zaire," *Journal of Infection* 21(1990):167–73.

51. A. E. Greenberg, W. Nsa, R. W. Ryder, et al., "*Plasmodium falciparum* malaria and perinatally acquired human immunodeficiency virus type I infection in Kinshasa, Zaire. A prospective, longitudinal cohort study of 587 children," *New England Journal of Medicine* 325(1991):105–09.

52. O. Muller, R. Moser, P. Guggenberger, and M. Alexander, "AIDS in Africa," *New England Journal of Medicine* 324(1991):847–48.

53. Muller and Moser, "The clinical and parasitological presentation."

54. Colebunders et al., "Incidence of malaria."

55. Greenberg et al., "*Plasmodium falciparum* malaria."

56. Ibid.

57. Colebunders et al., "Incidence of malaria."

58. Greenberg et al., "*Plasmodium falciparum* malaria."

59. J. B. Margolick, D. J. Volkman, T. M. Folks, and A. S. Fauci, "Amplification of HTLV-III/LAV infection by antigen-induced activation of T cells and direct suppression by virus of lymphocyte blastogenic responses," *Journal of Immunology* 138(1987):1719–23.

60. P. G. Smith, R. H. Morrow, and J. Chin, "Investigating interactions between HIV infection and tropical diseases." *International Journal of Epidemiology* 17(1988):705–07.

61. R. H. Morrow, R. L. Colebunders, and J. Chin, "Interactions of HIV infection with endemic tropical diseases," *AIDS* 3(1989):S79–S87.

62. Troye-Blomberg and Perlmann, "T cell functions."

63. Ho and Webster, "Immunology of human malaria."

64. Greenberg et al., "*Plasmodium falciparum* malaria."

65. Greenberg et al., "The association between malaria, blood transfusions, and HIV seropositivity."

66. A. Kochi, "The global tuberculosis situation and the new control strategy of the World Health Organisation," *Tubercle* 72(1991):1–6.

67. C. J. L. Murray, K. Styblo, and A. Rouillon, "Tuberculosis in developing

countries: Burden, intervention and cost," *Bulletin of the International Union against Tuberculosis and Lung Disease* 65(1)(March 1990).

68. P. Sudre, G. ten Dam, and A. Kochi, "Tuberculosis: A global overview of the situation today," *Bulletin of the World Health Organization* 70(2)(1992).

69. M. C. Raviglione, J. P. Narain, and A. Kochi, "HIV-associated tuberculosis in developing countries: Clinical features, diagnosis, and treatment," *Bulletin of the World Health Organization* (1992).

70. H. L. Reider, G. M. Cauthen, G. D. Kelly, et al., "Tuberculosis in the United States," *Journal of the American Medical Association* 262(1989):385–89.

71. H. L. Reider, G. M. Cauthen, G. W. Comstock, and D. E. Snider, Jr., "Epidemiology of tuberculosis in the United States," *Epidemiologic Review* 11(1989):79–88.

72. Centers for Disease Control, "Update: Tuberculosis elimination—United States," *Morbidity and Mortality Weekly Report* 39(1990):153–56.

73. Raviglione et al., "HIV-associated tuberculosis in developing countries."

74. Centers for Disease Control, *National HIV Seroprevalence Surveys: Summary of Results: Data from Serosurveillance Activities through 1989*, DHHS Publ. no. HIV/CID/9–90/006 (Washington, D.C.: Government Printing Office, 1990).

75. I. M. Onorato, E. McCray, and the Field Services Branch, "Prevalence of human immunodeficiency virus infection among patients attending tuberculosis clinics in the United States" *Journal of Infectious Diseases* 165(1992):8792.

76. Centers for Disease Control, Tuberculosis elimination—USA (August 1991).

77. R. L. Colebunders, R. W. Ryder, N. Nzilambi, et al., "HIV infection in patients with tuberculosis in Kinshasa, Zaire," *American Review of Respiratory Diseases* 139(1989):1082–85.

78. B. Standaert, F. Niragira, P. Kadende, and P. Piot, "The association of tuberculosis and HIV infection in Burundi," *AIDS Research and Human Retroviruses* 5(1989):247–51.

79. A. M. Elliot, N. Luo, G. Tembo, et al., "Impact of HIV on tuberculosis in Zambia: A cross-sectional study," *British Medical Journal* 301(1990):412–15.

80. P. Kelly, G. Burnham, and C. Radford, "HIV seropositivity and tuberculosis in a rural Malawi hospital," *Transactions of the Royal Society of Tropical Medicine and Hygiene* 84(1990):725–27.

81. H. E. J. Kool, D. Bloomkolk, P. A. Reeve, and S. A. Danner, "HIV seropositivity and tuberculosis in a large general hospital in Malawi," *Tropical and Geographical Medicine* 42(1990):128–32.

82. R. Long, M. Scalcini, J. Manfreda, et al., "Impact of human immunodeficiency virus type 1 on tuberculosis in rural Haiti," *American Review of Respiratory Diseases* 143(1991):69–73.

83. K. M. De Cock, E. Gnaore, G. Adjorlolo, et al., "Risk of tuberculosis in patients with HIV-1 and HIV-2 infections in Abidjan, Ivory Coast," *British Medical Journal* 302(1991):496–99.

84. Raviglione et al., "HIV-associated tuberculosis in developing countries."

85. A. D. Harris, "Tuberculosis and human immunodeficiency virus infection in developing countries," *Lancet* 335(1990):387–90.

86. P. A. Selwyn, D. Hartel, V. A. Lewis, et al., "A prospective study of risk of tuberculosis among intravenous drug users with human immunodeficiency virus infection," *New England Journal of Medicine* 320(1989):545–50.

87. M. M. Braun, N. Badi, R. W. Ryder, E. Baende, et al., "A retrospective cohort study of the risk of tuberculosis among women of childbearing age with HIV infection in Zaire." *American Review of Respiratory Diseases* 143(3)(1991): 501–04.

88. A. Kagame, J. Batungwanayo, S. Allen, et al., Prospective study of tuberculosis risk in a cohort of HIV seropositive women in Kigali, Rwanda, presented at the VII International Conference on AIDS, Florence, Italy, June 1992.

89. Centers for Disease Control, *National HIV Seroprevalence Surveys.*

90. Selwyn et al., "A prospective study of risk of tuberculosis."

91. P. Cathebras, J. A. Vohito, M. L. Yete, et al., "Tuberculose et infection par le virus de l'immunodéficience humaine en République Centrafricaine," *Médecine Tropicale* 48(1988):401–07.

92. C. P. Theuer, P. C. Hopewell, D. Elias, et al., "Human immunodeficiency virus infection in tuberculosis patients," *Journal of Infectious Diseases* 162(1)(1990):8–12.

93. T. Modilevsky, F. R. Sattler, and P. F. Barnes, "Mycobacterial disease in patients with human immunodeficiency virus infection," *Archives of Internal Medicine* 149(1989):2201–05.

94. R. E. Chaisson, G. F. Schecter, C. P. Theuer, et al., "Tuberculosis in patients with acquired immunodeficiency syndrome: Clinical features, response to therapy and survival," *American Review of Respiratory Diseases* 136(1987): 570–74.

95. Colebunders et al., "HIV infection in patients with tuberculosis."

96. Centers for Disease Control, *Tuberculosis Statistics—States and Cities*, DHHS Publication no. CDC85–8249 (Atlanta: U.S. Department of Health and Human Services 1985).

97. P. F. Barnes, A. B. Bloch, P. T. Davidson, et al., "Tuberculosis in patients with human immunodeficiency virus infection," *New England Journal of Medicine* 324(1991):1644–50.

98. J. Berenguer, S. Moreno, F. Laguna, et al., "Tuberculous meningitis in patients infected with the human immunodeficiency virus," *New England Journal of Medicine* 326(1992):668–72.

99. Murray et al., "Tuberculosis in developing countries."

100. J. Perrins, R. L. Colebunders, C. Karahunga, et al., "Increased mortality and tuberculosis treatment failure rate among human immunodeficiency virus (HIV) seropositive compared with HIV seronegative patients with pulmonary tuberculosis treated with 'standard' chemotherapy in Kinshasa, Zaire," *American Review of Respiratory Diseases* 144(1991):750–55.

101. C. F. Gilks, R. J. Brindle, L. S. Otieno, et al., "Extra-pulmonary and

disseminated tuberculosis in HIV-1 seropositive patients presenting to the acute medical services in Nairobi," *AIDS* 4(1990):981–85.

102. W. Rom, New York City Medical Center, statement, Associated Press News, February 1992.

103. "Purified Protein Derivative (PPD)-Tuberculin anergy and HIV infection," *Morbidity and Mortality Weekly Report* 140(RR-5):27–33. Guidelines for anergy testing and management of anergic persons at risk of tuberculosis.

104. American Thoracic Society/Centers for Disease Control, "Diagnostic standards and classification of tuberculosis," *American Review of Respiratory Diseases* 142(1990):725–35.

105. Long et al., "Impact of human immunodeficiency virus type 1 on tuberculosis in rural Haiti," ibid. 143(1991):69–73.

106. T. Modilevsky, F. R. Sattler, and P. F. Barnes, "Mycobacterial disease in patients with human immunodeficiency virus infection," *Archives of Internal Medicine* 149(1989):2201–05.

107. C. P. Theuer, P. C. Hopewell, D. Elias, et al., "Human immunodeficiency virus infection in tuberculosis patients," *Journal of Infectious Diseases* 162(1990):8–12.

108. E. Louie, L. B. Rice, and R. S. Holzman, "Tuberculosis in non-Haitian patients with acquired immunodeficiency syndrome," *Chest* 90(1986):542–45.

109. F. Kramer, T. Modilevsky, A. R. Waliany, et al., "Delayed diagnosis of tuberculosis in patients with human immunodeficiency virus infection," *American Journal of Medicine* 89(1990):451–56.

110. A. Kochi, "The global tuberculosis situation and the new control strategy of the World Health Organization," *Tubercle* 72(1991):1–6.

111. Y. Mukadi, J. Perriens, M. Kaboto, et al., Prolonged chemotherapy for tuberculosis following standard short course treatment among HIV-infected persons in Zaire, presented at the VII International Conference on AIDS, Florence, Italy, June 1991.

112. T. Mori and A. Kochi, Case Study on the Tuberculosis Control Programme of the United Republic of Tanzania (WHO-TUB Unit, in press).

113. K. Brudney and J. Dobkin, "Resurgent tuberculosis in New York City: HIV, homeless and the decline of tuberculosis control programs," *American Review of Respiratory Diseases* 144(1991):745–49.

114. P. Nunn, D. Kibuga, S. Gathua, et al., "Cutaneous hypersensitivity reactions due to thiacetazone in HIV-1 seropositive patients treated with tuberculosis," *Lancet* 337(1991):627–30.

115. C. A. Peloquin, "Shortages of antimycobacterial drugs," *New England Journal of Medicine* 326(1992):714.

116. A. Pablos-Méndez, M. C. Raviglione, B. Ruggero, and R. Ramase-Zuniga, "Drug resistant tuberculosis among the homeless in New York City," *New York State Journal of Medicine* 90(1990):351–55.

117. D. E. Snider and W. L. Roper, "The new tuberculosis," *New England Journal of Medicine* 332(1992):703–05.

118. Centers for Disease Control, "Tuberculosis and human immunodeficiency virus infections: Recommendations of the Advisory Committee for the

Elimination of Tuberculosis (ACET)," *Morbidity and Mortality Weekly Report* 38(1989):236–50.

119. H. Claremont, M. Johnson, J. Coberly, et al., Tolerance of short course tuberculosis chemoprophylaxis in HIV-infected individuals, presented at the VII International Conference on AIDS, Florence, Italy, June 1991.

5. HIV and Other Sexually Transmitted Diseases

1. J. N. Wasserheit, "Epidemiological synergy: Inter-relationships between HIV infection and other STDs," in *AIDS and Women's Reproductive Health,* ed. L. Chen et al. (New York: Plenum, 1992).

2. A. De Schryver and A. Meheus, "Epidemiology of sexually transmitted diseases: The global picture," *Bulletin of the World Health Organization* 68(1990):639–54; H. H. Handsfield. *Color Atlas and Synopsis of Sexually Transmitted Diseases* (New York: McGraw-Hill, 1992); O. Frank, "Sexual behaviour and disease transmission in sub-Saharan Africa: Past trends and future prospects," Paper prepared for IUSSP Anthropological Demography Committee Seminar on Anthropological Studies Relevant to Sexual Transmission of HIV, Sonderborg, Denmark, November 1990; R. C. Brunham and J. E. Embree, "Sexually transmitted diseases: Current and future dimensions of the problem in the Third World," in *Reproductive Tract Infections: Global Impact and Priorities for Women's Reproductive Health,* ed. A. Germain et al. (New York: Plenum, 1992).

3. R. M. May and R. M. Anderson, "Transmission dynamics of HIV infection," *Nature* 326(1987):137.

4. M. Over and P. Piot, "HIV infection and sexually transmitted diseases." (Washington, D.C.: Population, Health and Nutrition Division, World Bank, 1991).

5. R. C. Brunham and A. R. Ronald, "Epidemiology of sexually transmitted diseases in developing countries," in *Research Issues in Human Behavior and Sexually Transmitted Diseases in the AIDS Era,* ed. J. N. Wasserheit, S. O. Aral, and K. K. Holmes (Washington, D.C.: American Society for Microbiology, 1991).

6. A. A. Ehrhardt and J. N. Wasserheit, "Age, gender, and sexual risk behaviors for sexually transmitted diseases in the United States," in Wasserheit, Aral, and Holmes, *Research Issues in the AIDS Era.*

7. K. K. Holmes et al., "An estimate of the risk of men acquiring gonorrhea by sexual contact with infected females," *American Journal of Epidemiology* 91(1970):170; R. R. Hooper et al., "Cohort study of venereal disease. I: The risk of gonorrhea transmission from infected women to men," ibid. 108(1978):136; E. W. Hook III and H. H. Handsfield, "Gonococcal infections in the adult," in *Sexually Transmitted Diseases,* 2d ed., ed. K. K. Holmes et al. (New York: McGraw-Hill, 1990); F. N. Judson, "Sexually transmitted diseases: Gonorrhea," *Medical Clinics of North America* 74(6)(1990):1353–66.

8. P. F. Sparling, "Natural history of syphilis," in Holmes et al., *Sexually Transmitted Diseases.*

9. Frank, "Sexual behaviour and disease transmission."

10. Wasserheit, "Epidemiological synergy."

11. Over and Piot, "HIV infection and sexually transmitted diseases."

12. F. N. Judson et al., Fear of AIDS and incidence of gonorrhea, syphilis and hepatitis B, 1982–1990, presented at the VII International Conference on AIDS, Florence, Italy, June 1991.

13. Over and Piot, "HIV infection and sexually transmitted diseases."

14. A. De Schryver and A. Meheus, "Epidemiology of sexually transmitted diseases: The global picture," *Bulletin of the World Health Organization* 68(1990).

15. J. N. Wasserheit, "The significance and scope of reproductive tract infections among Third World women," *International Journal of Gynecology and Obstetrics* Suppl. 3(1989):145–68.

16. Over and Piot, "HIV infection and sexually transmitted diseases."

17. A. E. Washington et al., "The economic cost of pelvic inflammatory disease," *Journal of the American Medical Association* 255(1986):1735–38.

18. D. A. Grimes, "Death due to sexually transmitted diseases: The forgotten component of reproductive mortality," *Journal of the American Medical Association* 255(1986):1727–29.

19. L. Weström, "Incidence, prevalence and trends of acute inflammatory disease and its consequences in industrialized countries," *American Journal of Obstetrics and Gynecology* 138(1980):880–92; L. Weström and P. A. Mardh, "Acute pelvic inflammatory diseases," in Holmes et al., *Sexually Transmitted Diseases*; P. A. Mardh, "Ascending chlamydial infection in the female genital tract," in *Chlamydial Infections,* ed. J. D. Oriel et al. (Cambridge: Cambridge University Press, 1986); M. W. Adler, "Trends for gonorrhea and pelvic inflammatory disease in England and Wales in a defined population," *American Journal of Obstetrics and Gynecology* 138(1980):901–04.

20. Weström, "Incidence, prevalence and trends of acute inflammatory disease."

21. Population Information Program, Center for Communication Programs, Johns Hopkins University, Baltimore, U.S. (1983).

22. A. V. Ratnam et al., "Syphilis in pregnant women in Zambia," *British Journal of Venereal Diseases* 58(1982):355–58.

23. K. Atrash et al., "Ectopic pregnancy in the United States," *Morbidity and Mortality Weekly Report* 35(255)(1986):29–37.

24. Wasserheit, "The significance and scope of reproductive tract infections"; Washington et al., "The economic cost of pelvic inflammatory disease."

25. P. Piot and A. Meheus, "Epidémiologie des maladies sexuellement transmissibles dans les pays en developpement," *Annales de la Société Belge de Médecine Tropicale* 63(1983):87–110; S. K. Hira et al., "Congenital syphilis in Lusaka, II. Incidence at birth and potential risk among hospital deliveries," *East African Medical Journal* 59(1982):306–10.

26. M. Laga et al., "Epidemiology of ophthalmia neonatorum in Kenya," *Lancet* 2(1986):1145–48; F. P. Galega, "Gonococcal ophthalmia neonatorum: The case for prophylaxis in tropical Africa," *Bulletin of the World Health Organization* 62(1984):95–98.

27. S. Aral and K. K. Holmes, "Sexually transmitted diseases in the AIDS era," *Scientific American* 264(2):62–69.

28. Brunham and Embree, "Sexually transmitted diseases."

29. Brunham and Ronald, "Epidemiology of sexually transmitted diseases in developing countries."

30. Rwandan HIV Seroprevalence Study Group, *Lancet* 1(1989):941–43.

31. Wasserheit, "The significance and scope of reproductive tract infections among Third World women."

32. I. R. Sami, "Female circumcision with special reference to the Sudan," *Annals of Tropical Paediatrics* 6(1986):99–115; E. Tanganelli, "Implicazioni ginecologiche e osteiriche della circoncisione femminile in Somalia," *Minerva Ginecologica* 41(1989):469–74.

33. Frank, "Sexual behavior and disease transmission in sub-Saharan Africa."

34. V. Muntarbhorn, Rights of the child: Sale of children, UN Commission on Human Rights E/CN.4/1992/55 (February 1992).

35. Over and Piot, "HIV infection and sexually transmitted diseases."

36. G. Albrecht, J. Wells, and A. Valleron, HIV risk behaviors among adolescents/young adults in three countries, presented at the VII International Conference on AIDS, Florence, Italy, June 1991.

37. P. Piot and M. Laga, "Current approaches to sexually transmitted disease control in developing countries," in Wasserheit, Aral, and Holmes, *Research Issues in the AIDS Era.*

38. D. Woodhouse et al., "Street outreach for STD/HIV prevention—Colorado Springs, Colorado, 1987–1991," *Morbidity and Mortality Weekly Report* 41:6, 94–101.

39. M. Laga, A. Meheus, and P. Piot, "Epidemiology and control of gonococcal ophthalmia neonatorum," *Bulletin of the World Health Organization* 67(1989):471–78.

40. K. Holmes and S. Aral, "Behavioral interventions in developing countries," in Wasserheit, Aral, and Holmes, *Research Issues in the AIDS Era.*

41. R. Schilling et al., "Developing strategies for AIDS prevention research with black and Hispanic drug users," *Public Health Reports* 104(1)(Jan.–Feb. 1989):2–8.

42. C. Airhihenbuwa et al., "HIV/AIDS education and prevention among African-Americans: A focus on culture," *AIDS Education and Prevention* (in press).

43. F. Judson, Issues which relate to the role of STD control in the control of HIV/AIDS, WHO internal communication.

44. *AIDS in the World* survey, 1992.

6. The Demographic, Economic, and Social Impact of AIDS

1. S. Foster and S. Lucas, Socioeconomic aspects of HIV and AIDS in developing countries: A review and annotated bibliography (Department of Public Health and Policy, London School of Hygiene and Tropical Medicine, 1991).

2. E. Bos, M. T. Vu, and A. Levin, *World Population Projections, 1992–93 Edition* (Baltimore: Johns Hopkins University Press, forthcoming).

3. R. A. Bulatao and E. Bos, "Projecting the demographic impact of AIDS" (Population and Human Resources Department, World Bank, 1991).

4. R. A. Bulatao and E. Bos, "Projecting mortality for all countries," Policy, Planning, and Research Working Paper no. 337 (Population and Human Resources Department, World Bank, 1989).

5. E. Bos and R. Bulatao, "Projecting fertility for all countries," Policy, Research, and External Affairs Working Paper no. 500 (Population and Human Resources Department, World Bank, 1990).

6. World Bank, Seminar on AIDS and Population Policy, August 28, 1990 (background materials) (Washington, D.C., 1990).

7. L. Valleroy, J. Harris, and P. Way, "The impact of HIV-infection on child survival in the developing world," *AIDS* 4(7)(1990):667–72.

8. E. Bos, Projecting the number of AIDS orphans in one African country (Population and Human Resources Department, World Bank, 1991).

9. J. Armstrong, "Socioeconomic implications of AIDS in developing countries," *Finance and Development* 28(4)(1991):14–17.

10. K. M. De Cock et al., AIDS—The leading cause of adult death in a West African city (Abidjan), presented at the VI International Conference on AIDS, San Francisco, U.S., June 1990.

11. W. Carswell, G. Lloyd, and J. Howells, "Prevalence of HIV-1 in East African lorry drivers," *AIDS* 3(1989):759–61.

12. B. M. Nkowane, "The impact of HIV infection and AIDS on a primary industry: Mining (A case study of Zambia)," in *The Global Impact of AIDS*, ed. A. F. Fleming et al. (New York: Wiley-Liss, 1988).

13. E. Cohen, "Tourism and AIDS in Thailand," *Annals of Tourism Research* 15(1988):467–86.

14. S. Gillespie, "Potential impact of AIDS on farming systems: A case study from Rwanda," *Land Use Policy* 4(1989):301–12.

15. F. Davachi et al., "The economic impact on families of children with AIDS in Kinshasa, Zaire," in Fleming et al., *The Global Impact of AIDS*.

16. T. Barnett and P. Blaikie, *AIDS in Africa: Its Present and Future Impact* (London: Bellhaven Press, 1992).

17. O. Muller and N. Abbas, "The impact of AIDS mortality on children's education in Kampala, Uganda," *AIDS Care* 2(1)(1990):77–80.

18. A. Scitovsky, "The cost of AIDS: An agenda for research," *Health Policy* 11(1989):197–208.

19. D. S. Shepard, "Costs of AIDS in a developing area: Indirect and direct costs of AIDS in Puerto Rico," in *Economic Aspects of AIDS and HIV Infection*, ed. D. Schwefel et al. (Berlin: Springer-Verlag, 1990).

20. R. Tapia-Conyer et al., The economic impact of AIDS in Mexico, presented at the VI International Conference on AIDS, San Francisco, U.S., June 1990.

21. M. Viravaidya, S. Obremskey, and C. Myers, "The economic impact of

AIDS on Thailand," Harvard School of Public Health, Department of Population and International Health, Working Paper no. 4 (March 1992).

22. A. Whiteside, "AIDS in Southern Africa" (Economic Research Unit, University of Natal and Development Bank of Southern Africa, Durban, 1990).

23. M. Ainsworth, M. Over, and J. L. Lamboray, "Economic impact of AIDS in Africa," in *AIDS in Africa*, ed. M. Essex et al. (New York: Raven Press, forthcoming).

24. S. D. Foster, "Affordable clinical care for HIV related illness in developing countries," *Tropical Diseases Bulletin* 87(11)(1990):121–29.

25. S. E. Hassig et al., "An analysis of the economic impact of HIV infection among patients at Mamy Yemo Hospital, Kinshasa, Zaire," *AIDS* 4(1990):883–87.

26. A. Gray, Economic aspects of AIDS and HIV infection in the UK (Department of Public Health and Policy, London School of Hygiene and Tropical Medicine, 1991).

27. K. Tolley and M. Gyldmark, "The cost of treating AIDS and HIV positive patients in an attempt to standardise the cost model," Paper presented at Summer Meeting of HESG, Aberdeen, Scotland, 1991.

28. E. Smith, J. Klemm, and P. Pine, Differential eligibility for public health care financing programs by persons in various stages of HIV infection, Presented at the VI International Conference on AIDS, San Francisco, U.S., June 1990.

29. National Commission on AIDS, *America: Living with AIDS* (Washington, D.C., 1991).

30. American Council of Life Insurance and Health Insurance Association of America, "AIDS Related Claims Survey" (1991).

31. E. A. Preble, "Impact of HIV/AIDS on African children," *Social Science and Medicine* 31(6)(1990):671–80.

7. Achievements in Research

1. For a further discussion of both HIV-1 and HIV-2, see Françoise Barré-Sinoussi, "HIV virus variability" and "The epidemiology of HIV-2 infection" by Kevin De Cock.

2. A. S. Fauci, "Impact of biomedical research on the AIDS epidemic," in *Science Challenging AIDS*, ed. G. B. Rossi et al. (Basel: Karger, 1992), p. 5.

3. Ibid.

4. See Barré-Sinoussi, "HIV virus variability."

5. I. V. D. Weller, "Present outlook for clinical trials," in *Science Challenging AIDS*.

6. I. V. D. Weller, personal communication, 1991.

7. Fauci, "Impact of biomedical research."

8. Food and Drug Administration, *General Considerations for the Clinical Evaluation of Drugs*, HEW 77–3040 (Washington, D.C.: U.S. Government Printing Office, 1977).

9. The Law Center, College of Public and Community Service, University of Massachusetts, Boston, and the Multicultural AIDS Coalition, *Searching for*

Women: A Literature Review on Women, HIV and AIDS in the United States (Boston, 1992).

10. Communication from the American Foundation for AIDS Research (AMFAR), January, 1992.

11. F. Barin, S. M'Boup, F. Denis, et al., "Serological evidence for virus related to simian T-lymphotropic retrovirus III in residents of West Africa," *Lancet* 2(1985):1387–89.

12. F. Clavel, D. Guetard, F. Brun-Vezinet, et al., "Isolation of a new human retrovirus from West African patients with AIDS," *Science* 233(1986):343–46.

13. K. M. De Cock, F. Brun-Vezinet, "Epidemiology of HIV-2," *AIDS* 3(1989):S89–95.

14. K. M. De Cock, F. Brun-Vezinet, and B. Soro, "HIV-1 and HIV-2 infections and AIDS in West Africa," *AIDS* 5(1991):S21–28.

15. De Cock and Brun-Vezinet, "Epidemiology of HIV-2."

16. De Cock, Brun-Vezinet, and Soro, "HIV-1 and HIV-2 infections and AIDS in West Africa."

17. A. Wilkins, R. Hayes, P. Alonso, et al., "Risk factors for HIV-2 infection in The Gambia," *AIDS* 5(1991):1127–32.

18. L. H. Harrison, A. P. J. da Silva, H. D. Gayle, et al., "Risk factors for HIV-2 infection in Guinea Bissau," *Journal of Acquired Immune Deficiency Syndromes* 4(1991):1155–60.

19. A. Del Mistro, J. Chotard, A. J. Hall, et al., "HIV-1 and HIV-2 seroprevalence rates in mother-child pairs living in The Gambia (West Africa)," ibid. 5(1992):19–24.

20. A. G. Poulsen, B. B. Kvinesdal, P. Aaby, et al., "Lack of evidence of vertical transmission of human immunodeficiency virus type 2 in a sample of the general population in Bissau," ibid., pp. 25–30.

21. K. M. De Cock, K. Odehouri, R. L. Colebunders, et al., "A comparison of HIV-1 and HIV-2 infections in hospitalized patients in Abidjan, Côte d'Ivoire," *AIDS* 4(1990):443–48.

22. K. M. De Cock, E. Gnaore, G. Adjorlolo, et al., "Risk of tuberculosis in patients with HIV-I and HIV-II infections in Abidjan, Ivory Coast," *British Medical Journal* 302(1991):496–99.

23. J. Pepin, G. Morgan, D. Dunn, et al., "HIV-2-induced immunosuppression among asymptomatic West African prostitutes: Evidence that HIV-2 is pathogenic but less so than HIV-1," *AIDS* 5(1991):1165–72.

24. Del Mistro et al., "HIV-1 and HIV-2 seroprevalence rates in mother-child pairs."

25. De Cock and Brun-Vezinet, "Epidemiology of HIV-2."

26. Ibid.

27. Del Mistro et al., "HIV-1 and HIV-2 seroprevalence rates in mother-child pairs."

28. L. Thior, T. Siby, I. Traore, et al., L'histoire naturelle du VIH-2 au Sénégal: Cas cliniques au sein d'une cohorte de prostituées, presented at the VI International Conference on AIDS in Africa, Dakar, Senegal, December 1991.

29. Sebastian B. Lucas, personal communication, 1991.

8. National AIDS Programs

1. In this instance, the survey covered a period beginning in the mid-1980s. Thus, certain countries that have become divided since that time—in particular the USSR and Czechoslovakia—are included as single entities here.

2. Using a score applied to 40 indicators, the Index is meant to reflect the extent to which people enjoy cultural, social, economic, and political freedom; United Nations Development Program (UNDP), *Human Development Report 1991*, p. 20.

3. World Health Assembly, Resolution WHA 40. 26, Global Strategy for the Prevention and Control of AIDS, Geneva, WHO, 5 May 1987.

4. Ibid.

5. *WHO AIDS Series 1: Guidelines for the Development of National AIDS Control Programs* (Geneva, 1987–88).

6. J. Mann and K. Kay, "Confronting the pandemic: The World Health Organization's Global Programme on AIDS, 1986–1989," *AIDS* 5 Suppl. 1 (1991):S221–28.

7. K. S. M. Matomora, J.-L. Lamboray, et al., "Integration of AIDS program activities into national health systems," *AIDS* 5 Suppl. 1(1991):S193–96.

8. G. Lewis, J. Finlay, and R. Widdus, AIDS programmes in transition. *World Health Forum*, vol. 12 (1991).

9. See Pan American Health Organization (PAHO), "Nongovernmental Organizations," SPP15/5 (1990).

10. For a general description and elaboration of these NGO typologies, see David Korten, *Getting to the 21st Century* (West Hartford: Kumerian Press, 1990). For relevance to AIDS groups, see Tim Brodhead and Jeff O'Malley, "NGOs and Third World Development: Opportunities and Constraints," WHO/GPA/GMC(2)/ 89.5(1989), and the work of Pamela Hartigan at PAHO, especially "Non-Governmental Organizations."

11. Statistics were published in *AIDS & Society* 3(1), using the Inventory of Nongovernmental Organizations Working on AIDS in Countries That Receive Development Cooperation or Assistance, WHO/GPA/DIR/90.5.

12. J. Shepard, C. Cameron, G. Gizaw, et al., Rapid assessment of national AIDS programme costs, presented at the VI International Conference on AIDS, San Francisco, U.S., June 1990.

13. *AIDS in the World* survey and personal communication with National AIDS Program, Thailand.

14. D. Shepard and R. Bail, "Costs of care for persons with AIDS in Rwanda," consultants' report (Geneva, WHO Global Programme on AIDS, 1991).

15. WHO/Global Programme on AIDS, Review of six HIV/AIDS home care programmes in Uganda and Zambia (Geneva, 1991); B. W. Victor, *AIDS in a Caring Society* (Stockholm: Nordic School of Public Health and the Danish Research Council for Health Sciences, 1991).

16. C. Cameron and D. Schopper, Trip report and followup trip report. Costs of treatment of AIDS patients at Bamrasnaradura Hospital, Bangkok, Thailand, June and August 1990. In M. Viravaidya, S. Obremskey, and C. Myers, "The economic impact of AIDS on Thailand," Harvard School of Public Health, Department of Population and International Health, Working Paper no. 4 (March 1992).

17. C. Cameron and J. Shepard, "Resource allocation assessment of Swiss AIDS programme: Final report," Consultants' report (Geneva: WHO Global Programme on AIDS, 1990).

18. M. Bez, SIDA et Hôpital: Les chiffres clés (Paris: CISIH, Ministère des Affaires Sociales et de l'Intégration, September 1991).

19. U.S. Department of Health and Human Services, Health Care Financing Administration, Office of the Actuary, Baltimore, Md. (1992).

20. K. Davis, R. Bialek, C. Beyrer, et al., *Financing health care for persons with HIV disease: Policy options,* Technical report for the National Commission on AIDS, August 1991.

21. Robert Wood Johnson Foundation, *Challenges in Health Care: A Chartbook Perspective 1991.* (Princeton, N.J., 1991).

22. J. Iglehart, "Health policy report: Financing the struggle against AIDS," *New England Journal of Medicine* 317(3)(1987):180–184; J. Iglehart et al., "The socioeconomic impact of AIDS on health care systems," *Health Affairs* 6(3)(1987):137–47.

23. Robert Wood Johnson Foundation, *Challenges in Health Care.*

24. Viravaidya, Obremskey, and Myers, "The economic impact of AIDS on Thailand."

25. New York: Macmillan, 1987, p. xiii.

9. Prevention

1. N. Ferencic, P. Alexander, G. Slutkin, et al., Study to review effectiveness and coverage of current sex-work interventions in developing countries, presented at the VII International AIDS Conference, Florence, Italy, June 1991.

2. For futher discussion of the uses of information, see P. Brown, "AIDS and the Media," and P. Piotrow, "AIDS and Mass Persuasion," in Chapter 16.

3. F. Mhalu, K. Hirji, P. Ijumba, et al., "A cross-sectional study of a program for HIV infection control among public house workers," *Journal of Acquired Immune Deficiency Syndromes* 4(1991):290–96.

4. E. N. Ngugi, personal communication, 1992.

5. S. Hassig, AIDSTECH, personal communication, 1992.

6. R. Pleak and H. F. L. Meyer-Bahlberg, "Sexual behavior and AIDS knowledge of young male prostitutes in Manhattan," *Journal of Sex Research* 27(1990):557–87.

7. E. Van de Walle, "The social impact of AIDS in sub-Saharan Africa," *Milbank Quarterly* 68(1990):10–32.

8. J. O. Chikwem, S. D. Chikwem, and T. O. Ola, "Evaluation of public

awareness and attitudes to acquired immune deficiency syndrome (AIDS)," *Nigerian Medical Practitioner* 16(1988):159–63.

9. D. Wilson and A. Mehryar, "The role of the AIDS knowledge, attitudes, beliefs and practices research in sub-Saharan Africa," *AIDS* 5 Suppl. 1(1991):S177–81.

10. P. Selwyn, C. Feiner, C. Lipshutz, et al., "Knowledge about AIDS and high-risk behavior among IDUs in New York City," *AIDS* 1(1987):247–54.

11. P. Kleinman, D. Goldsmith, S. Friedman, et al., "Knowledge about behaviors affecting the spread of AIDS: A survey of IDUs and their associates in New York City," *International Journal of the Addictions* 25(1990):345–61.

12. C. S. Weisman, C. A. Nathanson, M. Ensminger, et al., "AIDS clients of a family planning clinic," *Family Planning Perspectives* 21(1989):213–17.

13. V. Seltzer, J. Rabin, and F. Benjamin, "Teenagers' awareness of the acquired immunodeficiency syndrome and the impact on their sexual behavior," *Obstetrics Gynecology* 74(1989):55–58.

14. M. J. Rotheram-Borus and C. Koopman, "Sexual risk behavior, AIDS knowledge, and beliefs about AIDS among predominantly minority gay and bisexual male adolescents," *AIDS Education and Prevention* 3(4)(1991):305–12.

15. P. Lorenzetti, P. Rossi, L. Armignacco, et al., "AIDS-related knowledge and behaviors among teenagers—Italy, 1990," *Morbidity and Mortality Weekly Report* 40(1990):214–21.

16. C. S. Landefeld, M. M. Chren, J. Shega, et al., "Students' sexual behavior, knowledge, and attitudes relating to the acquired immunodeficiency syndrome," *Journal of General Internal Medicine* 3:161–65.

17. L. Carroll, "Gender differences in AIDS knowledge among students in an Eastern University," *Social Science Research* 74:212–21.

18. S. B. Thomas, A. G. Gilliam, and C. G. Iwrey, "Knowledge about AIDS and reported risk behaviors among black college students," *Journal of American College Health* 38:61–66.

19. L. A. Gray and M. Saracino, "College students' attitudes, beliefs, and behaviors about AIDS: Implications for family life educators" (Corvallis, Ore.: Department of Counseling, College of Education, Oregon State University, 1990).

20. C. Abraham, P. Sheeran, D. Abrams, et al., "Young people learning about AIDS: A study of beliefs and information sources," *Health Education Research* 6(1991):19–29.

21. D. Romer and R. Hornik, "AIDS education for youth: An approach to choosing messages and channels," Center for International, Health, and Development Communication, University of Pennsylvania, Working Paper no. 127.

22. A. J. Ibanga, E. E. Williams, and I. J. Ibanga, Undergraduate students and AIDS: A study of knowledge, attitudes, and practices in Calabar, Nigeria, presented at the I International Conference on AIDS, Amsterdam, Netherlands, 1985.

23. H. G. Miller, C. F. Turner, and L. E. Moses, eds., *AIDS: The Second Decade* (Washington, D.C.: National Academy Press, 1990).

24. R. W. Hingson, L. Strunin, B. M. Berlin, and T. Heeren, "Beliefs about

AIDS, use of alcohol, drugs and unprotected anal sex among Massachusetts adolescents," *American Journal of Public Health* 80(1990):295–99.

25. S. T. Sugerman, A. C. Hergenroeder, M. R. Chacko, and G. S. Parcel, "Acquired immunodeficiency syndrome and adolescents: Knowledge, attitudes, and behaviors of runaway and homeless youths," *American Journal of Diseases in Children* 145(1991):431–35.

26. L. A. Kurdek and G. Siesky, "The nature and correlates of psychological adjustment in gay men with AIDS-related conditions," *Journal of Applied Social Psychology* 20(1990):846–60.

27. A. Prieur, "The dangers of love," in *Changing Sexual Behaviors in the Shadow of AIDS*, ed. M. Cohen (New York: Plenum, forthcoming).

28. K. Siegel, P. Grodsky, and A. Herman, "AIDS risk-reduction guideline: A review and analysis," *Journal of Community Health* 2(1986):233–43.

29. E. de Vroome, M. E. Paalman, T. G. Sandfort, et al., "AIDS in the Netherlands: The effects of several years of campaigning," *International Journal of STDs and AIDS* 1(1990):268–75.

30. K. de Vries, E. de Vroome, T. G. Sandfort, et al., The effectiveness of the 1989 multi-media safe sex campaign in the Netherlands, presented at the I European Conference on Effective Health Education, Rotterdam, Netherlands, December 1989.

31. P. Weatherburn, P. Davies, and A. Hunt, "The response to AIDS in the London gay community," in Cohen, *Changing Sexual Behaviors*.

32. B. Robert and S. Rosser, "Evaluation of the efficacy of AIDS education interventions for homosexually active men," *Health Education Research* 5(1990):299–308.

33. M. Cohen and T. Sandfort, Theory: A practical guide to synchronizing HIV prevention with stage of the HIV epidemic, presented at the V Conference on the Social Aspects of AIDS, London, U.K., March 1991.

34. R. Mullins, "Reading ability and the use of condoms," *Medical Journal of Australia* 151(1989):358–59.

35. J. Drosin, J. Price, J. Spilsbury, and W. Martin, Condom sales and protection through non-traditional outlets: An evaluation of the Zaire social marketing program, presented at the 1991 AIDS Prevention Conference, USAID, Rosslyn, Virginia, November 1991.

36. F. Wasserfallen and R. Staub, "The gay community response to AIDS in Switzerland," in Cohen, *Changing Sexual Behaviors*.

37. P. M'Pelé, personal communication, Congo, 1992.

38. R. C. Hornik, "Channel effectiveness in development communication programs" (Philadelphia: Annenberg School of Communications, 1991).

39. T. Edgar, S. Hammond, F. Lee, and S. Vicki, "The role of the mass media and interpersonal communication in promoting AIDS-related behavioral change," *AIDS Public Policy Journal* 4(1990):3–9.

40. E. Stoller and G. Rutherford, "Evaluation of AIDS prevention and control programs," *Current Science Ltd.* 3(1989):S289–96.

41. J. Martin, L. Dean, M. Barcia, and W. N. Hall, "The impact of AIDS on

a gay community: Changes in sexual behavior, substance use, and mental health," *American Journal of Community Psychology* 17(1987):269–93.

42. R. Stall and J. Paul, "Changes in sexual risk for infection with the HIV virus among gay and bisexual men in San Francisco," in Cohen, *Changing Sexual Behaviors*.

43. G. Dowsett, S. Kippax, R. W. Connell, and J. Crawford, "The contribution of the gay community to sexual behavior change among homosexually active men in Australia," ibid.

44. T. Myers, D. McLeod, and L. Calzavara, "Responses of gay and bisexual men to HIV/AIDS in Toronto, Canada: Community-based initiatives, AIDS education and sexual behavior," ibid.

45. D. Hausser, E. Zimmerman, F. Dubois-Arder, and F. Paccaud, "Evaluation of the AIDS prevention strategy in Switzerland" (Lausanne: Institut universitaire de médecine sociale et préventive, 1991).

46. H. J. A. van Haastrecht, J. A. R. van den Hoek, and R. A. Coutinho, "Evidence for a change in behavior among heterosexuals in Amsterdam under the influence of AIDS," *Genitourinary Medicine* 67:199–206.

47. K. Wellings, personal communication, 1992.

48. S. D. Cochran, J. Keidan, and A. Kalechstein, "Sexually transmitted diseases and acquired immunodeficiency syndrome (AIDS): Changes in risk reduction behaviors among young adults," *Sexually Transmitted Diseases* 17(1990):80–86.

49. E. de Vroome, T. Sandfort, and R. Tielman, Sources of information used and the adoption of safer sex among men, Presented at the VII International Conference on AIDS, Florence, Italy, June 1991.

50. J. de Wit, E. de Vroome, T. Sandfort, et al., "Effects of coping style and health locus of control on changes in sexual behavior in a cohort of homosexual men" (Gay and Lesbian Studies, University of Utrecht, Netherlands, 1990).

51. M. Ekstrand and T. Coates, "Maintenance of safer sexual behaviors and predictors of risky sex: The San Francisco Men's Health Study," *American Journal of Public Health* 80(1990):973–77.

52. M. Pollak and J. P. Moatti, HIV-risk perception and determinants of sexual behavior, Workshop of Sexual Behavior and Risk of HIV Infection, Brussels, Belgium, 1989.

53. N. Hessol, A. Lifton, P. O'Malley, et al., "Prevalence, incidence and progression of HIV infection in homosexual and bisexual men in hepatitis B vaccine trials, 1987–88," *American Journal of Epidemiology* 130(1989):1167–75.

54. M. Ross, B. Freedman, and R. Brew, "Changes in sexual behavior between 1986 and 1988 in matched samples of homosexually active men," *Community Health Studies* 8(1989):276–80.

55. J. Martin et al., "The impact of AIDS on a gay community."

56. van Haastrecht et al., "Evidence for a change in behavior among heterosexuals in Amsterdam under the influence of AIDS."

57. D. Serwadda, M. Wawer, S. Musgrave, and J. Konde-Lule, An assessment of the AIDS-related knowledge, attitudes, and practices in Rakai District, Uganda,

presented at the V International Conference on AIDS, Montreal, Canada, June 1989.

58. A. Prieur, "Norwegian gay men: Reasons for continued practice of unsafe sex," *AIDS Education and Prevention* 2(1990):109–15.

59. A. Hunt and P. Davies, "What is a sexual encounter?" in *AIDS: Responses, Interventions and Care*, ed. P. Aggleton, G. Hart, and P. Davies (London: Falmer Press, 1991).

60. M. Cohen, "Changing to safe sex: Personality, logic and habit," in Aggleton, Hart, and Davies, *AIDS: Responses, Interventions and Care*.

61. B. Spencer, Institutional barriers to condom promotion: The forgotten factor? presented at the V Conference on the Social Aspects of AIDS, London, U.K., March 1991.

62. R. Wallace, "A synergism of plagues: 'Planned shrinkage,' contagious housing destruction, and AIDS in the Bronx," *Environmental Research* 47(1988):1–33.

63. E. M. Ankrah, Women and AIDS in Africa: Socio-cultural issues of empowerment, presented at AIDS and Reproductive Health: Agenda for Research and Action, Bellagio, Italy, November 1990.

64. M. T. Bassett and M. Mhloyi, "Women and AIDS in Zimbabwe: The making of an epidemic," *International Journal of Health Services* 21:143–56.

65. See Chapter 16, "AIDS and Mass Persuasion."

66. D. Dwyer, R. Howard, J. Downie, and A. N. Cunningham, "The grim reaper campaign," *Medical Journal of Australia* 149(1988):49–50.

67. Ibid.

68. H. Nicholas, L. Glover, D. Parr, et al., The effect of a government AIDS media campaign on a general population, presented at the III International Conference on AIDS, Washington, D.C., June 1987.

69. *The World's Women, 1991* (New York: United Nations, 1991).

70. M. J. Rotheram-Borus, M. Rosario, and C. Koopman, "Minority youths at high risk: Gay males and runaways," in *Adolescent Stress: Causes and Consequences*, ed. M. Colten and S. Gore (New York: Aldine de Gruyter, 1991).

71. B. Goldman, "Health of Toronto's street kids disturbing, study reveals," *Canadian Medical Association Journal* 138(1988):1041–43.

72. Sugerman et al., "Acquired immunodeficiency syndrome and adolescents."

73. Goldman, "Health of Toronto's street kids disturbing."

74. C. B. Boyer and S. M. Kegeles, "AIDS risk and prevention among adolescents," *Social Science and Medicine* 33(1991):11–23.

75. R. Pleak and H. Meyer-Bahlberg, "Sexual behavior and AIDS knowledge of young male prostitutes in Manhattan," *Journal of Sex Research* 27(1990):557–87.

76. J. Ross, M. Rich, J. Molzen, and M. Pensak, *Family Planning Child Survival: 100 Developing Countries* (New York: U.S. Center for Population and Family Health, Columbia University, 1988).

77. Sugerman et al., "Acquired immunodeficiency syndrome and adolescents."

78. N. E. MacDonald, G. A. Wells, W. A. Fisher, et al., "High-risk STD/HIV: Behavior among college students," *Journal of the American Medical Association* 263(1990):3155–59.

79. J. Mantell and S. Schinke, "The crisis of AIDS for adolescents: The need for preventive risk-reduction interventions," in *Contemporary Perspectives on Crisis Intervention* (Bloomington: Indiana University Press, 1987).

80. M. J. Rotheram-Borus and C. Koopman, "AIDS and adolescents," in *Encyclopedia of Adolescence,* ed. R. M. Lerner, A. C. Petersen, and J. Brooks-Gunn (New York and London: Garland Publishing, 1991).

81. Gray and Saracino, "College students' attitudes, beliefs, and behaviors about AIDS."

82. D. Rosenthal, S. Moore, and I. Brumen, "Ethnic group differences in adolescents' responses to AIDS," *Australian Journal of Social Issues* 25(1990): 220–39.

83. W. Belschner, A. Engel, H. Henicz, and S. Muller-Doohm, Sexual behavior of adolescents against the backgrounds of AIDS (Research Group Health Promotion, University of Oldenburg, Germany, 1991).

84. L. W. Svenson and C. K. Varnhagen, "Knowledge, attitudes and behaviours related to AIDS among first-year university students," *Canadian Journal of Public Health* 81(1990):139–40.

85. E. Segest, O. Mygind, W. Jorgensen, and M. Bechgaard, "Free condoms in youth clubs in Copenhagen," *Journal of Adolescence* 13(1990):17–24.

86. M. K. Strader and M. L. Beaman, "Comparison of selected college students' and sexually transmitted disease clinic patients' knowledge about AIDS, risk behaviors and beliefs," *Journal of Advanced Nursing* 16(1991):584–89.

87. MacDonald et al., "High-risk STD/HIV."

88. C. R. Baffi, K. K. Shroeder, K. J. Redican, and L. McCluskey, "Factors influencing selected heterosexual male college students' condom use," *Journal of American College Health* 38(1989):137–41.

89. P. Aggleton and I. Warwick, Young people, adolescents and AIDS research, presented at the IV Conference on the Social Aspects of AIDS, London, U.K., April 1990.

90. Boyer and Kegeles, "AIDS risk and prevention."

91. C. Koopman, M. J. Rotheram-Borus, R. Henderson, et al., "Assessment of knowledge of AIDS and beliefs about AIDS prevention among adolescents," *AIDS Education and Prevention* 2(1990):58–69.

92. D. Romer and R. Hornik, "Using mass media for prevention of HIV infection among adolescents," in *Adolescents and AIDS: A Generation in Jeopardy,* ed. R. J. Clemente (Newbury Park, Calif.: Sage, 1992).

93. Aggleton and Warwick, Young people, adolescents and AIDS research.

94. Mantell and Schinke, "The crisis of AIDS for adolescents."

95. J. Brooks-Gunn and F. F. Furstenberg, Jr., "Coming of age in the era of AIDS: Puberty, sexuality, and contraception," *Milbank Quarterly* 68(1990):59–83.

96. S. Clift and D. Stears, "Moral perspectives and safer sex practice: Two themes in teaching about HIV and AIDS in secondary schools," in Aggleton, Hart, and Davies, *AIDS: Responses, Interventions and Care.*

97. R. Valdiserri, *Preventing AIDS: The Design of Effective Programs* (New Brunswick, N.J.: Rutgers University Press, 1989).

98. "Introduction: An overview of AIDS and women's health," in *AIDS and Women's Reproductive Health,* ed. L. C. Chen, J. Sepulveda-Amor, and S. J. Segal (New York: Plenum, 1992).

99. P. A. Selwyn, E. E. Schoenbaum, D. Davenny, et al., "Prospective study of human immunodeficiency virus infection and pregnancy outcomes in intravenous drug users," *Journal of the American Medical Association* 261 (1989):1289–94.

100. R. W. Ryder, V. L. Batter, M. Nsuami, et al., "Fertility rates in 238 HIV-1 seropositive women in Zaire followed for 3 years postpartum," AIDS 5(1991): 1521–27.

101. M. Potts, R. Anderson, and M. C. Boily, "Slowing the spread of human immunodeficiency virus in developing countries," *Lancet* 338(1991):608–13.

102. S. Day, "Prostitute women and AIDS: Anthropology," *AIDS* 2(1988):421–28.

103. D. Wilson, P. Chiroro, S. Lavelle, and C. Mutero, "Sex workers and client sex behaviour and condom use in Harare, Zimbabwe" (Department of Psychology, University of Zimbabwe, Harare, 1991).

104. Day, "Prostitute women and AIDS."

105. J. A. Inciardi, A. E. Pottieger, M. A. Forney, et al., "Prostitution, IV drug use, and sex-for-crack exchanges among serious delinquents: Risk for HIV infection," *Criminology* 29(1991):221–35.

106. W. Sittitrai, T. Brown, and S. Virulrak, "Patterns of bisexuality in Thailand," in *Bisexuality and HIV/AIDS: A Global Perspective,* ed. R. A. P. Tielman, Manuel Carballo, and A. C. Hendriks (Buffalo: Prometheus Books, 1991).

107. H. Miller, C. Turner, and L. Moses, "Interventions for female prostitutes," in idem, *AIDS: The Second Decade.*

108. J. Joseph, S. Montgomery, et al., "Magnitude and determinants of behavioral risk reduction: Longitudinal analysis of a cohort at risk for AIDS," *Psychology and Health* 1(1987):73–86.

109. S. Perry, L. Jacobsberg, and K. Fogel, "Orogenital transmission of human immunodeficiency virus (HIV)," *Annals of Internal Medicine* 111(11) (1989):951–52.

110. M. Boulton, "Review of the literature on bisexuality and HIV transmission," in Tielman, Carballo, and Hendriks, *Bisexuality and HIV/AIDS.*

111. Stall and Paul, "Changes in sexual risk for infection in San Francisco."

112. Dowsett et al., "The contribution of the gay community."

113. Boulton, "Review of the literature."

114. R. Hays, S. Kegeles, and T. Coates, "High HIV risk-taking among young gay men," *AIDS* 4(1990):901–07.

115. Sittitrai and Brown, "Patterns of bisexuality in Thailand."

116. I. Prochazka, R. Prusa, and J. Svoboda, "Men having sex with men: Behavioral changes in Czechoslovakia," in Cohen, *Changing Sexual Behaviors.*

117. B. Kumar, "Patterns of bisexuality in India," in Tielman, Carballo, and Hendriks, *Bisexuality and HIV/AIDS.*

118. M. E. Cohen, Using theoretical frameworks to evaluate HIV prevention programs, presented at the VII International Conference on AIDS, Florence, Italy, June 1991.

119. J. B. Brunet, Director, Centre Européen pour la Surveillance Epidémiologique du SIDA, personal communication, 1991.

120. Stall and Paul, "Changes in sexual risk for infection in San Francisco."

121. M. Bochow, "Reactions of the gay community to AIDS in East and West Berlin," in Cohen, *Changing Sexual Behaviors.*

122. Wasserfallen and Staub, "The gay community response."

123. M. D. Davis, U. Klemmer, and G. W. Dowsett, "Bisexually active men and beats: Theoretical and educational implications" (AIDS Council of New South Wales and MacQuarie University, Australia, December 1991).

124. M. Cohen, "Changing to safer sex: Personality, logic and habit," in Aggleton, Hart, and Davies, *AIDS: Responses, Interventions and Care.*

125. Robert and Rosser, "Evaluation of the efficacy of AIDS education."

126. E. de Vroome, T. Sandfort, and R. Tielman, Sources of information used and the adoption of safer sex among gay men, presented at the VII International Conference on AIDS, Florence, Italy, June 1991.

127. D. Ostrow, "AIDS prevention through effective education," *Daedalus* 118(1989):229–53.

128. Dowsett et al., "The contribution of the gay community."

129. C. Frutchey, "The role of community-based organizations in AIDS and STD prevention," in *Promoting Safer Sex*, ed. M. Paalman (Amsterdam: Swets Zeitlinger, 1989).

130. A. Roumeliotou, G. Tapoutsaki, G. Kallinikos, et al., Prevention of HIV infection in Greek registered prostitutes: A five-year study, presented at the VI International Conference on AIDS, San Francisco, U.S., June 1990.

131. E. N. Ngugi, F. A. Plummer, J. N. Simonsen, et al., "Prevention of transmission of human immunodeficiency virus in Africa: Effectiveness of condom promotion and health education among prostitutes," *Lancet* 2(8616)(1988):887–90.

132. F. Mhalu, K. Hirji, P. Ljumba, et al., "A cross-sectional study of a program for HIV infection control among public house workers," *Journal of Acquired Immune Deficiency Syndromes* 4(3)(1991):290–96.

133. R. Detels, P. English, B. R. Visscher, et al., "Seroconversion, sexual activity, and condom use among 2,915 HIV seronegative men followed for up to 2 years," ibid. 2(1)(1989):77–83.

134. M. A. Fischl, G. M. Dickinson, G. B. Scott, et al., "Evaluation of heterosexual partners, children, and household contacts of adults with AIDS," *Journal of the American Medical Association* 257(5)(1987):640–44.

135. de Vries et al., The effectiveness of the 1989 multi-media safe sex campaign in the Netherlands.

136. S. Tipping, Male approval and acceptance of condoms in diverse cultural settings: The SOMARC social marketing experience, presented at the National Family Planning and Reproductive Health Association Conference, Washington, D.C., 1991.

137. S. Hassig, AIDSTECH, personal communication, 1992.

138. M. J. Rotheram-Borus, C. Koopman, C. Haignere, and M. Davies, "Reducing HIV sexual risk behaviors among runaway adolescents," *Journal of the American Medical Association* 266(1991):1237–41.

139. R. O. Valdiserri, D. W. Lyter, L. C. Leviton, et al., "AIDS prevention in homosexual and bisexual men: Results of a randomized trial evaluating two risk reduction interventions," *AIDS* 3(1989):21–26.

140. J. Kelly, J. St. Lawrence, T. Brasfield, et al., "AIDS risk behavior patterns among gay men in small southern cities," *American Journal of Public Health* 80(1990):416–18.

141. L. Denelegi, J. Weber, and S. Toquato, "Drug users' AIDS-related knowledge, attitudes and behaviors before and after AIDS education sessions," *Public Health Reports* 105(1990):504–10.

142. S. Friedman, M. Levine, and K. Siegel, "AIDS: The formulation of a sociological perspective" (Chicago: Society for the Study of Social Problems, 1986).

143. S. Hassig, AIDSTECH, personal communication, 1992.

144. R. Fox, N. Odaka, R. Brookmeyer, and N. F. Polk, "Effect of HIV antibody disclosure on subsequent sexual activity in homosexual men," *AIDS* 1(1987):241–46.

145. N. R. Barling and S. M. Moore, "Adolescents' attitudes towards AIDS, precautions, and intention to use condoms," *Psychological Reports* (1990):883–90.

146. M. W. Ross, "Attitudes towards condoms and condom use: A review," *International Journal of STDs and AIDS* 3(1992):10–16.

147. Baffi et al., "Factors influencing male college students' condom use."

148. R. Fitzpatrick, J. McLean, M. Boulton, and G. Hart, "Factors influencing condom use in a sample of homosexually active men," *Genitourinary Medicine* 66(1990):346–50.

149. Robert and Rosser, "Evaluation of the efficacy of AIDS education."

150. Strader and Baeman, "Comparison of selected college students' and patients' knowledge about AIDS."

151. G. Ahmed, E. C. Liner, N. E. Williamson, and W. P. Schellstede, "Characteristics of condom use and associated problems: Experience in Bangladesh," *Contraception* 42(5)(1990):523–33.

152. Prieur, "Norwegian gay men."

153. D. Kleiber, M. Wilke, and E. Kreilkamp, AIDS and sex tourism (Sozialpädagogisches Institut Berlin, Germany, 1992).

154. L. Liskin, C. Wharton, R. Blackburn, and P. Kestelman, "Population reports: Condoms—now more than ever," *Population Reports* 18(1990).

155. D. Blairman, address at inter-agency consultation to discuss strategies for coordinating and improving global condom supply, Geneva, February 1990.

156. L. Schwab-Zabin, P. T. Piotrow, L. S. Liskin, and R. Weinick, "Lessons from family planning and their application to AIDS prevention" (Geneva: World Health Organization, 1990).

157. E. F. Jones, J. D. Forrest, N. Goldman, et al., "Teenage pregnancy in developed countries: Determinants and policy implications," *Family Planning Perspectives* 17(2)(1985):53–63.

158. Liskin et al., "Population reports."

159. D. Romer and R. Hornik, "Condom social marketing as an AIDS prevention strategy," Report prepared for the WHO Global Programme on AIDS, University of Pennsylvania, 1991.

160. P. Koder and E. L. Roberto, *Social Marketing* (New York: Free Press, 1989).

161. Ahmed et al., "Characteristics of condom use."

162. C. Baudry, "Le SIDA en questions," *50 Millions de Connommateurs* 2(1991):50–59.

163. M. D. Brown, "Spermicidal condoms," *Kansas Medicine* 89(4)(1988): 114–15.

164. S. Townsend, "Spermicides for family planning and disease prevention: An update," *Family Health International Network* 12(3)(1991).

165. K. Turjanmaa and T. Reunala, "Allergic reactions to rubber condoms," *Genitourinary Medicine* 65(6)(1989):402–03.

166. K. Turjanmaa and T. Reunala, "Condoms as a source of latex allergen and cause of contact urticaria," *Contact Dermatitis* 20(5)(1989):360–64.

167. R. Stube, B. Voeller, and A. Davidhazy, "High-speed cinematography of the initial break-point of latex condoms during the air burst test," *Contraception* 41(6)(1991):591–603.

168. M. J. Free, J. Hutchings, F. Lubis, and R. Natakusumah, "An assessment of burst strength distribution data for monitoring quality of condom stocks in developing countries," *Contraception* 33(3)(1986):285–99.

169. J. Gerofi, G. Shelley, and B. Donovan, "A study of the relationship between tensile testing of condoms and breakage in use," *Contraception* 43(2)(1991):177–85.

170. R. Foldesy, E. Carter, and B. Voeller, quoted in "Condom manufacturing standards improving," *Family Health International Network* 12(3)(1991).

171. Free et al., "An assessment of burst strength distribution data."

172. Ibid.

173. M. J. Free, personal communication, 1992.

174. L. J. Clark, R. P. Sherwin, and R. F. Baker, "Latex condom deterioration accelerated by environmental factors: I. Ozone," *Contraception* 39(3)(1989):245–51.

175. R. F. Baker, R. P. Sherwin, G. S. Bernstein, et al., "Precautions when lightning strikes during the monsoon: The effect of ozone on condoms" (letter), *Journal of the American Medical Association* 260(10)(1988)1404–05.

176. B. Voeller, A. Coulson, G. S. Bernstein, and R. M. Nakamura, "Mineral oil lubricants cause rapid deterioration of latex condoms," *Contraception* 39(1)(1989):95–102.

177. D. J. Martin, "A study of the deficiencies in the condom-use skills of gay men," *Public Health Reports* 105(6):638–40.

178. C. Chan-Chee, I. de Vincenzi, M. Sole-Pla, et al., "Use and misuse of condoms" (letter), *Genitourinary Medicine* 67(2)(1991):173.

179. G. A. Richwald, M. A. Wamsley, A. H. Coulson, and D. E. Morisky, "Are condom instructions readable? Results of a readability study," *Public Health Reports* 103(4)(1988):355–59.

180. R. M. Mullins, "Reading ability and the use of condoms" (letter), *Medical Journal of Australia* 151(6)(1989):358–59.

181. National Research Council; Committee on AIDS Research and the Behavioral, Social and Statistical Sciences; and Commission on the Behavioral and Social Sciences and Education, *AIDS: Sexual Behavior and Intravenous Drug Use*, ed. C. Turner, H. Miller, and L. Moses (Washington, D.C.: National Academy of Sciences, 1989).

182. The Law Center, College of Public and Community Service, University of Massachusetts, Boston, and the Multicultural AIDS Coalition, *Searching for Women: A Literature Review on Women, HIV and AIDS in the United States* (Boston, 1992).

183. Department of Epidemic Prevention, Ministry of Health, Epidemiology and Prevention of HIV/AIDS in China.

184. J. M. N. Ch'ien, B. C. Low, and F. C. Mau, Report on the Street Addicts Survey on AIDS Awareness (1991).

185. F. C. Mesquita, A. R. Moss, A. L. Reingold, et al., Pilot study of HIV antibody seroprevalence among injection drug users in the city of Santos, Sao Paulo State, Brazil, presented at the VII International Conference on AIDS, Florence, Italy, June 1991.

186. T. E. Feucht, R. C. Stephens, and S. W. Roman, "The sexual behavior of intravenous drug users: Assessing the risk of sexual transmission of HIV," *Journal of Drug Issues* 29(2)(1990):195–213.

187. Ibid.

188. P. W. Brickner, R. A. Torres, M. Barnes, et al., "Recommendations for control and prevention of human immunodeficiency virus (HIV) infection in injection drug users," *Annals of Internal Medicine* 110(19)(1989):833–37.

189. R. P. Brettle, "HIV and harm reduction for injecting drug users" (editorial review), *AIDS* 5(1991):125–36.

190. H. R. Guydish, A. Abramowitz, W. Woods, et al., "Changes in needle-sharing behavior among intravenous drug users: San Francisco, 1986–1988," *American Journal of Public Health* 80(8)(1990):995–97.

191. G. J. Hart, A. L. M. Carvell, N. Woodward, et al., "Evaluation of needle exchange in Central London: Behaviour change and anti-HIV status over one year," *AIDS* 3(1989):261–65.

192. C. F. Robert, J. J. Deglon, J. Wintsch, et al., "Behavioral changes in

intravenous drug users in Geneva: Rise and fall of HIV infection 1980–1989," *AIDS* 4(1990):657–60.

193. J. R. Robertson, C. A. Skidmore, and J. J. K. Roberts, "Infection in intravenous drug users: A follow-up study indicating changes in risk-taking behaviour," *British Journal of the Addictions* 83(1988):387–91.

194. S. Salmaso, S. Conti, H. Sasse, et al., "Drug use and HIV-1 infection: Report from the second Italian Multicenter Study," *Journal of Acquired Immune Deficiency Syndromes* 4(6)(1991):607–13.

195. K. Dolan, G. V. Stimson, and M. C. Donoghoe. Differences in HIV rates and risk behavior of drug injectors attending, and not attending, syringe exchanges in England, presented at the VI International Conference on AIDS, San Francisco, U.S., June 1990.

196. International Narcotics Control Board, Report of the International Narcotics Control Board, 1990.

197. Ministries of Health, Czech and Slovak Federal Republic, Short-term plan for the prevention and control of AIDS in Czechoslovakia (1990).

198. A. F. H. Britten, Role of League of Red Cross and Red Crescent Societies, WHO document GBSI/GPA/15E (Geneva, 1988).

199. A. F. H. Britten, Global blood safety initiative—Data provided by the League of Red Cross and Red Crescent Societies, WHO document GBSI/GPA/3E (Geneva, 1988).

200. J. Leikola, "How much blood for the world?" *Vox Sang* 54(1988):1–5.

201. WHO, Blood and blood products: Report by the Director-General, Executive Board document EB/79/7 Add. (Geneva, 1987).

202. Ibid.

203. J. Emmanuel and A. Britten, "Reducing HIV transmission through blood," in *Handbook for AIDS Prevention in Africa*, ed. P. Lamptey et al. (Durham, N.C.: Family Health International 1990).

204. Ibid.

205. Ibid.

206. Britten, Role of League of Red Cross and Red Crescent Societies.

207. A. F. H. Britten, "Worldwide supply of blood and blood products," *World Journal of Surgery* 11(1987):82–85.

208. WHO, Blood and blood products.

209. Britten, "Worldwide supply of blood and blood products."

210. WHO, Utilization and supply of human blood and blood products, Document A28/WP/6 (May 1975).

211. Ibid.

212. Britten, "Worldwide supply of blood and blood products."

213. M. G. Smith, "Propagation in tissue cultures of a cytopathogenic virus from human salivary gland virus (SGV) disease," *Proceedings of the Society for Experimental Biology and Medicine*, 92(1956):424–30.

214. W. P. Rowe, J. W. Hartley, S. Waterman, et al., "Cytopathogenic agent resembling human salivary gland virus recovered from tissue cultures of human adenoids," ibid., pp. 418–24.

215. T. H. Weller, J. C. Macauley, J. M. Craig, et al., "Isolation of intranuclear inclusion producing agents from infants with illnesses resembling cytomegatic inclusion disease," ibid. 94(1957):4–12.

216. B. J. Polesz, F. W. Ruscetti, A. F. Gazdar, et al., "Detection and isolation of type C retrovirus particles from fresh and cultured lymphocytes of a patient with cutaneous T-cell lymphoma," *Proceedings of the National Academy of Sciences* 77(1980):7415–19.

217. Y. Hinuma, K. Nagata, M. Hanaoka, et al., "Adult T-cell leukemia: Antigen in an ATL cell line and detection of antibodies to the antigen in human sera," ibid. 78(1981):6476–80.

218. V. S. Kalyanaraman, M. G. Sarngadharan, M. Robert-Guroff, et al., "A new subtype of human T-cell leukemia virus (HTLV-II) associated with a T-cell variant of hairy cell leukemia," *Science* 218(1982):571–73.

219. F. Barré-Sinoussi, J. C. Chermann, F. Rey, et al., "Isolation of a T-lymphotropic retrovirus from a patient at risk for Acquired Immune Deficiency Syndrome (AIDS)," *Science* 220(1983):868–70.

220. P. J. Kanki, F. Barin, S. M'Boup, et al., "New human T-lymphotropic virus type III (STLV-IIIAGM)," *Science* 232(1986):238–43.

221. F. Clavel, D. Guetard, F. Brun-Vezinet, et al., "Isolation of a new human retrovirus from West African patients with AIDS," *Science* 233(1986):344–46.

222. B. S. Blumberg, H. J. Alter, and S. Visnich. "A 'new' antigen in leukemia sera," *Journal of the American Medical Association* 191(1965):541–46.

223. A. M. Prince, "An antigen detected in the blood during the incubation period of serum hepatitis," *Proceedings of the National Academy of Sciences* 60(1968):814–21.

224. D. S. Dane, C. H. Cameron, and M. Briggs, "Virus-like particles in serum of patients with Australia antigen associated hepatitis," *Lancet* 2(1970):695–98.

225. Q. L. Choo, G. Kuo, A. J. Weiner, et al., "Isolation of a cDNA clone derived from a blood-borne non-A, non-B viral hepatitis genome," *Science* 244(1989):359–62.

226. M. Rizzetto, M. G. Canese, S. Arico, et al. "Immunofluorescence detection of a new antigen-antibody system (X/anti-X) associated to hepatitis B virus in liver and serum of HBsAg carriers," *Gut* 18(1977):997–1003.

227. WHO, Blood and blood products.

228. I. Ntita, K. Mulanga, C. Dulat, et al., "Risk of transfusion-associated HIV transmission in Kinshasa, Zaire," *AIDS* 5(4)(1991):437–39.

10. Providing Care

1. Report of the informal consultation on the needs of people with HIV infection and disease and their families, 4–6 September 1989 (Geneva: WHO Global Programme on AIDS, 1989).

2. C. Cameron and D. Schopper, "Issues for national consideration in the planning of AIDS patient care management," Consultants' report (Geneva: WHO Global Programme on AIDS, 1990).

3. D. Schopper and J. Walley, Care for AIDS patients in developing countries: A review (Geneva: WHO Global Programme on AIDS, 1990).

4. WHO Regional Office for Europe, AIDS service organizations into the 1990s: People's needs and the best response, Report on a WHO workshop, Vienna, 11–14 October 1990.

5. P. Exon, comp., *Strategy for Comprehensive Care and Support for People with HIV Infection in the European Region* (Copenhagen: WHO Regional Office for Europe, 1991).

6. L. Shore, comp., *Comprehensive Care for People Living with HIV/AIDS* (Copenhagen: WHO Regional Office for Europe, 1990).

7. B. W. Victor, *AIDS in a Caring Society* (Stockholm: Nordic School of Public Health and the Danish Research Council for Health Sciences, 1991).

8. J. P. Martin, "The array of community services for people with AIDS. Recommendations for research," *Caring* (November 1989).

9. J. Simon, E. Ratsma, E. P. Manjolo, and J. Trostle, Voices from the epidemic: A report of the needs assessment for community/home care, Report submitted to Malawi AIDS Control Programme (December 1991).

10. Coordinated care services for people living with HIV/AIDS, second meeting, WHO Regional Office for Europe (1990).

11. C. Cameron and J. Shepard, "Resource allocation assessment of Swiss AIDS programme: Final report," Consultants' report (Geneva: WHO Global Programme on AIDS, 1990).

12. F. Hellinger, "Forecasting the medical care costs of the HIV epidemic: 1991–1994," *Inquiry* 28(Fall 1991):213–25.

13. A. Scitovsky and M. Over, "AIDS: costs of care in the developed and developing world," *AIDS* 2(1988):S71–81.

14. S. Foster and S. Lucas, "Socioeconomic aspects of HIV and AIDS in developing countries," PHP Departmental Publication 3 (London School of Hygiene and Tropical Medicine, 1991).

15. Traditional medicine programme and Global Programme on AIDS, Report of the consultation on AIDS and traditional medicine: Prospects for involving traditional health practitioners, Francistown, Botswana, 23–27 July 1990 (Geneva: WHO, 1990).

16. Council of State and Territorial Epidemiologists, AIDS Program, Center for Infectious Diseases, CDC, "Revision of the CDC surveillance case definition for Acquired Immunodeficiency Syndrome," *Morbidity and Mortality Weekly Report* 36(1S)(1987):3–13.

17. Global Programme on AIDS, WHO review of six HIV/AIDS home care programmes in Uganda and Zambia (Geneva, 1991).

18. WHO, Guidelines for counselling people about Human Immunodeficiency Virus (Geneva, 1990).

19. E. Katabira and R. Wabitsch, "Management issues for patients with HIV infection in Africa," *AIDS* 5 Suppl. 1(1991):S149–55.

20. WHO, Clinical management guidelines for HIV infection in adults. GPA/NPS/90.1 (Geneva, 1990).

21. E. Katabira and R. Goodgame, eds., *AIDS Care: Diagnostic and Treatment Strategies for Health Workers* (AIDS control program, Ministry of Health, Republic of Uganda, 1989).

22. S. Foster, "Affordable clinical care for HIV related illness in developing countries," *Tropical Diseases Bulletin* 87(11)(1990):121–29.

23. N. Sewankambo, "Care of HIV-infected people in the developing world: Practical aspects," *AIDS* 3 Suppl. 1(1989):S195–99.

24. J. Hampton, Living positively with AIDS: The AIDS Support Organization (TASO), Uganda. Strategies for Hope, no. 1. ActionAIDS, AMFER, World in Need (1990).

25. World Bank, Population and Human Resources Operations Division, Southern Africa Department, Tanzania AIDS assessment and planning study (Washington, D.C., 1992, forthcoming).

26. N. Kaleeba, The AIDS Support Organization (TASO), personal communication, Entebbe, Uganda, October 1991.

27. Personal communication with participants in WHO Workshop on home and community based care, Entebbe, Uganda, October 1991.

28. The AIDS Support Organization. Field visit by C. Cameron to TASO Kampala center and home care visits, presented at WHO workshop on home and community based care, Entebbe, Uganda, October 1991.

29. K. Pallangyo and R. Laing, Background study on alternative approaches to managing the opportunistic illnesses of HIV-infected persons: Costs and burden on the Tanzanian health care system, Report prepared for the World Bank (September 1990).

30. A. Harries, "Tuberculosis and Human Immunodeficiency Virus infection in developing countries," *Lancet* 335(1990):387–90.

31. The care and support of children of HIV-infected parents (Geneva: WHO Global Programme on AIDS, 1991).

32. Y. Kouri et al., "Improving the cost-effectiveness of AIDS health care in San Juan, Puerto Rico," *Lancet* 337(1991):1397–99.

33. M. Drummond and L. Davies, "Treating AIDS: The economic issues," *Health Policy* 10(1988):1–19.

34. M. Drummond and L. Davies, eds., AIDS: The challenge for economic analysis, Report of a WHO meeting, University of Birmingham, U.K., 1989.

35. A. Hardy, K. Rauch, D. Echenber, et al., "The economic impact of the first 10,000 cases of acquired immunodeficiency syndrome in the United States," *Journal of the American Medical Association* 255(1986):209–11.

36. AIDS: The contribution of self-help groups to prevention and care. Report on a WHO workshop, Leuven, Belgium, WHO regional office for Europe (6–8 December 1989).

37. National Commission on AIDS, *America Living with AIDS* (Washington, D.C., 1991), p. 67.

38. J. Rowley, R. Anderson, and T. Wan Nt, "Reducing the spread of HIV infection in sub-Saharan Africa: Some demographic and economic implications," *AIDS* 4(1)(1990):47–56.

11. The Cost of AIDS Care and Prevention

1. K. Pallangyo and R. Laing, Background study on alternative approaches to managing the opportunistic illnesses of HIV-infected persons: Costs and burden on the Tanzanian health care system, Report prepared for the World Bank, September 1990.

2. D. Shepard and R. Bail, "Costs of care for persons with AIDS in Rwanda," consultants' report (Geneva: WHO Global Programme on AIDS, 1991).

3. World Bank, *World Development Report 1991* (New York: Oxford University Press, 1991).

4. Shepard and Bail, "Costs of care for persons with AIDS in Rwanda."

5. World Bank, *World Development Report 1991.*

6. A. Scitovsky and M. Over, "AIDS: Costs of care in the developed and developing world," *AIDS* 2(1988):S71–81.

7. A. Griffiths, "Implications of the medical and scientific aspects of HIV and AIDS for economic resourcing," in *The Global Impact of AIDS,* ed. A. Fleming et al. (New York: Wiley-Liss, 1988).

8. I. Campbell, Medical Advisor, Salvation Army International Headquarters, London, presentation to the Congressional Forum on HIV/AIDS, Washington, D.C., June 1992.

9. S. Foster, F. Chibamba, et al., "Cost of AIDS counselling and home based care at Monze District Hospital, Monze, Zambia, 1991," Paper presented at the WHO workshop on home and community-based care, Entebbe, Uganda, October 1991.

10. C. Cameron and D. Schopper, Trip report, Follow-up trip report. Costs of treatment of AIDS patients at Bamrasnaradura Hospital, Bangkok, Thailand, June and August 1990, in M. Viravaidya, S. Obremskey, and C. Myers, "The economic impact of AIDS on Thailand," Harvard School of Public Health, Department of Population and International Health. Working Paper no. 4 (March 1992).

11. Ibid.

12. Viravaidya, Obremskey, and Myers, "The economic impact of AIDS on Thailand."

13. Scitovsky and Over, "AIDS: Costs of care in the developed and developing world"; Y. Kouri, D. Shepard, et al., "Improving the cost-effectiveness of AIDS health care in San Juan, Puerto Rico," *Lancet* 337(1991):1397–99.

14. R. Tapia-Conyer, A. Martin, et al., The direct costs of AIDS: Current and projected resource requirements in Mexico (Mexico City and Durham, N.C.: CONASIDA and Family Health International, 1990).

15. T. Reach, A. Martin, and S. Forsythe, Hospice planning in Barbados, presented at the VI International Conference on AIDS, San Francisco, U.S., June 1990.

16. S. Foster and S. Lucas. "Socioeconomic aspects of HIV and AIDS in developing countries," PHI Departmental Publication 3, London School of Hygiene and Tropical Medicine, 1991.

17. Kouri et al., "Improving the cost-effectiveness of AIDS health care in San Juan, Puerto Rico."

18. B. W. Victor, *AIDS in a Caring Society* (Stockholm: Nordic School of Public Health and the Danish Research Council for Health Sciences, 1991).

19. Griffiths, "Implications of the medical and scientific aspects of HIV and AIDS."

20. F. Hellinger, "Forecasting the medical care costs of the HIV epidemic 1991–1994," *Inquiry* 28(Fall 1991):213–25.

21. Ibid.

22. M. Bez. "SIDA et Hôpital: Les chiffres clés" (Paris: CISIH, Ministère des Affaires Sociales et de l'Integration, 1991).

23. Ibid.

24. Hellinger, "Forecasting the medical care costs."

25. Ibid.

26. Ibid.

27. Bez, "SIDA et Hôpital."

28. Société de Pathologie Infectieuse de Langue Française (SPILF), consensus conferences on antimicrobial therapy, "Pneumocystosis in the HIV-infected patient, 11 May 1990," *Médecine des Maladies Infectieuses* 20, special issue (August–September 1990):318–21.

29. S. N. Cohen, "Infection with Pneumocystis carinii," in *Medical Microbiology and Infectious Diseases*, ed. A. I. Braude (Philadelphia: W. B. Saunders, 1981).

30. W. T. Hughes, S. Kuhn, S. Chaudhary, et al., "Successful chemoprophylaxis for Pneumocystis carinii pneumonia," *New England Journal of Medicine* 297(1977):1419.

31. W. Rozenbaum, The treatment of AIDS-related infections, presented at the II International Conference on AIDS, Paris, France, June 1986.

32. P. M. Girard, A. G. Simot, E. Bouvet, et al., "Prévention de la pneumocystose au cours de l'infection VIH," *Bulletin Epidémiologique Hébdomadaire* 14(1990).

33. SPILF, "Pneumocystosis in the HIV-infected patient, 11 May 1990."

34. Surveillance du SIDA en France (situation au 31 décembre 1991), *Bulletin Epidémiologique Hébdomadaire* 6(1992).

35. M. C. Delmas, C. Patris, J. Pillonel, et al., "Analyse de la survie des sujets attients de SIDA diagnostiqués dans les principaux hôpitaux parisiens," ibid. 5(1991).

36. A. Auperin, C. Chouald, V. Halley des Fontaines, et al., "Pneumocystosis carinii pneumonia in HIV-infected patients without specific prophylaxis: A study of social characteristics" (in press).

37. D. Merrien, F. Raffii, E. Billaud, et al., Pneumocystis carinii pneumonia in the era of prophylaxis, presented at the III European Conference on Clinical Aspects and Treatment of HIV infection, Paris, March 1992.

38. C. Michon, P. DeTruchis, L. Mier, et al., Pneumocystis carinii pneumo-

nia in 1989–1990: Who and why? presented at the VII International Conference on AIDS, Florence, Italy, June 1991.

9. Ibid.

40. Auperin et al., "Pneumocystosis carinii pneumonia in HIV-infected patients."

41. A. Fiori and A. Triomphe, "L'évaluation économique du coût et du traitement de la pneumocystose," *Médecine des Maladies Infectieuses* 20, special issue (August–September 1990):414–19.

42. W. Rozenbaum, M. Kadivar, S. Gharakhanian, et al., Trimethoprim–sulfamethoxazole vs. pentamidine inhalations for primary prophylaxis of Pneumocystis carinii pneumonia, presented at the VI International Conference on AIDS, San Francisco, U.S., June 1990.

43. C. Cameron and J. Shepard, "Resource allocation assessment of Swiss AIDS programme: Final report," consultants' report (Geneva: WHO Global Programme on AIDS, 1990).

44. A. Detsky and G. Naglie, "A clinician's guide to cost-effectiveness analysis," *Annals of Internal Medicine* 113(2)(1990):798–802.

45. J. Eisenberg, "Clinical economics: A guide to the economic analysis of clinical practices," *Journal of the American Medical Association* 262(20)(1989): 2879–86.

46. D. Jamison, Health sector priority review (draft), (Washington, D.C.: World Bank, 1991).

47. M. Drummond and L. Davies, "Treating AIDS: The economic issues," *Health Policy* 10(1988):1–19.

48. M. Drummond and L. Davies, eds., AIDS: The challenge for economic analysis, report of a WHO meeting, University of Birmingham, U.K., 1989.

49. Victor, *AIDS in a Caring Society.*

50. M. Carballo and D. Miller, "HIV counselling: Problems and opportunities in defining the new agenda for the 1990s," *AIDS Care* 1(1989).

51. Griffiths, "Implications of the medical and scientific aspects of HIV and AIDS."

52. E. Karabira and R. Wabitsch, "Management issues for patients with HIV infection in Africa," *AIDS* 5 Suppl. 1(1991):S149–55.

53. National Commission on AIDS, *America Living with AIDS* (Washington, D.C., 1991), pp. 70–73.

54. Dr. Eric van Praag, Chief, Health Care Services, WHO, Geneva, personal communication, January 1992.

55. World Bank, Population and Human Resources Operations Division, Southern Africa Department, *Tanzania AIDS Assessment and Planning Study* (Washington, D.C., forthcoming).

56. M. Over, S. Bertozzi, J. Chin, et al., "The direct and indirect cost of HIV infection in developing countries: The case of Zaire and Tanzania," in Fleming et al., *The Global Impact of AIDS.*

57. M. Viravaidya, S. Obremskey, and C. Myers, "The economic impact of

AIDS on Thailand," Harvard School of Public Health, Department of Population and International Health, Working Paper no. 4 (March 1992).

58. G. Ohi, Kai, and Kobayashi, "AIDS prevention in Japan and its cost-benefit aspects," *Health Policy* 8(1987):17–27.

13. AIDS and Human Rights

1. The Siracusa principles on the limitation and derogation provisions in the International Covenant on Civil and Political Rights, Annex to U.N. Doc. E/CN.4/1985/4, September 28, 1984.

2. G. Rosen, *History of Public Health* (New York: M.D. Publications, 1958).

3. Jones Merritt, "The constitutional balance between health and liberty," *Hastings Center Report* 16(6) (December 1986):2–10.

4. Cf. *Fay Godfrey* v. *United Kingdom* (No. 8542/79), and *Wain* v. *United Kingdom* (No. 10787/84).

5. P. Sieghart, *AIDS & Human Rights: A UK Perspective* (London: British Medical Association Foundation for AIDS, 1989).

6. K. Tomasevski, "Before AIDS, beyond AIDS: Human rights of people with communicable diseases," in *Human Rights in the Twenty-First Century: A Global Challenge*, ed. K. E. Mahoney and P. J. Mahoney (Dordrecht: Martinus Nijhoff, 1992).

7. Sub-Commission on Prevention of Discrimination and Protection of Minorities, Decision 1988/111 of 1 September 1988 and Resolution 1989/19 of 31 August 1989; and Commission on Human Rights, Decision 1990/65 of 7 March 1990.

8. Concise note by Mr. Luis Varela-Quiros pursuant to Sub-Commission decision 1988/11, U.N. Doc. E/CN.4/Sub.2/1989/5 (July 14, 1989); Discrimination against HIV-infected people or people with AIDS, Preliminary report prepared by Luis Varela-Quiros, Special Rapporteur, U.N. Doc. E/CN.4/Sub.2/1990/9 (August 2, 1990); and Discrimination against HIV-infected people or people with AIDS, Progress report by Mr. Luis Varela-Quiros, Special Rapporteur, U.N. Doc. E/CN.4/Sub.2/1991/10 (July 24, 1991).

9. Resolution of the European Parliament of 30 March 1989 on the fight against AIDS, *Official Journal of the European Communities* 158(26 June 1989):477.

10. K. Tomasevski, "Equality and non-discrimination: Action by the international community against AIDS-related discrimination," *7th International Colloquy on the European Convention on Human Rights, Copenhagen, Oslo, Lund, 30 May–2 June 1990*, Council of Europe, H/Coll.(90)14(1990).

11. Cf. *AIDS Discrimination in Canada. A Study of the Scope and Extent of Unfair Discrimination in Canada against Persons with AIDS, and Those Known or Feared to be HIV-positive*, Vancouver, Canada (1989).

12. *Report of the Working Panel on Discrimination and Other Legal Issues—HIV/AIDS*, Sydney, Australia (1989); *Epidemic of Fear. A survey of AIDS*

Discrimination in the 1980s and Policy Recommendations for the 1990s (New York: American Civil Liberties Union, 1990).

13. R. J. Blendon and K. Donelan, "Discrimination against people with AIDS. The public's perspective," *New England Journal of Medicine* 319(15)(1988):1022–26.

14. S. M. Kegeles, T. J. Coates, T. A. Christopher, et al., "Perceptions of AIDS: The continuing saga of AIDS-related stigma," *AIDS* 3 Suppl. 1 (1989):S253–58.

15. Cf. State of health in *Equality in Employment and Occupation. General Survey of the Reports on the Discrimination (Employment and Occupation) Convention (No. 111) and Recommendation (No. 111), 1958.* Report of the Committee of Experts on the Application of Conventions and Recommendations, International Labour Conference, 75th Session (1988):69–72.

16. "Conclusions of the Council and the Ministers for Health of the Member States, meeting with the Council, on 15 December 1988, concerning AIDS and the place of work" *Official Journal of the European Communities* 28 (1989):2–3.

17. Trebilcock, "AIDS and the workplace. Some policy pointers from international labour standards," *International Labour Review* 128(1)(1989):29–45.

18. Vogel, "Discrimination on the basis of HIV infection: An economic analysis," *Ohio State Law Journal* 49(1989):986–93.

19. N. J. Nusbaum, "Public health and the law: HIV antibody status and employment discrimination," *Journal of Acquired Immune Deficiency Syndromes* 2(1989):103–06.

20. Ohsfeldt and Gohmann, "Societal attitudes towards AIDS and AIDS-related health insurance regulations," *AIDS & Public Policy Journal* 4(3)(1989):159–63.

21. Levine, "AIDS: Public health and civil liberties," *Hastings Center Report,* special suppl. (December 1986):2.

22. C. Thomas, preface to *A Synopsis of State AIDS Laws Enacted during 1983–1987 Legislative Sessions* (October 1988).

23. H. E. Lewis, "Acquired Immunodeficiency Syndrome: State legislative activity," *Journal of the American Medical Association* 258(17)(1987):2410–14.

24. "Summary of legislative situation and policy on AIDS and HIV infection in Europe: September 1988," in *Health Legislation and Ethics in the Field of AIDS and HIV Infection. Report on an International Consultation, Oslo, 26–29 April 1988* (1989), pp. 20–22.

25. S. S. Fluss, "What can legislators do to combat AIDS?" *World Health Forum* 9(1988):365–69.

26. J. C. Petricciani, "Licensed tests for antibody to human T-lymphotropic virus type III," *Annals of Internal Medicine* 103(5)1985:726–29.

27. United Nations Commission on Human Rights, Consideration of the report of the mission which took place in Cuba in accordance with Commission decision 1988/106, U.N. Doc. E/CN.4/1989/46 (February 21, 1989), para. 131.

28. S. S. Fluss and Latto, "The coercive element in legislation for the control

of AIDS and HIV infection: Some recent developments," *AIDS & Public Policy Journal* 2(1987):11–20.

29. R. Bayer, *Private Acts, Social Consequences: AIDS and the Politics of Public Health* (London: Collier Macmillan, 1989).

30. I. J. Volinn, "Issues of definitions and their implications: AIDS and leprosy," *Social Sciences and Medicine* 29(10)(1989):1157–62.

31. Resolution on the VI International Conference on AIDS (San Francisco, U.S., June 1990), *Official Journal of the European Communities* C/38/83 (19 February 1990).

32. "Refusal to designate AIDS communicable upheld by New York State Appellate Court," *AIDS Policy & Law* 5(9)(1990):1–2.

33. A. S. Benenson, ed., *Control of Communicable Diseases in Man: An Official Report of the American Public Health Association* (Washington, D.C., 1985).

34. WHO, *Social and Health Aspects of Sexually Transmitted Diseases. Principles of Control Measures* (Geneva, 1977).

35. Richards and Bross, "Legal aspects of STD control: Public duties and private rights," in *Sexually Transmitted Diseases,* ed. K. K. Holmes et al. (New York: McGraw-Hill, 1990).

36. A. Brandt, "AIDS in historical perspective: Four lessons from the history of sexually transmitted diseases," *American Journal of Public Health* 78(4)(1988): 367–71.

37. WHO, *Venereal Disease Control. A Survey of Recent Legislation* (Geneva, 1975).

38. C. W. Hutt, *International Hygiene* (London: Methuen, 1927).

39. L. Gostin and W. J. Curran, "Legal control measures for AIDS: Reporting requirements, surveillance, quarantine, and regulation of public meeting places," *American Journal of Public Health* 77(2)(1987):214–18.

40. Cf. *Criteria that must be considered in planning and implementing HIV screening programmes. Report of the WHO Meeting on Criteria for HIV Screening Programmes,* Geneva, 20–21 May 1987, WHO/SPA/GLO/87.2; *Screening and testing in AIDS prevention and control programmes,* WHO/SPA/INF/88.1; and *Unlinked anonymous screening for the public health surveillance of HIV infections. Proposed international guidelines,* GPA/SFI/89.3.

41. Institute of Medicine and National Academy of Sciences, *Confronting AIDS* (Washington, D.C., 1986).

42. Z. Gussow, *Leprosy, Racism, and Public Health: Social Policy in Chronic Disease Control* (Boulder, Colo.: Westview Press, 1989).

43. D. J. Bibel, "Santayana's warning unheeded: The parallels of syphilis and Acquired Immune Deficiency Syndrome (AIDS)," *Sexually Transmitted Diseases* 16(4)(1989):201–09.

44. M. A. Field, "Testing for AIDS: Uses and abuses," *American Journal of Law and Medicine* 16(1–2)(1990):33–106.

45. Hunter, "AIDS prevention and civil liberties: The false security of mandatory testing," *AIDS & Public Policy Journal* 2(3)(Summer–Fall 1987):1–10.

46. W. Winkelstein, Jr. and Johnson, "Epidemiology: Overview," *AIDS* 4 Suppl. 1 (1990):S95–97.

47. *Weekly Epidemiological Record* 60(40)(1985):311.

48. "Functioning of the International Health Regulations for the period 1 January to 31 December 1985 (part I)," *Weekly Epidemiological Record* 61(50)(1986):389.

49. Cf. M. Duckett and A. J. Orkin, "AIDS-related migration and travel policies and restrictions: A global survey," *AIDS* 3 Suppl. 1 (1989):S231–52.

50. Cf. L. J. Nelson, "International travel restrictions and the AIDS epidemic," *American Journal of International Law* 81(1987):230–36; N. E. Allin, "The AIDS pandemic: International travel and immigration restrictions and the World Health Organization's response," *Virginia Journal of International Law* 28(1988):1043–64.

51. WHO, *Notification of Communicable Diseases. A Survey of Existing Legislation* (Geneva, 1959).

52. G. G. Griesser et al., eds., *Data Protection in Health Information Systems: Considerations and Guidelines* (New York and Amsterdam: Elsevier/North Holland, 1980).

53. *Convention for the protection of individuals with regard to automatic processing of personal data* (European Treaty Series, no. 108); *Regulations for automated medical data banks. Recommendation No. R (81) 1 adopted by the Committee of Ministers of the Council of Europe on 23 January 1981 and Explanatory Memorandum (1981); Protection of personal data used for scientific research and statistics. Recommendation No. R (83) 10 adopted by the Committee of Ministers of the Council of Europe on 23 September 1983 and Explanatory Memorandum (1984).*

54. Revised version of the guidelines for the regulation of computerized personal data files prepared by Louis Joinet, Special Rapporteur, U.N. Doc. E/CN.4/1990/72 (February 20, 1990).

55. H. Edgar and H. Sandomire, "Medical privacy issues in the age of AIDS: Legislative options," *American Journal of Law & Medicine* 16(1–2)(1989):155–210.

56. S. S. Fluss and Zeegers, "Reporting of AIDS and Human Immunodeficiency Virus (HIV) infection: A worldwide review of legislative and regulatory patterns and issues," *AIDS & Public Policy Journal* 5(1)(1989):32–36.

57. D. Crimp and A. Rolston, "AIDS demo graphics," *Diss. Abstr. Int.* [A]; 21(195)1990:1–12.

58. H. F. Hull, C. J. Bettinger, R. M. Gallaher, et al., "Comparison of HIV-antibody prevalence in patients consenting to and declining HIV-antibody testing in an STD clinic," *Journal of the American Medical Association* 260(7)(1988):935–38.

59. "Mandatory HIV reporting testing deterrent?" *CDC AIDS Weekly,* March 27, 1989:8.

60. G. Ohi, H. Terao, T. Hasegawa, et al., "Notification of HIV carriers: Possible effect on uptake of HIV testing," *Lancet* 2 (8617)(1988):947–49.

61. Gorgens, "The Third Epidemic. Special Report," *WorldAIDS* May 1989:11.

62. E. Sandstrom, "Public health approach to HIV infection in Sweden," in *AIDS in Children, Adolescents, and Heterosexual Adults*, ed. R. F. Schinazi and A. J. Nahmias (New York: Elsevier, 1988).

63. Illinois Public Health Act 85–925, House Bill 936 (1987).

64. Illinois Department of Public Health, Data for the first 12 months of mandatory pre-marital HIV testing (mimeo, undated).

65. Illinois Public Act 86–884, House Bill No. 18 (1989).

66. A. Gromyko, "European data on HIV-seropositivity surveys: Advantages and disadvantages of various HIV-surveillance strategies," *HIV Seropositivity and AIDS Prevention and Control, Moscow, 14–17 March 1989*, EUR/ICP/GPA 041, 67.

67. "Eastern Europe faces a Western epidemic," *New Scientist* April 8, 1989:25–26.

68. Explanatory memorandum to the Recommendation (89)14 on the ethical issues of HIV infection in the health care and social settings, Council of Europe, Strasbourg, 24 October 1989, paras. 154 and 163(iv).

69. Ashman, "Homosexuality and human rights," in *Second ILGA Pink Book: A Global View of Lesbian and Gay Liberation and Oppression* (1988).

70. Human rights and disability, Progress report prepared by Leandro Despouy, Special Rapporteur, U.N. Doc. E/CN.4/Sub.2/1988/11 (June 13, 1988).

71. Roden, "Educating through the law: The Los Angeles AIDS Discrimination Ordinance," *U.C.L.A. Law Review* 33(1986):1410.

72. "Anti-discrimination statutes in the states. State AIDS Reports," *Intergovernmental Health Policy Project* 5 (October–November 1988).

73. Ministerial Decision No. 291 for 1988 of 20 July 1988, para. 5.

74. "Anti-AIDS legislation defended," *The Nation* (Bangkok), September 22, 1989.

75. "Hearing draws strong support for AIDS Bill," *Bangkok Post*, November 24, 1989.

76. J.-C. Pomonti, "AIDS explosion threatens Thailand," *Le Monde*, August 21, 1991; reproduced in *Guardian Weekly* (Manchester, U.K.), September 8, 1991:16.

77. "Thailand moves to staunch the virus: Catch if catch can," *Far Eastern Economic Review* (February 13, 1992):30.

78. "High Court upholds isolation of HIV carriers," *The Herald* (Pajim Goa), December 9, 1989:1.

79. Memorandum of the Director of WHO Communicable Diseases Division to the Director-General, July 1983.

80. R. Sabatier, ed., *Blaming Others: Prejudice, Race and Worldwide AIDS* (London: Panos Institute, 1988).

81. "World AIDS Day 1991: World Health Organization appeals to world leaders to 'Share the challenge of HIV/AIDS,'" Address by Dr. Hiroshi Nakajima, Director-General. Press release WHO/UN 95 (November 29, 1991):1.

82. The Global Strategy for AIDS Prevention and Control, Doc. SPA/INF/87.1 (May 5, 1987), paras. 2–4.

83. Statement by the Secretary-General of the United Nations before the General Assembly. Press release SG/SM/816/GA/334 (October 20, 1987):3.

84. Statement of H. E. Javier Pérez de Cuellar, Secretary-General of the United Nations, on the occasion of World AIDS Day, December 1, 1988:5.

85. Social aspects of AIDS prevention and control, WHO/SPA/GLO/87.2 (Geneva, December 1987).

86. *Report of the Global Commission on AIDS*, Geneva, 29–31 March 1989, WHO Doc. GPA/GCA(1)/89.1, para. 19.6.

87. International Consultation on AIDS and Human Rights, Geneva, 26–28 July 1989, Final Document, U.N. Doc. HR/AIDS/1989/3, paras. 18(d) and 13.

88. Commission on Human Rights, *Non-discrimination in the field of health*, resolution 1989/11 of 2 March 1989, preamble.

89. World Health Assembly, *Global strategy for the prevention and control of AIDS*, resolution WHA40.26 of 15 May 1987, preamble.

90. World Health Assembly, *Avoidance of discrimination against HIV-infected persons and persons with AIDS*, resolution WHA41.24 of 13 May 1988, preamble.

91. Council of Europe, *Guidelines for the drawing up of a public health policy to fight AIDS*, Annex to Recommendation No. R (87)25 of 26 November 1987, paras. 2.1.2 and 2.1.3.

92. Explanatory memorandum to Recommendation No. 1116 (1989) of the Parliamentary Assembly on AIDS and human rights, Doc. 6104, at 13–14.

93. Council of Europe, Parliamentary Assembly, Recommendation 1080 (1988) on a coordinated European health policy to prevent the spread of AIDS in prisons of 30 June 1988, para. 14(iv).

94. International Consultation on AIDS and Human Rights, Final Document, Geneva, 26–28 July 1989, U.N. Doc. HR/AIDS/1989/3, para. 18(D).

95. M. Kirby, "AIDS—Legal issues," *AIDS 1988* 2 Suppl. 1 (1989):S212.

96. United Nations, *Commission on Human Rights. Report of the First Session*, U.N. Doc. E/259/1947, paras. 21–22.

97. T. van Boven, "Human rights and development: The UN experience," in *Human Rights and Development: International Views*, ed. D. P. Forsythe (London: MacMillan, 1989).

98. Second periodic reports submitted by States parties to the Covenant containing rights covered by Articles 10 to 12, in accordance with the second stage of the programme established by the Economic and Social Council in its resolution 1988 (LV), Addendum 24, Denmark, U.N. Doc. E/C.12/1988/4 of 10 February 1988, para. 130.

99. Second periodic reports submitted by States parties to the Covenant containing rights covered by Articles 10 to 12, in accordance with the second stage of the programme established by the Economic and Social Council in its resolution 1988 (LX), Addendum 24, The Netherlands, U.N. Doc. E/1986/4/Add.24, para. 330.

15. The Shape of the Pandemic

1. Centers for Disease Control, "Pneumocystis pneumonia—Los Angeles," *Morbidity and Mortality Weekly Report* 30(1981):250–52.

2. Centers for Disease Control, *HIV/AIDS Surveillance Report*, January 1992:1–16.

3. European Non-Aggregate Data Set (ENAADS), European Centre for the Epidemiological Monitoring of AIDS. This database includes reports for 98 percent of AIDS cases reported by the 32 countries of the European region, through December 1991.

4. J. M. Karon, T. J. Dondero, and J. W. Curran, "The projected incidence of AIDS and estimated prevalence of HIV infection in the United States," *Journal of Acquired Immune Deficiency Syndromes* 1(1988):542–50.

5. World Health Organization, *In Point of Fact* (Geneva, May 1991)(no. 74).

6. Centers for Disease Control, *HIV/AIDS Surveillance*.

7. ENAADS, European Centre for the Epidemiological Monitoring of AIDS.

8. Centers for Disease Control, "The second 100,000 cases of acquired immunodeficiency syndrome—United States, June 1981–December 1991," *Morbidity and Mortality Weekly Report* 41(1992):28–29.

9. B. Habibi, "Contamination des hémophiles par le VIH," *Concours Médical* 18(1991):113–18.

10. J. W. Ward, S. D. Holmberg, J. R. Allen, et al., "Transmission of human immunodeficiency virus by blood transfusions screened as negative for HIV antibody," *New England Journal of Medicine* 318(1988):473–78.

11. J. M. Karon and R. L. Berkelman, "The geographic and ethnic diversity of AIDS incidence trends in homosexual/bisexual men in the United States," *Journal of Acquired Immune Deficiency Syndromes* 4(1991):1179–89.

12. Centers for Disease Control, "Self-reported changes in sexual behaviors among homosexual and bisexual men from the San Francisco City Clinic cohort," *Morbidity and Mortality Weekly Report* 76(1987):685–89.

13. Centers for Disease Control, "Declining rates of rectal and pharyngeal gonorrhea in males—New York City," *Morbidity and Morality Weekly Report* 33(1984):295–97.

14. M. A. Fischl, D. D. Richman, M. H. Grieco, et al., "The efficacy of azidothymidine (AZT) in treatment of AIDS and AIDS-related complex," *New England Journal of Medicine* 317(1987):185–91.

15. R. Stall, M. Ekstrand, L. Pollack, L. McKusick, and T. J. Coates, "Relapse from safer sex: the next challenge for AIDS prevention efforts," *Journal of Acquired Immune Deficiency Syndromes* 3(1990):1181–87.

16. Centers for Disease Control, "Trends in gonorrhea in homosexually active men—King County, Washington, 1989," *Morbidity and Mortality Weekly Report* 38(1989):762–64.

17. L. A. Kingsley, H. Bacellar, S. Zhou, et al., Temporal trends in HIV seroconversion: A report from the Multicenter AIDS Cohort Study (MACS), presented at the VI International Conference on AIDS, San Francisco, U.S., June 1990.

18. M. A. Catchpole, "Sexually transmitted diseases in England and Wales," PHLS Communicable Disease Centre, *CDR Review* 2(1992):1–7; M. A. Waugh, "Resurgent gonorrhea in homosexual men," *Lancet* 337(1991):375; J. A. R. Van Den Hoek, G. J. P. Van Griesven, and R. A. Coutinho, "Increase in unsafe homosexual behavior," *Lancet* 336(1990):179–80.

19. P. A. Waight and E. Miller, "Incidence of HIV infection among homosexual men," *British Medical Journal* 303(1991):311.

20. L. Meyer, E. Couturier, and Y. Brossard, "Prévalence de l'infection VIH chez les patients consultants pour une suspicion de MST." *Bulletin Epidémiologique Hébdomadaire* 9(1992):40–42.

21. Centers for Disease Control, *HIV/AIDS Surveillance.*

22. ENAADS, European Centre for the Epidemiological Monitoring of AIDS.

23. Centers for Disease Control "Update: Acquired immunodeficiency syndrome associated with intravenous drug use—United States, 1988," *Morbidity and Mortality Weekly Report* 38(1989):165–70.

24. T. A. Green, J. M. Karon, and O. C. Nwanyanwu, "Changes in AIDS incidence trends in the United States," *Journal of Acquired Immune Deficiency Syndromes* (in press).

25. R. Berkelman, P. Fleming, T. Green, et al., The epidemic of AIDS in intravenous drug users (IVDUs) and their heterosexual partners in the southeastern United States, presented at the VI International Conference on AIDS, San Francisco, U.S., June 1990.

26. D. M. Allen, I. M. Onorato, and P. A. Sweeney, Seroprevalence of HIV infection in intravenous drug users (IVDUs) in the United States, presented at the VI International Conference on AIDS, San Francisco, U.S., June 1990.

27. R. J. Battjes, R. W. Pickens, and Z. Amsel, "HIV infection and AIDS risk behaviors among intravenous drug users entering methadone treatment centers in selected U.S. cities," *Journal of Acquired Immune Deficiency Syndromes* 4(1991):1148–54.

28. R. A. Hahn, I. M. Onorato, T. S. Jones, et al., "Prevalence of HIV infection among intravenous drug users in the United States," *Journal of the American Medical Association* 261(1989):2677–84.

29. Meyer et al., "Prévalence de l'infection VIH."

30. G. Papaevangelou, R. Ancelle-Park, and Y. Seyrer, HIV prevalence and risk factors among IDUs in the European community, presented at the VII International Conference on AIDS, Florence, Italy, June 1991.

31. A. Skidmore, J. R. Robertson, A. A. Robertson, et al., "After the epidemic: Follow-up of HIV seroprevalence and changing patterns of drug use," *British Medical Journal* 300(1990):219–23; PHLS AIDS Centre, "The unlinked anonymous HIV prevalence monitoring programme in England and Wales: Preliminary results," *CDR Review* 7(1991):69–76.

32. M. Zaccarelli, G. Rezza, E. Girardi, et al., "Monitoring HIV trends in injecting drug users: An Italian experience," *AIDS* 4(1990):1007–10.

33. Ibid.; J. A. Van Haastrecht, A. E. Johanna, J. A. R. Van Der Hoek, et al.,

"The course of the HIV epidemic among IDUs in Amsterdam, The Netherlands," *American Journal of Public Health* 81(1991):59–62.

34. W. Szata, HIV testing programmes in Poland, presented at the Prevalence and Incidence of HIV Infection in Europe Workshop, St. Maurice, France, November 1991.

35. Centers for Disease Control, *HIV/AIDS Surveillance.*

36. Waugh, "Resurgent gonorrhea."

37. Centers for Disease Control, "Update: Acquired immunodeficiency syndrome—United States, 1981–1990," *Morbidity and Mortality Weekly Report* 40(1991):358–69.

38. R. Brookmeyer, "Reconstruction and future trends of the AIDS epidemic in the United States," *Science* 235(1991):37–42.

39. R. Berkelman, P. Fleming, S. Chu, et al., Women and AIDS: The increasing role of heterosexual transmission in the United States, presented at the VII International Conference on AIDS, Florence, Italy, June 1991.

40. M. Gwinn, M. Pappaioanou, J. R. George, et al., "Prevalence of HIV infection in childbearing women in the United States," *Journal of the American Medical Association* 265(1991):1704–08.

41. PHLS AIDS Centre, "Unlinked anonymous HIV prevalence monitoring programme"; E. Couturier, Y. Brossard, C. Larsen, et al., "Prévalence de l'infection VIH chez les femmes enceintes de la region parisienne," *Bulletin Epidémiologique Hébdomadaire* 33(1991):139–40; G. Ippolito, F. Costa, M. Stegriano, et al., "Blind serosurveys of HIV antibodies in newborns in 92 Italian hospitals," *Journal of Acquired Immune Deficiency Syndromes* 4(1991):402–07.

42. M. E. St. Louis, G. A. Conway, C. R. Hayman, et al., "Human immunodeficiency virus infection in disadvantaged adolescents," *Journal of the American Medical Association* 266(1991):2387–91.

43. Centers for Disease Control, "HIV-related knowledge and behaviors among high school students—selected U.S. sites, 1989," *Morbidity and Mortality Weekly Report* 39(1990):385–89, 395–97.

44. R. M. Greenblatt, S. A. Lukehart, and F. A. Plummer, "Genital ulceration as a risk factor for human immunodeficiency virus infection," *AIDS* 2(1988):47–50.

45. R. T. Rolfs and A. K. Nakashima, "Epidemiology of primary and secondary syphilis in the United States, 1981 through 1989," *Journal of the American Medical Association* 264(1990):1432–37.

46. Centers for Disease Control, "Relationship of syphilis to drug use and prostitution," *Morbidity and Mortality Weekly Report* 37(1988):755–58; J. K. Andrus, D. W. Fleming, D. R. Harger, et al., "Partner notification: Can it control epidemic syphilis?" *Annals of Internal Medicine* 112(1990):539–43.

47. Centers for Disease Control, *HIV/AIDS Surveillance.*

48. Habibi, "Contamination des hémophiles."

49. *WHO Weekly Epidemiological Record* 65(1990):239–43.

50. M. C. Gwinn, M. Pappaioanou, J. R. George, et al., "Prevalence of HIV

infection in childbearing women in the United States," *Journal of the American Medical Association* 265(1991):1704–08.

51. Centers for Disease Control, unpublished data.

52. P. F. Barnes, A. B. Bloch, P. T. Davidson, et al., "Tuberculosis in patients with human immunodeficiency virus infection," *New England Journal of Medicine* 324(1991):1644–50; J. A. Jereb, G. D. Kelly, S. W. Dooley, et al., "Tuberculosis morbidity in the United States: Final data, 1990," in *CDC Surveillance Summaries*, December 1991, *Morbidity and Mortality Weekly Report* 40(No. SS-3)(1991):23–29.

53. Centers for Disease Control, "Tuberculosis and human immunodeficiency virus infection: Recommendations of the advisory committee for the elimination of tuberculosis (ACET)," *Morbidity and Mortality Weekly Report* 38(1989):243–50.

54. Centers for Disease Control, "Nosocomial transmission of multidrug resistant tuberculosis among HIV-infected persons—Florida and New York, 1988–1991," *Morbidity and Mortality Weekly Report* 40(1991):585–91.

55. L. Thiry, S. Sprecher-Goldberger, T. Jonekheer, et al., "Isolation of AIDS virus from cell-free breast milk of three healthy virus carriers," *Lancet* 2(1985):891–92; A. Ruff, J. Coberly, H. Farzadegan, et al., Detection of HIV-1 by PCR in breast milk, presented at the VII International Conference on AIDS, Florence, Italy, June 1991; M. Bucens, J. Armstrong, and M. Stuckey, Virological and electron microscopic evidence for postnatal HIV transmission via breast milk, presented at the IV International Conference on AIDS, Stockholm, Sweden, June 1988; N. Vonesch, F. Caprilli, H. A. Castiglione, et al., The human colostrum as a route of HIV-1 transmission, presented at the VII International Conference on AIDS, Florence, Italy, June 1991.

56. L. Belec, J. C. Bouquety, A. J. Georges, et al., "Antibodies to human immunodeficiency virus in the breast milk of healthy, seropositive women," *Pediatrics* 85(1990):1022–26; P. Van de Perre, D. G. Hitimana, and P. Lepage, "Human immunodeficiency virus antibodies of IgG, IgA, and IgM subclasses in milk of seropositive mothers," *Journal of Pediatrics* 113(1988):1039–41.

57. M. J. Oxtoby, "Human immunodeficiency virus and other viruses in human milk: Placing the issues in broader perspective," *Pediatric Infectious Disease Journal* 7(1988):825–35.

58. J. B. Ziegler, D. A. Cooper, R. Johnson, and J. Gold, "Postnatal transmission of AIDS associated retrovirus from mother to infant," *Lancet* 1(1985):896–99; P. Weinbreck, V. Loustaud, F. Denis, et al., "Postnatal transmission of HIV infection," *Lancet* 1(1988):482; P. Lepage, P. Van de Perre, M. Carael, et al., "Postnatal transmission of HIV from mother to child," *Lancet* 2(1987):400; E. R. Stiehm and P. Vink, "Transmission of human immunodeficiency virus infection by breastfeeding," *Journal of Pediatrics* 118(1991):410–12; J. B. Ziegler, G. J. Stewart, R. Penny, et al., Breast feeding and transmission of HIV from mother to infant, presented at the IV International Conference on AIDS, Stockholm, Sweden, June 1988; R. Colebunders, B. Kapita, W. Nekwei, et al., "Breast feeding and transmission of HIV," *Lancet* 2(1988):1487; M. Bucens, J. Armstrong, and M. Stuckey,

Virological and electron microscopic evidence for postnatal HIV transmission via breast milk, presented at the IV International Conference on AIDS, Stockholm, Sweden, June 1988.

59. S. K. Hira, U. G. Mangrola, C. Mwale, et al., "Apparent vertical transmission of human immunodeficiency virus type 1 by breast-feeding in Zambia," *Journal of Pediatrics* 117(1990):421–24.

60. P. Van de Perre, A. Simonon, P. Msellati, et al., Mother-to-infant postnatal transmission of HIV-1: A cohort study, presented at the VII International Conference on AIDS, Florence, Italy, June 1991.

61. H. Subhash, U. Mangrola, C. Mwale, et al., Breast feeding and HIV-1 transmission, presented at the V International Conference on AIDS, Montreal, Canada, June 1989.

62. C. Gabiano, P. A. Tovo, M. de Martino, et al., HIV-1 transmission rate in first born children to seropositive mothers and interfering factors, presented at the VII International Conference on AIDS, Florence, Italy, June 1991.

63. Colebunders et al., "Breastfeeding and transmission of HIV"; J. Kreiss, P. Datta, D. Willerford, et al., Vertical transmission of HIV in Nairobi: Correlation with maternal viral burden, presented at the VII International Conference on AIDS, Florence, Italy, June 1991; M. Lallemant, S. Lallemant-Le Coeur, L. Samba, et al., Assessing the risk for mother-infant HIV-1 transmission: A challenge in developing countries, presented at ibid.; R. A. Hague, J. Y. Q. Mok, L. MacCallum, et al., Do maternal factors influence the risk of vertical transmission of HIV? presented at ibid.; M. E. St. Louis, U. Kabagabo, C. Brown, et al., Maternal factors associated with perinatal HIV transmission, presented at ibid.

64. A. Briend, B. Wojtyniak, and M. G. M. Rowland, "Breast feeding, nutritional state, and child survival in rural Bangladesh," *British Medical Journal* 296(1988):879–82; A. Briend and A. Bari, "Breast feeding improves survival, but not nutritional status, of 12–35 months old children in rural Bangladesh," *European Journal of Clinical Nutrition* 43(1989):603–08.

65. J. P. Habicht, J. DaVanzo, and W. P. Butz, "Mother's milk and sewage: Their interactive effects on infant mortality," *Pediatrics* 81(1988):456–61.

66. R. G. Feachem and M. A. Koblinsky, "Interventions for the control of diarrhoeal diseases among young children: Promotion of breast-feeding," *Bulletin of the World Health Organization* 62(1984):271–91; J. M. Jason, P. Nieburg, J. S. Marks, et al., "Mortality and infectious disease associated with infant feeding practices in developing countries," *Pediatrics* 74(1984):702–27.

67. J. F. Lew, R. I. Glass, R. E. Gangarosa, et al., "Diarrheal deaths in the United States, 1979 through 1987," *Journal of the American Medical Association* 265(1991):3280–84.

68. Feachem and Koblinsky, "Interventions for the control of diarrhoeal diseases among young children."

69. A. S. Cunningham, D. B. Jelliffe, and E. F. P. Jelliffe, "Breast-feeding and health in the 1980s: A global epidemiologic review," *Journal of Pediatrics* 118(1991):659–66; Feachem and Koblinsky, "Interventions for the control of diarrhoeal diseases among young children."

70. H. Bauchner, J. M. Leventhal, and E. D. Shapiro, "Studies of breast milk and infections: How good is the evidence?" *Journal of the American Medical Association* 256(1986):887–92.

71. S. Diaz, G. Rodriguez, O. Peralta, et al., "Lactational amenorrhea and the recovery of ovulation and fertility in fully nursing Chilean women," *Contraception* 38(1988):53–67; B. A. Gross, "Breast-feeding and natural family planning," *International Journal of Fertility* 33 Suppl. (1988):24–31; R. L. Jackson, "Ecological breastfeeding and child spacing," *Clinical Pediatrics* 27(1988):373–77; B. Israngkura, K. I. Kennedy, B. Leelapatana, et al., "Breast feeding and return to ovulation in Bangkok," *International Journal of Gynaecology and Obstetrics* 30(1989):335–42.

72. M. Singarimbun and C. Manning, "Breastfeeding, amenorrhea and abstinence in a Javanese village," *Studies in Family Planning* 7(1976):175–79; G. A. Oni, "Breastfeeding: Its relationship with postpartum amenorrhea and postpartum sexual abstinence in a Nigerian community," *Social Science and Medicine* 24(1987):255–62.

73. S. Thapa, R. V. Short, and M. Potts, "Breast feeding, birth spacing and their effects on child survival," *Nature* 335(1988):679–82.

74. S. R. Millman and E. C. Cooksey, "Birth weight and the effects of birth spacing and breast feeding on infant mortality," *Studies in Family Planning* 18(1987):202–12; R. D. Retherford, M. K. Choe, S. Thapa, and B. B. Gubhaju, "To what extent does breastfeeding explain birth-interval effects on early childhood mortality?" *Demography* 26(1989):439–50.

75. K. Krasovec, "The implications of poor maternal nutritional status during pregnancy for future lactational performance," *Journal of Tropical Pediatrics* 37 Suppl. (1991):3–10.

76. Ibid.

77. S. J. Heymann, "Modelling the impact of breast feeding by HIV-infected women on child survival," *American Journal of Public Health* 80(1990):1305–09.

78. Ibid.; A. Nicoll, J. Z. J. Killewo, and C. Mgone, "HIV and infant feeding practices: Epidemiological implications for sub-Saharan African countries," *AIDS* 4(1990):661–65.

79. National Control of Diarrhoeal Diseases Project, "Impact of the national control of diarrhoeal diseases project on infant and child mortality in Dakahlia, Egypt," *Lancet* 2(1988):145–48.

80. B. F. Melville, "Can low income women in developing countries afford artificial feeding?" *Journal of Tropical Pediatrics* 37(1991):141–42.

81. A. E. Tozzi, P. Pezzotti, and D. Greco, "Does breast-feeding delay progression to AIDS in HIV-infected children?" *AIDS* 4(1990):1293–94.

82. V. V. Pokrovsky, I. Kuznetsova, and I. Cramova, Transmission of HIV infection from an infected infant to his mother by breast feeding, presented at the VI International Conference on AIDS, San Francisco, U.S., June 1990.

83. A. J. Ammann, "Is there an acquired immune deficiency syndrome in infants and children?" *Pediatrics* 72(1983):430–32; A. Rubinstein, M. Sicklick, A. Gupta, et al., "Acquired Immunodeficiency with reversed T4/T8 ratios in infants

born to promiscuous and drug addicted mothers," *Journal of the American Medical Association* 249(1983):2350–56; N. Lapointe, J. Michaud, D. Pekovik, et al., "Transplacental transmission of HTLV-III virus," *New England Journal of Medicine* (1985):312–25; G. B. Scott, B. E. Buck, J. G. Leterman, et al., "Acquired immunodeficiency syndrome in infants," *New England Journal of Medicine* 310(1984):76–81; M. J. Cowan, D. Hellmann, D. Chudwin, et al., "Maternal transmission of acquired immune deficiency syndrome," *Pediatrics* 73(1984):382–86; E. Vilmer, A. Fisher, C. Griscelli, et al., "Possible transmission of a Human Lymphotropic retrovirus (LAV) from mother to infant with AIDS," *Lancet* 2(1984):229–30; P. A. Thomas, H. W. Jaffe, T. J. Spira, et al., "Unexplained immunodeficiency in children," *Journal of the American Medical Association* (1984):252–644.

84. A. J. Ammann, "The acquired immunodeficiency syndrome in infants and children," *Annals of Internal Medicine* 103(1985):734–37; G. M. Shearer, "Other factors to consider in infantile AIDS," *New England Journal of Medicine* 311(1984):189–90.

85. S. Pahwa, M. Kaplan, S. Fikrig, et al., "Spectrum of human T-cell lymphotropic virus type III infection in children. Recognition of symptomatic, asymptomatic, and seronegative patients," *Journal of the American Medical Association* 255(1986):2299–2305.

86. J. Ninane, D. Moulin, M. De Bruyere, et al., "AIDS in two African children: One with fibrosarcoma of the liver," *European Journal of Pediatrics* 144(1985):385–90; A. Nemeth, S. Bygdeman, E. Sandström, et al., "Early case of acquired immunodeficiency syndrome in a child from Zaire," *Sexually Transmitted Diseases* 13(1986):111–13.

87. Centers for Disease Control, "Recommendations for assisting in the prevention of perinatal transmission of human T-lymphotropic virus type III/lymphadenopathy-associated virus and acquired immunodeficiency syndrome," *Morbidity and Mortality Weekly Report* 34(1985):721–31.

88. J. Chin, "Current and future dimensions of the HIV/AIDS pandemic in women and children," *Lancet* 336(1990):221–24.

89. M. Lallemant, S. Lallemant-Le Coeur, D. Cheynier, et al., "Mother-child transmission of HIV and infant survival in Brazzaville, Congo," *AIDS* 3(1989): 643–46; S. Blanche, C. Rouzioux, M. L. Guihard Moscato, et al., "A prospective study of infants born to women seropositive for human immunodeficiency virus type 1," *New England Journal of Medicine* 320(1989):1643–48; R. W. Ryder, W. Nsa, S. E. Hassig, et al., "Perinatal transmission of the human immunodeficiency virus type 1 to infants of seropositive women in Zaire," *New England Journal of Medicine* 320(1989):1637–42; M. Lallemant, S. Lallemant-Le Coeur, L. Samba, et al., Assessing the risk for mother-infant HIV-1 transmission: A challenge in developing countries, presented at the VII International Conference on AIDS, Florence, Italy, June 1991; P. Lepage, P. Van de Perre, P. Msellati, et al., Natural history of HIV-1 infection in children in Rwanda: A prospective cohort study, presented at ibid.; S. K. Hira, G. J. Kamanga, C. Mwale, et al., "Perinatal trans-

mission of HIV-1 in Zambia," *British Medical Journal* 299(1989):1250–52; P. Datta, J. Embree, J. O. Ndinya-Achola, et al., Perinatal HIV-1 transmission in Nairobi, Kenya: 5-year follow-up, presented at the VII International Conference on AIDS, Florence, Italy, June 1991; J. C. Bouquety, C. Lanckriet, R. M. Siopathis, et al., "Etude de la transmission périnatale d'HIV-1 à Bangui, RCA," *Lères Journées de Pédiatrie Africaines* (Bangui), January 1990; W. A. Andiman, B. J. Simpson, B. Olson, et al., "Rate of transmission of Human Immunodeficiency virus Type 1 Infection from mother to child and short-term outcome of neonatal infection. Results of a prospective cohort study," *American Journal of Diseases in Children* 144(1990):758–66; C. Hutto, W. P. Parks, S. Lai, et al., "A hospital-based prospective study of perinatal infection with human immunodeficiency virus type 1," *Journal of Pediatrics* 118(1991):347–53; M. M. Mayers, K. Davenny, E. E. Schoenbaum, et al., "A prospective study of infants of human immuno-deficiency virus seropositive and seronegative women with a history of intrave-nous drug use or of intravenous drug using sex partner, in the Bronx, New York City," *Pediatrics* 8(1991):1248–56; N. A. Halsey, R. Boulos, E. Holt, et al., "Trans-mission of HIV-1 infections from mothers to infants in Haiti. Impact on childhood mortality and malnutrition," *Journal of the American Medical Association* 264(1990):2088–92; European Collaborative Study, "Children born to women with HIV-1 infection: Natural history and risk of transmission," *Lancet* 337(1991):253–60.

90. C. Rouzioux, M. J. Mayaux, S. Blanche, et al., The materno-fetal trans-mission rates of HIV-1 and of HIV-2 in France, presented at the VIII International Conference on AIDS, Amsterdam, Netherlands, July 1992.

91. T. S. Sibailly, G. Adjorolo, H. Gayle, et al., Prospective study to compare HIV-1 and HIV-2 perinatal transmission in Abidjan, Ivory Coast, presented at ibid.

92. P. A. Pizzo, "Considerations for the evaluation of antiretroviral agents in infants and children infected with Human Immunodeficiency Virus: A perspec-tive from the National Cancer Institute," *Review of Infectious Diseases* 12(1990):S561–69.

93. E. Jovaisas, M. A. Koch, A. Schäfer, et al., "LAV/HTLV-III in 20 week fetus," *Lancet* 2(1985):1129; S. Sprecher, G. Soumenkoff, F. Puissant, and M. Degueldre, "Vertical transmission of HIV in 15-week fetus," *Lancet* 2(1986):288–89; S. H. Lewis, C. Reynolds-Kohler, H. E. Fox, and J. A. Nelson, "HIV-1 in tro-phoblastic and villous Hobauer cells, and haematological precursors in eight-week fetuses," *Lancet* 335(1990):565–68.

94. J. E. Embree, M. Braddick, P. Datta, et al., "Lack of correlation of mater-nal human immunodeficiency virus infection with neonatal malformations," *Pediatric Infectious Disease Journal* 8(1989):700–04.

95. A. Krivine, A. Yakudima, M. Le May, et al., "A comparative study of virus isolation, polymerase chain reaction, and antigen detection in children of mothers infected with human immunodeficiency virus," *Journal of Pediatrics* 116(1990):372–76; P. S. Weintrub, P. P. Ulrich, J. R. Edwards, et al., "Use of poly-merase chain reaction for the early detection of HIV infection in the infants of

HIV-seropositive women," *AIDS* 5(1991):881–84; A. Ehrnst, S. Lindgren, M. Dictor, et al., "HIV in pregnant women and their offspring: Evidence for late transmission," *Lancet* 338(1991):203–07.

96. J. J. Goedert, A. M. Dulièce, C. Amos, et al., "High risk of HIV-1 infection for first-born twins," *Lancet* 338(1991):1471–75.

97. European Cohort Study, "Risk factors for mother-to-child transmission of HIV-1," *Lancet* 339(1992):1007–12.

98. J. B. Ziegler, D. A. Cooper, R. O. Johnson, and J. Gold, "Postnatal transmission of AIDS-associated retrovirus from mother to infant," *Lancet* 1(1985): 896–98.

99. P. Lepage, P. Van de Perre, M. Carael, et al., "Postnatal transmission of HIV from mother to child," *Lancet* 2(1987):400; P. Weinbreck, V. Loustaud, F. Denis, et al., "Postnatal transmission of HIV infection," *Lancet* 1(1988):482; R. Colebunders, B. Kapita, W. Nekwei, et al., "Breastfeeding and transmission of HIV," *Lancet* 2(1988):1487; E. R. Steihm and P. Vink, "Transmission of human immunodeficiency virus infection by breast-feeding," *Journal of Pediatrics* (1991): 410–12.

100. R. L. Colebunders, B. Kapita, W. Nekwei, et al., Breast feeding and transmission of HIV, presented at the IV International Conference on AIDS, Stockholm, Sweden, June 1988; S. Hira, Breast feeding as a risk factor for HIV-1 transmission, presented at the V International AIDS Conference, Montreal, Canada, June 1990.

101. P. Van de Perre, A. Simono, P. Msellati, et al., "Postnatal transmission of human immunodeficiency virus type 1 from mother to infant," *New England Journal of Medicine* 325(1991):593–98.

102. P. Van de Perre, D. G. Hitimana, and P. Lepage, "Human immunodeficiency virus antibodies of IgG, IgA and IgM subclasses in milk of seropositive mothers," *Journal of Pediatrics* 113(1988):1039–41; L. Belec, J. C. Bouquety, A. J. Georges, et al., "Antibodies to human immunodeficiency virus in the breast milk of healthy, seropositive women," *Pediatrics* 85(1990):1022–26.

103. S. Blanche, M. Tardieu, A. M. Duliege, et al., "Longitudinal study of 94 symptomatic infants with perinatally acquired human immunodeficiency virus infection. Evidence for bimodal expression of clinical and biological symptoms," *American Journal of Diseases in Children* 144(1990):1210–15.

104. N. Malanda, N. Badi, L. Mundele, et al., Morbidity and mortality in successive births: Cohorts of children and their HIV (+) mothers in Zaire, presented at the VI International Conference on AIDS, San Francisco, U.S., June 1990.

105. European Cohort Study, "Risk factors for mother-to-child transmission"; S. Lindgren, B. Anzen, A. B. Bohlin, et al., "HIV and child-bearing: Clinical outcome and aspects of mother-to-infant transmission," *AIDS* 5(1991):1111–16.

106. M. E. St. Louis, U. Kabagabo, C. Brown, et al., Maternal factors associated with perinatal HIV transmission, presented at the VII International Conference on AIDS, Florence, Italy, June 1991.

107. J. Kreiss, P. Datta, D. Willerford, Vertical transmission of HIV in Nairobi: Correlation with maternal viral burden, presented at ibid.

108. R. Rossi, V. Moschese, P. A. Broliden, et al., "Presence of maternal antibodies to human immunodeficiency virus type 1 envelope glycoprotein gp 120 epitopes correlates with the uninfection status of children born to seropositive mothers," *Proceedings of the National Academy of Science* 86(1989):8055–58; J. J. Goedert, H. Mendenz, J. E. Drummond, et al., "Mother-to-infant transmission of human immunodeficiency virus type 1: Association with prematurity or low anti-gp 120," *Lancet* 2(1989):1351–54; Y. Devash, T. A. Calvelli, D. G. Wood, et al., "Vertical transmission of human immunodeficiency virus is correlated with the absence of high-affinity/avidity maternal antibodies to the gp 120 principal neutralizing domain," *Proceedings of the National Academy of Science* 87(1990):3445–49.

109. B. S. Parekh, N. Shaffer, C. P. Pau, et al., "Lack of correlation between maternal antibodies to V3 loop peptides of gp120 and perinatal HIV-1 transmission. The NYC Perinatal HIV Transmission Collaborative Study," *AIDS* 5(1991):1179–84.

110. Ryder et al., "Perinatal transmission of the human immunodeficiency virus type 1."

111. S. M. Wolinsky, C. M. Wike, B. T. Korber, et al., "Selective transmission of human immunodeficiency virus type-1 variants from mothers to infants," *Science* 28(255)(1992):1134–37.

112. P. A. Selwyn, E. E. Schoenbaum, K. Davenny, et al., "Prospective study of human immunodeficiency virus infection and pregnancy outcomes in intravenous drug users," *Journal of the American Medical Association* 261(1989):1289–94; A. Berrebi, W. E. Kobuch, J. Puel, et al., "Influence of pregnancy on human immunodeficiency virus disease," *European Journal of Obstetrics, Gynecology and Reproductive Biology* 37(1990):211–17.

113. M. Temmerman, F. A. Plummer, N. B. Mirza, et al., "Infection with HIV as a risk factor for adverse obstetrical outcome," *AIDS* 4(1990):1087–93.

114. P. Miotti, G. Kiomba, N. Odaka, et al., Timing of excess mortality in children of HIV-infected African mothers, presented at the VII International Conference on AIDS, Florence, Italy, June 1991.

115. P. Lepage, F. Dabis, D. Hitimana, et al., "Perinatal transmission of HIV-1: Lack of impact of maternal HIV infection on characteristics of live births and on neonatal mortality in Kigali, Rwanda," *AIDS* 5(1991):295–300.

116. F. Hecht, "Counseling the HIV-positive woman regarding pregnancy," *Journal of the American Medical Association* 257(1987):3361.

117. Selwyn et al., "Prospective study of human immunodeficiency virus infection."

118. S. Lallemant-Le Coeur, L. Samba, P. M'Pelé, et al., Prise en charge clinique et psycho-sociale de longue-durée des couples mère-enfants suivis dans le cadre d'une étude de la transmission verticale d'HIV-1: Enseignements pour la mise en place d'une procédure de conseil prénatal à Brazzaville, Congo, presented at the V International Conference on AIDS in Africa, Kinshasa, Zaire, October 1990.

119. L. Sherr et al., *HIV and AIDS in Mothers and Babies: A Guide to Counselling* (Cambridge, Mass.: Blackwell Scientific Publications, 1991).

120. A. M. Prince, H. Reesink, D. Pascual, et al., "Prevention of HIV infection by passive immunization with HIV immunoglobulin," *AIDS Research and Human Retroviruses* 7(12)(1991):971–73.

121. L. S. Cook, L. A. Koutsky, and K. K. Holmes, "Circumcision and sexually transmitted diseases," *American Journal of Epidemiology* 134(1991):781.

122. N. Touchette, "HIV-1 link prompts circumspection on circumcision," *Journal of National Institutes of Health Research* 3(1991):44–46.

123. J. Bongaarts, P. Reining, P. Way, and F. Conant, "The relationship between male circumcision and HIV infection in African populations," *AIDS* 3(1989):373–77; S. Moses, J. E. Gradley, N. J. D. Nagelkerke, et al., "Geographical patterns of male circumcision practices in Africa: Association with HIV seroprevalence," *International Journal of Epidemiology* 19(1990):693–97.

124. J. N. Simonsen, D. W. Cameron, M. N. Gakinya, et al., "Human immunodeficiency virus infection in men with sexually transmitted diseases," *New England Journal of Medicine* 319(1988):274–78.

125. S. K. Hira, H. Kamanga, R. Macuacua, et al., "Genital ulcers and male circumcision as risk factors for acquiring HIV-1 in Zambia" (letter), *Journal of Infectious Diseases* 3(1990):584–85.

126. M. Carael, P. H. Van de Perre, P. H. Lepage, et al., "Human immunodeficiency virus transmission among heterosexual couples in Central Africa," *AIDS* 2(1988):201–05.

127. W. D. Cameron, N. J. Simonsen, L. J. D'Costa, et al., "Female to male transmission of human immunodeficiency virus type 1: Risk factors for seroconversion in men," *Lancet* 2(1989):403–07.

128. Simonsen et al., "Human immunodeficiency virus infection."

129. M. Becker and J. Joseph, "AIDS and behavioral change to reduce risk: A review," *American Journal of Public Health* 78(1988):394–411; R. Stall, T. J. Coates, and C. Hoff, "Behavioral risk reduction for HIV infection among gay and bisexual men: A review of results from the United States," *American Psychologist* 43(11)(1988):878–85; S. Doll, F. Judson, D. Ostrow, et al., "Sexual behavior before AIDS: The hepatitis B studies of homosexual and bisexual men," *AIDS* 4(11)(1990):1067–73.

130. M. Ekstrand and T. Coates, "Maintenance of safer sexual behaviors and predictors of risky sex: The San Francisco Health Study," *American Journal of Public Health* 80(1990):973–77.

131. R. Stall, M. Ekstrand, L. Pollack, et al., "Relapse from safer sex: The next challenge for AIDS prevention efforts," *Journal of Acquired Immune Deficiency Syndromes* 3(12)(1990):1181–87.

132. R. Stall, M. Ekstrand, L. Bye, et al., Relapse from safe sex among gay and bisexual men in San Francisco: The Communication Technologies Surveys. Unpublished manuscript.

133. K. R. O'Reilly, D. L. Higgins, C. Galavotti, and J. Sheridan, Relapse from safer sex among homosexual men: Evidence from four cohorts in the AIDS Com-

munity Demonstration Projects, presented at the V International Conference on AIDS, San Francisco, U.S., June 1990.

134. G. Hart, M. Boulton, R. Fitzpatrick, et al., "'Relapse' to unsafe sexual behavior amongst gay men: A critique of recent behavioural HIV/AIDS research," *Sociology of Health and Illness* 14(1992):216–30.

135. S. Kippax, G. W. Dowsett, M. Davis, et al., *Social Aspects of the Prevention of AIDS*, 1991 Sustaining Safe Sex Survey—Technical Report for the Australian Federation of AIDS Organisations and the AIDS Council of New South Wales (Sydney: Macquarie University, AIDS Research Unit, 1991).

136. J. B. F. deWit, G. J. P. van Griensven, G. Kok, et al., "Serial cross-sectional and longitudinal changes in sexual behavior among homosexual men in Amsterdam 1984–88," *American Journal of Public Health* (in press).

137. L. A. Kingsley, S. Y. L. Zhou, H. Bacellar, et al., "Temporal trends in human immunodeficiency virus type 1 seroconversion 1984–1989," *American Journal of Epidemiology* 134(4)(1991):331–39.

138. P. A. Waight and E. Miller, "Incidence of HIV infection among homosexual men," *British Medical Journal* 303 (311)(1991).

139. J. B. F. deWit, E. de Vroome, G. J. P. van Griensven, et al., Increase in the incidence of HIV infections in relation to higher levels of unsafe sexual behavior, in a cohort of homosexual men in Amsterdam. Unpublished manuscript.

140. Surveillance Branch, AIDS Office, San Francisco Department of Public Health, HIV incidence and prevalence in San Francisco in 1992: Summary report from an HIV Consensus Meeting, February 1992.

141. Kingsley et al., "Temporal trends in human immunodeficiency virus"; Waight and Miller, "Incidence of HIV infection"; B. Willoughby, M. Schecter, K. Craib, et al., Characteristics of recent seroconverters in a cohort of homosexual men: Who are the prevention failures? presented at the VI International Conference on AIDS, San Francisco, U.S., June 1990.

142. J. A. Kelly, J. S. St. Lawrence, and T. L. Brasfield, "Predictors of vulnerability to AIDS risk behavior relapse," *Journal of Consulting and Clinical Psychology* 59(1)(1991):163–66; Stall et al., "Relapse from safer sex."

143. O'Reilly et al., "Relapse from safer sex among homosexual men"; Willoughby et al., "Characteristics of recent seroconverters"; Kelly et al., "Predictors of vulnerability"; R. Bolton, J. Vincke, R. Mak, and E. Dennehy, "Alcohol and risky sex: In search of an elusive connection," *Medical Anthropology* 65(1992).

144. O'Reilly et al., "Relapse from safer sex among homosexual men"; Kelly et al., "Predictors of vulnerability"; A. Prieur. "The Dangers of Love," in *Changing Sexual Behaviors in the Shadow of AIDS: A Survey of Gay and Bisexual Behavior in Communities throughout the World*, ed. M. Cohen (New York: Plenum, 1992).

145. R. Valdiserri. *Preventing AIDS: The Design of Effective Programs* (New Brunswick, N.J.: Rutgers University Press, 1989); Stall et al., "Relapse from safer sex"; T. G. M. Sandfort, E. M. M. de Vroome, G. J. P. van Griensven, and R. A. P. Tielman, "Factors predicting consistent condom use among homosexual men: An exploratory analysis," *Psychology and Human Sexuality* (in press).

146. J. L. Chin, The Increasing Impact of the HIV/AIDS Pandemic on Women and Children, Paper presented at the American Public Health Association meeting, Atlanta, Georgia, November 1991.

147. This critique is more fully elaborated in E. Reid, "Placing women at the center of the analysis," in *Women and AIDS: Strategies for the Future* (1991); and J. Hamblin and E. Reid, "Women, the HIV epidemic and human rights," paper prepared for the International Workshop on AIDS: A Question of Rights and Humanity, The Hague, May 1991. See also D. Worth, "Sexual decision-making and AIDS: Why condom promotion among vulnerable women is likely to fail," *Studies in Family Planning* 20(November/December 1989):6; Z. Stein, "HIV prevention: The need for methods women can use," *American Journal of Public Health* 80(1990):460–62; and K. Carovano, "More than mothers and whores: Redefining the AIDS prevention needs of women," *International Journal of Health Services* 21(1)(1991):131–42.

148. J. Jacobson, "Women's reproductive health: The silent emergency," *WorldWatch Paper* 102 (June 1991).

149. Stein, "HIV Prevention: The need for methods women can use"; N. J. Alexander, "Sexual transmission of human immunodeficiency virus: Virus entry into the male and female genital tract," *Fertility and Sterility* 54(1990):1–18; "Barriers and boundaries" (editorial), *Lancet* 335(1990):1497–98.

150. R. McNamara, *Female Genital Health and the Risk of HIV Transmission*, UNDP Issues, Paper no. 4 (1992).

151. M. Mongola, Interview for *Reflections on the Impact of the HIV Epidemic*, 1991 (UNDP, forthcoming).

152. E. Reid, "Placing Women at the centre of the analysis," in *Women and AIDS: Strategies for the Future* (Canadian International Development Agency 1991).

153. S. Baldwin and J. Twigg, "Women and community care—Reflections on a debate," in *Women's Issues in Social Politics*, ed. M. Maclean and D. Groves (London: Routledge, 1991).

154. World Health Organization, Global Programme on AIDS, *Report of the Meeting on Research Priorities Relating to Women and HIV/AIDS*, GPA/DIR/91.2 (Geneva, 1991); Stein, "HIV prevention."

155. Josef Decosas and Violette Pendeault, The demographic AIDS trap for women in Africa, presented at the VII International Workshop on AIDS: A Question of Rights and Humanity, The Hague, May 1991.

156. United Nations, *Adolescent Reproductive Behavior* (New York, 1989).

157. "Barriers and boundaries," *Lancet*.

158. N. O'Farrell and I. Windsor, "Sexual behavior in HIV-1 seropositive Zulu men and women in Durban, South Africa," letter to the editor, *JAI Syndromes* 4(1991):1258–59; M. J. Wawer, D. Serwadda, S. D. Musgrave, et al., "Dynamics of the spread of HIV-1 infection in a rural district of Uganda," *British Medical Journal* 303(1991):1303–06; D. Cohen, *AIDS in Uganda*, report on a programming mission for UNDP Fifth Cycle Support to Uganda (1992).

159. C. Miller and M. Gardner, "AIDS and mucosal immunity: Usefulness of

the SIV macaque model of genital mucosal transmission," *Journal of Acquired Immune Deficiency Syndromes* 4(1991):1169–92.

160. United Nations Development Program (UNDP), *Report of the Informal Consultation on Behavior Change, Dalar* (1991), forthcoming; B. Willmore and S. Ray, *AIDS: An Issue for Every Woman,* Proceedings of the Women and AIDS Support Network Conference, Harare, Zimbabwe, 1989; E. Reid, "Two voices," in *World Health* (Geneva: WHO, 1990).

161. Willmore and Ray, *AIDS: An Issue for Every Woman.*

162. Ibid.; M. Mongola, Interview for *Reflections on the Impact of the HIV Epidemic,* 1991 (UNDP, forthcoming).

163. E. A. Preble, "Impact of HIV/AIDS on African children," *Social Science and Medicine* 31(6)(1990):671–80.

164. UNICEF, *Children and AIDS: The Impending Calamity* (1990).

165. Anti-Slavery International, *Anti-Slavery Reporter,* series VII, vol. 3(7)(1991):8.

166. T. N. Naik, S. Sarkar and H. L. Singh, "Intravenous drug users—A new high-risk group for HIV infection in India," *AIDS* 5(1)(1991):117–18.

167. P. Portegies, J. de Gans, J. M. Lange, et al., "Declining incidence of AIDS dementia complex after introduction of zidovudine treatment," 299(1989):819–21. (Published erratum appears in *British Medical Journal* 299[6708][1989]:1141.)

168. O. A. Selnes, E. Miller, J. C. McArthur, et al., "HIV-1 infection: No evidence of cognitive decline during the asymptomatic stages," *Neurology* 40(1990):204–08; O. A. Selnes, J. C. McArthur, W. Royal, et al., "HIV-1 infection and intravenous drug use: Longitudinal neuropsychological evaluation of asymptomatic subjects," *Neurology* (1992, in press).

169. World Health Organization, *Report of the Second Consultation on the Neuropsychiatric Aspects of HIV-1 Infection* (Geneva, January 1990).

170. J. M. Pluda, R. Yarchoan, E. S. Jaffe, et al., "Development of non-Hodgkin's lymphoma in a cohort of patients with severe human immunodeficiency virus (HIV) on long-term antiretroviral therapy," *Annals of Internal Medicine* 113(1990):276–82; M. Rosenblum, R. Levy, and D. Bredesen, "Overview of AIDS in the nervous system," in *AIDS and the Nervous System,* ed. M. Rosenblum, M. Levy, and D. Bredesen (New York: Raven Press, 1988).

171. Rosenblum et al., "Overview of AIDS in nervous system."

172. Ibid.; J. F. Kurtze. "The epidemiology of neurologic disease in clinical neurology," in *Clinical Neurology,* ed. A. B. Baker and L. H. Baker (Philadelphia: Harper & Row, 1986).

16. Shaping the Response

1. K. Choopanya, S. Vanichiseni, D. C. Des Jarlais, et al., "Risk factors and HIV seropositivity among injecting drug users in Bangkok," *AIDS* 5(1991):1509–13.

2. R. P. Brettle, "HIV and harm reduction for injection drug users," *AIDS* 5(1991):125–36.

3. Ibid.

4. J. R. Robertson et al., "Epidemic of AIDS-related virus (HTLV-III/LAV) infection among intravenous drug abusers," *British Medical Journal* 26(5)(1986): 515–29.

5. Brettle, "HIV and harm reduction."

6. F. Facy, E. Le Huede, and H. D. Ramirez, "Drug addicts and syringe sharing in France: Epidemiological study 1988," *International Journal of the Addictions* 26(5)(1991):515–29.

7. P. Espinoza et al., Has the open sale of syringes modified the syringe exchanging habits of drug addicts? presented at the IV International Conference on AIDS, Stockholm, Sweden, June 1988.

8. K. Stewart, G. Sattler, and K. Hedge, The implementation of waste disposal strategies for needle and syringe exchange programs, presented at the III International Conference on the Reduction of Drug Related Harm, Melbourne, Australia, March 1992.

9. D. Lowe, B. Milechman, R. Cotton, et al., Maximizing return rates and safe disposal of injection equipment in Australian needle and syringe exchange programs, presented at the VI International Conference on AIDS, San Francisco, U.S., June 1990.

10. WHO Global Programme on AIDS, "Country watch," *AIDS Health Promotion Exchange* 2(1991):12.

11. R. Tsai, E. H. Goh, P. Webeck, and V. Mullins, "Prevention of human immunodeficiency virus infection among intravenous drug users in New South Wales, Australia: The needles and syringes distribution programme through retail pharmacies," *Asia-Pacific Journal of Public Health* 2(4)(1988):245–51.

12. D. C. Des Jarlais and S. R. Friedman, "AIDS and legal access to sterile drug injection equipment," *Annals of the American Academy of Political and Social Science* (1992, in press).

13. D. S. G. Sloan, "Community pharmacies and the prevention of AIDS among injecting drug misusers," *British Medical Journal* 299 (6714) (1989):1525–26.

14. M. E. Rodriguez and M. D. Anglin, "The epidemiology of illicit drug use in Spain," *Bulletin on Narcotics* 39(1987):67–74.

15. WHO Global Programme on AIDS, "Country watch."

16. E. Buning, cited in G. V. Stimson, "Syringe-exchange programmes for injecting drug users," *AIDS* 3(1989):253–60.

17. Sloan, "Community pharmacies."

18. The Exchange Machine was developed by Scarabee Systems and Technology of Rotterdam, as reported in *International Working Group on AIDS and IV Drug Use: The Newsletter* 4(3)(1989):29.

19. Des Jarlais and Friedman, "AIDS and legal access."

20. H. Stover, "Slot machines and exchange programmes an important HIV-prevention measure," *International Working Group on AIDS and IV Drug Use: The Newsletter* 4(3)(1989):12–13.

21. Netherlands Ministry of Welfare, Health and Cultural Affairs and Ministry of Justice, The Drug Abuse Situation in the Netherlands (September 1991).

22. A. Wodak, "Country report," *International Working Group on AIDS and IV Drug Use: The Newsletter* 4(3)(1989):4.

23. Stover, "Slot machines and exchange programmes."

24. Intergovernmental Committee on AIDS, A report on HIV/AIDS Activities in Australia 1990–91, compiled by the AIDS Policy and Programs Branch of the Commonwealth Department of Health, Housing and Community Services, Australia (February 1992).

25. Ibid.

26. A. Wodak, St. Vincent's Hospital, Alcohol and Drug Service, Sydney, Australia, personal communication, 1992.

27. Ibid.

28. J. K. Watters, University of California, San Francisco, personal communication.

29. L. D. Wenger and L. D. Moore, Needle exchange and user self-organization in San Francisco: An ethnographic study, presented at the III International Conference on the Reduction of Drug Related Harm, Melbourne, Australia, March 1992.

30. Ministries of Health, Czech and Slovak Federal Republic, Short-Term Plan for the Prevention and Control of AIDS in Czechoslovakia (1991).

31. Australian National AIDS and Injecting Drug Use Study, *Neither a borrower nor a lender be,* First Report of the Australian National AIDS and Injecting Drug Use Study, 1989 Data Collection (Sydney, 1991).

32. L. Wenger, Prevention Point Research Group, Oakland, Calif., personal communication, 1992.

33. H. Hagan, D. C. Des Jarlais, D. Purchase, et al., Lower HIV seroprevalence, declining HBV incidence, and safer injection in relation to the Tacoma syringe exchange, presented at the VII International Conference on AIDS, Florence, Italy, June 1991.

34. C. Bardoux, E. Buning, A. Leentvaar-Kuijpers, et al., Declining incidence of acute hepatitis B among drug users in Amsterdam may indicate a change in risk behavior, presented at the V International Conference on AIDS, Montreal, Canada, June 1989.

35. F. Taylor, "Decline in hepatitis B cases," *American Journal of Public Health* 81(2)(1991):221–22.

36. G. J. Hart, N. Woodward, A. M. Johnson, et al., "Prevalence of HIV, Hepatitis B and associated risk behaviours in clients of a needle exchange in central London," *AIDS* 5(1991):543–47.

37. G. J. Hart, A. L. M. Carvell, N. Woodward, et al., "Evaluation of needle exchange in central London: Behavior change and anti-HIV status over one year," *AIDS* 3(1989):261–65.

38. J. A. R. Van Den Hoek, H. J. A. van Haastrecht, and R. A. Coutinho, "Risk reduction among intravenous drug users in Amsterdam under the influence of AIDS," *American Journal of Public Health* 79(10)(1989):1355–57.

39. W. Heckman, "HIV prevention among IVDUs in the Federal Republic of Germany: Stability and change," *International Journal of the Addictions* 26(12)(1991):1321–31.

40. J. K. Watters, Y. T. Cheng, G. L. Clark, and J. Lorvick, Syringe exchange in San Francisco: Preliminary findings, presented at the VII International Conference on AIDS, Florence, Italy, June 1991.

41. Hart et al., "Prevalence of HIV."

42. M. C. Donoghoe, K. A. Dolan, and G. V. Stimson, Changes in injectors' HIV risk behaviour and syringe supply in the U.K., 1987–90, presented at the VII International Conference on AIDS, Florence, Italy, June 1991.

43. Watters et al., "Syringe exchange in San Francisco."

44. J. Kelsall and N. Crofts, How methadone works as a harm reduction strategy for blood-borne infections among injecting drug users, presented at the III International Conference on the Reduction of Drug Related Harm, Melbourne, Australia, March 1992.

45. E. C. Buning, "Effects of the Amsterdam needle and syringe exchange," *International Journal of the Addictions* 26(12)(1991):1303–11.

46. E. Kaplan, Yale University, personal communication, 1992.

47. Hagan et al., "Lower HIV seroprevalence."

48. Ibid.

49. H. J. A. van Haastrecht et al., "The course of the HIV epidemic among intravenous drug users in Amsterdam, the Netherlands," *American Journal of Public Health* 81(1)(1991):59–62.

50. B. Lungberg and B. Christensson, Still no HIV epidemic among local drug users at four year follow-up of the first Swedish syringe exchange program, presented at the VII International Conference on AIDS, Florence, Italy, June 1991.

51. Hart et al., "Evaluation of needle exchange in central London."

52. R. Newcombe, The Liverpool syringe exchange scheme for drug injectors: Initial evidence of effectiveness in HIV infection, presented at the I International Conference on the Global Impact of AIDS, London, March 1988.

53. A. Wodak et al., "Antibodies to the human immunodeficiency virus in needles and syringes used by intravenous drug abusers," *Medical Journal of Australia* 147(1987):275–76.

54. J. Guydish et al., Detecting HIV antibodies in needle exchange syringes, presented at the VII International Conference on AIDS, Florence, Italy, June 1991; R. Heimer, E. C. Cadman, and E. H. Kaplan, Detection of HIV proviral DNA in the needles of intravenous drug users in the City of New Haven Needle Exchange Program, presented at ibid; M. G. Baker, M. I. Tobias, and H. Brady, Detection of HIV antibodies in used syringes in New Zealand, presented at ibid.

55. B. Ljungberg, B. Christensson, K. Tunving, et al., "HIV prevention among injection drug users: Three years of experience from a syringe exchange program in Sweden," *Journal of Acquired Immune Deficiency Syndromes* 4(1991):890–95.

56. K. I. Kall and R. G. Olin, "HIV status and changes in risk behaviour among intravenous drug users in Stockholm 1987–1988," *AIDS* 4(1990):153–57.

57. B. Christensson and B. Ljungberg, "Syringe exchange for prevention of

HIV infection in Sweden: Practical experiences and community reactions," *International Journal of the Addictions* 26(12)(1991):1293–1302.

58. F. Mesquita, Secretaria de Higiene e Saúde, Santos AIDS Reference Center, Brazil, personal communication, 1992.

59. C. Hankins, Montreal General Hospital, Canada, personal communication, 1992.

60. G. Tembo, E. Van Praag, H. Mutambo, et al., Sentinel Surveillance of HIV Infection in Zambia, presented at the V International Conference: AIDS in Africa, Kinshasa, Zaire, October 1990.

61. WHO Global Programme on AIDS, Current and future dimensions of the HIV/AIDS pandemic: A capsule summary (Geneva, 1991).

62. J. Chin and J. M. Mann, "Global patterns and prevalence of AIDS and HIV infection," *AIDS* 2 Suppl. 1 (1988):S247–52.

63. World Health Organization Global Programme on AIDS, "Cumulative cases of HIV infection worldwide: Estimate for 1990, projection for 2000," in M. J. Oxtoby and H. D. Gayle, "AIDS in women and children," *Outlook* 8(4)(1990):2–6.

64. B. B. North, "Effectiveness of Vaginal Contraceptives in Prevention of Sexually Transmitted Diseases," in *Heterosexual Transmission of AIDS*, ed. N. J. Alexander, H. L. Gabelnick, and J. M. Spieler (New York: Wiley-Liss, 1990).

65. International Prophylactics, Inc. (IP), "Questions and Answers about Bikini Condom: The Condom Worn by Women" (brochure) (Princeton, N.J.: IP).

66. M. A. Leeper, Presentation to the U.S. Food and Drug Administration (USFDA) Obstetrics and Gynecology Devices Panel at USFDA Hearing, Washington, D.C., January 1992.

67. M. Conant, D. Hardy, J. Sernatinger, et al., "Condoms prevent transmission of AIDS-associated retrovirus" (letter), *Journal of American Medical Association* 255(13)(1986):1706.

68. W. L. Drew, M. Blair, R. C. Miner, and M. Conant, "Evaluation of the virus permeability of a new condom for women," *Sexually Transmitted Diseases* 17(2) (April–June 1990):110–112.

69. B. Voeller et al., "Gas, dye and viral transport through polyurethane condoms" (letter), *Journal of the American Medical Association* 266(1991):2986–87.

70. M. A. Leeper, "Preliminary evaluation of Reality, a condom for women," *AIDS Care* 2(3)(1990):287–90; M. A. Leeper and M. Conrardy, "Preliminary evaluation of Reality, a condom for women to wear," *Advances in Contraception* 5(4)(1989):229–35.

71. G. Farr, Presentation to the U.S. Food and Drug Administration (USFDA) Obstetrics and Gynecology Devices Panel at USFDA Hearing, Washington, D.C., January 1992.

72. M. Goldman, A. R. Pebley, C. F. Westoff, and L. E. Paul, "Contraceptive failure rates in Latin America," *International Family Planning Perspectives* 9(2)(1983):50–57; J. Trussel and K. Kost, "Contraceptive failure in the United

States: A critical review of the literature," *Studies in Family Planning* 18(5)(1987):237–83.

73. Trussel and Kost, "Contraceptive Failure in the United States"; J. Trussel, R. A. Hatcher, and W. Cates, Jr., "Contraceptive failure in the United States: An update," *Studies in Family Planning* 21(1)(1990):51–54.

74. M. A. Leeper, Update on the WPC-333 (Reality) female condom, presented at the VI International Conference on AIDS, San Francisco, U.S., June 1990; G. Shangold, D. Soper, D. Shoupe, et al., Report on the Study to Evaluate the Prevention of Trichomoniasis and Chlamydia Reinfection by Compliant Use of WPC-333 (Reality) Female Condom (1991).

75. L. Liskin, C. Wharton, R. Blackburn, and P. Kestelman, "Condoms—now more than ever," *Population Reports* (Population Information Program, Johns Hopkins Center for Communication Programs), Series H, no. 8 (1990).

76. M. Monny-Lobé, J.-P. Tchupo, T. Turk, et al., *Acceptability of the Female Condom among a High-Risk Population in Cameroon* (Durham, N.C.: Family Health International, 1991).

77. D. E. Soper, "Evaluation of the effects of a female condom on the female lower genital tract," *Contraception* 44(1991):21–29.

78. W. Bounds, J. Guillebaud, L. Stewart, and S. Steele, "A female condom (Femshield): A study of its user-acceptability," *British Journal of Family Planning* 14(1988):83–87; H. Lehto and L.-L. Seppänen, Femidom User Acceptability Study in Finland 1990–91: Summary Report (1991); F. N. Mur, Madrid User Study (1991); J. Ruminjo, E. G. Mwathe, N. Thagana, et al., *Consumer Preference and Functionality Study of the Reality Female Condom in a Low Risk Population in Kenya* (Durham, N.C.: Family Health International, 1991); C. Sakondhavat, *Consumer Preference Study of the Female Condom in a Sexually Active Population at Risk of Contracting AIDS: Khon Kaen, Thailand. Final Report* (Khon Kaen, Thailand: Khon Kaen University, 1989); C. Sakondhavat, *Consumer Preference Study of Modified Female Condom in a Sexually Active Population at Risk of Contracting AIDS* (Khon Kaen, Thailand: Khon Kaen University, 1990).

79. Bounds et al., "A female condom (Femshield)"; Mur, Madrid User Study; Ruminjo et al., *Consumer Preference and Functionality Study*; Sakondhavat, *Consumer Preference Study of the Female Condom* and *Consumer Preference Study of the Modified Female Condom*.

80. Sakondhavat, *Consumer Preference Study of the Female Condom* and *Consumer Preference Study of the Modified Female Condom*.

81. Sakondhavat, *Consumer Preference Study of the Modified Female Condom*.

82. Bounds et al., "A female condom (Femshield)"; Lehto and Seppänen, Femidon User Acceptability Study; Mur, Madrid User Study.

83. Monny-Lobé et al., *Acceptability of the Female Condom*.

84. Bounds et al., "A female condom (Femshield)"; Lehto and Seppänen, Femidon User Acceptability Study; Mur, Madrid User Study; T. Tansathit and S. Cheevakej, *Femshield Acceptability Study among Family Planning Acceptors (A Pilot Study)* (Thailand: Chiang Mai University, 1990, mimeo).

85. Monny-Lobé et al., *Acceptability of the Female Condom*; Ruminjo et

al., *Consumer Preference and Functionality Study*; Sakondhavat, *Consumer Preference Study of the Modified Female Condom*; Tansathit and Cheevakej, *Femshield Acceptability Study*.

86. Bounds et al., "A female condom (Femshield)"; Lehto and Seppänen, Femidon User Acceptability Study.

87. Ruminjo et al., *Consumer Preference and Functionality Study*; Sakondhavat, *Consumer Preference Study of the Female Condom* and *Consumer Preference Study of the Modified Female Condom*.

88. Ruminjo et al., *Consumer Preference and Functionality Study*.

89. Monny-Lobé et al., *Acceptability of the Female Condom*.

90. Liskin et al., "Condoms—Now more than ever."

91. J. Shelton, "USAID supports research on the female condom: Part of agency's population program," Press release (January 31, 1992).

92. Monny-Lobé et al., *Acceptability of the Female Condom*; Ruminjo et al., *Consumer Preference and Functionality Study*.

93. S. Townsend, "Female condom—New barrier device soon to be available," *Network* 12(2)(1991):18–21, 27.

94. Ibid.

95. M. E. Guinan, "Female condoms, an urgent need," *Journal of American Medical Women Association* 46(4)(1991):131, 134.

96. World Health Organization (WHO), *Report of the consultation on partner notification for preventing HIV transmission*, WHO/GPA/ESR/89.2 (Geneva, 1989); WHO Global Programme on AIDS and Programme of STD, *Consensus statement from consultation on partner notification for preventing HIV transmission* (Geneva, January 1989); Centers for Disease Control, "Partner notification for preventing human immunodeficiency virus (HIV) infection—Colorado, Idaho, South Carolina, Virginia," *Morbidity and Mortality Weekly Report* 37(1989):393–96, 401–02; Association of State and Territorial Health Officials, National Association of County Health Officials, U.S. Conference of Local Health Officers, *Guide to Public Health Practice: HIV Partner Notification Strategies* (Washington, D.C.: Public Health Foundation, 1988).

97. WHO, *Report of the consultation on partner notification*; WHO Global Programme on AIDS and Programme of STD, *Consensus Statement*; D. Miller and A. J. Pinching, "HIV tests and counselling: Current issues," *AIDS* 3(suppl. 1)(1989):S187–93; M. W. Adler and A. M. Johnson, "Contact tracing for HIV infection," *British Medical Journal* 296(1988):1420–21; J. J. Potterat, N. E. Spencer, D. E. Woodhouse, and J. B. Muth, "Partner notification in the control of human immunodeficiency virus infection," *American Journal of Public Health* 29(1989):874–75; L. Gostin and W. J. Curran, "AIDS screening confidentiality and the duty to warn," *American Journal of Public Health* 77(1987):361–65; K. E. Toomey and W. Cates, "Partner notification for the prevention of HIV infection," *AIDS* 3(suppl. 1)(1989):S57–62; J. E. Osborn, "AIDS: Politics and science," *New England Journal of Medicine* 318(1988):444–47; R. Bayer and K. E. Toomey, "HIV prevention and the two faces of partner notification: Policy, politics and ethics," *American Journal of Public Health* (in press).

98. J. J. Eron and M. S. Hirsch, "New anti-HIV-1 therapies and combinations:

Current data and prospects," *AIDS* 4(suppl. 1)(1990):S193–200; J. Feinberg and J. Mills, "Treatment of opportunistic infections," *AIDS* 4(suppl. 1)(1990):S209–15.

99. Toomey and Cates, "Partner notification."

100. K. Porter, Communicable Disease Surveillance Centre, U.K. Public Health Laboratory Service, London, U.K., personal communication, 1992.

101. R. A. Keenlyside, A. Hawkins, A. M. Johnson, and M. W. Adler, "Attitudes to contact tracing and partner notification for persons with HIV infection among health advisers and consultants in genito-urinary medicine in the U.K.," *British Medical Journal* (in press).

102. A. Stroobant, Institute of Hygiene and Epidemiology, Epidemiology Unit, Brussels, Belgium, personal communication, 1992.

103. S. De Witt, Clinique des Maladies Infectieuses, Hôpital de Saint Pierre, Brussels, Belgium, personal communication, 1992.

104. N. Clumeck, Director, AIDS Activities, Hôpital de Saint Pierre, Brussels, Belgium, personal communication, 1992.

105. WHO-EC Collaborating Centre on AIDS, *AIDS Surveillance in Europe. 1991 Quarterly Report no. 31* (Paris, 1991).

106. J. Gieseke, K. Ramstedt, F. Granath, et al., "Efficacy of partner notification for HIV infection," *Lancet* 338(1991):1096–1100; J. Gieseke, K. Ramstedt, F. Granath, et al., "Partner notification as a tool for research in HIV epidemiology," *AIDS* 61(1992):101–07.

107. Stroobant, personal communication.

108. V. Hasseltveldt, National Institute for Public Health, Oslo, Norway, personal communication, 1992.

109. WHO, *Report of the consultation on partner notification*; J. E. Kristofferson, Case contact tracing and testing in HIV infection, presented at the IV International Conference on AIDS, Stockholm, Sweden, June 1988.

110. H. Briehm, Reykjavik City Hospital Department of Medicine, Reykjavik, Iceland, personal communication, 1992.

111. M. Melbye, Department of Epidemiology, State Serum Institute, Copenhagen, Denmark, personal communication, 1992.

112. WHO Regional Office for Europe, HIV/AIDS in Central and Eastern Europe: Epidemiology, prevention and control (24 July 1991).

113. WHO, *Report of the consultation on partner notification*.

114. A. Vass, Department of Public Health and Epidemiology, Ministry of Welfare of the Republic, Budapest, Hungary, personal communication, 1992.

115. G. Walter, Chief, Department of Epidemiology and Microbiology, Ministry of Health of the Czech Republic, Prague, Czechoslovakia, personal communication, 1992.

116. WHO, *Report of the consultation on partner notification*.

117. J. Kohut, "Country still groping to provide care: China," *Boston Globe,* June 15, 1991.

118. WHO, *Report of the consultation on partner notification*.

119. T. C. Quinn, J. P. Narian, and F. R. K. Zacarias, "AIDS in the Americas: A public health priority for the region," *AIDS* 4(1990):709–24.

120. J. Hospetales, Caribbean Epidemiology Centre, Pan American Health Organisation, Port of Spain, Trinidad and Tobago, personal communication, 1992.

121. C. Cholmondley, Caribbean Epidemiology Centre, Pan American Health Organisation, Port of Spain, Trinidad and Tobago, personal communication, 1992.

122. P. Figueroa, Epidemiology Unit, Ministry of Health, Kingston, Jamaica, personal communication, 1992.

123. WHO, *Report of the consultation on partner notification.*

124. Quinn et al., "AIDS in the Americas"; E. J. Perez-Stable, "Cuba's response to the HIV epidemic," *American Journal of Public Health* 81(1991):563–66.

125. Perez-Stable, "Cuba's response."

126. R. S. Remis, Centre for AIDS Studies, DSC Montreal General Hospital, Quebec, Canada, personal communication, 1992.

127. Ibid.

128. Toomey and Cates, "Partner notification."

129. M. L. Rekert, L. Knowles, D. Spencer, and B. Pengelly, Patient referral or provider referral: Which do patients prefer? presented at the VI International Conference on AIDS, San Francisco, U.S., June 1990.

130. Potterat et al., "Partner notification in the control"; G. W. Rutherford, J. M. Woo, D. P. Neal, et al., "Partner notification and the control of human immunodeficiency virus infection," *Sexually Transmitted Diseases* 2(1992):107–10; R. F. Wykoff, J. L. Jones, S. T. Longshore, et al., "Notification of the sex and needle sharing partners of individuals with human immunodeficiency virus in rural South Carolina: 30-month experience," *Sexually Transmitted Diseases* 18(1991):217–20.

131. Potterat et al., "Partner notification in the control"; Rutherford et al., "Partner notification and the control of human immunodeficiency virus"; J. L. Jones, R. F. Wykoff, S. L. Hollis, et al., "Partner acceptability of health department notification of HIV exposure, South Carolina," *Journal of the American Medical Association* 264(1990):1284–86.

132. G. Marks, J. L. Richardson, and N. Maldonado, "Self-disclosure of HIV infection to sexual partners," *American Journal of Public Health* 81(1991):1321–22; G. Marks, J. L. Richardson, M. Ruiz, and N. Maldonado, "HIV-infected men's practices in notifying past sexual partners of infection risk," *Public Health Reports* 107(1992):100–05; D. J. Schnell and D. L. Higgins, Disclosure of HIV test results to male sex partners among men who have sex with men (manuscript submitted for publication).

133. S. E. Landis, V. J. Schoenback, D. J. Weber, et al., "Results of a randomized trial of partner notification in cases of HIV infection in North Carolina," *New England Journal of Medicine* 326(1992):101–06.

134. K. E. Toomey, unpublished data.

135. WHO, *Report of the consultation on partner notification.*

136. Ibid.

137. Ibid; Toomey and Cates, "Partner notification."

138. Keenlyside et al., "Attitudes to contact tracing."

139. Bayer and Toomey, "HIV prevention."

140. See, e.g., R. Shilts, *And the Band Played On* (New York: St. Martin's Press, 1987; London: Penguin Books, 1988); S. Watney, *Policing Desire: Pornography, AIDS, and the Media* (Minneapolis: University of Minnesota Press, 1989); S. Panem, *The AIDS Bureaucracy* (Cambridge, Mass.: Harvard University Press, 1988).

141. D. C. Colby and T. E. Cook, "Epidemics and agendas: The politics of nightly news coverage of AIDS," *Journal of Health Politics, Policy and Law* 16(1991):215–49.

142. See, e.g., J. Kitzinger and D. Miller, *In Black and White*, Medical Research Council Working Paper 27 (Glasgow University Media Group, 1991); S.-A. Kambamba et al., PSI project PEM-SIDA, Kinshasa, Zaire, presented at the VI International Conference on AIDS in Africa, Dakar, December 1991.

143. J. Street, "British government policy on AIDS," *Parliamentary Affairs* 41(1988):490–508.

144. V. Berridge, "AIDS, the media and health policy," *Health Education Journal* 50(1991):179–85.

145. Interview with Simon Watney, London, December 1991.

146. J. Kinsella, *Covering the Plague* (New Brunswick, N.J.: Rugters University Press, 1990).

147. See, e.g., S. Watney, "AIDS, Moral panic theory and homophobia," in *Social Aspects of AIDS*, ed. P. Aggleton and H. Homans (Lewes, U.K.: Falmer Press, 1988); K. Wellings, "Perceptions of risk—Media treatment of AIDS," ibid.; R. Sabatier et al., *Blaming Others: Prejudice, Race and Worldwide AIDS* (London and Washington, D.C.: Panos Institute, 1988); M. Pitts and H. Jackson, "AIDS and the press: An analysis of the coverage of AIDS by Zimbabwe newspapers," *AIDS Care* 1(1989):77–83.

148. Wellings, "Perceptions of risk."

149. Pitts and Jackson, "AIDS and the press."

150. *Ghanaian Times* (Accra), quoted in *New York Times*, April 15, 1987.

151. S. Ramos, consultant to ABIA, the Brazilian Interdisciplinary Association for AIDS, Rio de Janeiro, letter to author, 1991.

152. C. Patton, "Inventing 'African AIDS'," *New Formations* 10(1990):25–40.

153. Sabatier et al., *Blaming Others.*

154. Pitts and Jackson, "AIDS and the press."

155. T. Cook, Notes for the Next Epidemic, Part One: Lessons from the News Coverage of AIDS, Discussion Paper D12, Harvard University John F. Kennedy School of Government (1991); T. Netter, The media and AIDS: A global perspective (1992, in press).

156. Panem, *The AIDS Bureaucracy*; Berridge, "AIDS, the media and health policy"; C. Herzlich and J. Peirret, "The construction of a social phenomenon: AIDS in the French press," *Social Science and Medicine* 29(1989):1235–42.

157. Berridge, "AIDS, the media and health policy."

158. Ibid.

159. Colby and Cook, "Epidemics and agendas."

160. Berridge, "AIDS, the media and health policy."

161. *Washington Post*, December 22, 1991; interviews with CDC staff, January 1992.

162. G. Philo, *Seeing and Believing* (London: Routledge, 1990)

163. Ibid.

164. Quoted in article in *Africa Now*, February 1987.

165. Jean Pape, Address to NIAID's IV International Conference on AIDS Vaccine Development, Marco Island, Florida, October 1991.

166. See, e.g., *Times of Zambia*, March 3, 1988.

167. *Travel Trade Gazette*, November 2, 1989; *Annals of Tourism Research* 15(1988):467–86.

168. Interview with D. Miller, Glasgow Media Group.

169. C. Mouli and S. Nyirenda, The impact of mass-media promotion of Kemron as the new miracle AIDS cure on the AIDS prevention effort in Zambia (Copperbelt Health Education Project, P.O. Box 23567, Kitwe, Zambia, 1990).

170. F. Kroger, AIDS—Health communication's greatest challenge. Case studies of effective health communication programs, presented at the 1991 Health Communication Day, Johns Hopkins University Center for Communication Programs, Baltimore, Md., October 1991; R. G. Parker, AIDS education and health promotion in Brazil: Lessons from the past and prospects for the future (1990).

171. K. Bosompra, "Dissemination of health information among rural dwellers in Africa: A Ghanaian experience," *Social Science and Medicine* 29(9)(1989): 1133–40; H. Bagarukayo, KAP study on AIDS among school pupils in Kabale District, Uganda, presented at the VII International Conference on AIDS, Florence, Italy, June 1991; C. A. Church and J. Geller, "Lights! Camera! Action! Promoting family planning with TV, video, and film," *Population Reports* (Population Information Program, Johns Hopkins Center for Communication Programs), Series J, no. 38 (1989); P. T. Piotrow, J. G. Rimon II, K. E. Winnard, et al., "Mass-media family planning promotion in three Nigerian cities," *Studies in Family Planning* 21(5)(1990):265–74; J. Convisser, "The Zaire mass media project: A model AIDS prevention project," in *PSI Special Reports*, ed. H. Crowley and B. Derr (Population Services International, 1991).

172. Sabatier et al., *Blaming Others*.

173. Church and Geller, "Lights! Camera! Action!"; L. Liskin, C. A. Church, and P. T. Piotrow, "AIDS education—A beginning," *Population Reports* (Population Information Program, Johns Hopkins Center for Communication Programs), Series L, no. 8 (1989).

174. M. V. Jimenez and L. S. Bond, paper presented at the VI International Conference on AIDS, San Francisco, U.S., June 1990; B. Birchmeier, J. E. Richard, D. Hausser, et al., AIDS in Swiss newspapers: Reporting of preventive events and designing the image of AIDS, presented at the V International Conference on AIDS, Montreal, Canada, June 1989; L. Guzman, B. Rico, C. Magis, and G. Rangel, AIDS and the Mexican press, ibid.; D. Lupton, "AIDS and the popular media: A new perspective at Florence," *AIDS Care* 3(4)(1991):447–49.

175. Liskin et al., "AIDS education."

176. Church and Geller, "Lights! Camera! Action!"

177. J. T. Bertrand, P. Russell-Brown, and E. G. Landry, Evaluation of the Caribbean Contraceptive Social Marketing Project in three countries (1985); J. G. Rimon II and C. L. Lettenmaier, *Trip Report: Strategic Options for IEC Interventions in Kenya* (Baltimore: Population Communication Services of the Johns Hopkins University, 1990).

178. J. G. Rimon II, D. L. Kincaid, and E. W. Whitney, *Trip Report: Philippines* (Baltimore: Population Communication Services of the Johns Hopkins University, 1980).

179. Social Planning, Analysis, and Administration Consultants, Final report: SIS/IEC center impact evaluation study (Cairo, 1988).

180. H. Koné and K. F. Yao, Projet Panafricain de Supports Imprimés en Matière de Planification Familiale, Notes et Etudes de CERCOM, no. 1 (Université Nationale de Côte d'Ivoire, Centre d'Enseignement et de Recherche en Communication, 1989).

181. Population Communication Services of the Johns Hopkins University, *Final Report: Generic Condom Promotion in Colombia (LA-COL-01)* (Baltimore: Population Communication Services, Johns Hopkins University, and PRO-FAMILIA, 1986).

182. P. Twivy, "Comment on changing attitudes to condoms through advertising," *Family Planning Today* 4 (1988):4.

183. R. Tebere, "Uganda: Condoms provoke an AIDS storm," *New African* 282(1991):27.

184. J. P. Baggaley, "Perceived effectiveness of international AIDS campaigns," *Health Education Research, Theory & Practice* (1)(1988):7–17.

185. A. Payne Merritt, D. L. Kincaid, M. Lujan, et al., Mass-media AIDS prevention campaign in Lima, Peru, presented at the 117th Annual Meeting of the American Public Health Association (APHA), Chicago, Ill., 1989; Population Communication Services, *Final Report (LA-COL-01)*.

186. L. Sherr, Long and short term impact of the U.K. government health education campaign on AIDS (1988).

187. D. Serwadda, M. Wawer, S. Musgrave, et al., An assessment of AIDS related knowledge, attitudes, and practices (KAP) in Rakai District, Uganda, presented at the V International Conference on AIDS, Montreal, Canada, June 1989.

188. Parker, "AIDS education and health promotion."

189. Liskin et al., "Condoms—Now more than ever."

190. Population Services International, Dual strategy in Zaire promotes condom use for AIDS protection (1990).

191. G. Ojeda, R. Vernon, and R. Murad, *IEC Service Delivery and Condom Distribution through Family Planning Organizations for AIDS and STD Prevention. (Final Report)* (Bogota: Asociación ProBienestar de la Familia Colombiana and the Population Council, 1989).

192. B. Makanjuola, "Living with AIDS," *West Africa*, 1991:14–20.

193. O. B. Ayowa, J. E. Brown, and R. C. Brown, L'éducation publique sur le

SIDA à Kananga, Zaire, 1987–1990; correspondence with Okako Bibi Ayowa, L'Institut Médical Chrétien du Kasai (1991).

194. Academy for Educational Development (AED) *AIDSCOM Communication from Behavior Change Task Force, 27–28 March 1991* (Washington, D.C.: Academy for Educational Development, 1991).

195. L. Sherr and J. Green, Evaluation of health education in Britain, presented at the III International Conference on AIDS, Washington, D.C., June 1987.

196. D. J. Wilson and C. Wilson, An AIDS information strategy in Zimbabwe, presented at the I International Conference on Information and Education on AIDS, Ixtapa, Mexico, October 1988.

197. Serwadda et al., "An assessment of AIDS related knowledge."

198. Liskin et al., "AIDS education."

199. S. McCombie, Preliminary statistics for the Ugandan film *It's Not Easy*, Annenberg School of Communication, University of Pennsylvania, personal communication, January 1992.

200. R. F. Soames Job, "Effective and ineffective use of fear in health promotion campaigns," *Australian Journal of Public Health* 78(2)(1988):163–67.

201. A. Morlet, J. J. Guinan, I. Diefenthaler, and J. Gold, "The impact of the 'Grim Reaper' National AIDS Educational Campaign on the Albion Street (AIDS) Centre and the AIDS Hotline," *Medical Journal of Australia* 148(6)(1988):282–86.

202. O. Ogunyankin and M. K. Jinadu, Evaluation of AIDS education through mass media, presented at the VI International Conference on AIDS, San Francisco, U.S., June 1990.

203. D. Hausser, University of Lausanne, Condom use in Switzerland, personal communication, October 1990; F. Dubois-Arber, P. Lehmann, D. Hausser, and F. Gutz-Willer, *Evaluation des campagnes de prévention du SIDA en Suisse: deuxième rapport de synthèse 1988*, Cah. Rech. Doc. IUMSP, no. 39 (Lausanne, Switzerland: Institut Universitaire de Médecine Sociale et Préventive, 1989); J. F. Martin and P.-A. Michaud, "AIDS education in Switzerland: Implementing strategies to reach groups with high risk behaviours, particularly youth," *Health Education Research Theory and Practice* 3(1)(1988):105–12.

204. M. Ramah, J. L. Izazola, M. Ramos, and J. L. Valdespino, Condom promotion to gay men in Mexico: Why focusing on lifestyle of target group may not work, presented at the V International Conference on AIDS, Montreal, Canada, June 1989.

205. L. Cole, Family Health International, "Condoms—Because You Care" campaign, personal communication, January 1991.

206. J. Sepulveda, J. A. Izazola, J. L. Valdespino, et al., Massive campaign for AIDS education, achievements and problems, presented at the V International Conference on AIDS, Montreal, Canada, June 1989.

207. Payne Merritt, "Mass-media AIDS prevention campaign."

208. Convisser, "The Zaire mass media project."

209. L. Ward, "Drama: An effective way to educate about AIDS," *Social Casework* 69(6)(1988):3936; M. Helquist and G. Sealy, Rural AIDS education and theatre project in Trinidad and Tobago (unpublished, 1989); C. Evian, Popular

theatre and community AIDS education, presented at the IV International AIDS Education Conference, Puerto Rico, August 1990; and personal correspondence with Clie Evian, City Health Department, 1477 Johannesburg 2000, South Africa.

210. Family Health International, "North Carolina: AIDSTECH Project," *Network* 11(1)(1989):12–13.

211. R. A. Goodman, ed., "Effectiveness in disease and injury prevention: Characteristics of parents who discuss AIDS with their children—US, 1989," *Morbidity and Mortality Weekly Report* 40(46)(1991):789–91.

212. M. E. Gallen, L. Liskin, and N. Kak, "Men—New focus for family planning programs," *Population Reports* (Population Information Program, Johns Hopkins Center for Communication Programs), Series J, no. 33 (1986); P. E. Hollerbach, *Power in Families, Communication and Fertility Decision-Making*, Center for Policy Studies Working Paper no. 53 (New York: Population Council, 1990); L. Rainwater, *And the Poor Get Children: Sex, Contraception, and Family Planning in the Working Class* (Chicago: Quadrangle Books, 1960); United Nations, Economic and Social Commission for Asia and the Pacific (ESCAP), "Family planning communication programmes and their impact on husband-wife communication," and "Husband-wife communication: Measurement and correlation with family planning," in *Husband-Wife Communication and Practice of Family Planning* (Bangkok: ESCAP, 1974).

213. M. E. Gallen and W. Rinehart, "Operations research: Lessons for policy and programs," *Population Reports* (Population Information Program, Johns Hopkins Center for Communication Programs), Series J, no. 31 (1986); D. L. Kincaid, J. R. J. Elias, P. Coleman, and F. Segura, *Getting the Message: The Communication for Young People Project*, AIDS Evaluation Special Study no. 56 (Washington, D.C.: Agency for International Development, 1988); R. J. Lapham and W. P. Mauldin, "Contraception prevalence: The influence of organized family planning programs," *Studies in Family Planning* 16(3)(1985):117–37; Population Communication Services, *Annual Report: FY87* (Baltimore: Johns Hopkins University, 1988) and *Annual Report: FY88* (Baltimore: Johns Hopkins University, 1989); R. E. Rice and C. K. Atkins, eds., *Public Communication Campaigns*, 2d ed. (Newbury Park, Calif.: Sage, 1989).

214. Kroger, "AIDS—Health communication's greatest challenge."

215. M. E. Carillo, S. M. Toavar, P. B. Cipriano, et al., AIDS hotline: Model in a developing country, presented at the VI International Conference on AIDS, San Francisco, U.S., June 1990.

216. S. Maayan, D. Engelhard, S. Boger, et al., "Epidemiological observations in the AIDS clinic at the Hadassah University Hospital in Jerusalem," *Israel Journal of Medical Sciences* 25(6)(1989):309–13.

217. P. T. Piotrow and R. C. Meyer, "Promoting family planning: Findings from operations research and program research: The MORE Project International Conference on Operations Research," in *Operations Research: Helping Family Planning Programs Work Better* (New York: John Wiley and Sons, 1991).

218. M. S. Boone, J. U. Farley, and S. J. Samuel, "A cross-country study of commercial contraceptive sales programs: Factors that lead to success," *Studies in Family Planning* 16(1)(1985):96–102.

219. P. Zuegin, F. Dubois-Arber, D. Hausser, and R. Lehmann, Sexual behaviour of young adults and the effect of AIDS-prevention campaigns in Switzerland, presented at the V International Conference on AIDS, Montreal, Canada, June 1989.

220. PSI Marketing Associates, Social marketing of contraceptives: Briefing book (unpublished, 1990).

221. Kincaid et al., *Getting the Message.*

222. A. Bandura, *Social Foundations of Thought and Action* (Englewood Cliffs, N.J.: Prentice-Hall, 1986); M. Sabido, Towards the social use of soap opera: Mexico's experience with the reinforcement of social values through TV soap operas, presented at the Annual Conference of the International Institute of Communications, Strasbourg, France, September 1981; A. Singhal and E. Rogers, "Pro-social television for development in India," in *Public Communication Campaigns,* ed. R. Rice and C. Atkin (Newbury Park, Calif.: Sage, 1989).

223. Kincaid et al., *Getting the Message;* Piotrow et al., "Mass-media family planning"; S. H. Yun, D. L. Kincaid, Y. Yaser, and G. Ozler, The national family planning IEC campaign of Turkey (unpublished, 1990); McCombie, Preliminary statistics for the Ugandan film; Convisser, "The Zaire mass media project."

224. McCombie, Preliminary statistics for the Ugandan film.

225. Convisser, "The Zaire mass media project."

226. P. Mubiana, A research survey conducted in Ndola and Kitwe to assess a radiodrama play called *Nishilakamoru* (1991).

227. M. M. Dayrit, O. T. Monzon, V. Basaca-Sevilla, and C. G. Hayes, "Emerging patterns of HIV infection and control in the Philippines," *Western Journal of Medicine* 147(6)(1987):723–25.

228. Ayowa et al., "L'éducation publique."

229. Kincaid et al., *Getting the Message.*

230. J. G. Rimon II, "Leveraging messages and corporations: The Philippine experience," *Integration* (Japanese Organization for International Cooperation in Family Planning [JOICFP]) 22(1989):37–44.

231. Population Communication Services (PCS) of The Johns Hopkins University, *Nigeria Family Health Services Project Information Education and Communication (IEC) Component: Year Two Activities, April 1989 to March 1990* (Baltimore: PCS, 1991).

232. Ayowa et al., "L'éducation publique."

233. Convisser, "The Zaire mass media project."

234. C. Gray, "Myths about AIDS continue to flourish," *Canadian Medical Association Journal* 138(8)(1988):733, 735.

235. Convisser, "The Zaire mass media project."

236. M. Paalman and K. de Vries, *Condom Promotion in the Netherlands: Strategy and Implementation* (Utrecht: Dutch STD Foundation, 1988).

237. P. Lehmann, D. Hausser, B. Somaini, and F. Gutzwiller, "Campaign against AIDS in Switzerland: Evaluation of a nationwide education programme," *British Medical Journal* 295(6606)(1987):1118–20.

238. Population Services International (PSI), *Annual Report* (Washington, D.C.: PSI, 1989).

239. S. Tipping, The Futures Group, Changes in condom promotion in the 1980s, sales of social marketing condoms, personal communication, September 1990 and April 1991; G. O'Sullivan, the Futures Group, Morocco social marketing project, personal communication, December 1990.

240. H. Hughes, "Ze Cabro-Macho does it safely: Building an AIDS awareness campaign among Brazil's construction workers," *AIDS Action* (4)(1988):2–3.

241. Payne Merritt et al., "Mass media AIDS prevention campaign."

242. Academy for Educational Development, Evaluation of the impact on U.S. audiences of a dramatic presentation designed for continental African audiences, AIDSCOM Research Note no. 1, August 1991.

243. Ibid.

244. V. R. Prewitt, "Health beliefs and AIDS educational materials," *Family and Community Health* 12(2)(1989):65–76.

245. D. F. Stone, It's not easy, presented at the VI International Conference on AIDS, San Francisco, U.S., June 1990.

246. Parker, "AIDS education and health promotion."

247. Gray, "Myths about AIDS."

248. M. Kapila and K. Wellings, "The U.K. public education campaign—Evaluation and evolution," unpublished manuscript (1989).

249. Ibid.

250. R. B. De Jong, Netherlands condom advertising campaign, Radio Nederland Training Centre Workshop, 1991.

251. D. L. Kincaid, S. H. Yun, P. T. Piotrow, et al., "Turkey's mass media family planning campaign," in *Impact of Organizations on Mass Media Health Behavior Campaigns,* ed. T. E. Backer, E. M. Rogers, and R. Denniston (in press, 1992).

252. P. T. Piotrow, D. L. Kincaid, M. J. Hindin, et al., Changing men's attitudes and behavior: The Zimbabwe male motivation project (Johns Hopkins University Center for Communication Programs, 1992).

253. R. Bayer, *Private Acts, Social Consequences: AIDS and the Politics of Public Health* (New York: Free Press, 1989).

254. D. W. Lyter, "The role of HIV testing in AIDS prevention programs," in R. O. Valeliseni, *Preventing AIDS* (New Brunswick, N.J.: Rutgers University Press, 1989).

255. G. Frankenberg, "Germany: The uneasy triumph of pragmatism," in *AIDS in the Industrialized Democracies,* ed. D. L. Kirp and R. Bayer (New Brunswick, N.J.: Rutgers University Press, 1992).

256. M. Steffen, "France: Social solidarity and scientific expertise," in Kirp and Bayer, *AIDS in the Industrialized Democracies.*

257. Bayer, *Private Acts, Social Consequences.*

258. J. K. van Wijngaarden, "The Netherlands: AIDS in a consensual society," in Kirp and Bayer, *AIDS in the Industrialized Democracies.*

259. R. Bayer and L. Gostin, "Legal and ethical issues in AIDS," in *Current Issues in AIDS: Vol. 2,* ed. M. S. Gottlieb et al. (Chichester, U.K.: John Wiley & Sons, 1989).

260. Centers for Disease Control, "Education and foster care for children infected with human T-lymphotrophic virus type III/Lymphadenopathy-associated virus," *Morbidity and Mortality Weekly Report* 34(1985):517–21.

261. Centers for Disease Control, "Recommendations for preventing transmission of infection with human T-lymphotrophic virus type III/lymphadenopathy-associated virus in the workplace," *Morbidity and Mortality Weekly Report* 34(1985):681–86, 691–95.

262. World Health Organization Global Programme on AIDS, Report of the meeting on criteria for HIV screening programmes, WHO/SPA/GLO/87.2.

263. R. Bayer and C. Healton, "Controlling AIDS in Cuba: The logic of quarantine," *New England Journal of Medicine*, April 13, 1989:1022–24.

264. T. Hammett, "AIDS in correctional facilities: 1988 update," *Issues and Practices in Criminal Justice*, June 1989.

265. J. Ballard, "Australia: Participation and innovation in a federal system," in Kirp and Bayer, *AIDS in the Industrialized Democracies.*

266. B. Henriksson and H. Ytterberg, "Sweden: The power of the moral(istic) left," in Kirp and Bayer, *AIDS in the Industrialized Democracies.*

267. Steffen, "France: Social solidarity."

268. E. Albaek, "Denmark: AIDS and the political pink triangle," in Kirp and Bayer, *AIDS in the Industrialized Democracies.*

269. Bayer and Gostin, "Legal and ethical issues."

270. J. Colombotos et al., Physicians, nurses, and AIDS: Preliminary findings from a national study (Washington, D.C.: Agency for Health Care Policy and Research, 1991).

271. R. Blendon, K. Donelan, and R. A. Knox, "Public opinion and AIDS: Lessons for the second decade," *Journal of the American Medical Association* 267(7)(1992):981–86.

272. L. Gostin, "HIV-Infected physicians and the practice of seriously invasive procedures," *Hastings Center Report* 19(1)(1989):32–39.

273. Centers for Disease Control, "Possible transmission of human immunodeficiency virus to a patient during an invasive dental procedure," *Morbidity and Mortality Weekly Report* 39(1990):489–93.

274. Centers for Disease Control, "Update: Transmission of HIV infection during invasive dental procedures—Florida," *Morbidity and Mortality Weekly Report* 40(1991):377–80.

275. A. Caplan, "Make a leap of faith? It's an AIDS dilemma," *St. Paul Press*, June 23, 1991.

276. American Medical Association, Statement on HIV infected physicians (January 17, 1991).

277. Blendon et al., "Public opinion and AIDS."

278. M. Angell, "A dual approach to the AIDS epidemic," *New England Journal of Medicine* 324(1991):1498–1500.

279. M. Barnes et al., "The HIV-infected heath care professional: Employment policies and public health," *Law, Medicine & Health Care* 18(4)(1990):311–30.

280. Centers for Disease Control, "Recommendations for preventing trans-

mission of human immunodeficiency virus and hepatitis B virus to patients during exposure-prone invasive procedures," *Morbidity and Mortality Weekly Report* 40(RR-8)(1991):1–7.

281. Centers for Disease Control, Proposed guidelines for providing HIV testing services to inpatients and outpatients in acute-care hospital settings (September 17, 1991, mimeo).

282. L. Jones, "HIV infection labeled as STD; board to clarify testing policy," *American Medical News*, December 14, 1990:3.

283. Colombotos et al., "Physicians, nurses, and AIDS." .

284. C. Levine and R. Bayer, "The ethics of screening for early intervention in HIV disease," *American Journal of Public Health* 79(12)(1989):1661–67.

285. Colombotos et al., "Physicians, nurses, and AIDS."

286. A. M. Comeau, J. A. Harris, K. McIntosh, et al., "Polymerase chain reaction in detecting HIV-infection among seropositive infants: Relation to clinical status and age and to results of other assays," *Journal of Acquired Immune Deficiency Syndromes* 5(3)(1992):271–78.

287. Working Group on PCP Prophylaxis in Children, "Guidelines for prophylaxis against pneumocystis carinii pneumonia for children infected with human immunodeficiency virus," *Morbidity and Mortality Weekly Report* 40(RR-2)(1991):1–13.

288. Institute of Medicine, *HIV Screening of Pregnant Women and Newborns* (Washington, D.C.: National Academy Press, 1991).

289. Task Force on Pediatric AIDS, American Academy of Pediatrics, "Prenatal human immunodeficiency (HIV) testing," *American Academy of Pediatrics News*, February 1992:20.

290. C. Turner, H. C. Miller, and L. E. Moses, eds., *AIDS Sexual Behavior and Intravenous Drug Use* (Washington, D.C.: National Academy Press, 1989).

291. R. Bayer, L. H. Lumey, and L. Wan, "The American, British, and Dutch responses to unlinked anonymous HIV seroprevalence studies: An international comparison," *AIDS* 4(1990):283–90.

292. Government of Canada, Federal AIDS Centre, Guidelines in ethical and legal conditions in anonymous unlinked HIV seroprevalence research (1988).

293. World Health Organization Global Programme on AIDS, Unlinked anonymous screening for public health surveillance of HIV infections: Proposed international guidelines (1989).

294. Albaek, "Denmark: AIDS and the political pink triangle."

295. Henriksson and Ytterberg, "Sweden: The power of the moral(istic) left."

296. K. Henry, K. Willenbring, and K. Crossleg, "Human immunodeficiency virus antibody testing: A description of practices and policies at U.S. infectious-disease-teaching hospitals and Minnesota hospitals," *Journal of the American Medical Association* 259(12)(1988):1819–22.

297. Albaek, "Denmark: AIDS and the political pink triangle."

298. E. Feldman, "Japan: AIDS as a 'non-issue,'" in Kirp and Bayer, *AIDS in the Industrialized Democracies*.

299. D. M. Rayside and E. A. Lindquist, "Canada: Community activism,

federalism, and the new politics of disease," in Bayer and Kirp, *AIDS in the Industrialized Democracies*.

17. Policy and Program Issues

1. U.S. National Commission on AIDS, *Report: HIV Disease in Correctional Facilities* (Washington, D.C.: National Institute of Justice, 1990).

2. G. P. Wormser, L. B. Krupp, J. P. Hanrahan, et al., "Acquired immune deficiency syndrome in male prisoners: New insights into an emerging syndrome," *Annals of Internal Medicine* 98(1983):297–393.

3. T. W. Harding, "AIDS in prison," *Lancet* 2(1987):1260–63.

4. WHO, *Drug Abusers in Prisons: Managing Their Health Problems*, WHO Regional Publications, European Series no. 27 (The Hague, 1988).

5. U.S. National Commission on AIDS, *Report*.

6. S. A. Chambuso, AIDS in prison: The Tanzanian experience, presented at a seminar on prison medicine, International Committee of the Red Cross, Port Louis, Mauritius, 1991.

7. "Health care for prisoners: Implications of 'Kalk's refusal,'" editorial, *Lancet* 337(1991):647–48; T. W. Harding, "Can prison medicine be ethical?" *Journal of Irish Colleges of Physicians and Surgeons* 20(1991):2621–25.

8. Wormser et al., "Acquired immune deficiency syndrome in male prisoners."

9. Council of Europe, Parliamentary Assembly, Recommendation 1080 on a coordinated European policy to prevent the spread of AIDS in prisons, Strasbourg (1988).

10. "A European committee looks at degrading treatment in custody," editorial, *Lancet* 338(1991):1559–60.

11. T. M. Hammett and M. Saira, *1989 Update: AIDS in Correctional Facilities* (Washington, D.C.: National Institute of Justice, 1990); cited in E. Kantor, *AIDS and HIV Infection in Prisoners: Epidemiology and Transmission*, AIDS Knowledge Base Text (San Francisco General Hospital, 1991).

12. Report of the AIDS and Housing Project, *Survey into Levels of Satisfaction among Tenants Housed because of Their HIV Infection* (London: Josef Rowntree Foundation, 1992).

13. S. Leckie, *From Housing Needs to Housing Rights: An Analysis of the Right to Housing under International Human Rights Law* (London: International Institute for Environment and Development, 1992).

14. Report of the AIDS and Housing Project, *Survey into Levels of Satisfaction*; A. Hendriks and S. Leckie, *AIDS and Housing Rights in Western Europe: A Comparative Study of the Netherlands, Spain and the United Kingdom* (London: the National AIDS Trust, 1991).

15. Leckie, *From Housing Needs to Housing Rights*.

16. Hendriks and Leckie, *AIDS and Housing Rights*.

17. Report of the AIDS and Housing Project, *Survey into Levels of Satisfaction*.

18. R. Cohen and L. S. Wiseberg, *Double Jeopardy—Threat to Life and Human Rights* (Cambridge, Mass.: Human Rights Internet, March 1990).

19. L. Schweitzer, "Welkom in Simonszhuis," *Amsterdam Drug Tijdschrift*, April 1991:6.

20. Anonymous, "AIDS more prevalent among homeless," *San Francisco Chronicle* (June 18, 1991).

21. Hendriks and Leckie, *AIDS and Housing Rights*; Cohen and Wiseberg, *Double Jeopardy*.

22. Hendriks and Leckie, *AIDS and Housing Rights*.

23. Ibid.

24. Ibid.

25. Ibid.

26. See, e.g., D. Altman, *AIDS in the Mind of America* (New York: Anchor Press/Doubleday, 1986); C. Perrow and M. Guillen, *The AIDS Disaster* (New Haven: Yale University Press, 1990); and R. Padgug and G. Oppenheimer, "Riding the tiger: AIDS and the gay community," in *AIDS: The Making of a Chronic Disease*, ed. E. Fee and D. Fox (Berkeley: University of California Press, 1992).

27. As analyzed by the Global AIDS Policy Coalition in its overall 1992 *AIDS in the World* database.

28. See D. Altman, "The Primacy of Politics: Organizing around AIDS" *AIDS* 5 Suppl. 2 (1991):S231–38.

29. See J. O'Malley, "WHO/GPA support to NGOs in the early 1990s," unpublished manuscript (1990).

30. See, e.g., J. Zita Grover's remarks in the "AIDS and Democracy" round-table, in *Democracy*, ed. B. Wallis (Seattle: Bay Press, 1990).

31. This argument is dealt with at greater length in T. Klouda, "Getting the obvious to stick: Linking sexual health, HIV and STDs to global issues of poverty and development," BMA Conference on Sexual Health, Cambridge (March 1991, in press).

32. USAID, *HIV Infection and AIDS: A report to Congress on the USAID Program for the Prevention and Control* (Washington, D.C., May 1991); Statement by R. Cobb, Deputy Assistant Administrator, Bureau for Africa, Agency for International Development on A.I.D. and the HIV/AIDS Pandemic in Africa before the Subcommittee on Africa, Committee on Foreign Affairs, U.S. House of Representatives, Washington, D.C., November 6, 1991; AIDS Technical Support Project Amendment (AIDS Technical Support, 1991); USAID HIV/AIDS Prevention Program: Financial Year 1990 Funding Summary (August 5, 1991).

33. B. W. Victor, AIDS in a caring society: Practice and policy. Ph.D. diss., Nordic School of Public Health, Gothenburg, 1991; Nils Gussing Development Consulting Services, Norwegian Red Cross International AIDS Programmes (Geneva, 1991).

34. UNESCO paper delivered to the Venice Appeal in June 1991.

35. World Bank, The Bank's agenda for action on AIDS in Africa: A review of implementation (April 1991); A. Hamilton (Director PHRD, World Bank), testimony to the U.S. Presidential Commission on the HIV epidemic, 1988; AIDS

components in World Bank Projects, internal Bank document (1991); J. Clinton and N. Fernandez, *International AIDS Grantmaking* (New York: Funders Concerned about AIDS, December 1991).

36. M. A. Fischl, D. D. Richman, M. H. Grieco, et al., "The efficacy of azidothymidine (AZT) in the treatment of patients with AIDS and AIDS-related complex: A double-blind, placebo-controlled trial," *New England Journal of Medicine* 317(1987):185–91.

37. Personal communication from the Wellcome Foundation, London, United Kingdom, (December 13, 1991).

38. Policy Statement of the American Public Health Association, *American Journal of Public Health* 81(1991):250.

39. Communications from the Wellcome Foundation to *AIDS in the World*, January–April 1992.

40. M. D. Stein, J. Piette, V. Mor, et al., "Differences in access to Zidovudine (AZT) among symptomatic HIV-infected persons," *Journal of General Internal Medicine* 6(1991):35–40.

41. *Treatment Issues: The Gay Men's Health Crisis Newsletter of Experimental AIDS Therapies*, December 1991.

42. *America Living with AIDS: Report of the National Commission on AIDS in the USA* (1991).

43. *American Journal of Public Health*, 1991.

44. Ibid.

45. N. Gilmore, "The Impact of AIDS on drug availability and accessibility," *AIDS* 1992 (in press).

46. Ibid.

47. *Scrip World Pharmaceuticals News, Review Issue* (Richmond, U.K.: PJB Publications, Ltd., 1991), p. 22.

48. R. L. Sivard, *World Military and Social Expenditures, 1991* (Washington, D.C.: World Priorities, 1991).

18. The Next Epidemic

1. J. Lederberg, "Medical science, infectious disease, and the unity of mankind," *Journal of the American Medical Association* 260 (1988):684–85.

2. M. B. Oldstone, "Viruses can cause disease in the absence of morphological evidence of cell injury: Implications for uncovering new diseases in the future," *Journal of Infectious Diseases* 159(1989):384–89.

3. S. Z. Salahuddin, D. V. Ablashi, P. D. Markham, et al., "Isolation of a new virus, HBLV, in patients with lymphoproliferative disorder," *Science* 234(1986):596–601.

4. S. O. Aral and K. K. Holmes, "Sexually transmitted disease in the AIDS era," *Scientific American* 264(1991):62–69.

5. Centers for Disease Control, "Imported dengue—United States, 1989," *Morbidity and Mortality Weekly Report* 39(1990):741–42.

6. W. H. Thompson and C. B. Gunderson, in *California Serogroup Viruses*, ed. C. H. Calisher and W. H. Thompson (New York: Alan R. Liss, 1983).

7. B. Beaty, personal communication, 1990.

8. M. Domingo, L. Ferrer, M. Pumarola, et al., "Morbillivirus in dolphins" (letter), *Nature* 348(1990):21.

9. S. Kennedy, J. A. Smyth, and S. J. McCullough, et al., "Confirmation of cause of recent seal deaths," *Nature* 335(1988):404.

10. S. Morse, Report to the conference on emerging viruses, The Evolution of Viruses and Viral Diseases, National Institutes of Health, May 1989.

11. K. Johnson, Report to ibid.

12. Centers for Disease Control, *Morbidity and Mortality Weekly Report*, June 22, 1990.

13. P. B. Jahrling, T. W. Geisbert, P. W. Dalgard, et al., "Preliminary report: Isolation of ebola virus from monkeys imported to the USA," *Lancet* 335(1990):502–05.

14. J. I. Esteban, J. C. Lopez-Talavera, J. Genesca, et al., "High rate of infectivity and liver disease in blood donors with antibodies to hepatitis C virus," *Annals of Internal Medicine* 115(1991):443–49.

15. J. Hayashi, K. Nakashima, W. Kajiyana, et al., "Prevalence of antibody hepatitis C virus in hemodialysis patients," *American Journal of Epidemiology*, 134(1991):651–57.

16. P. S. Sarma and J. Gruber, "Human T-cell lymphotrophic viruses in human diseases," *Journal of the National Cancer Institute* 82(1990):1100–06.

17. K. N. Ward, J. J. Gray, and S. Efstathiou, "Brief report: Primary human herpesvirus 6 infection in a patient following liver transplantation from a sero-positive donor," *Journal of Medical Virology* 28(1989):69–72.

18. J. B. Page, S. H. Lai, D. D. Chitwood, et al., "HTLV-I/II seropositivity and death from AIDS among HIV-1 seropositive intravenous drug users," *Lancet* 355(1990):1439–41.

19. H. Lee, P. Swanson, V. S. Shorty, et al., "High rate of HTLV-II infection in seropositive intravenous drug users in New Orleans," *Science* 244(1989):471–75.

20. D. C. Des Jarlais, Risk reduction and stabilization of HIV seroprevalence among drug injectors in New York City and Bangkok, Thailand, presented to the VII International Conference on AIDS, Florence, Italy, June 1991.

21. WHO, "Implementation of the global strategy for health for all by the year 2000, second evaluation: Eighth report of the world health situation," Document A - 45/3 (March 1992).

22. Ibid.

23. M. D. Grmek, *History of AIDS* (Princeton: Princeton University Press, 1990).

24. R. C. Gallo, *Virus Hunting* (New York: Basic Books, 1991).

25. B. J. Beaty, D. R. Sundin, L. J. Chandler, et al., "Evolution of Bunyaviruses by genome reassortment in dually infected mosquitoes *(Aedes triseriatus),*" *Science* 230(1985):548–50.

26. L. J. Chandler, G. Hogge, M. Endres, et al., "Reassortment of La Crosse and Tahyna bunyaviruses in Aedes triseriatus mosquitos," *Virus Research* 20(1991):181–91.

27. A. El Hussein, R. F. Ramig, F. R. Holbrook, et al., "Asynchronous mixed infection of Culicoides variipennis with bluetongue virus serotypes 10 and 17," *Journal of General Virology* 70(1989):3355–62.

28. L. J. Chandler, B. J. Beaty, G. D. Baldridge, et al., "Heterologous reassortment of bunyaviruses in Aedes triseriatus mosquitoes and transovarial and oral transmission of newly evolved genotypes," *Journal of General Virology* 71(1990):1045.

29. T. H. Weller, "Science, society, and changing viral-host relationships," *Hospital Practice* March 30, 1988:113–20.

30. H. M. Temin, *Journal of Acquired Immunodeficiency Syndromes* 2(1989):1.

31. S. Yokoyama, C. Chung, T. Gojobori, et al., "Molecular evolution of the human immunodeficiency and related viruses," *Molecular Biology and Evolution* 5(1988):237–57.

32. J. Holland, Report to the conference on emerging viruses, The Evolution of Viruses and Viral Diseases, National Institutes of Health, May 1989.

33. Ibid.

34. M. A. McClure, M. S. Johnson, D. F. Feng, et al., "Sequence comparisons of retroviral proteins: Relative rates of change and general phylogeny," *Proceedings of the National Academy of Sciences* 85(1988):2469–73.

35. Ibid.

36. J. H. Strauss and E. G. Strauss, "Evolution of RNA viruses," *Annual Review of Microbiology* 42(1988):657–83.

37. Ibid.

38. M. LeGuern and J. A. Levy, "Human immunodeficiency virus (HIV) type 1 can superinfect HIV-2-infected cells: Pseudotype virions produced with expanded cellular host range," *Proceedings of the National Academy of Sciences* 89(1992):363–67.

39. R. Isfort, D. Jones, R. Kost, et al., "Retroviruses insertion into herpesvirus in vitro and in vivo," *Proceedings of the National Academy of Sciences* 89(1992):991–95.

40. J. Fenkel, Report to the conference on emerging viruses, The Evolution of Viruses and Viral Diseases, National Institutes of Health, May 1989.

41. W. Reeves, Report to ibid.

42. J. McCormick, personal communication.

About the Editors

Jonathan M. Mann, M.D., M.P.H., is the General Editor of *AIDS in the World*, Professor of Epidemiology and International Health at the Harvard School of Public Health, Director of the International AIDS Center of the Harvard AIDS Institute, and Chair of the VIIIth International Conference on AIDS/III STD World Congress. Dr. Mann received his B.A. from Harvard College, his M.D. from Washington University in St. Louis, and his M.P.H. from the Harvard School of Public Health. From 1975 to 1984, Dr. Mann was State Epidemiologist and Assistant Director of the Department of Public Health in New Mexico. From 1984 to 1986, he directed Projet SIDA, a collaborative AIDS research project involving the U.S. Centers for Disease Control, the U.S. National Institute of Allergy and Infectious Diseases, the Institute of Tropical Medicine in Antwerp, Belgium, and the Ministry of Health, Republic of Zaire. From 1987 to 1990 he was Director of the World Health Organization Global Programme on AIDS. Dr. Mann has written numerous articles on AIDS and other health issues.

Daniel J. M. Tarantola, M.D., is the Scientific Editor of *AIDS in the World* and a Research Associate at the International AIDS Center, Harvard School of Public Health. He received his medical degree from Paris University, where he did postgraduate training in nephrology. After participating in emergency and rural health development programs for voluntary organizations in Africa and Latin America in the early 1970s, Dr. Tarantola helped create Médecins sans Frontières, a French-based medical relief organization. From 1974 to 1977, he worked with and then led the WHO smallpox eradication campaign in Bangladesh. He also participated in the early stages of WHO global initiatives, including childhood immunization and control of diarrheal disease and acute respiratory infections in Asia and the Pacific. In 1987, Dr. Tarantola helped create the WHO Global Programme on AIDS, heading its National AIDS Programs unit. From late 1990, Dr. Tarantola worked with WHO disaster relief programs for health services in Asia, Africa, and the Middle East before moving to the Harvard School of Public Health in 1991.

Thomas W. Netter is the Managing Editor of *AIDS in the World*. He received his B.A. in English literature and history from the University of Pittsburgh. From 1977 to 1984, he was a domestic and foreign correspondent for the Associated Press. He has worked as a print and broadcast journalist, writing for newspapers in the United States, Canada, and Europe, including the *New York Times* and the

International Herald Tribune. He has covered a wide variety of international issues ranging from political upheavals and arms control to the environment, trade, finance, human rights, and health. From 1987 to 1990, Mr. Netter helped establish the Public Information Office of the WHO Global Programme on AIDS, developed a global media strategy for AIDS, and planned and coordinated public information campaigns on other health issues. He has worked as a communications consultant and editor at the Harvard School of Public Health since 1991.

Acknowledgments

The Editors gratefully acknowledge the following people and organizations for their contributions to *AIDS in the World*. Without their help, and that of many other friends and colleagues throughout the world who gave their time and attention, this book could not have been written.

Authors and contributors: Peter Aggleton, Dennis Altman, The Appropriate Health Resources and Technologies Action Group (AHRTAG), Jill Armstrong, Mike Bailey, Mariella Baldo, Tony Barnett, Françoise Barré-Sinoussi, Ronald Bayer, Robert Beal, Nancy Berezin, Robert Bernstein, Robert J. Biggar, Piers Blaikie, Eduard Bos, Uwe Brinkmann, Anthony Britten, Phyllida Brown, Françoise Brun-Vezinet, Jean-Baptiste Brunet, Jorge Cabral, Charles Cameron, Ian Campbell, Patricia Case, Christopher Castle, Clement Chela, Mitchell E. Cohen, James W. Curran, Kevin De Cock, Don C. Des Jarlais, Shelby Dietrich, Gary Dowsett, Jay Drosin, Maria Ekstrand, Jonathan Elford, Eka Esu-Williams, Joel Finlay, Mindy Fullilove, Laurie Garrett, Shahin Gharakhanian, Larry Gostin, Alan E. Greenberg, Jon M. Greenberg, Sofia Gruskin, Ian Gust, Timothy W. Harding, Mark Harrington, Graham Hart, Susan Hassig, Aart Hendriks, Jody Heymann, Sean Hosein, Hilary Hughes, Noerine Kaleeba, Lazare Kaptue, John M. Karon, Richard A. Keenlyside, Jeffrey Kelly, Michael Kirby, David L. Kirp, Tony Klouda, Marc Lallemant, Sophie Lallemant-Le Coeur, Normand Lapointe, Maureen Law, Zita Lazzarini, Laurie S. Liskin, Mario Maj, Carsten Mantel, Carola Marte, Justin C. McArthur, Rita C. Meyer, Marvellous Mhloyi, David Miller, Hans Moerkerk, Oliver Morton, Pierre M'Pelé, Declan Murphy, Jean-Yves Nau, Banakpo Ngagele, Justin Nguma, Franck Nouchi, Jeff O'Malley, June E. Osborn, Cheryl Overs, Anne Petitgirard, Margaret Phillips, Phyllis T. Piotrow, Lane Porter, Richard Rector, Elizabeth Reid, Richard Rothenberg, Rachel Royce, Willy Rozenbaum, Chuanchom Sakondhavat, Georgette Schaller, Helen Schietinger, Julia Shepard, Laurence Slutsker, Ron Stall, Karen Stanecki, Street Kids International, Suzanne Thomas, Katarina Tomasevski, Kathleen E. Toomey, Gottfried van Griensven, Ana Vasconcelos, Robert Wachter, Rodrick Wallace, Judith N. Wasserheit, Peter O. Way, Bruce Weniger, Diane Widdus, Ramnik J. Xavier, Debrework Zewdie, Bernard A. Zulu, Anthony Zwi.

Advisers, reviewers, and contacts in international organizations: Calle Almedal, Rosemarie Ancelle, Sandra Anderson, Sue Armstrong, Nilton Arnt, Mariella

Baldo, Kazem Behbehani, Gabriel Bez, Kapita Bila, Dennis Blairman, Dorothy Blake, Eric Blas, Ralph Bolton, David Brandling-Bennett, Diego Buriot, Tony Burton, Manuel Carballo, Lincoln Chen, Jim Chin, Daniel Defert, Timothy Dondero, Albina du Boisrouvray, Karen Edstrom, Svein Erik Ekeid, Jean Emmanuel, Gunila Ernberg, Jose Esparza, Nina Ferencic, Peter Figueroa, Harvey Fineberg, Susan Foster, Phyllis Freeman, Gerald Friedland, Pat Friel, Nidgel Gibbs, Norbert Gilmore, Robert Grose, Neal Halsey, Birgit Hansen, Jeffrey Harris, Susan Hassig, Alan Haworth, David Heymann, Allan Hill, Susan Holck, David Hunter, Pol Jansegers, Steve Jones, Frank Judson, Marc Karam, Joan Kaufman, Lev Khodakevich, Michael Kirby, Arata Kochi, Jukka Koistinen, Steve Kraus, Richard Laing, Jean-Louis Lamboray, Peter Lamptey, Aldo Landi, Michel Lavollay, Gary Lloyd, Alan Lopez, William Lyerly, Jean-Elie Malkin, Marie-Paule Mann, Anne Martin, Elizabeth Matenga, Joseph McCormick, Anthony Measham, Michael Merson, Sheila Mitchell, Kaiya Montaocean, Jan-Olof Morfeldt, Chip Myers, Ben Nkowane, Jeff O'Malley, Gloria Ornelas Hall, Mead Over, Georg Petersen, Peter Piot, Gilles Poumerol, Mario Raviglione, Thomas Rehle, Michael Reich, Astrid Richardson, Marie-Paule Roudil, Robin Ryder, Jean-Paul Ryst, Michèle Ryst, Renée Sabatier, Norman Sartorius, Jaime Sepúlveda Amor, Suzanne Shafner-Cherney, Don Shepard, Werasit Sittitrai, Yvonne Sliep, Gary Slutkin, Abdulramane Sow, Mikel Stempke, Philippe Sudre, Mark Szczeniowski, Hiko Tamashiro, Suzanne Thomas, Erik van Praag, Monica Vernette, Rudolf Wabitsh, Judith N. Wasserheit, John Watters, John Wickett, Roy Widdus, Roslaw Widy-Wirski, Brigid Willmore, Fernando Zacarias, Laurent Zessler. Other contributors, advisors, and reviewers cannot be individually acknowledged here because of regulations within their respective institutions of affiliation.

Delphi respondents: Anthony Adams, Michael Adler, Uwe Brinkmann, Euclides Castilho, Kenneth Castro, Roy Chan, Peter Drotman, Josef Estermann, Donato Greco, Jacob K. John, Ann Marie Kimball, Samuel Okware, Jean William Pape, Vadim V. Pokrovsky, Thomas Quinn, Martin Schechter, David Sokal, Peter O. Way, and other respondents who have asked that their names be withheld.

Members of National AIDS Commissions, staff of Ministries of Health, in particular of National AIDS Programs, other government services, and non-governmental organizations of the following countries/areas have contributed information to surveys conducted by *AIDS in the World*: Argentina, Australia, Austria, Belgium, Belize, Bermuda, Brazil, Cameroon, Canada, Chile, China, Colombia, Congo, Costa Rica, Côte d'Ivoire, Egypt, Ethiopia, Federation of Czech and Slovak Republics, Fiji, France, Germany, Guinea-Bissau, Haiti, Hong Kong, India, Indonesia, Ireland, Israel, Italy, Jamaica, Japan, Malaysia, Mexico, Morocco, the Netherlands, New Zealand, Nigeria, Norway, Pakistan, Papua New Guinea, Philippines, Poland, Puerto Rico, Republic of South Africa, Rwanda, St. Lucia, Senegal, Sweden, Switzerland, Thailand, Trinidad and Tobago, Uganda, USSR/CIS, United Kingdom, United Republic of Tanzania, United States, Zambia, Zimbabwe.

Assistant editor: Amy Wollin Benjamin.

Core staff assistants: Sharon E. Walcott, Jen Wang.

Epidemiological analysis and data management: Sara Back, Carsten Mantel.

Data management assistants: Susan Andrade, Francine Grodstein, Neena Jain, Nakul Jerath, Wahed Khan, Eva Lepisto, Gurinder Shahi, Robert Simon.

Research assistants: Gabrielle Bercy, Michelle Bowdler, Lucia Cargill, Paul Coplan, Debra Efroymson, Naomasa Hirota, Nakul Jerath, Roya Kohani, Jennifer Kohn, Kayla Laserson, Mia MacDonald, Maria Madison, Catherine Meikle, Lisa Moore, Mark Mullins, Nehal Neamatullah, Nawal Nour, Joas Rugemalila, Gurinder Shahi, Robert Simon, Meena Thayu, Lucy Wilson, Gina Wingood.

Editorial assistants: Gino DelGuercio, Beth Fertig, Jill Hannum, Peter Wrobel.

Other staff assistants: Marcy Bailey-Adams, Gregory Gunter, Donny Jones, Lida Kagan, Ruth Kagan, Kris Kalil, Anna Manresa, Julie Rioux, Ann Sussman, Matthew Woods.

Translation assistance: Catherine Horrigan, Kayla Laserson, Robert Simon, Arnaud Tarantola, Jen Wang.

The Editors also wish to acknowledge the following organizations for their help in providing or reviewing information presented here: Agence Nationale de Recherches sur le SIDA (France), AIDS Coalition to Unleash Power (ACT-UP), Association François-Xavier Bagnoud, Australian International Development Assistance Bureau, Centre Nationale de la Recherche Scientifique (France), Department of Community Services and Health (Australia), Department of Health/Research Development Division (United Kingdom), EC Commission AIDS Program, Family Health International, German Federal Ministry for Research and Health, Health and Welfare Department's National Health Research and Development Programme (Canada), Institut National de la Recherche Agronomique (France), Institut Pasteur (France), International Federation of Red Cross and Red Crescent Societies, International Planned Parenthood Federation, Istituto Superiore di Sanità/Virology Department (Italy), John Snow Inc., Medical and Health Research Program, Ministry of Health and Welfare/Health Services Bureau/Infectious Diseases Control Office (Japan), National Institutes of Health (United States), Office de Recherche Scientifique dans les Territoires d'Outre-mer (France), Pan American Health Organization, PANOS Institute, Pharmaceutical Manufacturers Association (United States), Salvation Army, Save the Children Fund, Swedish Agency for Research Cooperation with Developing Countries, Swedish Council for Medical Research, Swiss Federal Office of Public Health/AIDS Unit, United Nations Children's Fund, United Nations Development Program, United Nations Educational, Scientific, and Cultural Organization, U.S. Agency for International Development, U.S. Bureau of the Census, U.S. Centers for Disease Control, U.S. Food and Drug Administration, World Bank, World Federation of Hemophilia, World Health Organization.

The report draws on statistical information from databases created by the Population Crisis Committee, United Nations Development Program, United Nations Population Fund, U.S. Bureau of the Census, World Bank, World Health Organization, Medline and AIDSline; special thanks are also extended to the staff of the Countway Library of the Harvard Medical School.

The participation of the above persons or organizations does not imply their endorsement of all statements presented in AIDS in the World, 1992.

Index

AIDS-related CNS lymphomas, 682
AIDS-related programs: diversity, 784–785; effectiveness, 788–801; funding patterns, 790–794; needs to be addressed, 788. *See also* AIDS service organizations (ASOs); Nongovernmental organizations (NGOs)
AIDS service organizations (ASOs), 306–311, 774–787; activities of, 309; communities and, 776–778; counseling, 822; emergence, 775–776; funding, 783; future, 786–787; governments and, 778–781, 785; network building, 780; number, 308, 784–785; professionalism, 84; strategies, 781–783. *See also* Community-based response; Nongovernmental organizations (NGOs)
AIDS Support Organization, The. *See* The AIDS Support Organization
AIDS Technical Support Project (AIDSTECH), USAID, 401, 803
Albania, 47, 111
Alzheimer's disease, 230, 678, 683
American Foundation for AIDS Research (AMFAR), 516
American Medical Association (AMA), 752, 754–755
American Public Health Association, 813
American Red Cross, 70, 422
American Society of Tropical Medicine and Hygiene (ASTMH), 838
Americans with Disabilities Act (ADA), 544, 782
Amnesty International, 540
Amsterdam: homelessness in, 771; IDUs in, 689, 696, 697
Anemia, malaria-caused, 148
Angola, 38
Anti-AIDS clubs, 359
Antibodies, mother-to-child transmission and, 638–639
Antidiscrimination legislation, 561–567
Antiretroviral therapy, dementia and, 679–680
Antiviral drugs: research achievements, 233–239; virus mutation and, 835–836
Argentina: AZT treatment costs, 813, 818; nondiscrimination legislation, 562
Asia: AIDS reporting, 114, 116; blood transfusion, 69–70, 422; breast feeding

and fertility, 619–620; commercial sex workers, HIV infection in, 53; health care, 450, 455; HIV infection projections, 4; homosexual men, HIV infection in, 55–56; IDUs, HIV infection in, 56; model predictions of AIDS spread, 26; nondiscrimination legislation, 563; partner notification, 714–715; pregnant women, HIV infection in, 65–66; prevention expenditures, 478; STD clinic patients, HIV infection in, 62; USAID funding, 802–803. *See also specific locations*; North East Asia GAA; Southeast Asia GAA
ASOs. *See* AIDS service organizations
Associacão Brasileira Interdisciplinar de AIDS (ABIA), 744–745, 780
Association de Lutte contre le SIDA, 779
Association François-Xavier Bagnoud, vii, ix–x
Australia, 117, 405; ASOs, 782; AZT treatment costs, 813, 818; blood transfusion services, 425; HIV-infected prisoners, 766; HIV testing, 750; IDUs, 418; intervention programs, 351; mass media, 738, 743, 745; NAPs, 295, 296; national health care system, 315; NGOs, 307, 780, 781, 782; safe sex among gay men, 654; syringe access, 685, 687–691, 692, 695, 697
AZT (Zidovudine), 609; access to, 812–820; ACT-UP and, 238–240; children and, 642–645; costs of, 812–815; dementia and, 679–680; Foscavir® and, 242; paying for, 815–818; research achievements, 233–239; supportive health care services and, 818; treatment with, 642–643
AZT/ddI treatments, 234

Bactrim®, for PCP, 240
Bangladesh, 395, 400, 619
Bantsimba, 644
Barbados, 715, 734
BCG vaccine, 162–163
Behavior. *See* Safe sex; Sexual behavior
Belgium, 798–799; ASOs, 780; AZT treatment costs, 818; heterosexual transmission, 612–613; partner notification, 709

CARITAS Internationalis, 516
CDC. *See* Centers for Disease Control
CD4, synthetic, 234–235
CD4 counts: cost of, 818; perinatal transmission and, 638
CD4+ lymphocytes, HIV variability and, 272–273
Center for Communication Programs, Johns Hopkins University, 395
Center for International Research (CIR), U.S. Bureau of the Census, 41
Centers for Disease Control (CDC) (U.S.), 750; AIDS and hemophilia, 421, 438, 444, 446; breast-feeding guidelines, 617; health care cost estimates, 495; HIV testing and screening, 753, 754–755; partner notification evaluation, 717–718; planned research funding, 267; sex ratios of HIV infection, 83; tuberculosis statistics, 160
Central African Republic, 634
Central America: health care, 465–466, 493; transmission, 122–124. *See also* Latin America GAA
Central Europe, 535, 711. *See also specific locations*
Central nervous system (CNS) infections, 681
Cervical cancer, AIDS interactions with, 143, 144–146
Chancroid, 174, 178
Child mortality rate (CMR): AIDS and, 127, 131, 208–209; breast feeding and, 621
Children: AZT and, 642–643, 664; blood transfusions, in Romania, 712; in developing countries, 293–294; diagnosis of AIDS, 113; discrimination against, 543–544; economic impacts and, 220, 221; health care, 673–674, 676–677; health care costs, 673; HIV/AIDS impacts, 293–294, 667–674; HIV infection, 90, 614–615, 667–677; HIV-1 and HIV-2 infection, 276; of IDUs, adoption of, 642; information and education programs, 670; malaria, 146–147; mortality, 127, 131, 208–209, 210, 211; orphaned by AIDS, 90, 210, 220, 225, 463, 465, 642, 667, 671–673, 786; physical needs, 675–

676; projections, 2, 131–132, 700; psychological effects, 670, 672, 676; responses to, 669, 674–677; sexuality of, 670–671; social impacts of AIDS and, 225; symptomless, treatment of, 644; transmission from mother to, 585–586, 614, 627, 629–645; vulnerability, 373–374, 668, 673. *See also* Adolescents; Infants; Pediatric AIDS
Chile, 289–291, 782–783, 806
Chimpanzees, vaccine development and, 249, 251–252
China, 56, 97, 410, 714
Chlamydia, 172–173; female condoms and, 702; HIV interaction with, 178; reproductive system and, 180–181; transmission of, 176, 177
Chorio-amniotitis, mother-to-child transmission and, 639
Circumcision, 447–452
Clinical trials, drug approval process and, 236–237
Clotting factor products, 442, 446
CNS. *See* Central nervous system
Coalition building, 282, 305–311
Cocaine, injection of, 410
Colombia, 734, 735
Commercial sex workers: estimated number, by GAA, 376; female condom use, 703; government policies and, 344–345; HIV prevalence and incidence, by GAA, 52–55; programs targeted at, 330, 372–381; safe sex and, 344–345; sale of children as, 184; STDs and, 175, 180–183, 187; trading sex for drugs by, 377
Commission of European Communities. *See* EEC
Commitment, to NAPs, 282, 286–294
Community-based response: ASOs and, 776–778; effectiveness, 4, 791; programs, 772–774; resistance to, 774; USAID and, 803–804. *See also* AIDS service organizations (ASOs)
Community norms, AIDS prevention and, 339, 343
Comores, 562
Complacency, 322–333
Condoms, 187, 330, 390–406; adolescents and, 356; in anti-AIDS kits for IDUs,

690; breakage, 395, 404–405; commercial sex workers and, 373, 381; demand, 395–396; design, 402, 404; distribution, 397–400; effectiveness, 391; female, 661, 700–707; gay men and, 386, 391; logistics of providing, 397, 398–399, 406–407; lubricants and, 395, 402; mass media and, 734–735, 736, 739, 740–741; plastic and latex, 396, 402, 403; for prisoners, 767, 769; promotion, 400–401, 734–735, 736, 743, 744–745, 746; quality issues, 402–404; reading levels of instructions, 405; suppliers in Africa, 399; use, 186, 391, 392–394, 395; women and, 650–660, 700

Congo, 289, 335, 351, 636

Conjunctivitis, gonococcal, 181, 188

Contact tracing. *See* Partner notification

Contagion, fear of, 542, 562–563

Contain-and-control public health strategy, 281

Contraception, 641, 702

Contraceptive Research and Development Program (CONRAD), 702

Cooperation-and-inclusion public health strategy, 281

Core groups, 174, 176–177; sexually transmitted diseases and, 52; targeting for STD prevention and control, 185–187. *See also* High-risk groups; Risk

Corporations, support of Global AIDS strategy by, 517

Costa Rica, 715–716

Costs: blood transfusions, 423, 425; dementia diagnosis, 682; HIV testing, 346, 434–435, 560; PCP prevention, 498; prevention and control, 478–482, 496–509, 669, 687; research, 260–264, 265. *See also* Health care costs

Côte d'Ivoire, 114, 218, 425, 734; HIV infection, 2, 34, 35, 40, 44–47, 276, 277; mother-to-child transmission, 636; partner notification, 713; urban-rural differentials in HIV infection, 77

Council of Europe: housing, 771, 772; human rights and, 561, 568, 569; notification of communicable diseases and, 558; recommendations about HIV infection in prisoners, 764

Counseling, 452–454; 820–824; effectiveness, 822–823; on mother-to-child transmission, 641–643; providers, 821–822; TASO and, 458–459

Crack cocaine, 166, 179, 377, 410

Crude death rate (CDR), AIDS and, 204–205

Cuba, 91; HIV screening, 552, 750; legislation, 547; partner notification, 716, 720

Cumulative estimates and projections: AIDS cases, by GAA, 27–30, 110, 128, 129, 130; AIDS cases in children, by GAA, 129; AIDS deaths, by GAA, 125; HIV infections, by GAA, 27, 105, 107; HIV infections in children, by GAA, 106; incidence, defined, 12–13; prevalence, defined, 13

Cytokines, 244

Cytotoxic T-cell lymphocytes (CTL), 639

Czechoslovakia, 34, 116, 712

Czech Republic, IDUs in, 417, 420, 693

Czech and Slovak Federal Republic, 284, 285

Daniel, Herbert, 780

Danish International Development Agency (DANIDA), 514

ddC, 233–234, 642

ddI, 233–234, 642, 644

Death rates, 372

Dehomosexualization, of AIDS, 388–389

Delphi method, 25; defined, 26; projections to year 2000, 106, 107, 128, 130

Dementia, 678–683; health care and diagnostic facilities and, 682; public policy and, 680–681

Demographic impacts of AIDS, 199–212; death rate, 204–205; dependency ratio, 209–210; infant and child mortality, 200, 208–209; interventions and, 210–212; life expectancy at birth, 205–207; modeling, 199–203; population growth, 203–204

Denmark, 425, 607, 689; HIV testing, 751, 758–759; human rights and, 572; IDUs, 611; ODA contributions, 520, 524, 527; partner notification, 711

Deutsche AIDS-Hilfe, 766, 783

IDUs, HIV infection in, 56; legislation, 548–549; mother-to-child transmission, 634; national AIDS prevention and control programs, 535; partner notification, 707–713; prevention expenditures, 478; prisoners, HIV infection in, 762, 766. *See also* Eastern Europe GAA; Western Europe GAA; *specific locations*

European Community (EC), 260–261, 772

European Parliament, 541, 548–549

Extrapulmonary tuberculosis, 156–157

Families, extended, in Africa: health care services and, 456–457; home health care for, 461

Family Health International, 702, 793

FDA. *See* U.S. Food and Drug Administration

Fear of AIDS contagion, 542, 562–563

Federation of Czech and Slovak Republics, 607. *See also* Czechoslovakia; Czech Republic; Czech and Slovak Federal Republic; Slovak Republic

Female condoms, 661, 700–707; acceptability, 703–705; design, 700–701, 703, 704; evaluation, 706–707; marketing and distribution, 703–705

Femidom®, 701

Fertility: AIDS and, 203–204; breast feeding and, 619–620; STDs and, 181

Fiji, 2, 289

Financing. *See* Funding

Finland, 425, 607, 710

Foscavir®, 242

France, 83, 84, 116; ASOs, 781–782, 785; blood transfusion, 425; community responses, 773; condom use, 400–401, 404–405; health care costs, 494, 495–496; health insurance, 815, 818; HIV population estimates, 47; HIV testing, 751, 755; homosexual/bisexual men, 609; IDUs, 417, 687, 688; mother-to-child transmission, 634, 636; NAP, 296; national health care system, 315; ODA contributions, 524; partner notification, 709; PCP, 497–499; prisoners, HIV infection in, 762; research spending, 261;

transmission through homosexual/bisexual men, 383

French Polynesia, 117

Funding: for AIDS health care, 5–6, 313–317; for AIDS service organizations, 783; bilateral, by country, 512–513, 522, 532; of Global AIDS Strategy, 511–535; multilateral, by country, 512–513, 520–521; for NAPs, 283, 311–317, 787–801; ODA agencies, 524; from OECD and OPEC members, 526–527; per capita, by country, 525; for prevention programs, 5–6, 311–313, 522; priorities, 799–801; research, 260–264, 265; by World Bank, 529

GAA. *See* Geographic Areas of Affinity (GAAs)

Gay Group, 744

Gay and Lesbian Anti-Violence Project, 563

Gay men: activism, 388–389; antagonism toward, 562–563, 722–723; ASOs and, 775, 777, 783, 785; de-identification of AIDS with, 388–389; HIV prevalence and incidence in, by GAA, 55–56; IDUs, 610; prevention programs for, 337, 381–390; rights of, 389–390; safe sex and, 383–384, 386, 653–657. *See also* Homosexual/bisexual transmission

Gay Men's Health Crisis (GMHC), 385, 775, 785

Gender ratios. *See* Sex ratios

Gender-specific issues, 657–667. *See also* Women

Genetic structure and variability of HIV, 267–275

Genital herpes, 173, 176, 178

Genital secretions, STDs and, 176

Genital ulcer disease (GUD), 178, 650, 651, 652

Genital warts, 174

Geographic Areas of Affinity (GAAs): cumulative AIDS cases by, 110, 128, 129, 130; cumulative AIDS deaths by, 125; cumulative HIV infections by, 27–30, 105, 107; cumulative pediatric AIDS cases by, 129; cumulative pediatric HIV

Health services, 330, 337–338
Hemophilia, 606; comprehensive care, 443; defined, 442; estimated number of newborns with, 441; financial assistance for HIV-infected people with, 445; HIV incidence and prevalence in persons with, 438; national and international response, 444; prevention and, 438–446; transmission and, 421, 606; treatment products, 443–444; world pattern, 442
Hepatitis B virus, 695–696, 702, 834
Heroin, 410
Herpes simplex virus (HSV), 178
Heterosexual transmission, 15, 612–614, 777, 783; in the Caribbean, 91; in Europe, 118; by GAA, 30, 52–55; in Latin America, 124; in Southeast Asia, 98; in South East Mediterranean, 96; of STDs, 174–177; in sub-Saharan Africa, 89; in U.S., 118, 122
High-risk groups, 185–187, 554. See also Core groups
HIV: genetic structure, 267–268; genetic variability, 269–272; life cycle, 233; research achievements and, 229, 267–275
HIV-1 infection: diagnosis, 274; malaria and, 143–148; mutation, 835, 837; in sub-Saharan Africa, 89; transmission routes, 276; variability, 267, 269, 274
HIV-2 infection: diagnosis, 274; epidemiology, 275–277; geographic variation, in Africa, 79; latency period, 276; mother-to-child transmission, 636; mutation, 835, 837; in sub-Saharan Africa, 89; transmission, 275–277; variability, 267, 269, 274
HIV/AIDS Prevention in Africa program, 804
HIV dementia. See Dementia
HIV genome, composition of, 268–271
HIV incidence: cumulative, by GAA, 27, 29, 105; defined, 12–13; estimation methods, 25–27; by GAA, 19–22, 30; global projections, 101–108; leveling off of, 81–82; male-female ratio, by GAA, 31; peaking of, 33, 82; projections by GAA, 101–108
HIV screening: of health service users, by country, 555; of high-risk groups, by country, 554; at international borders, 347; mass, 552–557; of migrants, by country, 556; by occupational categories, by country, 557; of travelers, by country, 556. See also HIV testing
HIV testing: behavior change and, 748–750; blind, 757; clinical, 754–757; costs, 346, 434–435, 560; dementia and, 680–681; in developing countries, 434–435, 450; discrimination and, 747, 750–754; epidemiology and, 750, 757–758; ethical considerations, 547, 747–759; groups targeted for, 552–557; of IDUs, 414; mandatory, 346–347, 551–557, 749, 751, 752–753, 757; pregnancy and, 755–756; premarital, 560; of prisoners, 764, 765; safety and, 749, 750–754; tuberculosis screening and, 753–754. See also HIV screening
HIV transmission. See Bisexual transmission; Heterosexual transmission; Homosexual/bisexual transmission; Sexual transmission
Hodgkin's disease, 143
Hoffmann–La Roche, 234
Home health care. See Health care
Homelessness, 771–772
Homosexual/bisexual transmission, 15, 505, 605, 607–609; in Canada, 122; in Europe, 116, 607, 609; by GAA, 30–31; intervention programs and, 381–390; in Latin America, 122–124; risk reduction, 653–557; in U.S., 118. See also Gay men; Lesbians
Honduras, 34
Hospices, 465, 773–774
Hospital costs: comparative, 484; in France, 495–496; in Rwanda, 485–486, 487; in Thailand, 489–492. See also Health care costs
Hot Rubber condom campaign, 401, 736
Housing, AIDS-related issues and, 769–774
HTLV-1, 636, 834
HTLV-2, 834
Human Freedom Index, 286
Humanistic Institute for Cooperation with Developing Countries (HIVOS), 516
Human papillomavirus (HPV), 144, 173–174

Human rights, 537–573; activism and, 567–573; country ranking criteria, 540; disease classification and, 548–551; disease reporting and, 558–559; HIV/AIDS prevention and care and, 538–541, 564–566; HIV/AIDS-related violence, 562–563; HIV testing and, 547, 552–557, 751–753; international policies, 564–566; legislation and, 543–548; litigation and, 570–572; nondiscrimination and, 561–567; partner notification and, 720; patterns, 541–548; prisoners and, 761–762; public health measures and, 538–541; responses, 567–573; UNESCO and, 809; violations, 570–572. *See also* Discrimination

Hungary, 116, 712

Iceland, 710–711
IDUs. *See* Injection drug users
Immigration regulations, 551
Immunomodulators, 244
Incidence, defined, 12–13
Index of Individual Vulnerability, 580–581
India, 98–99, 114; HIV infection, 2, 15, 26, 35–36, 53, 56; NAP, 295, 296; national vulnerability, 597; nondiscrimination legislation, 567; partner notification, 714; street children, 673
Infant mortality, 200, 208–209
Infants: breast feeding of, 616–629; diagnosis in, 632–634, 636–643; hemophilia in, 441; HIV infection of, 614–615; HIV testing of, 756–757; perinatal transmission and, 629–645. *See also* Pediatric AIDS
Infectious diseases: AIDS interactions with, 133–163; breast versus bottle feeding and, 617–618, 619
Influenza, 835
Information and education programs, 325, 330–337; barriers to success, 330–331; channels, 335–337; educational materials, 808; via entertainment, 741–742, 746; Karate Kids, 362–363; mass media and, 732, 733–734; messages, 331–335; on mother-to-child transmission, 641–643; for prisoners, 766; for women, 659.

See also Prevention and control programs
Injection drug users (IDUs): adoption of children of, 642; defined, 410–411; denial issues, 420; drugs used, by country, 408; gaps in programs targeting, 419–420; harm reduction strategies, 414, 418–419, 685–699, 768; HIV-2 infection in, 834; HIV prevalence and incidence in, 56, 697–698; HIV testing of, by country, 415; homosexual/bisexual men, 610; individual needs, 411–414; numbers, 408–409, 411; pregnancy in, 641; prevention and control programs, 406–420; in prison, 762–763, 767–768; social and cultural issues, 414–419; syringe access, 685–699, 767–768; syringe sharing, 412, 419–420, 696; trading sex for drugs, 377; transmission, 15, 583–584, 606, 609–612; treatment programs, 611, 696–697; vulnerability, 420, 583–584
Injection-related diseases, syringe access and, 695–696
Insurance: health, 224–225, 815; industry, AIDS and, 224–225; life, 224–225
Integrated primary health care (PHC), 192
International Consultation on AIDS and Human Rights, 569
International Council of AIDS Service Organizations (ICASO), 782
International Covenant on Economic, Social and Cultural Rights, 772
International Federation of Red Cross and Red Crescent Societies, 358, 422, 436, 461, 805–807
International Health Regulations, 554–555
International Labour Organization (ILO), ODA contributions by, 517, 528
International Planned Parenthood Federation (IPPF), 397
International Society of Blood Transfusion (ISBT), 436
International Steering Committee for People with HIV and AIDS, 782
Intervention programs. *See* Prevention and control programs
Intravenous drug users (IVDUs), 410. *See also* Injection drug users (IDUs)

Investigational New Drug (IND) application, 236
Ireland, 289
Isoniazid, 162
Israel, 114
Issue attention cycle, 725–726
Italy, 83, 116; ASOs, 780; community responses, 774; HIV infection rates in prisoners, 762; homosexual/bisexual transmission, 607; IDUs, 610–611; mother-to-child transmission, 634; partner notification, 709

Jamaica, 289, 290, 715
Japan, 19, 97, 114; HIV testing, 560; national health care system, 315; nondiscrimination legislation, 563; partner notification, 714
Job Corps, 67, 83, 613
Johns Hopkins University, Center for Communication Programs, 395, 741
Journalism, AIDS and, 720–732

KABP (knowledge, attitudes, behaviors, and practices), 59
Kaposi's sarcoma, 134, 135–139
Karate Kids, 360–361
Kenya, 114, 460; circumcision, 650, 651–652; female condom use, 704; HIV/AIDS impacts, 292; HIV seroprevalence, 34, 74; media coverage of AIDS, 729–730; mother-to-child transmission, 640
Kinshasa, Zaire, 4, 34
Kramer, Larry, 238
Kuwait, 527, 563

Lagos, 35
Language. See Terminology
Latency period, HIV-1 and HIV-2 infection and, 276
Latin America GAA: AIDS cases, 87–88, 109; AIDS deaths, 47, 87–88, 125; AIDS reporting, 112–113, 114, 122, 124; anti-AIDS clubs, 359; ASOs, 777; blood donors, 69; breast feeding and fertility, 620; commercial sex workers, 53; cumulative HIV infection, 105–108; female condom use, 702; funding of AIDS programs, 6; GAA classification, 19; health care costs, 506; HIV infection, 4, 28, 32, 53, 55, 56, 61–62, 65, 69, 87–88; homosexual men, 55; partner notification, 715–716; pediatric AIDS, 32; pregnant women, 65; STD clinic patients, 61–62; transmission modes, 31; USAID funding, 802. See also Central America; South America; specific locations
League of Red Cross and Red Crescent Societies. See International Federation of Red Cross and Red Crescent Societies
Legalistic responses, 792
Legislation: human rights and, 543–548; nondiscrimination, 561
Lesbians: AIDS activities, 388–389; ASOs and, 775, 777, 784; violence directed against, 562–563; risk of infection, 382
Life expectancy: after AIDS diagnosis, 679; at birth, AIDS and, 205–207
Life insurance, 224–225
Litigation, human rights and, 543–545, 570–572
London, 84; community responses, 773; HIV seroprevalence in IDUs, 697; homosexual/bisexual men, 609; syringe access, 696. See also United Kingdom
London Lighthouse, 773
Los Angeles, 561, 607, 608
Low-intensity wars, 38–39

Malaria, 133, 143–148
Malawi, 114, 203, 640, 795–796
Malaysia, 785
Male-to-female ratios. See Sex ratios
Malnutrition, 220
Mangabey monkeys, vaccine development and, 249
Manhattan Project, vaccine development and, 250–252

Mass media, 720–732; AIDS as disease of, 732, 733–747; behavior change and, 740–741; coverage patterns, 722–725; discussion, 739–740; effectiveness, 733–747; emotional response and, 737–739; entertainment, 741–742, 746; future coverage of AIDS, 732; impacts, 721–722, 723, 727–730; information and education, 335–337; issue attention cycle and, 725–726; NGOs and, 744–745; number of news items, 721, 725; political opposition to, 734–735; promotional material pretesting, 737; public service announcements, 735; reproductive health information, 733–734; standards, 742–744; targeted populations, 350, 735–736

Media: electronic, 335–337; print, 335–337; television, 733. *See also* Mass media

Medical care. *See* Health care

Medical care costs. *See* Health care costs

Medicines. *See* Therapeutic drugs

Mediterranean. *See* South East Mediterranean GAA

Men, life expectancy of, 207

Merck, 234

Methadone, 419, 768

Mexico, 114; health care costs, 493; HIV infection, 3, 36; HIV testing, 750; mass media, 738, 739, 740; NGOs, 307; partner notification, 716; prevention programs for youth, 360

Middle East: blood units collected, 422; reported AIDS cases, 114, 116; USAID funding, 802–803

Migrants, HIV screening of, by country, 556

Military conflict, 38–39, 182

Minorities, 772

Models, of demographic impacts of AIDS, 200–201

Monkeys, rhesus, vaccine development and, 249–250, 251

Morocco, 313

Mortality: AIDS and, 4, 204–205, 206; by GAA, 125, 130, 131, 132; HIV-1 and HIV-2 infection and, 276; in industrialized countries, 126–127; infant and child, 200, 208–209; by January 1, 1992, 124–127; projections, 131–132; rate, 204–205; tuberculosis and, 157, 158

Mother-to-child transmission, 585–586, 614; breast feeding and, 616–629, 636, 637; cohort studies, 635; factors affecting, 627. *See also* Perinatal transmission

Mozambique, 38

MSWM (men who have sex with men). *See* Gay men; Homosexual/bisexual transmission

Multicenter AIDS Cohort Study (MACS), 655, 656, 678

Multilateral-bilateral funding, 518–519, 523, 791

Multilateral funding, 512–513, 517–519, 520–521

Multiple epidemics, 81

Mutated viruses, 832

Mycobacterium tuberculosis, 149–163, 616

NAPs. *See* National AIDS programs

National AIDS advisory committees, 286–294, 791

National AIDS Hotline, 721, 730

National AIDS Information Clearinghouse, 306, 775

National AIDS Network, 782

National AIDS program managers, survey of, 289–291

National AIDS programs (NAPs), 279–324; coalition-building, 282, 305–311; commitment to, 282, 286–294; evaluating, 5–6, 282, 284–286, 297–300, 791; funding, 5–6, 283, 311–317, 787–801; mandatory testing and, 749; NGOs and, 305–311; priorities, 792–794; resource allocation, 483; staff turnover and burnout, 301–305; STD programs and, 189, 192, 301–304; structures, 300–301; survey of, 284–285; vulnerability and, 588–589, 590

National Council for International Health (NCIH), 804

National Gay and Lesbian Task Force, 562–563

National health care systems, 224, 315, 318–319

National Institute on Drug Abuse, 718

National Institutes of Health, 267

Needle-exchange programs, 415–416. *See also* Syringe access
Needle sharing. *See* Syringe sharing
Neisseria gonorrhoeae infections. *See* Gonorrhoeae
Nepal, 799
Netherlands, 116, 654; ASOs, 780, 781; behavior change, 383; funding, 520, 804–805; HIV testing, 749, 751, 755, 758; homosexual/bisexual transmission, 607; human rights and, 572; IDUs, 414, 611, 689, 692; information and education programs, 334; intervention programs, 351; mass media, 736, 743, 745; NAP, 296
Netherlands Organization for International Development, 805
Networking, by AIDS service organizations, 781–782
Neurosyphilis, 178
New Caledonia, 117
New York City: AIDS mortality, 124; health care costs, 501; HIV seroprevalence, 34, 370, 700; homelessness, 771; homosexual/bisexual men, 383, 607, 608, 609; IDUs, 610; pregnancy decisions, 370; prisoner education program, 766; South Bronx, 348–349; tuberculosis epidemic, 160–161
New Zealand, 85, 117, 289, 687, 688; HIV seroprevalence in IDUs, 698; national health care system, 315
NGOs. *See* Nongovernmental organizations
Nicaragua, 114
Niger, 809
Nigeria, 35, 289; commercial sex workers, 382–383; IDUs, 420; NAP, 295, 296; per-capita prevention expenditures, 482
Nondiscrimination legislation, 561–567
Nongonococcal urethritis (NGU), 172–173
Nongovernmental organizations (NGOs): condom marketing, 401; experience, 794–796; funding, 313, 516, 792–794; mass media and, 744–745; NAPs and, 291, 305–311; number, by year, 308; potential impacts, 797–799; responses, 308, 358–359, 772–774, 788, 792–794; USAID and, 804; WHO and, 783. *See also* AIDS service organizations (ASOs)

Non-Hodgkin's lymphoma (NHL), 134, 139–143
North America GAA: AIDS cases, 83, 109; AIDS deaths, 83; cumulative HIV infection, 105–108; funding, 5–6; health care systems, 465–466, 495, 506; HIV infection, 32, 83, 762, 763; 1992 HIV infection, 28; ODA contributions, 515; partner notification, 716–718; pediatric AIDS infections, 32; prevention expenditures, 478, 479; prisoners, 762, 763; reporting, 112–113; safe sex, 384, 654; transmission modes, 15, 30, 31. *See also specific locations*
North Carolina, 717
North East Asia GAA: AIDS cases, 96–98, 109; AIDS deaths, 96–98; cumulative HIV infection, 105–108; health care costs, 506; HIV infection, 96–98, 105–108; prevention expenditures, 478; reporting, 112–113; transmission modes, 30. *See also specific locations*
Norway: NAP, 296, 689; ODA contributions, 520, 527; partner notification, 710
Norwegian Red Cross Society (NRCS), 516, 805–807
Notification requirements, human rights and, 558–559

Occupational categories, HIV screening of, by country, 557
Oceania GAA: AIDS cases, 85–87, 109; AIDS deaths, 85–87; funding, 6; health care costs, 506; HIV infection, 4, 85–87, 105–108; prevention expenditures, 479; reporting, 112–113; transmission modes, 30, 31
ODA. *See* Offical development assistance
OECD (Organization for Economic Cooperation and Development), 515, 526–527
Official development assistance (ODA): bilateral funding, 518, 523–524, 528, 532, 793; funding by, 524, 787; Global AIDS Strategy funding and, 511–519; multilateral-bilateral funding, 518–519, 523, 793; multilateral funding, 515–517; from OECD and OPEC, 524, 526–527; official agencies, 514–515

OPEC (Organization of Petroleum Exporting Countries), 515, 526–527
Opportunistic infections (OIs), 240–246
Orphans. *See* AIDS orphans
Overseas Development Authority (ODA) (U.K.), 514

Pacific Islands, 2, 35, 117, 619–620
Pakistan, 313, 425
Panama, 806
Pan American Health Organization (PAHO), 122, 306, 825
PANOS Institute, 568
Papua New Guinea, 2, 85, 117, 289, 735
Paraguay, 2, 35, 114
Partner negotiation, 335
Partner notification, 707–720; in Africa, 713–714; in Asia, 714–715; in the Caribbean, 715–716; in Europe, 707–713; evaluated, 718–720; human rights and, 720; in Latin America, 715–716; in North America, 716–718; patient referral, 707, 709, 710, 713, 714, 717, 719; provider referral, 707, 709–712, 714–717, 719, 720
Patient referral, 707, 709, 710, 713, 714, 717, 719
PCP. *See Pneumocystis carinii* pneumonia
Pediatric AIDS: cumulative cases, by GAA, 106, 129; deaths, by GAA, 125, 128, 131; by GAA, 31–32, 129; HIV testing and, 756; reporting, 113; transmission and, 614. *See also* Children; Infants; Mother-to-child transmission; Perinatal transmission
Pelvic inflammatory disease (PID), 180
Pentamidine, aerosolized, for PCP, 240
Perinatal transmission, 629–645; cohort studies, 635; critical moment, 636–637; diagnosis, 632–634; education and counseling, 641–643; factors affecting, 627; history, 630–631; pregnancy term and, 640; prevention, 643–645; risks, 633–636, 638–639. *See also* Children; Infants; Mother-to-child transmission; Pediatric AIDS
Perinatal vaccination, 249, 253
Peru, 735, 739, 743

Pharmacies, syringe access through, 688–689
Philippines, 114, 289, 290, 734, 736, 743, 744
Placental barrier, integrity of, 639
Plants and plant extracts, as alternative AIDS therapies, 244–245
Plasma, 421, 426–427, 443–444. *See also* Blood and blood products; Blood transfusions
Plasmapheresis, 427
Plasmodium falciparum, 143–148
Pneumocystis carinii pneumonia (PCP): drug therapy for, 642; in France, 497–499; frequency, 498; prevention costs, 496, 498; prophylaxis, 240, 242
Point prevalence, 12
Poland, 116; community responses, 771; HIV infection, 2, 34–35, 612, 712; IDUs, 612, 686
Policy: AIDS prevention and, 343–344; dementia and, 680–681
Polymerase chain reaction (PCR), 274–275, 756, 826
Population estimates, general, 47
Population groups: age and sex patterns of HIV infection, 76; geographic variation, 79–81; HIV incidence and prevalence data, 37–47, 71–81; specific STD interventions, 187–189; urban-rural differentials, 76–79. *See also* Blood donors; Commercial sex workers; Gay men; Injection drug users; Lesbians; Pregnant women; Women
Population growth projections, 203–204
Population Services International (PSI), 401
PPD test, for tuberculosis, 159
Preclinical testing, drug approval process and, 236
Pregnancy: course of HIV infection in, 640; critical moment of transmission in, 636–637; female condoms and, 702; HIV infection and, 365–371; HIV screening and, 755–756; perinatal transmission, 629–645; STDs and, 180–181; therapeutic trials and, 643–645
Pregnant women: HIV prevalence and incidence in, by GAA, 64–67; as surrogates for general population, 64

Prevalence, 12–13, 605–606

Prevention and control programs, 4–6, 325–447, 792; Action for Youth project, 358–359; for adolescents and young adults, 352–365; AIDS and Reproductive Health Network, 366; for bisexual males, 387, 390; blood safety, 421–436; for children, 673–677; for commercial sex workers, 372–381, 389; condoms, 390–406; costs, 478–482, 496–509, 669, 687; demographic impacts and, 210–212; empowerment for, 571; funding, 5–6, 311–313; in gay communities, 381–390; for general population, 350–352; global approach to, 447; health and social services, 330, 337–338; hemophilia and, 438–446; homosexual practices and, 381–390; human rights and, 564–566; IDUs and, 406–420; information and education, 325, 330–337; international support for, 801–811; medical care-to-prevention spending ratios, 506; NAPs and, 483; NGOs and, 797–799; per-capita expenditures for, 479; in prisons, 767–769; reproductive health and, 365–372; social environment and, 330, 338–348; STD control programs and, 179–193; street children programs, 360–361; targeted populations for, 349–365; vulnerability and, 579; women and, 657–667. See also Information and education programs

Prevention and control terminology, human rights and, 539

Primary health care (PHC), 192, 677, 794

Primary prophylaxis, 240

Prisoners: discrimination and, 569, 570; health care, 766–767; HIV/AIDS policy, 761–769; HIV infection rates, 762; HIV testing, 764, 765; human rights and, 761–762; IDU, 762–763, 767–768; information and education programs, 766; preventive services, 767–769; segregation, 764; tuberculosis, 768–769; women, 768

Private voluntary organizations. See Non-governmental organizations

Progressive multifocal leukoencephalopathy (PML), 682

Prophylactic vaccination, 249, 253

Prostitutes. See Commercial sex workers

Provider referral, 707, 709–712, 714–717, 719, 720

Psychological needs, of children, 670, 672, 676

Psychosocial needs, of AIDS patients, 452–454

Public health measures: contain-and-control versus cooperation-and-inclusion, 281; disease notification, 558–559; HIV testing and surveillance, 551–552; human rights and, 538–541

Public opinion, 542, 739

Public service announcements, 735

Puerto Rico, 465, 493, 610

Pulmonary tuberculosis, 156

Reality®, 701

Red Cross. See International Federation of Red Cross and Red Crescent Societies

Reproductive system: adolescents and, 369; issues, 374–375; STDs and, 180–181

Research: achievements, 229–277; annual official assistance outside country, 263, 265; antiviral therapy, 233–239; behavioral, 259–266; epidemiological, 257–259, 275–277; funding, 260–264, 265; future, 264–267; HIV-2 infection, 275–277; HIV virus variability and, 267–275; opportunistic infections, 240–246; papers indexed by Medline, 257, 258–259, 267, 268–270; vaccine development, 247–257; women and, 663–665

Reticuloendotheliosis virus, 837

Retrovir®, 233, 812, 813, 818

Retroviral genomes, composition of, 267–268

Reverse transcriptase (RT), 233–234

Reverse transcriptase (RT) inhibitors, 233–234, 235

Rifampin, for tuberculosis, 161

Risk: core groups, 52, 174, 176–177, 185–187; groups, 13, 185–187, 554; high-risk groups, 185–187, 554; HIV testing and, 749, 750–754; partner notification and, 708; of perinatal transmission, 633, 638–639; reduction of, 653–657; sexual

Risk (cont.)
    behavior and, 76, 188; of tuberculosis,
        155–156; to women, 76, 382, 700
RNA, virus mutation and, 836
Rockefeller Foundation, 793–794
Romania, 93, 116, 606; partner
    notification, 712; pediatric AIDS cases,
    614; spread of HIV, 35
Rural areas: economic impacts, 219–221;
    household impacts, 196–197; urban-
    rural differentials, 76–79
Russia, 116. See also Soviet Union
Rwanda, 114; breast feeding, 618; circum-
    cision, 650; critical moment of perinatal
    transmission in, 637; family home
    health care, 461; health care, 459, 460,
    463, 469, 485–486, 487; health care fund-
    ing, 314, 317, 806; HIV seroprevalence
    survey, 40, 43–44, 181; malaria, 145,
    146; pregnancy in HIV-infected women,
    640; urban-rural differentials, 76–77
Ryan White Care Act, 782

Safe sex: adolescents and, 353, 355; bar-
    riers to, 331; commercial sex workers
    and, 344–345, 373–374, 378–379; gay
    men and, 383–384, 386, 653–657; hemo-
    philiacs and, 439, 442. See also Sexual
    behavior
St. Lucia, 715
San Francisco: community responses, 774;
    health care costs, 501; homelessness,
    771; homosexual/bisexual men, 383,
    607, 654, 655–656; IDUs, 419, 691–692,
    695; recognition of AIDS, 386; spread of
    HIV, 36
São Paulo, Brazil, 2, 34
Saudi Arabia, 111, 557
Scandinavia, 710, 712, 719
Scotland, 611, 686, 687, 693, 730
Sectoral impacts of HIV/AIDS, 213–218.
    See also specific sectors
Senegal, 425, 727
Sentinel populations, 51
Seroconversion Surveillance Project, 438
Service sector of economy, 219
Sex education, 186–187, 359–361
Sex ratios: of HIV infection, 30, 76; by

GAA, 31; in Oceania, 87; of reported
    AIDS cases, 124; in U.S., 83
Sexual behavior: of children, 670–671; cir-
    cumcision and, 650–651; fidelity, 659;
    HIV risk and, 76, 82; HIV testing and,
    748–750; information and education
    and, 330–331; mass media and, 740–741;
    partner negotiation, 335; serial monog-
    amy, 334; STDs and, 183; trading sex
    for drugs, 377; vulnerability and, 578,
    581–582; women and, 659–660. See also
    Safe sex
Sexually transmitted diseases (STDs), 165–
    193, 301–302; antimicrobial-resistant
    pathogen strains of, 166; cervical cancer
    and, 145; circumcision and, 646; clinics,
    56–64, 190–191, 375, 378; control of,
    179–193, 303–304; core groups and, 52,
    174, 176–177, 186; in developing coun-
    tries, 167–168; disease classification
    and, 550–551; female condoms and, 700;
    global epidemiology of, 166–174;
    HIV/AIDS and, 56–64, 178, 301–304,
    613–614; as indicators of high-risk sex-
    ual behavior, 185–186; partner
    notification and, 707–720; placental bar-
    rier and, 639; population-specific inter-
    ventions, 187–189; reproductive system
    and, 180–181; transmission of, 174–177;
    women and, 659, 661
Sexually transmitted infections (STIs),
    165n
Sexual risk reduction. See Safe sex
Sexual transmission: by GAA, 30–32; vul-
    nerability and, 582–583. See also Hetero-
    sexual transmission; Homosexual/bisex-
    ual transmission
Silver nitrate eye prophylaxis, for new-
    borns, 188
Simian immunodeficiency virus (SIV), 835
SIV-MAC, 249, 275
Slim disease, 433
Slovak Republic, 750
Smallpox, 825
Social and behavioral studies, 260
Social impacts of AIDS, 195–199, 225–226
Social services: discrimination in, 543–
    545; health care services and, 456–458;
    needs, 451, 454; prevention programs,

737, 745; ODA contributions, 514, 520; partner notification, 708–709; prisoners, HIV infection in, 765, 766; safe sex among gay men, 654, 655; STDs, 166, 172; syphilis, 166; syringe access, 696; targeted mass media, 737. *See also* London

United Nations: projected study of AIDS-related discrimination, 541; public health estimates, 835

United Nations Children's Fund (UNICEF), 465, 515, 528, 668, 793

United Nations Commission on Human Rights, 184, 568, 571–572

United Nations Committee on Economic, Social and Cultural Rights, 572, 772

United Nations Congress on Crime Prevention and Treatment of Offenders, 761

United Nations Development Program (UNDP), 286, 436, 515, 528, 793

United Nations Educational, Scientific and Cultural Organization (UNESCO), 517, 528, 807–809

United Nations General Assembly, 228

United Nations Population Division, 517, 528

United Nations Population Fund (UNFPA), 515, 528

United Nations Sub-Committee on the Prevention of Discrimination and Protection of Minorities, 772

United States: AIDS Litigation Project, 543–545; annual official assistance, 263; ASOs, 775, 781, 782; blood transfusions, 70–71, 425, 426, 432; breast feeding, 619; condoms, 405, 705; drug approval process, 236–237; entry restrictions, 558–559; Fair Housing Amendments Act, 773; general population estimates, 47; health care, 315–317, 318–319, 322, 465–466; health care costs, 222, 224, 493–495, 501, 506, 813; health insurance, 224, 815; hemophilia, 444–445; heterosexual transmission, 612–614; HIV/AIDS, 3, 34, 36–37, 47, 63–64, 66–67, 83, 114, 118–122, 605–616; HIV testing, 559–560, 561, 750, 751, 753, 754–755, 756, 757, 758; homosexual/bisexual men, 605, 607–609, 653–657; housing discrimination, 773; IDUs, 56, 63–64, 414, 415, 609–612, 698; legislation, 543, 547; media, 723, 730, 732, 739–740, 744; multiethnic STD strategies, 188; NAP, 295, 296; National Affordable Housing Act, 773; nondiscrimination legislation, 561; non-Hodgkin's lymphoma, 140–141; ODA contributions, 515, 520, 524, 528; partner notification, 717–718, 719; PID in, 180; research spending, 261; STDs, 63–64, 166, 179, 188; syringe access, 685, 692; therapeutic protocols, 645; tuberculosis, 149, 152–154

U.S. Agency for International Development (USAID), 41, 267, 397, 401, 514, 705–706, 737, 794, 801–804, 825

U.S. Bureau of the Census, Center for International Research (CIR), 41; Periodic Update on HIV/AIDS Surveillance Data Base, 37n, 41

U.S. Family of Seroprevalence Surveys, U.S. Public Health Service, 47, 50, 51, 56, 66, 67, 83

U.S. Food and Drug Administration (FDA), 234, 236–237, 238–240, 705, 819

Upper genital tract infection, 180

Urban areas: decay of, 348–349; migration to, STDs and, 180–181; urban-rural differentials, 76–79; viral infections and, 834–835; youth intervention programs in, 353, 360–361

Urethritis, 180

Uruguay, 806

USSR. *See* Soviet Union

Vaccine development, 248; approaches, 249–257; expectations, 254–256; Manhattan Project, 250–252; perinatal, 249, 253; research achievements, 247–257

Verhoef, Hans-Paul, 558–559

VIDEX®, 233

Violence: community projects and, 774; HIV/AIDS-related, 562–563, 769–770

Viral DNA, 268

Viral escape phenomena, 273

Viral infections: emerging, 826–839; mutation, 835–837; pre-AIDS, 826; preparation for, 837–839; recent epidemics,

Viral infections *(cont.)*
826–832; spread, 830–831, 833–835;
STDs, 166. *See also* Sexually transmitted diseases (STDs); *specific diseases*
Volunteer organizations. *See* AIDS activism; AIDS service organizations (ASOs); Nongovernmental organizations (NGOs)
Vulnerability, 6, 577–602; biological, 577; of children, 373–374, 668, 673; collective, 580, 590–602; defined, 578; empowerment and, 578–579; epidemiological, 577; IDUs and, 420; indexes, 594; individual, 578–589, 598–599; mandatory screening and, 346; national assessment of, 590–598; reduction, 566–589; sexual transmission and, 582–583; social status and, 590–591; societal, 592–597; transmission and, 582–586; of women, 373–374

Wales, 611, 765, 766
War, 38–39, 182
West Africa, 79
Western Europe GAA: AIDS cases, 83–85, 109; behavior change, 385; funding of AIDS-related health care costs, 224; health care costs, 506; HIV deaths, 83–85; HIV infection, 83–85, 105–108; ODA contributions, 515; partner notification, 712–713; prevention expenditures, 478, 479; reporting, 112–113; transmission modes, 15, 31, 607
WHO. *See* World Health Organization; World Health Organization, Global Programme on AIDS
Women: AZT access, 815; breast feeding, 616–629; cervical cancer, 144–146; *Chlamydia trachomatis* infection, 173; condoms and, 397, 659–660, 661; counseling, 459; in developing countries, 293–294; discussions with partners, 661–662; empowerment, 345, 348, 374–375; experimental therapeutic protocols and, 645; female condoms, 700–707; gender-specific issues, 657–667; heterosexual transmission and, 613; high- and low-transmission, 638; HIV infection, 2, 29–30, 659; HIV-1 and HIV-2 infection, 277;

information and education, 659, 736; intervention, 361, 659–667; life expectancy, 207; mother-to-child transmission, 365–366, 373–375, 585–586, 614, 629–645; narratives and, 666; in prison, 768; research and, 257–259, 663–665; risk, 76, 700; social impacts, 224–225; STDs and, 176, 183–184, 188; trading sex for drugs by, 377; transmission modes, 118; vulnerability, 373–374. *See also* Perinatal transmission; Pregnancy; Pregnant women
World Bank, 292, 515, 528, 529, 793, 809–811
World Federation of Hemophilia (WFH), 438, 444, 446
World Health Assembly, 297, 554
World Health Organization (WHO), 825; AIDS orphans projections, 672; ASOs and, 781; blood screening survey, 433; blood transfusions survey, 427; breast feeding guidelines, 616–617; counseling and, 820–821; definition of health, 8; definition of health care needs, 452; dementia and, 680; disease classification and, 549–550; Expanded Program on Immunization, 162; HIV/AIDS projections, 605, 700; HIV epidemiological classification, 15; HIV testing and, 554; housing response, 772; initial response to AIDS, 567; NAPs and, 296–297; NGOs identified, 307; prisoners and, 761, 764, 766; reporting to, 109–113; tuberculosis control, 149–150, 159; vaccine trial sites and, 249; WHO-EC Collaborating Center, 47. *See also* Global AIDS Strategy
World Health Organization, Global Programme on AIDS (WHO/GPA), 296, 436, 519–524, 750, 802; funding by, 792–793; HIV testing and, 757; human rights and, 567–569; multilateral contributions, 520–521; NGOs and ASOs and, 307, 783, 787; recognition of AIDS, 790–791; support by, 519–523, 787
World Hemophilia AIDS Center (WHAC), 438–439, 443, 446
World Organization of the Scout Movement (WOSM), 358

Young adults: Action for Youth project, 358–359; dependency ratio and, 209; economic impacts, 218; programs targeting, 352–365; STDs and, 175, 180, 186, 187. *See also* Adolescents

Young Men's/Young Women's Christian Association (YMCA/YWCA), 358

Yugoslavia, 35, 712

Zaire, 111, 114, 833; blood and blood products, 68, 433–434; community programs, 4; condom promotion, 400, 401, 736; health care expenditures, 223; HIV infection, 34, 35; information and education, 335, 741, 742, 743; malaria, 144–147; mother-to-child transmission, 638; prevention program for commercial sex workers, 330; World Bank and, 528

Zambia, 114; anti-AIDS clubs, 359; blood unit costs, 425; breast feeding, 618; circumcision, 650; funding, 806; HIV infection, 618, 700, 763; home health care, 453, 461, 462, 463, 488–489; malaria, 145, 146; mass media, 730, 742; NGOs, 306, 781, 782; prisoners, 763; women, 700

Zidovudine. *See* AZT

Zimbabwe, 38, 781; blood transfusions, 425, 427; health care, 456, 459; mass media, 723, 737, 745; NGOs, 307

This book was composed in Linotype-Hell's Trump Medieval (Postscript) by Technologies 'N Typography (Merrimac, MA) on a Dell 486p/66 PC in Ventura Publisher. It was printed and bound by Courier Corporation (Westford, MA). The paper is acid-free and was manufactured by the P. H. Glatfelter Paper Company (Spring Grove, PA). The book was designed by Joyce Weston.